Handbook of Obstetrics, Gynecology, and Primary Care

HANDBOOK OF OBSTETRICS, GYNECOLOGY, AND PRIMARY CARE

FREDERICK P. ZUSPAN, MD
Professor and Chairman Emeritus,
Department of Obstetrics and Gynecology,
The Ohio State University College of Medicine;
Ohio State University Medical Center,
Columbus, Ohio

EDWARD J. QUILLIGAN, MD
Professor Emeritus,
Department of Obstetrics and Gynecology,
University of California, Irvine,
College of Medicine,
Irvine, California;
UCI Medical Center,
Orange, California

Associate Editors

MICHAEL L. BLUMENFELD, MD
Associate Professor,
Department of Obstetrics and Gynecology;
Director, Division of General Obstetrics and Gynecology,
The Ohio State University College of Medicine;
Ohio State University Medical Center,
Columbus, Ohio

CYNTHIA B. EVANS, MD
Assistant Professor,
Department of Obstetrics and Gynecology,
The Ohio State University College of Medicine;
Ohio State University Medical Center,
Columbus, Ohio

MOON H. KIM, MD
Richard L. Meiling Chair and Professor,
Department of Obstetrics and Gynecology,
The Ohio State University College of Medicine;
Ohio State University Medical Center,
Columbus, Ohio

a Mosby handbook

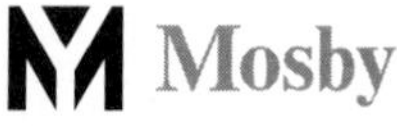

St. Louis Baltimore Boston Carlsbad
Chicago Minneapolis New York Philadelphia Portland
London Milan Sydney Tokyo Toronto

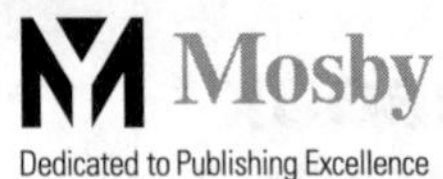

Printed in the United States of America

Mosby–Year Book, Inc.
11830 Westline Industrial Drive
St. Louis, Missouri 63146

International Standard Book Number 0-8151-99317

99 00 01/9 8 7 6 5 4 3

Contributors

Thomas J. Albert, Jr, MD
Assistant Professor,
Department of Obstetrics and Gynecology,
Louisiana State University Medical Center,
New Orleans, Louisiana

William B. Armstrong, MD
Assistant Professor,
Department of Otolaryngology–Head and Neck Surgery,
University of California, Irvine,
College of Medicine,
Irvine, California;
UCI Medical Center,
Orange, California

Kevin A. Ault, MD
Assistant Professor,
Department of Obstetrics and Gynecology,
University of Iowa Hospitals and Clinics,
Iowa City, Iowa

John J. Bergan, MD, FACS, FRCS (Hon), Eng
Professor of Surgery,
Loma Linda University Medical Center,
Loma Linda, California;
Clinical Professor of Surgery,
University of California, San Diego,
San Diego, California;
Clinical Professor of Surgery,
Uniformed Services University of the Health Sciences,
Bethesda, Maryland

Michael L. Blumenfeld, MD
Associate Professor,
Department of Obstetrics and Gynecology;
Director, Division of General Obstetrics and Gynecology,
The Ohio State University College of Medicine;
Ohio State University Medical Center,
Columbus, Ohio

John G. Boutselis, MD
Professor Emeritus,
Department of Obstetrics and Gynecology,
The Ohio State University College of Medicine;
Ohio State University Medical Center,
Columbus, Ohio

Jeffrey G. Boyle, MD
Des Moines Perinatal Center, PC,
West Des Moines, Iowa;
Director, Perinatal Diagnostic Center,
Mercy Hospital Medical Center,
Des Moines, Iowa

William E. Burak, Jr, MD
Assistant Professor,
Division of Surgical Oncology,
Department of Surgery,
The Ohio State University College of Medicine;
The Arthur G. James Cancer Hospital and Research Institute,
Columbus, Ohio

Renee M. Caputo, MD
Assistant Professor;
Director, Section of Urogynecology,
Department of Obstetrics and Gynecology,
The Ohio State University College of Medicine;
Ohio State University Medical Center,
Columbus, Ohio

Douglas Cesario, BS
Newport Beach, California

Thomas C. Cesario, MD
Dean, College of Medicine;
Professor,
University of California, Irvine,
Irvine, California;
UCI Medical Center,
Orange, California

Larry J. Copeland, MD
Professor and Chair,
Department of Obstetrics and Gynecology,
The Ohio State University College of Medicine;
Director, Gynecologic Oncology,
The Arthur G. James Cancer Hospital and Research Institute,
Columbus, Ohio

Leandro Cordero, MD
Professor, Pediatrics and Obstetrics,
The Ohio State University College of Medicine;
Director, Newborn Services,
Department of Pediatrics,
Ohio State University Medical Center,
Columbus, Ohio

Vicki C. Darrow, MD
Assistant Professor;
Director, General Obstetrics and Gynecology,
Department of Obstetrics and Gynecology,
University of California, Irvine,
College of Medicine,
Irvine, California;
UCI Medical Center,
Orange, California

John M. Davison, MD
Professor of Obstetric Medicine,
Department of Obstetrics and Gynecology,
University of Newcastle;
Consultant Obstetrician and Gynecologist,
Royal Victoria Infirmary,
Newcastle upon Tyne, United Kingdom

Christopher M. deGroot, MD
Associate Professor,
Department of Psychiatry,
East Carolina University School of Medicine;
Pitt County Memorial Hospital,
Greenville, North Carolina

Cynthia B. Evans, MD
Assistant Professor,
Department of Obstetrics and Gynecology,
The Ohio State University College of Medicine;
Ohio State University Medical Center,
Columbus, Ohio

William B. Farrar, MD, FACS
Associate Professor,
Department of Surgery;
Director, Division of Surgical Oncology,
The Ohio State University College of Medicine;
Director of Medical Affairs,
The Arthur G. James Cancer Hospital and Research Institute,
Columbus, Ohio

Pamela M. Foy, BS, RDMS
Clinical Coordinator of Ultrasound Services,
Department of Obstetrics and Gynecology,
The Ohio State University College of Medicine,
Columbus, Ohio

Chad I. Friedman, MD
Associate Professor,
Department of Obstetrics and Gynecology/Reproductive Endocrinology,
The Ohio State University College of Medicine,
Columbus, Ohio

John J. Fromkes, MD
Associate Professor;
Director, Division of Gastroenterology,
Department of Internal Medicine,
The Ohio State University College of Medicine;
Ohio State University Medical Center,
Columbus, Ohio

Steven G. Gabbe, MD
Professor and Chairman,
Department of Obstetrics and Gynecology,
University of Washington Medical Center,
Seattle, Washington

Vance O. Gardner, MD
Associate Clinical Professor,
Department of Orthopaedic Surgery,
University of California, Irvine,
College of Medicine,
Irvine, California;
Gardner & White Spine Institute,
Orange, California

Nancy E. Gin, MD
Assistant Clinical Professor,
Department of Internal Medicine,
University of California, Irvine,
College of Medicine,
Irvine, California

Mitchel P. Goldman, MD
Assistant Clinical Professor,
Department of Medicine/Dermatology,
University of California, San Diego Medical Center,
LaJolla, California

Michael C. Gordon, MD
Staff Perinatologist,
Department of Obstetrics and Gynecology,
Wilford Hall Medical Center,
San Antonio, Texas

Chris Harter, RN, IBCLC, CLE
Former Lactation Nurse Consultant;
Former Staff Development Coordinator,
Department of Women/Infant Nursing,
The Ohio State University Medical Center;
Breastfeeding Specialist,
Physicians for Women's Health,
Columbus, Ohio

Geri D. Hewitt, MD
Assistant Clinical Professor,
Department of Obstetrics and Gynecology,
The Ohio State University College of Medicine;
Ohio State University Medical Center;
Columbus Children's Hospital,
Columbus, Ohio

John C. Hoefs, MD
Associate Professor,
Department of Gastroenterology,
University of California, Irvine,
College of Medicine,
Irvine, California;
Director, Liver Disease Program,
UCI Medical Center,
Orange, California

F. Allan Hubbell, MD, MSPH
Chief, Division of General Internal Medicine and Primary Care,
University of California, Irvine,
College of Medicine,
Irvine, California;
UCI Medical Center,
Orange, California

Jay D. Iams, MD
Frederick P. Zuspan Professor,
Department of Obstetrics and Gynecology,
The Ohio State University College of Medicine;
Vice Chairman,
Department of Obstetrics and Gynecology,
Ohio State University Medical Center,
Columbus, Ohio

Rebecca D. Jackson, MD
Associate Professor,
Division of Endocrinology, Diabetes, and Metabolism,
Department of Internal Medicine,
The Ohio State University College of Medicine;
Ohio State University Medical Center,
Columbus, Ohio

Elizabeth A. Kennard, MD
Assistant Professor,
Department of Obstetrics and Gynecology,
The Ohio State University College of Medicine;
Ohio State University Medical Center,
Columbus, Ohio

David B. Keschner, MD
Resident, Department of Otolaryngology–Head and Neck Surgery,
University of California, Irvine,
College of Medicine,
Irvine, California;
Resident, Department of Otolaryngology–Head and Neck Surgery,
UCI Medical Center,
Orange, California

Moon H. Kim, MD
Richard L. Meiling Chair and Professor,
Department of Obstetrics and Gynecology,
The Ohio State University College of Medicine;
Ohio State University Medical Center,
Columbus, Ohio

Gregor J. Koobatian, MD
Clinical Instructor,
Department of Medicine–Gastroenterology and Hepatology,
University of California, Irvine,
College of Medicine,
Irvine, California;
Clinical Instructor,
Department of Medicine–Gastroenterology and Hepatology,
UCI Medical Center,
Orange, California

Mark B. Landon, MD
Associate Professor,
Department of Obstetrics and Gynecology,
The Ohio State University College of Medicine;
Vice Chairman,
Department of Obstetrics and Gynecology,
Ohio State University Medical Center,
Columbus, Ohio

George S. Lewandowski, MD
Clinical Assistant Professor,
Department of Obstetrics and Gynecology,
The Ohio State University College of Medicine;
The Arthur G. James Cancer Hospital and Research Institute,
Columbus, Ohio

James S. Ma, MD
Clinical Associate,
Department of Gastroenterology,
University of California, Irvine,
College of Medicine,
Irvine, California;
Attending Physician,
Department of Gastroenterology,
Mullikan Medical Center,
Los Angeles, California

Thomas Y. Ma, MD, PhD
Associate Professor,
Department of Medicine/Gastroenterology,
University of California, Irvine,
College of Medicine,
Irvine, California;
Veterans Administration Medical Center, Long Beach,
Long Beach, California

Christopher L. Mabee, MD
Clinical Instructor,
Division of Gastroenterology,
Department of Internal Medicine,
The Ohio State University College of Medicine;
Ohio State University Medical Center,
Columbus, Ohio

Carol A. Major, MD
Assistant Professor,
Department of Obstetrics and Gynecology,
University of California, Irvine,
College of Medicine,
Irvine, California;
UCI Medical Center
Orange, California

Douglas J. Marchant, MD
Adjunct Professor,
Department of Obstetrics and Gynecology,
Brown University;
Director, Breast Health Center,
Women and Infants Hospital,
Providence, Rhode Island;
Emeritus Professor of Surgery;
Emeritus Professor of Obstetrics and Gynecology,
Tufts University School of Medicine,
Boston, Massachusetts

John S. McDonald, MD
Professor and Chair,
Department of Anesthesiology,
The Ohio State University College of Medicine;
Ohio State University Medical Center,
Columbus, Ohio

Hooshang Meshkinpour, MD
Professor,
Department of Medicine,
University of California, Irvine,
College of Medicine,
Irvine, California;
Associate Chief,
Division of Gastroenterology,
Department of Medicine,
UCI Medical Center,
Orange, California

Jorge H. Mestman, MD
Professor,
Department of Medicine;
Director,
USC Center for Diabetes and Metabolic Diseases,
University of Southern California;
Chief, Diabetes,
Department of Medicine,
USC University Hospital,
Los Angeles, California

Randy R. Miller, MD
Associate Professor, Clinical Pediatrics,
Department of Pediatrics,
The Ohio State University College of Medicine;
Director of Nurseries,
Columbus Children's Hospital,
Columbus, Ohio

James L. Nicklin, MD
Clinical Fellow,
Department of Obstetrics and Gynecology,
The Ohio State University College of Medicine;
Clinical Fellow,
Department of Gynecologic Oncology,
The Arthur G. James Cancer Hospital and Research Institute,
Columbus, Ohio

Richard O'Shaughnessy, MD
Professor,
Department of Obstetrics and Gynecology,
The Ohio State University College of Medicine;
Ohio State University Medical Center,
Columbus, Ohio

Stephen F. Pariser, MD
Professor, Clinical Psychiatry and Obstetrics and Gynecology,
Department of Psychiatry,
The Ohio State University College of Medicine;
Director, Women's Mood Disorder Clinic,
Ohio State University Medical Center,
Columbus, Ohio

Maureen O'Brien Platt, MS, RD/LD
Department of Obstetrics and Gynecology,
Ohio State University Medical Center,
Columbus, Ohio

Pamela E. Prete, MD
Professor-in-Residence,
University of California, Irvine,
College of Medicine,
Irvine, California;
Chief, Rheumatology Section,
Department of Medical Service,
Veterans Administration Medical Center, Long Beach,
Long Beach, California

Edward J. Quilligan, MD
Professor Emeritus,
Department of Obstetrics and Gynecology,
University of California, Irvine,
College of Medicine,
Irvine, California;
UCI Medical Center,
Orange, California

Rosemary E. Reiss, MD
Associate Professor, Clinical Obstetrics and Gynecology,
Division of Maternal-Fetal Medicine,
Department of Obstetrics and Gynecology,
The Ohio State University College of Medicine;
Director, Clinical Obstetrics,
Ohio State University Medical Center,
Columbus, Ohio

Philip Samuels, MD
Associate Professor,
Department of Obstetrics and Gynecology,
The Ohio State University College of Medicine;
Director, Maternal–Fetal Medicine Fellowship Program,
Ohio State University Medical Center,
Columbus, Ohio

Beth Ann Schmalz, MS, CGC
Genetic Counselor,
Department of Obstetrics and Gynecology,
The Ohio State University College of Medicine;
Genetic Counselor,
Regional Genetic Center,
Columbus Children's Hospital,
Columbus, Ohio

Cynthia Shellhaas, MD
Assistant Professor,
Department of Obstetrics and Gynecology,
The Ohio State University College of Medicine;
Ohio State University Medical Center,
Columbus, Ohio

Phillip Shubert, MD
Assistant Professor,
Department of Obstetrics and Gynecology,
The Ohio State University College of Medicine;
Ohio State University Medical Center,
Columbus, Ohio

Stephen L. Stern, MD
Associate Professor,
Department of Psychiatry,
The Ohio State University College of Medicine;
Director, Mood Disorders Clinic,
Ohio State University Medical Center,
Columbus, Ohio

Julianne Stoody Toohey, MD
Assistant Clinical Professor,
Department of Obstetrics and Gynecology,
University of California, Irvine,
College of Medicine,
Irvine, California;
UCI Medical Center,
Orange, California

Wayne C. Trout, MD
Assistant Professor,
Department of Obstetrics and Gynecology,
The Ohio State University College of Medicine;
Ohio State University Medical Center,
Columbus, Ohio

Luis Vaccarello, MD
Assistant Professor,
Department of Obstetrics and Gynecology,
The Ohio State University College of Medicine;
The Arthur G. James Cancer Hospital and Research Institute,
Columbus, Ohio

Sandra R. Valaitis, MD
Assistant Professor;
Director, Urogynecology Unit,
Department of Obstetrics and Gynecology,
University of Chicago,
Chicago Lying-In Hospital,
Chicago, Illinois

Stanley van den Noort, MD
Professor and Chairman,
Department of Neurology,
University of California, Irvine,
College of Medicine,
Irvine, California;
Neurologist,
UCI Medical Center,
Orange, California

David A. Wininger, MD
Assistant Professor, Clinical Internal Medicine,
Department of Internal Medicine,
The Ohio State University College of Medicine,
Columbus, Ohio

Diana Yao, MD
Clinical Associate,
Department of Gastroenterology,
University of California, Irvine,
College of Medicine,
Irvine, California;
Attending Physician,
Department of Gastroenterology,
Veterans Administration Medical Center, Long Beach,
Long Beach, California

Frederick P. Zuspan, MD
Professor and Chairman Emeritus,
Department of Obstetrics and Gynecology,
The Ohio State University College of Medicine;
Ohio State University Medical Center,
Columbus, Ohio

Kathryn Zuspan, MD
Clinical Assistant Professor,
Department of Anesthesia,
University of Minnesota;
Anesthesiologist,
Hennepin County Medical Center,
Minneapolis, Minnesota;
Fairview Southdale Hospital,
Edina, Minnesota

Foreword

What a reversal of roles to be asked to write a foreword to a book by my mentors–and, of course, not just any mentors, but two of the founding fathers of modern obstetrics and gynecology in the United States. Drs. Zuspan and Quilligan were among those leaders who brought our specialty out of the age of anecdote and into the world of science and evidence-based clinical medicine. They have always been innovative and insightful into the clinical needs of our patients and the educational needs of our physicians. Today, when the publication of a new medical book usually means a journey into a specialty that is applicable to few patients and to an even more limited number of physicians, this book is unique in its approach by providing material that applies to all female patients and all physicians providing their care.

Few forces carry the impact of the dollar that pays for health care. Socioeconomic factors have affected the way health care is provided, resulting in changes that few of us anticipated. Although many of these changes may have been perceived in the health care community as detrimental to the well-being of our patients and their health care providers, one change in particular may be extraordinarily positive. That change is the response to a demand for a more comprehensive approach to the entire patient. Obstetricians/gynecologists are now committed to becoming knowledgeable about primary care, and primary care physicians are similarly committed to, at the least, covering the gynecologic aspects of women's health care, and in the case of more and more family physicians, to providing obstetric care as well. This book–a single, comprehensive resource for all such physicians–is a timely and critical contribution.

Having Drs. Zuspan and Quilligan edit such a text not only recognizes the value of their insight into the need for this effort, but also pairs two of the individuals most able to recruit the best possible authors for each subject from around the country. Anyone who has ever worked with these two giants knows one can never say no to such a request. With their influence and the connections that they have developed over the years, Drs. Zuspan and Quilligan were able to muster an impressive and varied group of authors to tackle this most ambitious project. These authors not only tackled the project, they mastered it as well.

Our patients have been blessed by the commitment of Drs. Zuspan and Quilligan to their overall health and well-being. We, as colleagues, have been equally blessed by their commitment to ensuring that we are knowledgeable and current. They have been tireless in their dedication to this commitment, and it has not ceased with their alleged retirements. This is a fitting addition to one of the later, but certainly not the last, chapters in their contributions. I hope all of you appreciate it as much as I do.

Thomas J. Garite, MD

Professor and Chairman,
Department of Obstetrics and Gynecology,
University of California, Irvine,
College of Medicine,
Irvine, California

Preface

Our expectation is that anyone who provides health care for a woman will find this handbook useful. It is actually three books in one: gynecology, obstetrics, and primary care. It is not intended to be a complete reference, but rather a book that can be used for the day-to-day care of patients. It is a quick guide to a specific problem the patient presents to the health care team. We made great efforts to cover topics that OB/GYNs and primary care physicians face daily with their patients.

To obtain information quickly, Part I: Gynecology, is organized alphabetically from Amenorrhea to Vulvar and Vaginal Carcinoma. Likewise, the chapters in Part III: Primary Care, range from AIDS to Varicose Veins. Part II: Obstetrics, follows the chronologic order of pregnancy, starting with the anatomic and physical changes of pregnancy and ending with resuscitation of the newborn. Interspersed throughout the part are chapters dealing with complications and medical conditions that may present during pregnancy. In addition, the algorithms throughout the book will provide information on evaluation, approach, management, and diagnosis at a glance.

Many hours and significant individual effort have gone into this publication. We could not have organized the book and maintained deadlines without the help of our section editors: Moon Kim, Michael Blumenfeld, and Cindy Evans. We truly appreciate their hard work as well as that of each chapter author. You would not be holding this book without the help of our able staff: Tracy Fox and Beverly Cochran at OSU and Mary Tiong at UCI. We could never have gone the distance without our Developmental Editor and coach at Mosby, Ellen Baker Geisel. A special thanks goes to her, as she kept us on our toes while keeping us laughing. Thanks, also, to Susie Baxter, Carol Sullivan Weis, Karen Rehwinkel, Dave Graybill, and Jen Marmarinos at Mosby.

We hope that this book will be useful to you in your daily patient-care activities.

Frederick P. Zuspan, MD
Edward J. Quilligan, MD

Preface

Contents

PART I: GYNECOLOGY
Moon H. Kim and Michael Blumenfeld, Editors

1. **Amenorrhea: Primary and Secondary, 3**
   Moon H. Kim
2. **Breast Disease, 10**
   MALIGNANT, 10
   William B. Farrar and William E. Burak, Jr.
   BENIGN, 21
   Douglas J. Marchant
3. **Cervical Cancer, 26**
   George S. Lewandowski and Luis Vaccarello
4. **Contraception, 34**
   Geri D. Hewitt
5. **Dysmenorrhea, 41**
   Elizabeth A. Kennard
6. **Ectopic Pregnancy, 44**
   Moon H. Kim
7. **Endometriosis, 52**
   Elizabeth A. Kennard
8. **Gestational Trophoblastic Disease, 55**
   Larry J. Copeland and James L. Nicklin
9. **Hirsutism, 64**
   Chad I. Friedman
10. **Infertility, 74**
    Moon H. Kim

11. Lower Genital Tract Infections, 83
Wayne C. Trout

12. Menopause, 91
Cynthia B. Evans

13. Mood Disorders, 97
Stephen L. Stern and Stephen F. Pariser

14. Nutrition and Menopause, 110
Maureen O'Brien Platt

15. Osteoporosis, 115
Rebecca D. Jackson

16. Ovarian Cancer, 124
James L. Nicklin and Larry J. Copeland

17. Papillomavirus Infections and the Abnormal Pap Smear, 134
George S. Lewandowski

18. Pelvic Inflammatory Disease and Its Sequelae, 140
Wayne C. Trout

19. Pelvic Masses—Benign, 147
Michael L. Blumenfeld

20. Pelvic Pain—Chronic, 156
John S. McDonald

21. Pelvic Floor Support, 163
Renee M. Caputo

22. Premenstrual Syndrome, 172
Cynthia B. Evans

23. Sexual Dysfunction, 178
Stephen F. Pariser

24. Sterilization, 184
Geri D. Hewitt

25. Urinary Dysfunction, 186
Renee M. Caputo

26. Uterine Bleeding—Abnormal, 199
Chad I. Friedman

27. **Uterine Cancers, 209**
Luis Vaccarello

28. **Vulvar and Vaginal Carcinoma, 216**
Luis Vaccarello and George S. Lewandowski

PART II: OBSTETRICS
Cynthia B. Evans, Editor

29. **Anatomic and Physiologic Changes in Pregnancy, 227**
Wayne C. Trout

30. **Preconceptional, Prenatal, and Postpartum Care, 232**
Cynthia B. Evans

31. **Nutrition and Pregnancy, 236**
Maureen O'Brien Platt

32. **Prenatal Diagnosis and Teratology, 240**
Thomas J. Albert, Jr.

33. **Genetics, 251**
Beth Ann Schmalz

34. **Ultrasound, 257**
NORMAL, 257
Jeffrey G. Boyle and Pamela M. Foy
ABNORMAL, 272
Pamela M. Foy and Steven G. Gabbe

35. **Antenatal Testing, 282**
Cynthia Shellhaas

36. **Medical Diseases in Pregnancy, 287**
CARCINOMA OF THE CERVIX, 287
John G. Boutselis
CARDIAC AND PULMONARY DISEASES, 293
Michael C. Gordon
DIABETES, 310
Mark B. Landon
ENDOCRINE ABNORMALITIES, 315
Mark B. Landon
HEMATOLOGIC COMPLICATIONS, 320
Philip Samuels
AUTOIMMUNE DISEASE, 332
Rosemary E. Reiss
HEPATIC AND GASTROINTESTINAL DISEASE, 341
Christopher L. Mabee and John J. Fromkes

CHRONIC HYPERTENSION, 351
Frederick P. Zuspan
RENAL COMPLICATIONS, 358
John M. Davison

37. Perinatal Infections and Immunizations, 366
Kevin A. Ault

38. Common Dermatologic Disorders, 375
Michael C. Gordon and Mark B. Landon

39. Premature Birth, 384
Jay D. Iams

40. Abnormal Cervical Competence, 397
Jay D. Iams

41. Third Trimester Bleeding, 403
Rosemary E. Reiss

42. Alloimmunization, 413
Richard O'Shaughnessy

43. Thromboembolic Disease, 419
Jeffrey G. Boyle

44. Intrauterine Growth Restriction, 426
Steven G. Gabbe

45. Preeclampsia/Eclampsia, 430
Frederick P. Zuspan

46. Postterm/Postdate Pregnancy, 437
Frederick P. Zuspan

47. Medical Emergencies in Obstetrics, 442
Wayne C. Trout

48. Malpresentation, 450
Geri D. Hewitt

49. Multiple Gestations, 459
Jeffrey G. Boyle

50. Fetal Heart Rate Monitoring, 466
Edward J. Quilligan

51. Obstetric Anesthesia, 470
Kathryn Zuspan

52. Breastfeeding, 474
Chris Harter

53. Adolescent Pregnancy, 482
Geri D. Hewitt

54. Substance Abuse in Pregnancy, 485
Phillip Shubert

55. Resuscitation of the Newborn, 489
Leandro Cordero and Randy R. Miller

PART III: PRIMARY CARE
Edward J. Quilligan, Editor

56. AIDS, 499
David A. Wininger

57. The Annual Examination, 506
Vicki C. Darrow and F. Allan Hubbell

58. Anxiety Reaction, 519
Christopher M. deGroot

59. Arthritis and Related Musculoskeletal Disorders, 527
Pamela E. Prete

60. Backache, 536
Vance O. Gardner

61. Cholecystitis, 543
Gregor J. Koobatian and John C. Hoefs

62. Connective Tissue Diseases, 548
Pamela E. Prete

63. Cystitis and Pyelonephritis, 558
Sandra R. Valaitis

64. Diarrhea—Chronic, 563
James S. Ma and Thomas Y. Ma

65. Domestic Violence and the Physician Response, 572
Julianne Stoody Toohey and Carol A. Major

66. Gastritis—Chronic and Acute, 578
Hooshang Meshkinpour

67. Headaches, 581
Stanley van den Noort

68. Hypertension, 586
Nancy E. Gin

69. Influenza, 594
Thomas C. Cesario

70. Laryngitis and Pharyngitis, 599
David B. Keschner and William B. Armstrong

71. Nutrition, 608
Diana Yao and Thomas Y. Ma

72. Peptic Ulcer Disease, 617
Hooshang Meshkinpour

73. Pneumonia: Viral and Bacterial, 627
Thomas C. Cesario and Douglas A. Cesario

74. Thyroid Disorders, 634
Jorge H. Mestman
HYPERTHYROIDISM, 634
HYPOTHYROIDISM, 639

75. Varicose Veins, 643
Mitchel P. Goldman and John J. Bergan

Index, 649

Handbook of Obstetrics, Gynecology, and Primary Care

PART I

Gynecology

Moon H. Kim and Michael L. Blumenfeld, Editors

1

Amenorrhea: Primary and Secondary

Moon H. Kim

Clinically, amenorrhea may be defined as the absence of menstrual bleeding. The absence of menstruation for more than 3 months is considered abnormal in previously menstruating women and is called *secondary amenorrhea. Primary amenorrhea* is the absence of menarche by the age of 16 years. *Amenorrhea* is not a diagnostic term, but rather a clinical manifestation associated with various functional and organic disorders.

Normal menstruation is the end point of an ovulatory cycle delicately regulated by the hypothalamic-pituitary-ovarian axis. Amenorrhea occurs in certain physiologic conditions such as pregnancy and lactation and during the premenarchal and postmenopausal years. Therefore it is essential that such conditions be ruled out when evaluating amenorrhea.

PATHOPHYSIOLOGY

The normal menstrual cycle is a physiologic result of the hormonal interplay of the hypothalamus, pituitary gland, ovary, and endometrium. Thus an understanding of endocrinologic changes is important in the diagnosis and management of amenorrhea. The following points are some of the key events in an ovulatory cycle:

1. Pulsatile secretion of gonadotropin-releasing hormone (GnRH) results in pulsatile secretion of the follicle-stimulating hormone (FSH) and the luteinizing hormone (LH).
2. FSH stimulates growth and development of the follicles.
3. Increased secretion of estradiol at midcycle results in positive feedback release of LH.
4. An increase in progesterone production by the luteinized granulosa cells augments the LH surge, which triggers the rupture of a mature follicle.
5. Following release of the oocyte, the ruptured follicle forms the corpus luteum, which has a life span of approximately 14 days and secretes progesterone.

Any alteration in these regulatory steps or the absence of oocytes in the ovary will result in amenorrhea.

DIAGNOSTIC EVALUATION

In conducting a careful history and physical examination, one may find it helpful to focus the diagnostic evaluation on disorders of the hypothalamus, pituitary, ovary, or outflow tract.

As Fig. 1-1 shows, the initial step in the workup of amenorrheic women starts with the exclusion of pregnancy, measurement of serum prolactin (PRL) and TSH levels, and assessment of endogenous estrogen production. The latter can be achieved by a progestin challenge because progestin effect is noted only on endometrium primed by estrogens. Diagnostic procedures include the following:

1. Progestin challenge (medroxyprogesterone acetate 10 mg daily for 5 days): Absence of withdrawal bleeding indicates a hypoestrogenic state or end organ failure/outflow obstruction.
2. Hypothalamic/pituitary evaluation: Measurement of serum levels of FSH, LH, PRL, TSH, and estradiol (E_2).
3. Androgenic evaluation: Measurement of serum testosterone and DHEA-S levels.
4. Karyotyping: Conducted when serum FSH level is high (>40 mIU/ml) in patients with absence of menarche or suspected premature ovarian failure.
5. Autoimmune disorder evaluation: Antinuclear antibody, microsomal antibody titer, etc.
6. Radiologic evaluation: Coned-down view of the sella turcica, CT, or MRI when a pituitary tumor is suspected.

With carefully directed evaluation, patients with amenorrhea will fall into one of the following five diagnostic categories: (1) anovulation, (2) hyperprolactinemia and/or pituitary or CNS tumors, (3) hypogonadotropic hypogonadism, (4) end organ/outflow defect, and (5) ovarian failure (Fig. 1-1).

Anovulation

Amenorrheic women who bleed to a progestin challenge are most likely to be anovulatory with estrogen production. Although their hypothalamic-pituitary-ovarian axis does not function cyclically with resulting ovulation, estrogen production (either from ovaries or from peripheral conversion of androstenedione) is sufficient to stimulate the endometrium. Depending on clinical presentation, the following additional tests may be ordered.

1. Hyperandrogenic state: serum testosterone and DHEA-S. Androstenedione, 17-OH progesterone, FSH, and LH, if needed.
2. Thyroid disorders: serum TSH, thyroid function tests.
3. Adrenal disorders, ovarian tumors: DHEA-S, cortisol, 17-OH progesterone.

Hyperprolactinemia/Pituitary Tumors

Prolactin secretion is primarily controlled by the inhibitory mechanism of dopamine, and to a lesser extent by gamma-aminobutyric acid (GABA). Any disruption in this inhibitory mechanism results in hyperprolactine-

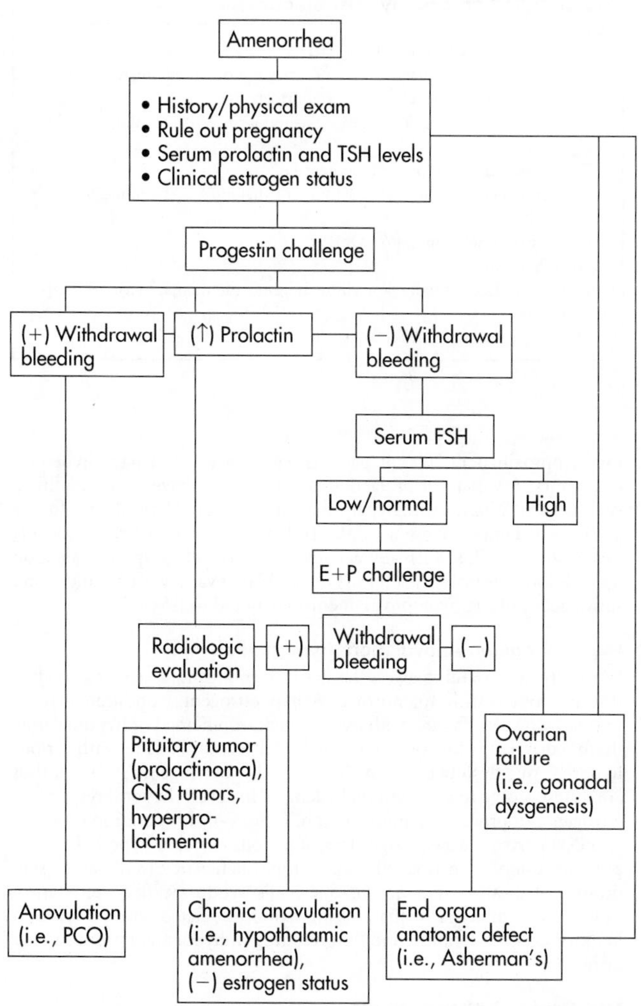

FIG. 1-1 Evaluation of amenorrhea.

BOX 1-1
Etiologic Factors: Hyperprolactinemia

Hormonal agents: Estrogen, OCs, TRH
CNS lesions: Craniopharyngioma, pituitary tumor, granulomatous lesions (i.e., sarcoidosis), stalk resection, trauma, etc.
Dopamine receptor-blocking agents: Phenothiazines, haloperidol, metoclopramide
Dopamine reuptake blocker: Nomifensine
Dopamine depleting agents: Reserpine, methyldopa, monoamine oxidase inhibitors
Dopamine turnover inhibitor: Opiates
Hypothyroidism
Ectopic prolactin production: Bronchogenic carcinoma, renal cell carcinoma
Others: Pregnancy, exercise, stress, etc.

mia. Approximately 30% of patients with amenorrhea have hyperprolactinemia. A variety of prolactin-releasing factors have been identified, such as TRH. Women with hyperprolactinemia should be evaluated for the presence of a microadenoma or macroadenoma, generally a slow-growing, benign tumor. This is usually accomplished by radiographic evaluation (coned-down view of sella turcica, CT, or MRI). A variety of conditions and substances causing hyperprolactinemia are noted in Box 1-1.

Hypoestrogenic Anovulation (Hypogonadism)

Clinically, it is useful to assess the status of endogenous estrogen production in women with amenorrhea. A hypoestrogenic condition may be caused by ovarian failure (with hypergonadotropinemia) or hypothalamic dysfunction (with low or low normal FSH levels). Patients with serious hypothalamic dysfunction usually are in a hypoestrogenic state and thus are unresponsive to a progestin challenge. However, they will respond to estrogen and progestin administration. Causes of this condition include anorexia nervosa, stress, weight loss, strenuous exercise, hypothalamic or pituitary tumor, and isolated gonadotropin deficiency (Kallmann's syndrome). Although uncommon, Sheehan's syndrome (hypopituitarism caused by pituitary ischemia and infarction associated with postpartum hemorrhage) is a serious condition resulting in hypogonadotropic amenorrhea.

End-Organ/Outflow Defects

Two general types of anatomic defects of the outflow tract that can cause amenorrhea are congenital malformation of the müllerian duct and acquired anatomic defects. Most of these are diagnosed by physical examination, history, ultrasonography, or MRI.

Congenital anomalies

1. *Müllerian agenesis:* Second most common cause of primary amenorrhea
   a. *46,XX*–Rokitansky-Küster-Hauser syndrome: The uterus and vagina are absent but the ovaries and sexual hair are normal. Urinary tract anomalies such as renal agenesis or pelvic kidney are common (25%-40%).
   b. *46,XY*–Androgen insensitivity syndrome (testicular feminization): X-linked recessive defect of the androgen receptors. The müllerian system (i.e., uterus and tubes) is absent, and a blind, pouched vagina is present. The gonads are testes, usually located in the inguinal canal, labia, or peritoneal cavity. Well-developed breasts and scanty sexual hair growth are typical. Testosterone level is elevated to the male range (>3 ng/ml). An increased risk of malignant transformation of the gonads requires gonadectomy after pubertal development.
2. *Müllerian fusion anomalies:* Transverse septum of the vagina occurs because of failure of the müllerian duct to fuse with the urogenital sinus. Uterine development is usually normal. The septum is located in the mid or upper vagina (85%) or in the lower third of the vagina (15%). No increased incidence of urinary tract anomalies is noted in women with transverse vaginal septum. Congenital absence of the cervix or stenosis is rare. An imperforate hymen is another fusion anomaly.

Acquired anomalies

Asherman's syndrome is characterized by intrauterine synechiae, mostly caused by traumatic D & Cs for abortion or postpartum hemorrhage. Rarely, metroplasty, C-section, myomectomy, or infection such as tuberculosis may be causes. A carefully obtained history will suggest an acquired defect, and diagnosis is confirmed by hysterogram or hysteroscopy. Cervical and vaginal stenosis are also acquired anomalies.

Ovarian Failure

Women with amenorrhea who do not respond to a progestin challenge but bleed after estrogen and progestin administration are estrogen deficient. When serum FSH levels are greater than 40 mIU/ml, gonadal failure is diagnosed. It can be caused by gonadal dysgenesis (GD), premature ovarian failure, gonadotropin-resistant ovary (Savage syndrome), or iatrogenic injury of the ovary.

GD is the most common cause of primary amenorrhea, and these women typically have infantile sexual development. Various somatic anomalies are associated with different types of GD, ranging from normal development to the classic stigmata of Turner's syndrome (i.e., short structure, neck webbing, cubitus valgus, and shieldlike chest). Cardiac anomalies (particularly coarctation of the aorta) and renal anomalies are seen in 15% to 20% of the cases. Chromosomal nondisjunction is usually the etiology. A karyotype must be ordered to rule out the presence of a Y cell line because of the increased risk of malignancy in the dysgenetic gonad with Y chromosome.

Premature ovarian failure (POF) should be considered in women younger than 40 who develop amenorrhea and elevated gonadotropin levels. Women with POF usually have symptoms of estrogen deficiency, such as hot flush and vaginal dryness. Etiologies include idiopathic premature follicular depletion, chromosomal anomalies (karyotyping needed for the nulligravida patient younger than the age of 30), autoimmune disorders (antibody studies are needed, such as ANA, thyroid, and ovarian), and rare enzyme deficiency as in galactosemia. Iatrogenic causes such as radiation or chemotherapy or viral infection should also be considered.

Gonadotropin-resistant ovary syndrome (Savage syndrome) is rare. It is characterized by elevated FSH and LH levels, poor response to HMG therapy, and ovarian tissue showing unstimulated follicles. The cause is unknown, but it is presumed that gonadotropin-receptor deficiency is a possible cause.

TREATMENT

Therapeutic approaches to amenorrhea depend on the diagnoses, associated disorders, patient age, and the patient's desire for conception. Because amenorrhea represents a symptom, its management varies greatly and should be individualized. Although treatment may be mainly for symptomatic relief, one must attempt to identify and eliminate any specific etiology.

Anovulation

For those trying to conceive, induction of ovulation with clomiphene citrate or HMG is indicated. In patients not desiring to conceive, a cyclic progestin (i.e., medroxyprogesterone acetate 10 mg daily for 5 days) or oral contraceptives should be used to prevent endometrial hyperplasia or dysfunctional uterine bleeding. For those with hyperandrogenism (i.e, polycystic ovary syndrome), the use of oral contraceptives may offer regular menstruation and suppression of ovarian androgen production. Adrenal hyperandrogenism can be managed with corticosteroids (i.e., dexamethasone 0.5 mg daily or prednisone 5 to 7.5 mg daily). Although androgen levels can be normalized, anovulation may persist. In such cases, a combination of oral contraceptives and corticosteroids may be effective.

Hyperprolactinemia/Pituitary Tumors

Bromocriptine (dopamine agonist) treatment for hyperprolactinemia and pituitary tumors is very effective and can be given orally or vaginally. The main side effects include nausea and vomiting. In over 90% of cases treated, normal menses are restored along with improvement of galactorrhea. Prolactin-secreting tumors (prolactinomas) are the most common tumors of the pituitary; they may present no clinical problem and are benign and slow-growing. Modern management of these tumors is primarily medical. Even macroadenomas (greater than 1 cm) can be treated with bromocriptine. With this agent, reduction of tumor size and normalization of menstrual cycles are well documented. When suprasellar extension causes neurologic manifestations not responsive to bromocriptine therapy, transsphenoidal surgery is recommended. Radiation therapy is rarely indicated.

Hypoestrogenic Anovulation/Amenorrhea

One must exclude ovarian failure (high FSH level) before considering therapeutic options for hypoestrogenic patients. Serum FSH levels are usually low or low normal. Ovulation and menses can be restored with use of gonadotropins or pulsatile administration of gonadotropin-releasing hormone. Generally, patients with hypoestrogenemia do not respond to clomiphene citrate. Ovulation induction is recommended solely for the purpose of treating infertility. When fertility is not a concern, cyclic estrogen-progestin (as in estrogen replacement therapy) may be recommended to prevent long-term effects of estrogen deficiency on bone density and atrophic changes of the reproductive tract.

Treatment of psychoemotional conditions such as anorexia nervosa or stress should be carefully coordinated with psychologists or psychiatrists. Likewise, patients with amenorrhea caused by weight loss or strenuous exercise will benefit from appropriate counseling.

End-Organ/Outflow Defects

The common congenital anomalies of the genital tract are müllerian agenesis and müllerian fusion anomalies. The former includes Rokitansky-Küster-Hauser syndrome and androgen insensitivity syndrome (or testicular feminization) in which no müllerian differentiation occurred and thus menstruation cannot be restored. Treatment goals may be to create a neovagina for sexual function and to provide counseling. Using nonsurgical dilation, a satisfactory neovagina can be expected in over 80% of the cases. Surgical management to create a neovagina should be reserved for those patients who fail a nonsurgical technique or who refuse the nonsurgical approach. In patients with androgen insensitivity syndrome (a karyotype of 46,XY), gonadectomy must be done because of the risk of malignant tumor. Müllerian fusion anomalies resulting in transverse septum of the vagina or imperforate hymen should be managed surgically by excising the obstructing lesion. Treatment for Asherman's syndrome, the most common acquired anomaly, is surgery with hysteroscopic lysis of adhesions. Postoperative administration of high-dose estrogen is recommended to stimulate regeneration of the endometrium.

Ovarian Failure

Patients with POF have hypergonadotropinemia and hypoestrogenemia. Such patients should be karyotyped to rule out the presence of a Y cell line that would place them at an increased risk of developing dysgerminomas or gonadoblastomas, in which case gonadectomy must be considered. All patients with POF should be advised to start hormone replacement therapy (cyclic estrogen-progestin). Patients with Turner's syndrome (a 45,X gonadal dysgenesis) may also have Hashimoto's thyroiditis, which should be treated. These patients may be able to conceive with the use of donor oocytes and assisted reproductive technology (ART) (in vitro fertilization [IVF] or gamete intrafallopian transfer [GIFT]).

KEY POINTS

1 Amenorrhea is a clinical manifestation associated with various functional and organic disorders that cause a significant alteration in the hypothalamic-pituitary-ovarian axis.

2 Five categories of amenorrhea include anovulation (eugonadotropic or euestrogenic), hyperprolactinemia with or without pituitary tumor, hypogonadotropic hypogonadism, end organ/outflow defect, and ovarian failure (hypergonadotropic and hypoestrogenic).

3 The presence of endogenous estrogen production suggests a functional capacity of the hypothalamic-pituitary-ovarian axis.

4 Hyperprolactinemia is present in 20% to 30% of amenorrheic women and should be evaluated.

5 Therapeutic approaches to amenorrhea depend on the diagnoses, associated disorders, patient age, and the patient's desire for conception.

SUGGESTED READINGS

Doody KM, Carr BR: Amenorrhea, *Obstet Gynecol Clin North Am* 17:361, 1990.

Ho Yeun B, ed: New concepts in the induction of ovulation: *Seminars in Reprod Endocrin,* vol 8, 1990.

Speroff L, Glass RH, Kase NG: Amenorrhea. In: *Clinical gynecologic endocrinology and infertility,* ed 5, Baltimore, 1994, Williams and Wilkins, p 401.

2

Breast Disease

Malignant

WILLIAM B. FARRAR AND WILLIAM E. BURAK, JR.

Cancer of the breast remains a significant health issue despite recent advances resulting in earlier diagnosis and management. Approximately one in nine U.S. women will develop breast cancer, accounting for the second most common cause of cancer-related death. Although it is primarily a disease of older women, breast cancer can affect any age group and is characterized as having a wide variation in its clinical course.

PATHOPHYSIOLOGY

Primary tumors of the breast should be classified as invasive or noninvasive, depending on whether the basement membrane of the mammary ducts has been violated by the tumor cells. Noninvasive, or intraductal, tumors include ductal carcinoma in situ (DCIS) or lobular carcinoma in situ (LCIS), depending on the cell of origin. Invasive *ductal* carcinoma is the most common type of invasive breast malignancy, arising from the epithelial cells that line the mammary ducts. Histologically, varying degrees of DCIS and a surrounding fibrotic response are evident. There are several subtypes of invasive ductal carcinoma including tubular, medullary, papillary, and colloid (mucinous). Invasive *lobular* carcinoma accounts for 3% to 4% of invasive breast cancers and originates from the mammary lobules. These malignancies have a unique histologic appearance characterized by small cells in a linear arrangement (Indian-filing) with a tendency to grow around ducts and lobules (targeted growth).

Although the exact etiology of breast cancer remains uncertain, genetics, hormones, and dietary factors probably play a significant role in carcinogenesis. Extensive research evaluating the role of risk factors for breast cancer continues; however, the findings have not translated into major clinical advances in early detection. Major risk factors include a personal risk of breast cancer, a first-degree relative with breast cancer, and biopsy-proved proliferative breast disease. Minor risk factors include age at menarche, age at which first child is born, and hormone (estrogen) use. These factors are useful in assessing overall risk and should be discussed with patients to help individualize their follow-up. Although a personal history of breast cancer is the strongest risk factor, a first-degree relative with breast cancer places the patient at a risk up to three times greater than that of the general population. True hereditary breast cancer is present in only 5% of all breast cancer cases, whereas the sporadic type accounts for more than 80%. A previous breast biopsy that showed proliferative breast disease also places the patient at increased risk, especially if atypical hyperplasia was present. Patients with atypia **and** a family history have a relative risk of 8.9, which approaches the risk of patients with in situ carcinoma.

With the discovery of the hereditary breast cancer genes BRCA-1 and BRCA-2, one will soon be able to assess an individual patient's risk of developing breast cancer should she be found to have a mutation in one of these genes. Unfortunately, the vast majority of nonhereditary cases of breast cancer do not involve BRCA-1 and BRCA-2 mutations.

DIAGNOSIS

Most patients with breast cancer will have a palpable mass or a mammographic abnormality (Fig. 2-1). Because mammography has proved to be effective in reducing breast cancer mortality in postmenopausal women, it has become widely used as a screening tool in addition to breast self-exam and examination by a physician.

The American Cancer Society guidelines for screening include breast self-exam after age 20, baseline mammogram at age 35 if there is a family history for breast cancer, mammogram every 1 to 2 years for women ages

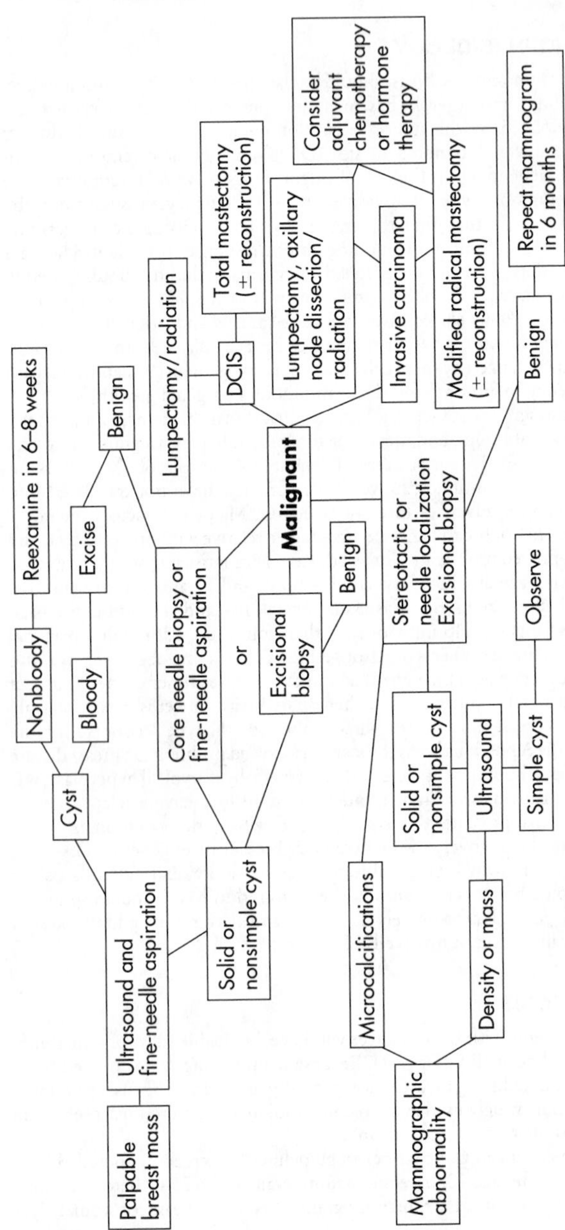

FIG. 2-1 Workup and management of patient with a breast mass.

40 to 49, and annual mammogram for those over age 50. Additionally, professional physical examination of the breast should be performed every 3 years between the ages of 20 and 40, and annually thereafter. These are only guidelines, and individual patients may require modification based on risk-factor analysis. With the inception of new screening programs and the use of these guidelines, earlier and smaller tumors are being diagnosed, resulting in more conservative breast surgery being performed and improved survival rates.

Patients being evaluated for a breast mass require a thorough history, which should include the length of time the palpable abnormality has been present, whether it changes in size during the menstrual cycle, any associated pain or tenderness, and the presence of major or minor risk factors. A painless mass that does not change in size during the menstrual cycle is the most common presentation of a malignancy. Bloody nipple discharge may also be present, although this is more commonly associated with benign disease. The physical examination should be centered around the breast mass, but it is also important to rule out synchronous breast lesions. It should also be determined whether there is fixation of the mass to the underlying chest wall or skin involvement. It is often difficult to discern a dominant mass in patients with fibrocystic changes. In most cases, a dominant nodule will be firmer, with distinct borders, whereas fibrocystic changes tend to be more diffuse and ill-defined. The axillary and supraclavicular nodes should also be palpated, however this is not always an accurate predictor of microscopic node involvement.

Once it is determined that a discrete mass is present, the first step in diagnosis is a thin-needle aspiration of the area in question. If fluid is obtained, three important criteria must be met: (1) the fluid must not be bloody, (2) the mass must completely resolve, and (3) the mass must not reappear on re-examination in 4 to 6 weeks. If the fluid is bloody or not completely drained, excisional biopsy is indicated. If the cyst reappears 4 to 6 weeks after the aspiration, it should be reaspirated. This can be performed two to three times before open excisional biopsy is required. If the mass is not cystic, the patient should undergo an open excisional biopsy, usually under local anesthesia. An alternative method of evaluating a highly suspicious, solid mass is through the use of a core-needle biopsy or fine-needle aspiration (FNA). If the core-needle biopsy permits the diagnosis of a malignancy, an excisional biopsy before definitive treatment is unnecessary. Because accurate results depend on the expertise and experience of the cytologist evaluating the FNA, most surgeons prefer to have a tissue diagnosis before initiating therapy. A negative FNA or core-needle biopsy should be followed by an excisional biopsy to ensure adequate tissue sampling. Before excisional biopsy, a mammogram should be performed not only to evaluate the mass in question but to be certain no other areas of the breast are suspicious. Even if the mammogram is completely negative, the dominant mass requires open biopsy because 10% to 15% of breast cancers are not seen on routine mammogram. Any other suspicious area on the mammogram can then be biopsied at the same time (Fig. 2-2).

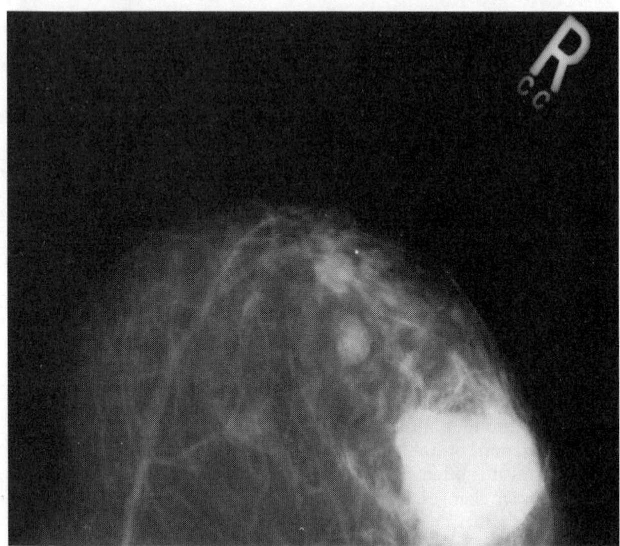

FIG. 2-2 Mammogram of a postmenopausal woman with a large, palpable mass (invasive ductal carcinoma). Note the other lesions, which were not palpable but proved to be additional foci of cancer, demonstrating the value of mammography in evaluating the remainder of the breast before surgery.

Mammographic abnormalities that are suggestive of malignancy are classified as either masses or microcalcifications. If a mass is present on mammography, it can usually be determined by ultrasound examination whether it is cystic or solid; often these two technologies complement one another. If a mass does not meet the sonographic criteria for a simple cyst, or if microcalcifications are present on mammogram, biopsy is warranted. Stereotactic core-needle biopsy or needle localization surgical biopsy are both acceptable biopsy methods. Stereotactic biopsy, done under mammographic guidance, has the advantage of being less "invasive" than a needle localization surgical biopsy, but adequate sampling of the suspicious lesion is required. If atypia is present on a stereotactic biopsy, an open biopsy is necessary to rule out a malignancy. Alternatively, needle localization biopsy involves the radiologist's placing a thin "guide wire" directly into or in close proximity to the mass or microcalcifications under mammographic guidance. The breast tissue near the tip of the wire is then removed surgically, usually under local anesthesia.

DIFFERENTIAL DIAGNOSIS

The differential diagnosis of a palpable breast mass includes a fibroadenoma, which is more common in the younger age group (ages 20 to 30), and fibrocystic mastopathy, seen in premenopausal and perimenopausal women. A fibroadenoma is best described as "rubbery" in consistency, with well-circumscribed borders. Complete excision is both diagnostic and therapeutic. There is no evidence that fibroadenomas will regress with time, therefore if not excised they may be a continued source of confusion. Fibrocystic mastopathy can present in a variety of fashions, including a palpable mass or mammographic abnormality.

Occasionally breast cancer will present with signs of skin erythema and edema (peau d'orange), mimicking a breast abscess. Should this occur in a nonlactating female, a full-thickness biopsy is required to rule out an inflammatory carcinoma. Paget's disease of the breast presents with eczematous changes of the nipple, indicating the presence of a subareolar malignancy, which can be either an intraductal or invasive cancer.

STAGING

The staging of breast cancer relies on both clinical and pathologic criteria that are helpful both in treatment and prognosis. The current staging method is the TNM system, similar to the TNM system used in other malignancies (Box 2-1). Physical examination and histologic confirmation are essential for accurate staging. Physical examination should include an estimate as to tumor size (**T**, tumor), relative mobility or fixation to the underlying pectoral fascia, or skin involvement (ulceration, erythema, and edema). Skin dimpling and pagetoid changes in the nipple do not indicate skin involvement unless accompanied by signs of ulceration, erythema, or edema.

Physical examination can be used to assess the axillary lymph node status (**N**, nodes), however it is not an accurate assessment and requires histologic evaluation of the lymph nodes obtained at the time of lumpectomy or mastectomy. A clinically "negative" axilla may contain histologically positive lymph nodes in up to 30% of patients.

Evidence of distant metastasis (**M**, metastasis) should be obtained through a careful history, physical exam, and the selective use of imaging studies. Since the most common sites of metastases are bone, lung, and liver, a chest x-ray and liver function tests are appropriate. A bone scan can be obtained, however its yield in the asymptomatic patient is extremely low. It can serve as a useful baseline study in the event that skeletal pain does develop in the follow-up period. Patients who initially have symptoms suggestive of metastatic disease benefit from the use of selected imaging studies (i.e., CT studies of the chest, abdomen, and brain).

TREATMENT

Noninvasive Carcinoma

DCIS

DCIS can present as a breast mass, either palpable or discovered on a mammogram. Additionally, it may be present (microscopic) in breast tissue surrounding a benign lesion discovered incidentally with a biopsy. By definition, DCIS is noninvasive, so metastasis outside of the breast is not

BOX 2-1

Breast TNM Classification

PRIMARY TUMOR (T)

TX Primary tumor cannot be assessed
T0 No evidence of primary tumor
Tis Carcinoma in situ
T1 Tumor 2 cm or less in greatest dimension
T2 Tumor >2 cm, but ≤5 cm in greatest dimension
T3 Tumor >5 cm in greatest dimension
T4 Tumor of any size with direct extension to chest wall or skin

REGIONAL LYMPH NODES (N)

N0 No regional axillary lymph node metastasis
N1 Metastasis to movable ipsilateral axillary lymph node(s)
N2 Metastasis to fixed ipsilateral axillary lymph node(s)
N3 Metastasis to ipsilateral internal mammary lymph node(s)

DISTANT METASTASIS

M0 No distant metastasis
M1 Distant metastasis

STAGE GROUPING

Stage 0	Tis	N0	M0
Stage I	T1	N0	M0
Stage II	T0, T1	N1	M0
	T2	N0, N1	M0
	T3	N0	M0
Stage III	T0, T1	N2	M0
	T2	N2	M0
	T3	N1, N2	M0
	T4	Any N	M0
	Any T	N3	M0
Stage IV	Any T	Any N	M1

Modified from the American Joint Committee on Cancer: *Manual for staging of cancer,* ed 4, Philadelphia, 1992, JB Lippincott.

found unless there are areas of microinvasion that go unrecognized. Patients with DCIS should be treated with lumpectomy followed by radiation therapy to the breast because their lifetime risk of developing an invasive cancer in that breast now approaches 30%. Radiation decreases the recurrence rate when instituted after complete excision with negative margins. Axillary dissection is not indicated unless an accompanying invasive cancer is present. Diffuse, extensive DCIS often requires total mastectomy.

Follow-up requires frequent physical exams as well as annual mammograms; these patients are at extremely high risk for the development of invasive cancer and should be followed in high-risk clinics.

LCIS

LCIS is a diagnosis usually made coincidentally when examining breast tissue for another reason. It does not present as a mass and is not evident on mammogram. Patients with LCIS are at a lifetime risk of 17% to 37% for developing *invasive ductal carcinoma* in either breast. Because of these factors, LCIS is not considered an early stage of breast cancer, but rather a marker for subsequent cancer development. Therefore patients with an LCIS diagnosis should be followed in a high-risk clinic with frequent (6 months) exams and annual mammography, and should be considered for enrollment into breast cancer prevention trials. An alternative treatment that can be offered to selected patients involves bilateral simple mastectomy with immediate reconstruction.

Invasive Carcinoma

Once the diagnosis of an invasive malignancy is made, a chest x-ray, baseline liver function tests, and a bone scan should be obtained. These baseline tests are obtained in case the patient later develops symptoms suggestive of metastatic disease, allowing a comparative study to be done.

Surgical options

Following the diagnosis of invasive cancer, treatment options should be completely discussed with the patient. A surgeon, radiation therapist, and plastic surgeon should be included in the discussions; the more information provided to the patient, the better opportunity she will have to make an educated decision. The final decision should not be influenced by the specific bias of the surgeon or other physician. Surgery remains the initial treatment for AJCC stage I, II, and some stage III breast cancers. In stage I and most stage II cancers, surgical options include a modified radical mastectomy or a lumpectomy with axillary dissection followed by breast irradiation. For large stage II and stage III tumors, modified radical mastectomy is the procedure of choice. Patients with advanced locoregional disease (including inflammatory cancer) may benefit from preoperative (neoadjuvant) chemotherapy and postoperative radiation therapy to maximize local control.

For early stage cancers (stage I and II), modified radical mastectomy or lumpectomy with axillary dissection should both be considered viable options. Several prospective studies have shown that these procedures both result in the same long-term survival rate, despite an increased local recurrence rate in patients treated with lumpectomy and axillary dissection.

There are several contraindications to lumpectomy and axillary dissection, such as multicentric cancer, retroareolar tumor location, and large tumor size in relation to breast size. Since the goal of breast-sparing surgery is to achieve an optimal cosmetic result, a lumpectomy that results in a less than desirable appearance should be avoided. Patients with small breasts are often poor candidates for lumpectomy and axillary dissection because lumpectomy followed by radiation produces a suboptimal cosmetic result. Therefore no absolute tumor size is an absolute contraindication, but the relative size should be considered. Additionally, patients with large breasts are not ideal candidates because the cosmetic appearance after radiation is often poor.

If a modified radical mastectomy is chosen, immediate reconstruction can be offered to selected patients. Those with advanced locoregional disease are not good candidates because local recurrence rates are high and postoperative radiation therapy may be necessary. Otherwise the options for immediate reconstruction include saline tissue expanders and implants or autologous tissue transfer with either a latissmus dorsi or rectus abdominus (TRAM) myocutaneous flap. Consultation with a plastic surgeon should be obtained before surgery so the patient can make an educated decision.

Adjuvant therapy

The rationale for adjuvant systemic therapy is based on the premise that many patients with early breast cancer have undetectable metastases that, if left unaddressed, would result in recurrence. Even though these micrometastases may not be clinically detectable, their presence is suggested by the natural history of many patients treated with surgery alone. There are two forms of systemic therapy used in adjuvant therapy–chemotherapy and hormonal therapy. When determining which early stage breast cancer patients will benefit from this additional treatment, it is useful to classify patients as pre- or postmenopausal, and node positive or node negative.

It is well accepted that premenopausal node-positive patients benefit from adjuvant chemotherapy. The 1985 NIH Consensus Panel concluded that adjuvant chemotherapy prolonged survival in this group of patients and should be considered the standard of care. The combination of cyclophosphamide, methotrexate (or adriamycin), and 5-flourouracil is the regimen of choice. Recently there has been increased interest in more dose-intensive chemotherapy for selected node-positive patients. Peters and colleagues report using high-dose chemotherapy with bone marrow transplant in premenopausal women with greater than 10 positive lymph nodes. The outcome of this nonrandomized trial resulted in a survival advantage in treated patients when compared with historical controls. This treatment is presently being evaluated in a larger group of patients in multicenter, randomized trials.

Premenopausal node-positive patients with positive estrogen receptors should be considered for treatment with hormonal therapy following chemotherapy because this may delay recurrence, although a survival advantage has been difficult to document in large clinical trials. It should be emphasized that this advantage, while statistically significant, is modest and has not proved to be associated with an improvement in overall survival. Unfortunately not all node-negative patients benefit from this therapy, so a tremendous amount of effort has gone into identifying "high risk" node-negative patients who might benefit. Tumor size, estrogen receptor content, DNA analysis, grade, and blood vessel invasion are taken into consideration in assessing risk of recurrence. Adjuvant chemotherapy is not without toxicity, so the clinician ideally would want to treat the group that would receive the most benefit. As more clinical trials are completed, treatment strategies will become more standardized.

Postmenopausal node-positive breast cancer patients generally are less likely to enjoy the same benefits of chemotherapy as the premenopausal group. Therefore hormonal therapy has been used in the adjuvant setting in postmenopausal hormone receptor–positive patients. Tamoxifen clearly improves disease-free survival in these patients in many studies, however only two trials have shown an overall survival advantage. Tamoxifen has been used in postmenopausal node-negative estrogen receptor–positive patients with a modest but significant improvement in disease-free survival. Chemotherapy is not effective in this setting.

Follow-up

Patients with early stage breast cancer should be followed for the remainder of their life because recurrences are seen as much as 15 to 20 years after diagnosis. These patients are also at increased risk of developing a second breast cancer. Therefore follow-up is aimed at detecting recurrence and screening the remaining breast tissue for malignancy. Patients should be followed at 3-month intervals for the first 2 to 3 years, and at 6-month intervals thereafter. Any new symptoms of bone pain, headaches, or neurologic changes should prompt an immediate workup. Otherwise, chest x-rays and liver function tests are performed during regular follow-up exams. Additionally, all patients should have annual mammograms to evaluate for local recurrence or a new cancer. The use of serum tumor markers (CEA, CA15-3) is controversial, but may help detect a metastatic lesion before development of symptoms.

Treatment of Metastatic Disease

The goal of systemic therapy for metastatic breast cancer is to improve quality of life and, if possible, prolong survival. Conventional therapy provides palliation to selected patients, however a survival benefit has been difficult to document. Conventional treatment can be either hormonal therapy or chemotherapy, depending on the patient's age, severity of symptoms, and hormone status of the primary tumor. Postmenopausal patients with estrogen or progesterone receptor–positive tumors who have non–life-threatening recurrences are good candidates for hormonal therapy, usually tamoxifen. If a response is seen and the patient subsequently progresses, a second-line hormone therapy should be instituted, usually a progestin or aromatase inhibitor. Response rates of up to 60% to 70% can be expected with hormonal therapy.

Chemotherapy is generally used in younger, hormone-unresponsive women or in a patient with life-threatening metastases, where a quicker response is needed. Conventional chemotherapy consists of the same agents used in adjuvant treatment: cyclophosphamide, 5-fluorouracil, and adriamycin or methotrexate. Taxol is also effective in this setting. Response rates range from 20% to 50%, with an average duration of 6 months.

High-dose chemotherapy with autologous bone marrow rescue (following conventional "induction" therapy) is becoming increasingly popular in the treatment of metastatic disease. Complete response rates are seen in 25% to 60% of patients, many of which are durable. With improved hematopoietic growth factors and the use of peripheral stem cells (as opposed to bone marrow), the morbidity and mortality of this procedure will hopefully be far outweighed by the benefit.

KEY POINTS

1 In the United States, approximately one in nine women will develop breast cancer during their lifetime.

2 Major risk factors include a personal risk of breast cancer, a first-degree relative with breast cancer, and biopsy-proved proliferative breast disease.

3 Solid, palpable breast masses should undergo biopsy regardless of patient age or mammographic findings.

4 Noninvasive ductal carcinoma (DCIS) accounts for more than 20% of mammographically detected cancers and is treated with lumpectomy followed by breast radiation.

5 The initial treatment of early stage breast cancer consists of lumpectomy, axillary dissection, and radiation or modified radical mastectomy.

6 Locally advanced breast cancer is usually treated with systemic chemotherapy followed by surgery.

7 For breast cancer metastasized to lung, bone, liver, and brain, treatment involves systemic chemotherapy or hormonal therapy. Symptomatic bone or brain metastases often require radiation therapy for effective palliation.

SUGGESTED READINGS

Fisher B et al: Lumpectomy compared with lumpectomy and radiation therapy for the treatment of intraductal breast cancer, *N Engl J Med* 328:1581-1586, 1993.

Kennedy MJ et al: High-dose chemotherapy with reinfusion of purged autologous bone marrow following dose-intense induction as initial therapy of metastatic breast cancer, *J Natl Cancer Inst* 83:920-926, 1991.

Peters WP et al: High dose chemotherapy with autologous bone marrow transplantation as consolidation after standard-dose adjuvant therapy for high-risk primary breast cancer, *J Clin Oncol* 11:1132-1143, 1993.

Benign

Douglas J. Marchant

Benign breast disease is more common than breast cancer, although the latter receives the most attention. The majority of patients complain of pain, a mass, or nipple discharge (Table 2-1). Frequently, these women receive inappropriate treatment because the symptoms are subjective and the findings often nonspecific. Special problems, including nipple discharge and mastitis, may occur during pregnancy and lactation.

Making the correct diagnosis and recommending appropriate treatment is complicated by a lack of basic knowledge about the descriptive and analytic epidemiology of these conditions, including the following:

1. No mass is obviously benign.
2. Nipple discharge seldom is associated with breast cancer; 85% to 90% of the cases are associated with benign breast disease.
3. Inflammation, unless associated with lactation, is unusual.

TABLE 2-1
Benign Breast Disease Versus Cancer

Factor	Benign breast disease	Breast cancer
SYMPTOMS AND PHYSICAL EXAMINATION		
Pain	Common	Uncommon
Nipple discharge	Common	Uncommon
Mass	Common	Common
DIAGNOSTIC STUDIES		
Mammogram	Seldom helpful	May confirm diagnosis and rule out occult lesion
Ultrasound	Helpful to differentiate cyst versus solid mass	Seldom helpful
FNA	May be helpful if there is a specific diagnosis	Helpful if positive
Pap smear	Seldom helpful	Helpful if positive
TREATMENT		
Surgery	Rarely	Multidisciplinary approach (surgery, radiation therapy, oncology)
Symptomatic	Usually	Rarely (palliation)
Specific	Rarely	Usually
Successful	Usually, but not always	Depends on stage of disease

4. Pain is an extremely subjective complaint. Experience has shown that correct diagnosis and successful treatment are directly proportional to the time spent with the patient. Frequently the pain is referred.

COMMON BENIGN NEOPLASMS

Common benign neoplasms for the most part represent palpable masses discovered during the reproductive years. The etiology is unknown, however fibroadenomas and phyllode tumors begin their development soon after menarche. A fibroadenoma is usually a single, painless, dominant mass. However, ultrasound evaluation of each breast may reveal multiple, nonpalpable lesions. Fibroadenoma is the most common lesion in the adolescent. Phyllodes are rare. The distinction between benign and malignant tumors depends on the mitotic activity of the lesion. Benign phyllode tumors are treated by repeat wide, local excision. Usually this can be accomplished with minimal cosmetic deformity.

The adenoma is a variant of the fibroadenoma and is composed of adenomatous or glandular elements. Specific types include adenoma of the nipple and lactational adenoma, which is discovered during pregnancy or lactation.

A lipoma may occur during the reproductive period but is most commonly found postmenopausally.

The intraductal papilloma usually is associated with nipple discharge (either clear, serosanguinous, or bloody). Most of these lesions are benign, but occasionally they will contain areas of intraductal carcinoma or frankly invasive tumor.

Patients who have bloody nipple discharge must be investigated, with one exception. Bloody nipple discharge, occasionally bilateral, is not unusual during pregnancy, particularly during the latter weeks of gestation. Bleeding is the result of disruption of blood vessels because of the rapid increase in functioning breast tissue in preparation for lactation. The discharge disappears following delivery. In non-pregnant patients, the duct must be located and surgically removed.

Palpable lesions must be considered cancer until proved otherwise. No lesion is obviously benign. The single exception is the mass discovered during adolescence. Palpable lesions also cannot be considered benign on the basis of their physical features (i.e., round, smooth, mobile, and nontender). For the young patient with a single, palpable mass, elective surgical removal is indicated. This usually is performed under local anesthesia. Patients with multiple palpable lesions present a therapeutic dilemma. Usually the largest and most symptomatic lesions are removed, thus confirming the diagnosis and avoiding multiple incisions. An alternative is fine-needle aspiration (FNA), provided that a specific diagnosis is given (i.e., consistent with fibroadenoma versus normal breast tissue). For mammographically discovered occult lesions, ultrasound evaluation may be used to assess stability. If there is any question concerning the diagnosis, open biopsy should be performed.

Occasionally, histologic evaluation of biopsy material will indicate atypical changes such as ductal hyperplasia with atypical changes and sclerosing adenosis. Management depends on the degree of atypia, which increases the risk for subsequent breast cancer 3 to 5 times.

FIBROCYSTIC CHANGES

The term *fibrocystic changes* represents a heterogeneous group of symptoms and clinical findings that surface during the late reproductive years–typically after age 35. Patients may experience a sudden onset of a painful, tender "mass" in one or both breasts. Physical examination reveals a dominant mass, and diagnosis of a simple cyst is confirmed either by ultrasound or aspiration. Therapeutic decisions become more complicated in the patient with multiple dominant masses, which are often asymptomatic and bilateral. Mammography often reveals multiple densities that on ultrasound represent simple cysts. These findings are not associated with the later development of carcinoma. Treatment often consists of reassurance, the occasional aspiration of a painful cyst, and follow-up ultrasound evaluation to confirm the diagnosis.

Mastodynia presents a major diagnostic challenge. It is a subjective complaint, and the origin of the pain may or may not be in the breast parenchyma. Cyclic mastalgia, discomfort occurring immediately before menses, is not uncommon. Patients usually seek treatment only when the discomfort occurs throughout the menstrual cycle or consistently in one breast. Many of these patients have referred pain, and careful examination will reveal that the tenderness is in the anterior chest wall. Symptomatic relief usually is proportional to the time spent with the patient, including obtaining a detailed history with specific reference to the details of physical activities, followed by a careful physical examination in multiple positions.

A number of treatment regimens have been recommended, none of which are entirely successful. These have included use of various hormones and vitamins, and restriction of methylxanthines. Recent evidence suggests that there is no relationship between caffeine and fibrocystic changes. On the other hand, if the patient "feels better" after restriction of these substances, one should not discourage continued abstinence.

INFLAMMATION

The most common inflammation of the breast is mastitis, either puerperal or nonpuerperal (i.e., squamous metaplasia). The etiology of puerperal mastitis is unknown, however a contribution by the infant, usually related to "cracked" nipples, has been suggested. Initial symptoms include a localized area of inflammation and tenderness and slight elevation of temperature. Treatment includes continuation of breastfeeding and use of appropriate antibiotics. Penicillin or one of its derivatives is the treatment of choice. If the patient does not respond and the tenderness and fever persist, a breast abscess should be suspected. Treatment is adequate drainage under general anesthesia, and antibiotics should be continued in full therapeutic doses for 7 to 10 days.

Occasionally patients present with nonlactational mastitis where periodic drainage occurs in the vicinity of the nipple areolar complex. Treatment with antibiotics and incision and drainage are unsuccessful. This condition is known as *squamous metaplasia.* It is not clear whether the infection occurs initially, followed by squamous metaplasia and intermittent discharge, or whether squamous metaplasia occurs first and is followed by infection. In either event, treatment is complete excision of the involved duct system.

NIPPLE DISCHARGE

Nipple discharge is either physiologic or pathologic. In the majority of cases the patient can be immediately reassured that cancer is unlikely. Approximately 10% to 12% of patients with breast cancer have associated nipple discharge.

A careful and detailed history is essential to make the proper diagnosis. Is the discharge produced only at the time of breast self-examination or when the nipple is squeezed? Does it occur with sexual stimulation? Does the patient take medication? Has she ever been pregnant? What are her physical activities? Most patients can describe the character of the discharge, however "bloody" nipple discharge when placed on a gauze pad often is black or green and no blood cells are found on microscopic evaluation.

Physiologic discharges occur after ovulation in some patients and also with sexual stimulation and medications, including oral contraceptives. The most common cause of physiologic discharge is duct ectasia. The discharge usually is bilateral and from several ducts. The classic symptom is bilateral, grayish to greenish-black discharge from multiple openings on the nipple. It may be unilateral. There is no specific treatment. Usually the discharge disappears within a few months. Surgical treatment is not indicated.

Three types of nipple discharge must be further evaluated: milky discharge, serous or bloody discharge, and postmenopausal discharge.

Galactorrhea is the spontaneous secretion of milky discharge not immediately associated with a pregnancy. Usually it is persistent and voluminous. Elevated prolactin levels may be associated with galactorrhea. Physiologic causes of hyperprolactinemia include breast stimulation, coitus, eating, exercise, pregnancy, sleep, and stress. Hyperprolactinemia also may be a result of pathologic factors, including brain and pituitary disorders, encephalitis, and pituitary microadenomas or macroadenomas. In addition, a number of pharmacologic agents may produce hyperprolactinemia.

Prolactin is secreted in a sleep-related circadian rhythm with maximum release between 3 AM and 5 AM. Therefore serum samples should be obtained in a fasting state between 8 AM and noon. A serum prolactin level greater than 20 ng/ml may be abnormal and should be further evaluated. Most of these patients should be referred to a reproductive endocrinologist for additional diagnostic studies and treatment. A quick diagnostic study in the office includes microscopic examination of the discharge that may reveal refractile fat globules, confirming the diagnosis of true galactorrhea.

Serous or bloody nipple discharge must be investigated and may be caused by a benign intraductal papilloma. However, carcinoma can occur in 10% to 15% of these patients. Treatment is excision of the involved duct.

Postmenopausal nipple discharge must be viewed with suspicion. Careful examination of the breast may reveal a mass or other findings consistent with carcinoma. Appropriate diagnostic studies include a mammogram and in most cases an open biopsy.

KEY POINTS

1 Breast discomfort usually is associated with fibrocystic changes.

2 The most common breast infection is puerperal mastitis, however the possibility of recurrent squamous metaplasia must not be overlooked in the non-pregnant patient.

3 Nipple discharge seldom is associated with breast cancer, however galactorrhea, serous or bloody discharge, and postmenopausal discharge should be carefully evaluated to rule out carcinoma, and in the case of galactorrhea, pituitary disorders.

4 No mass is obviously benign and, except for the teenager, each should be carefully evaluated to rule out carcinoma.

5 For most disorders the definitive treatment is surgical; however, for certain types of nipple discharge and mastodynia, symptomatic treatment and reassurance constitute appropriate therapy.

SUGGESTED READINGS

Fentiman IS: Mastalgia mostly merits masterly inactivity (Editorial), *Br J Clin Pract* 46:158, 1992.

Lafreniere R: Bloody nipple discharge during pregnancy: a rationale for conservative treatment, *J Surg Oncol* 43:228, 1990.

Leis HP Jr: Gross breast cysts: significance of apocrine type, identification by cyst fluid analysis and management, *Breast Dis* 6:185, 1993.

Marchant DJ: Breast diseases and the gynecologist, *Curr Prob Obstet, Gynecol, Infertil* 15:12, 1992.

3

Cervical Cancer

George S. Lewandowski and Luis Vaccarello

Management of cervical cancer should address screening, diagnosis, staging, and treatment. The impact of cervical cytologic screening is reflected in the 1997 American Cancer Society estimates that in the United States, 65,000 new cases of carcinoma in situ will be found, 14,500 new cases of cervical cancer will be diagnosed, and 4800 women will die of this disease each year. Effective screening with early diagnosis undoubtedly offers the best chance at eliminating cervical cancer.

DIAGNOSIS

Some women ultimately found to have cervical cancer seek treatment for abnormal, often postcoital, vaginal bleeding. Others will have undergone biopsy during evaluation of an abnormal Pap smear or when an abnormal lesion is demonstrated on exam. Although colposcopy is a great aid in the assessment of abnormal subclinical cervical lesions, biopsy should be performed on gross lesions at the time of discovery. Before biopsy, the clinician should carefully note the size, shape, and location of the abnormal areas. This approach is of particular importance if loop excision is chosen to provide the biopsy material, since orientation of the specimen and completeness of excision may have a significant effect on treatment decisions. It is important that frankly invasive cancer unequivocally demonstrated on biopsy **should not** be followed by loop excision or cone biopsy. These modalities should be reserved for cases in which the precise histopathologic diagnosis is unclear after biopsy.

Each patient's outcome will ultimately be determined by the extent of cancer spread (stage), its histologic appearance, and its biologic behavior. Once a diagnosis has been established by biopsy, staging and treatment should be quickly initiated and directed by an individual or team experienced in managing gynecologic malignancy.

PRETREATMENT EVALUATION

Staging

An accurate assessment of the extent of malignancy spread is crucial to treatment planning and estimating prognosis. The International Federation of Obstetrics and Gynecology (FIGO) has adopted and periodically revised definitions for the staging of gynecologic cancer. Revised FIGO guidelines for staging cervical cancer were published in 1995 (Box 3-1).

BOX 3-1

Summary of 1995 FIGO Staging for Cervical Cancer

Stage I	Invasive cancer confined to the cervix
IA	Invasive cancer identified microscopically
IA1	Stromal invasion 3 mm or less; width 7 mm or less
IA2	Stromal invasion between 3 and 5 mm; width 7 mm or less
IB	Invasive cancer greater than 5 mm in depth or 7 mm in width *or any size* lesion diagnosed on gross examination
IB1	Clinical lesion 4 cm or less in size
IB2	Clinical lesion greater than 4 cm in size
Stage II	Invasive cancer beyond cervix; not to the pelvic wall and not to the distal third of the vagina
IIA	No parametrial involvement (disease confined to upper two-thirds of the vagina)
IIB	Parametrial involvement
Stage III	Extension to the pelvic wall and/or the distal third of the vagina
IIIA	No extension to the pelvic wall (disease involves the distal third of the vagina)
IIIB	Extension to the pelvic wall (includes hydronephrosis and nonfunctioning kidney)
Stage IV	Extension beyond the true pelvis
IVA	Involves bladder or rectal mucosa
IVB	Spread to distant organs

The FIGO assignment of stage is based on a clinical examination and the evaluation of all pertinent histologic material. Since FIGO has chosen to allow only studies that are available worldwide, some important information (CT scan and MRI results) that would be available at many clinical centers is not formally allowed in the staging process (Box 3-2).

Disallowing advanced radiographic or surgical evaluation increases the likelihood of underestimating small or microscopic disease in the lymph system or within solid organs. The Gynecologic Oncology Group (GOG) recognizes the effect that this could have on the results of contemporary research and many GOG protocols allow the use of pretreatment CT scans and may require a retroperitoneal staging surgery with resection of pelvic and paraortic lymph nodes as a condition for eligibility. In clinical stage I and stage IIA disease, patients treated with radical hysterectomy are eligible for clinical trials only after the demonstration of nodal status via transperitoneal lymphadenectomy. Thus although all patients are assigned a pretreatment FIGO stage, entry onto GOG trials often requires the histologic confirmation of lymph node status, thus instituting a de facto surgical staging.

BOX 3-2
Staging Modalities Used in Cervical Cancer

ALLOWED BY FIGO

Physical examination
- General survey including lymphatics
- Vaginal examination
- Bimanual rectovaginal exam (consider exam under anesthesia)

Radiographic examinations
- Intravenous pyelogram (IVP)
- Barium enema
- Chest x-ray
- Skeletal x-rays

Procedures
- Biopsy (includes colposcopy, endocervical curretage, hysteroscopy, and conization)
- Cystoscopy
- Proctosigmoidoscopy

NOT ALLOWED BY FIGO

CT
MRI
Lymphangiography
Ultrasound
Radionucleotide imaging
Laparoscopy
Staging laparotomy

General Health Assessment

A comprehensive survey of the patient's overall health constitutes an important pretherapy consideration. Although studies suggest that age alone is a poor predictor of a patient's tolerance for therapy, other co-morbid conditions significantly affect the development and completion of a treatment plan.

Histology

Over the past 50 years, cytologic screening and the treatment of cervical dysplasia led to a decrease in the incidence of squamous cervical cancer. However, the relative occurrence of adenocarcinoma of the cervix appears to be rising, approaching 30% of all cases at some institutions.

The small-cell neuroendocrine cervical tumor has been identified. Although its histologic features are similar to small-cell cervical squamous cancer, immunocytochemistry can be used to differentiate between the two. The distinction is important because neuroendocrine lesions are more aggressive and both therapy and prognosis are affected by this accurate determination.

THERAPY

Treatment decisions in cervical cancer are based primarily on clinical stage (Fig. 3-1). Obviously, no mature, prospectively obtained patient management data can exist that is based on the 1995 FIGO classification.

Microinvasion (Stage IA1)

A microinvasive lesion is a squamous lesion that extends below the cervical basement membrane and yet carries a minimal risk of nodal metastasis. It therefore exceeds carcinoma in situ, or high-grade squamous intraepithelial lesion, but has little risk of systemic spread. Varying definitions of microinvasion have been proposed. Notably, all require a cervical cone biopsy with clear margins to establish a diagnosis of microinvasion. In spite of its wide use, loop excision technology has not been specifically addressed in the definition, even though several studies suggest that an appropriately performed loop excision provides similar information to a cervical cone biopsy.

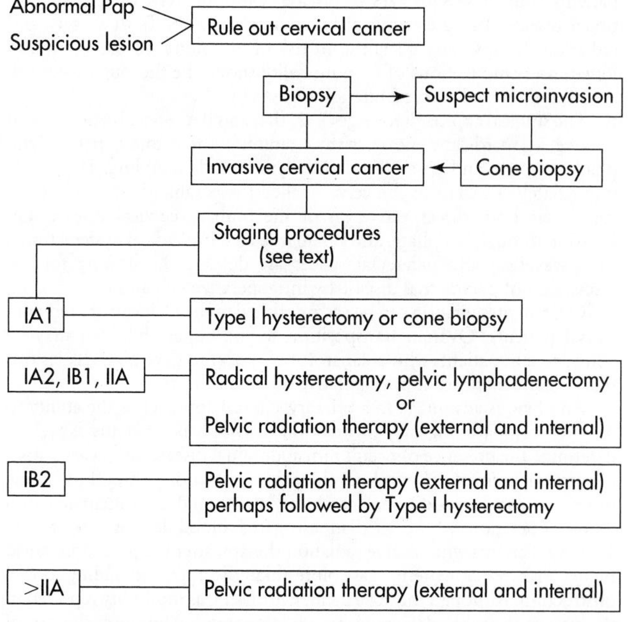

FIG. 3-1 Initial management options in cervical cancer.

The debate that surrounds the definition of microinvasion carries over into its management. Although it appears that hysterectomy (either vaginal or abdominal) constitutes sufficient treatment for microinvasive squamous cancer (FIGO Stage IA1), cervical conization with careful follow-up has been proposed as a reasonable alternative. Although some previously held definitions of microinvasion would encompass FIGO Stage IA2, many physicians would be uncomfortable managing a IA2 lesion without hysterectomy and some would propose an even more radical approach.

As noted previously, the definition of squamous microinvasion cannot be applied to cervical adenocarcinoma. In cases where hysterectomy has been performed shortly after a cone with clear margins has demonstrated adenocarcinoma in situ, residual disease can frequently be found. This implies a risk of multifocal disease not found in squamous microinvasion. Thus the management of cervical adenocarcinoma in situ remains controversial.

Early Stage Invasive Disease (Stages IA2, IB1, and IIA)

Since pelvic nodal metastases are found in about 15% of stages IA2, IB1, and IIA patients, management of these nodes constitutes an important issue. The anticipated 5-year survival rate of about 85% to 90% suggests that acceptable radiotherapeutic and surgical strategies exist that are useful in patients with these substages of disease. Unfortunately, the presence of nodal disease decreases survival by as much as 50%. Both surgery and radiation therapy carry a significant risk of morbidity, so the short- and long-term complications of each modality should be thoroughly considered and discussed before initiation of therapy.

The surgical approach to stages IA2, IB1, and IIA cervical cancer would involve a laparotomy along with a radical hysterectomy, pelvic lymphadenectomy, and possible paraortic lymph node sampling. The tissues immediately adjacent to the cervix–called the parametria–are at risk for spread via both direct extension of the primary cervical disease and invasion through lymphatic and vascular spaces. In a radical hysterectomy, the paravesical and pararectal spaces are developed, allowing for the assessment of parametrial disease by intraoperative palpation.

Ovarian preservation can be accomplished in the majority of premenopausal patients. Ovarian transposition to the upper abdomen may be considered in patients who at laparotomy appear to have high-risk lesions that might benefit from postoperative radiation therapy.

An obvious advantage to a primary surgical approach is the ability to provide histopathological confirmation of lymph node status as well as determine the presence of occult intraabdominal disease. Surgical complications include events such as bleeding, infection, thromboembolic disorders, and the additional morbidity that could be anticipated in a 4-hour operation whose median estimated blood loss is reported at 1100 ml. Patients who receive radiation therapy after the procedure are at higher risk for long-term gastrointestinal disorders, including bowel obstruction. Although the 50% incidence of serious morbidity reported in the past is probably decreased by contemporary techniques, the use of radical hysterectomy and radiation therapy should be reserved for patients with high risk for recurrence. Transabdominal lymphadenectomy for cervical cancer without radical hysterectomy should be avoided. In patients who will be involved in a clinical trial, a pelvic and paraortic lymphadenectomy can be performed using a retroperitoneal approach with lower risk of postoperative gastrointestinal complications.

Bulky Cervical Disease (Stage IB2)

The 1995 FIGO staging modification that divides macroscopically visible cervical lesions (stage IB) into stages IB1 and IB2 is a recognition that bulky tumors confined to the cervix present an additional treatment challenge. Lesions now classified as IB2 were formerly referred to as *bulky* or *barrel-shaped* IB lesions. The treatment controversy that surrounds these tumors recognizes that increased tumor volume within the cervical primary increases the likelihood of nodal metastases. Relatively poor oxygenation to these tumors may increase their resistance to radiotherapy. As a result, a combination of radiation therapy followed with an extrafascial hysterectomy has been proposed in an effort to combine modalities while minimizing morbidity. The GOG has attempted to identify optimal therapy with GOG Protocol 71–randomizing eligible patients to traditional pelvic radiation (external beam plus two brachytherapy implants) or a combined approach using similar external beam therapy and a single implant, followed by an extrafascial hysterectomy. Although the data has not fully matured, there is a significant recurrence rate and lower survival probability than with nonbulky lesions, supporting the concept of a more aggressive approach. Results of this study and other trials are needed to clearly define a treatment plan.

Advanced Pelvic Disease (Stages IIB, III, and IVA)

Radiation therapy constitutes the primary modality of therapy in women whose cervical cancer extends beyond the cervix and upper vagina at the time of staging. A treatment plan should be developed that usually starts with external beam radiation therapy (teletherapy) and finishes with use of internal brachytherapy implants. To maximize the antitumor effect, the course of therapy should be completed with as few days without treatment as side effects will allow.

External radiation therapy is administered according to a predetermined prescription that defines a total dose given to a specific field by a route and over a time interval that will allow the delivery of regular fractions. Issues that are crucial to the success of radiation therapy include tumor radiosensitivity, the tolerance of surrounding normal tissues, and the intent of the therapeutic intervention (i.e., long-term curve versus short-term palliation).

A generic treatment plan to treat advanced cervical cancer begins with external beam radiation. The total teletherapy dose ranges from 45 to 50 Gy delivered in 1.8 to 2.0 Gy fractions over 5 to 6 weeks. The machine's voltage, the route of delivery (ports), and pelvic fields are defined, which ideally sterilizes tumor within the pelvic lymph nodes and shrinks the central tumor. The reduction in tumor size from effective external beam therapy should facilitate placement of the internal radiation therapy device closer to the central mass. Ultimately this would suggest a higher likelihood of cure with lower morbidity from treatment. Although techniques are used to block the delivery of radiation to tissues not involved with tumor, some organs cannot be excluded. As a result, the side effects and complications of pelvic radiation therapy include diarrhea, colitis, small and large bowel obstruction, gastrointestinal and genitourinary fistulae, and suppression of irradiated pelvic bone marrow. Care in developing and executing a treatment plan can lower the incidence of these conditions but will not eliminate their occurrence.

A number of compounds are being investigated in an effort to improve outcome in advanced cervical cancer. Chemotherapeutic agents (cisplatinum, 5-fluorouracil, hydroxyurea), antibiotics (metronidazole), and other drugs (WR-2721) are currently in use or have been used with radiation therapy in clinical trials in an effort to improve tumor cell sensitivity to radiation. Any inherent antitumor effect that the compound carries would be of additional theoretical benefit. Unfortunately, each of these agents also has side effects with the potential to interrupt the radiation treatment plan, and they are most properly used in the setting of a clinical trial.

Advanced Extrapelvic Disease

The delivery of radiation therapy to paraortic nodes that contain metastatic cancer is an area of controversy and ongoing research. Although some contend that up to 25% of patients may be salvaged in this setting, the delivery of radiation through the relatively immobile duodenum and distal ileum provides a setting with a significant risk of bowel obstruction.

Extranodal cervical cancer that can be demonstrated beyond the pelvis has a very poor prognosis. Treatment must be individualized. A plan should address both short-term local control of disease and relief from those symptoms likely to result from the metastatic spread. Radiotherapy to specific metastases, chemotherapy, and limited surgery may play a role in this setting.

Recurrent Cervical Cancer

The suspicion of recurrent cervical cancer should be evaluated quickly and thoroughly by a physician experienced in managing this condition. A thorough examination and careful biopsies confirming the recurrence should be followed by a chest x-ray and CT scan of the abdomen and pelvis to assess the extent of disease.

For local pelvic recurrences following radical hysterectomy, radiation therapy should be instituted. The prior radical pelvic dissection increases the risk of bowel obstruction and fistula formation, yet the potential for salvage will ordinarily outweigh these risks. Several small series quote survival rates that range from 5% to 53% in patients treated with radiation therapy for central pelvic recurrence following radical hysterectomy.

Patients with a central recurrence following radiation therapy for cervical cancer should be evaluated for pelvic exenteration. Patients without obvious extrapelvic disease on exam, abdominopelvic CT scan, and chest x-ray should be counseled regarding an exenterative procedure. A total pelvic exenteration includes a radical hysterectomy, cystectomy, and resection of the rectosigmoid, and requires diversion of the urinary and fecal streams. Although newer techniques hold promise for continent urinary diversion and low rectal reanastomosis to maintain the continuity of the GI tract, the patient should be prepared for the possibility of living with both urinary and fecal stomas. Vaginal reconstruction with musculocutaneous flaps should be considered either at the time of exenteration or at a second procedure.

Those patients in whom exenteration is successfully completed would be expected to have a 5-year survival rate of about 50%. There may be, however, significant physical and psychological sequelae from the procedure, so ongoing support from a knowledgeable team is crucial to the long-term recovery of patients following exenteration.

Cancer of the Cervix in Pregnancy

Cancer of the cervix in pregnancy is discussed in Chapter 36.

KEY POINTS

1 In developed countries, the use of Pap smear screening has led to a decrease in the incidence of invasive cervical cancer.

2 Diagnosis is not based on a Pap smear alone, *biopsy is required.*

3 Staging has both clinical and pathologic components.

4 Some modalities available in developed countries (CT, MRI) are not allowed in the FIGO classification.

5 Most cervical cancers are of squamous histology; the incidence of adenocarcinoma is now rising.

6 Therapy has its basis in stage grouping.

SUGGESTED READINGS

Christopherson WA: The spread and staging of cervical cancer. In Sciarra JJ ed: *Gynecology and obstetrics,* vol 4, Philadelphia, 1992, JB Lippincott, pp 1-14.

Fanning J, Hilgers RD, Palabrica C: Surgical stapling technique for radical hysterectomy, *Gynecol Oncol* 55:179-184, 1994.

Fiorica JV et al: Morbidity and survival patterns in patients after radical hysterectomy and postoperative adjuvant pelvic radiotherapy, *Gynecol Oncol* 36:343-347, 1990.

Parker SL et al: Cancer statistics, 1997, *CA Cancer J Clin* 47:527, 1997.

Shepherd JH (International Federation of Obstetrics and Gynecology). Staging announcement: FIGO staging of gynecologic cancers; cervical and vulva, *Int J Gynecol Cancer* 5:319, 1995.

Stehman FB et al: Carcinoma of the cervix treated with irradiation therapy. I. A multivariate analysis of prognostic variables in the Gyncologic Oncology Group, *Cancer* 67:2776-2785, 1991.

Stehman FB et al: Uterine cervix. In Hoskins WJ, Perez CA, Young RC: *Principles and practice of gynecologic oncology,* ed 2, Philadelphia, 1997, Lippincott-Raven, pp 785-858.

Wagner H Jr, Keys HM: Basic principles of radiation therapy. In Copeland L, ed: *Textbook of gynecology,* Philadelphia, 1993, WB Saunders, pp 897-913.

4

Contraception

Geri D. Hewitt

Approximately 50% of pregnancies in the United States are unintended and more than half of these are aborted. From ages 20 to 34, American women have the highest proportion of pregnancies aborted in the world. To combat this high rate of unintended pregnancies, patients must have access to and education about various forms of contraception. In particular, clinicians need to convey information regarding the cost, risks, benefits, methods of action, failure rates, and proper usage of different contraceptive methods.

ORAL CONTRACEPTION

Oral contraceptive agents are the most commonly used form of birth control among never-married women in the United States. Combination oral contraceptive pills (OCPs) contain two components, an estrogen and a progestin. They are given daily for three weeks, followed by one "pill-free" week when the patient takes a placebo and should have withdrawal bleeding. OCPs work by inhibiting ovulation by suppressing FSH and LH secretion, producing an endometrium that is inhospitable to implantation, and changing the cervical mucus so that it becomes resistant to sperm penetration. OCPs have a 3% first-year user failure rate.

Low-dose preparations (<50 mg of ethinyl estradiol) are extremely safe in properly selected patients. However, several absolute contraindications to OCP use exist: (1) thrombophlebitis, thromboembolic disorders, or CVA; (2) active liver disease with impaired liver function; (3) breast cancer; (4) undiagnosed abnormal vaginal bleeding; (5) known or suspected pregnancy; and (6) smokers over the age of 35.

Relative contraindications that require prudent clinical judgment before initiating OCP use include (1) migraine headaches, (2) hypertension, (3) diabetes mellitus, (4) elective surgery, (5) epilepsy, (6) obstructive jaundice in pregnancy, (7) sickle cell disease, and, (8) gallbladder disease.

Despite the effectiveness of OCPs, compliance remains an obstacle for many patients, and noncompliance leads to pill failure and unintended pregnancies. There are three major factors that affect compliance and that clinicians should address with their patients: (1) OCPs effects on cancer, cardiovascular disease, and fertility; (2) side effects such as breakthrough bleeding, amenorrhea, nausea, headache, and weight gain; (3) inadequate information on pill taking or complicated pill packaging or package inserts.

Breakthrough bleeding (BTB) is a common side effect occurring in 10% to 30% of patients in the first month on OCPs and usually resolves by the third month of pill use. Early in the course of OCP use, BTB is caused by the thinning of the endometrium in response to the progestin component of the pill and is most successfully managed by adequate counseling before initiating pill use. It does not represent a decrease in OCP effectiveness. Later than three months, BTB is most likely a result of progestin-induced decidualization of the endometrium, which can lead to asynchronous bleeding. If the bleeding occurs in the third week of the pill pack, the patient can stop taking the pills, wait 7 days and then initiate a new cycle pack. Another approach is to have the patient take estradiol 2 mg or conjugate estrogen 1.25 mg for 7 days when the bleeding starts, regardless of where she is in her cycle. Having the patient "double up" on her pills is ineffective and will make the problem worse.

Because the progestin component of OCPs leads to thinning of the endometrium, many women have very light periods or may even experience amenorrhea. This is not harmful, and when the patient resumes ovulation after discontinuing the OCPs, the endometrium will return to normal.

There are no studies that show that low-dose OCPs cause weight gain. Other commonly experienced side effects that patients may experience include breast tenderness and nausea, both of which resolve with time.

Long-term use of OCPs does not affect fertility, and there is no benefit from having patients take a break from their OCPs. If a patient does conceive on OCPs, she is at no increased risk of congenital anomalies. The only risk of conceiving immediately after discontinuing OCP use is difficulty in dating the pregnancy. There is no increased risk of spontaneous abortion, ectopic pregnancy, or birth defects. Currently there is no evidence that OCP use in pubertal girls has any negative impact on growth and development. Some experts advocate the use of the progestin-only minipill by lactating women, which has been shown in some studies to improve breast milk quantity and nutritional quality.

Many patients have concerns about the association between use of OCPs and cancer. OCPs decrease the risk of both endometrial and epithelial ovarian cancer. OCP use for at least 12 months decreases the risk of endometrial cancer by 50%. The risk of developing epithelial ovarian cancer in OCP users is decreased by 40% when compared with nonusers. Some concern exists regarding an increased incidence of cervical dysplasia and cervical cancer in OCP users. However, many confounding variables, including age of first intercourse, number of sexual partners, use of barrier contraception, exposure to HPV, and smoking, make it difficult to draw firm conclusions on the risk of cervical cancer or dysplasia and OCP use. Because of that concern, it is important to perform annual Pap smears in OCP users. OCPs have not been shown to increase the risk of liver cancer.

In addition to protection against endometrial and epithelial ovarian cancers, there are numerous other noncontraceptive benefits of OCPs. These include a decreased incidence of benign breast disease, ectopic pregnancy, PID, endometriosis, and ovarian cysts, as well as more regular menses with less flow, dysmenorrhea, and anemia and a delayed onset of osteoporosis. OCPs are frequently used for purposes other than contraception. They have been successfully used to treat dysmenorrhea, anovulatory dysfunctional uterine bleeding, acne, and hirsutism. OCPs are also effective in decreasing the risk of recurrent ovarian cysts, providing hormonal therapy to amenorrheic patients, and providing prophylaxis against the recurrence of endometriosis when taken continuously.

BARRIER METHODS

Barrier methods of contraception include diaphragms, cervical caps, spermicides, and condoms. They decrease the risk of PID and STDs by 50%.

Diaphragms are round, flat latex devices that are placed in the vagina up against the cervix. They are used in conjunction with spermicide and must be properly fitted by a clinician. They are very safe with few side effects. Infrequently, patients may experience irritation from the latex or spermicide. Urinary tract infections (UTIs) are more common in diaphragm users than OCP users, and patients should be encouraged to void after intercourse. Patients with recurrent UTIs should have their diaphragms checked for proper fit and may require single-dose prophylactic antibiotics at the time of intercourse. Failure rates with the diaphragm vary anywhere from 2% to 23%, with a typical failure rate after 1 year of use of about 18%. The lowest failure rates are seen in highly motivated, older, married women. The diaphragm should be inserted into the vagina, after placing a teaspoonful of spermicide in the dome of the diaphragm, no longer than 6 hours before intercourse. The diaphragm should be kept in place at least 6 hours after intercourse and for no longer than 24 hours. An applicatorful of additional spermicide should be placed in the vagina before each additional episode of intercourse while the diaphragm is in place. There is currently no data on diaphragm use and transmission of the HIV virus.

The cervical cap is used more widely in Europe than in the United States. Its efficacy is equal to that of the diaphragm. Advantages over the diaphragm are that the cervical cap can be used without a spermicide and it can be left in place for up to 36 hours. However, the cervical cap is more difficult to properly fit and insert. It should be inserted at least 20 minutes and no more than 4 hours before intercourse and should be left in place after intercourse for at least 6 hours.

Spermicides are agents that inactivate sperm in the vagina before the sperm can move into the upper genital tract. They are often used in combination with diaphragms, cervical caps, or condoms, and do provide some protection against pregnancy when used alone. Spermicides have a typical failure rate of about 20% and should be inserted 10 to 30 minutes before sexual intercourse and again before each episode of intercourse. An advantage of spermicides is their availability over the counter at a relatively inexpensive cost. Also, they confer some protection against STDs. An allergic reaction may occur in up to 5% of spermicide users. Spermicide use has not been shown to increase the risk of spontaneous abortion or congenital anomalies.

Condoms provide effective contraception as well as protection from STDs. Ninety-nine percent of condoms sold are made of latex and provide protection against STDs, including HIV. Condoms have a typical failure rate of approximately 12% after 1 year of use. Inconsistent or improper use accounts for most condom failures, with breakage rates ranging from 1 to 12 per 100 acts of vaginal intercourse. Patients should be given specific instructions on the proper use of condoms. Oil-based lubricants should be avoided because they will weaken the integrity of the latex. Vaginal medications may also affect condom integrity. All patients at risk for STDs should be encouraged to use latex condoms with any other additional form of contraception they may be practicing.

Female condoms are pouches that line the vagina. They also provide protection from STDs, including HIV, as well as contraception. Female condoms are readily available over the counter; however, they are more expensive than male condoms and more cumbersome to use.

LONG-ACTING PROGESTINS

Norplant and Depo-Provera are two types of long-acting, reversible contraception currently available in the United States. Both methods employ progestins that provide contraception by inhibiting ovulation, thickening cervical mucus, and causing the endometrium to become atrophic.

The Norplant system consists of six silastic rods that contain the progestin levonorgestrel. The progestin diffuses through the rods where it is absorbed by the circulatory system and produces its contraceptive effect. The system should be inserted during the first five days of the menses to ensure that the patient is not pregnant. It is effective within 24 hours of insertion and remains effective for up to 5 years. Norplant is highly protective against pregnancy with a user failure rate of 0.2% during the first year of use.

Norplant has many advantages in addition to its low failure rate. It is also a very safe form of contraception that once placed requires very little patient motivation and is reversible when removed. It does not impair fertility long term. Norplant is cost-effective when left in place for 5 years and can be placed immediately postpartum, even in breastfeeding women. Norplant can be safely used in patients with contraindications to estrogen-containing oral contraceptions. There are no patient weight limitations with the current Norplant system.

The biggest disadvantage of Norplant is the unpredictable vaginal bleeding experienced in up to 80% of patients during the first year as a result of the progestin effect on the endometrium. Bleeding patterns are highly variable and can range from amenorrhea to daily spotting. Some patients do have regular menstrual cycles because one third of cycles on Norplant are ovulatory. Also, placement and removal of the rods requires a minor surgical procedure by trained personnel. The Norplant rods can be seen under the skin in some patients, and Norplant does not provide any protection against STDs. There are no significant metabolic or lipoprotein profile changes in Norplant users.

Absolute contraindications to Norplant use include active thrombophlebitis or thromboembolic disease, undiagnosed genital bleeding, active liver disease, liver tumors, and breast cancer. Relative contraindications to Norplant include cigarette smoking in women more than 35 years old, a history of ectopic pregnancy, hypercholesterolemia, severe acne, hypertension, a history of cardiovascular disease, gallbladder disease, migraine headaches, depression, immunocompromised patients, and concomitant use of medications that induce microsomal liver enzymes.

Pregnancy rates during the first year after Norplant removal are comparable to that of women not using contraception. There is no increase in adverse pregnancy outcomes after removal of the Norplant system. Reported side effects of Norplant include headache, acne, weight gain or loss, mastalgia, hyperpigmentation over the implants, hirsutism, depression, mood changes, anxiety, nervousness, ovarian cyst formation, and galactorrhea.

Depo-Provera is another long-acting, reversible form of contraception that involves an intramuscular injection of medroxyprogesterone acetate. The dose is 150 mg every 3 months and, if given during the first five days of the menstrual cycle, is effective immediately.

The advantages of Depo-Provera are that it is very safe and reliable, with a typical user failure rate of 0.3% during the first year. Also, once the patient is injected, compliance is not a problem. Depo-Provera increases breast milk production in lactating women and although measurable at low levels in breast milk, produces no adverse effects on infant growth and development. Noncontraceptive health benefits of Depo-Provera include decreased risk of endometrial cancer, reduced menstrual flow and anemia, less PID, decreased endometriosis, and decreased risk of ectopic pregnancy.

Because of the progestational effect on the endometrium, 30% of Depo-Provera users do report irregular bleeding during the first year of use. The majority of patients, however, become amenorrheic after several injections. Other reported side effects include breast tenderness, weight gain, and depression. Some studies have demonstrated an adverse change in lipoprotein levels in Depo-Provera users. Nevertheless, no change is seen in coagulation factors or carbohydrate metabolism. The return of fertility is delayed about nine months after the last injection of Depo-Provera, although there is no impact on long-term fertility.

INTRAUTERINE DEVICE

Two types of IUDs are currently available in the United States, the Paraguard or copper IUD (TCU-308A) and the Progestasert IUD that releases progesterone. Both provide safe, reversible contraception with a first-year user failure rate of approximately 3%. The Paraguard IUD is effective for up to 10 years. The Progestasert IUD must be replaced annually.

IUDs exert their contraceptive action in the uterine cavity by producing an intrauterine environment that is spermicidal so that very few sperm reach the ovum in the fallopian tube. The copper IUD may enhance a sterile inflammatory response in the endometrium. Copper may also be spermicidal. The progestin-releasing IUD causes the endometrium to become decidualized, with atrophy of the glands. This inhibits sperm capitation and survival, as well as implantation. In women using IUDs, assays for β-HCG show that fertilization occurs in less than 1% of menstrual cycles. IUDs are not an abortifacient.

Patient selection for IUD use should be limited to patients at a low risk for STDs, such as patients in a mutually monogamous sexual relationship. These patients are not at increased risk of PID with IUD use. IUD-related infections are limited to the time of insertion and are generally polymicrobial. Patients should have negative cervical cultures before IUD insertion. Patients with a history of heavy menstrual bleeding or dysmenorrhea may notice a worsening of their symptoms with the copper IUD and may be better candidates for the progesterone IUD. Up to 15% of women discontinue IUD use secondary to menstrual problems. Other contraindications to IUD use include abnormalities of the uterine cavity, an immunosuppressed state, an increased risk of endocarditis, and uterine cavities that sound less than 6 cm or greater than 10 cm. Patients with allergies to copper or Wilson's disease should choose the progesterone IUD.

IUD users are not at increased risk of ectopic pregnancy. Their risk compared to noncontraceptors is decreased by 50%. If a patient does conceive with an IUD in place, the risk of ectopic pregnancy is 3% to 4% and the risk of spontaneous abortion is 50%. After the IUD is removed, there is no impairment to fertility and no increased rate of adverse pregnancy outcomes.

An IUD can be inserted at any time during the menstrual cycle. However, many clinicians like to insert them at the time of menses when the open cervical os may facilitate insertion and there is assurance that the patient is not pregnant. Expulsion rates of 10% can be expected in the first year of use. IUDs can safely be placed 4 to 8 weeks post partum. Doxycycline 100 mg orally can be given 1 hour before insertion to decrease the risk of insertion-related infection. Patients with mitral valve prolapse (MVP) should receive prophylactic antibiotics at the time of insertion.

PERIODIC ABSTINENCE OR "RHYTHM"

Couples using periodic abstinence or the "rhythm" method avoid pregnancy by abstaining from intercourse during the fertile times of the menstrual cycle. This method is best suited for highly motivated couples and has a typical first-year user failure rate of approximately 20%. The average couple using the method properly must abstain from intercourse 17 days each cycle. Approximately 1% of reproductive-age women in the United States use periodic abstinence.

Periodic abstinence is most effective when multiple indicators of fertility are used in combination. These include counting cycle days, assessing cervical mucus changes, and measuring basal body temperatures. If a woman has regular menstrual cycles, she may estimate her fertile period by recording the length of six cycles and then subtracting 18 days from the shortest cycle and 11 days from the longest cycle. Assessment of cervical mucus is also called the *Billings method.* Patients are taught to appreciate the midcycle estrogen-induced changes in cervical mucus, namely an increase in the amount of clear, thin, stringy mucus. Abstinence should be initiated when the change in the mucus is first noted and continued until the fourth day after the last day of the clear mucus. A woman's basal body temperature (BBT) rises about 0.2° to 0.4° C or 0.4° to 0.8° F after ovulation in response to the increasing levels of progesterone. Patients using the BBT method should abstain from intercourse until the night of the third day of a shift in temperature.

EMERGENCY CONTRACEPTION

Exposure to unprotected intercourse increases the risk of pregnancy and STDs. Patients at risk should be offered emergency contraception and counseled about possible STDs. Oral contraceptives can be used for emergency contraception and if given within 72 hours of intercourse have a 2% failure rate. One popular regimen is Ovral, two pills taken by mouth and then repeated 12 hours later. Side effects include nausea, vomiting, breast tenderness, headache, and dizziness. Patients with contraindications to OCPs should not be given this type of emergency contraception.

For patients at low risk for STDs, an IUD may be inserted as emergency contraception and if used within 5 days of intercourse has a failure rate of 0.1%. Both types of emergency contraception are believed to work by interfering with implantation.

KEY POINTS

1. Oral contraceptive pills work by inhibiting ovulation, making the endometrium inhospitable to implantation, and thickening cervical mucus.
2. Noncontraceptive health benefits of OCPs include a decreased risk of endometrial and epithelial ovarian cancer; decreased incidence of benign breast disease, ectopic pregnancy, PID, endometriosis, and ovarian cysts; and more regular menstrual cycles with less flow and dysmenorrhea.
3. Barrier methods of contraception include spermicides, condoms, diaphragms, and cervical caps and are known to decrease the transmission of STDs.
4. IUDs work by creating an intrauterine environment that is spermicidal. They are not abortifacients.
5. Periodic abstinence relies on couples avoiding intercourse during the fertile times of the cycle, which is predicted by monitoring cycle length, cervical mucus changes, and basal body temperature.
6. Oral contraceptive pills can be used for emergency contraception and have a 2% failure rate if given within 72 hours of intercourse.

SUGGESTED READINGS

American College of Obstetricians and Gynecologists: ACOG Technical Bulletin 198, Washington, DC, October, 1994.

The Cancer and Steroid Hormone Study of the CDC and NICHD: The reduction in risk of ovarian cancer associated with oral contraceptive use, *New Engl J Med* 316:650, 1987.

The Cancer and Steroid Hormone Study of the CDC and NICHD: Combination oral contraceptive use and the risk of endometrial cancer, *JAMA* 257:796, 1987.

Lee NC, Rubin GL, Borucki R: The intrauterine device and pelvic inflammatory disease revisited: new results from the Women's Health Study, *Obstet Gynecol* 72:1, 1988.

Rushton L, Jones DR: Oral contraceptive use and breast cancer risk: a method analysis of variations with age at diagnosis, parity, and total duration of oral contraceptive use, *Br J Obstet Gynaecol* 99:239, 1992.

Speroff L, Darney P: *A clinical guide for contraception,* Baltimore, 1992, Williams and Wilkins.

Speroff L, Glass RH, Kase NG: *Clinical gynecologic endocrinology and infertility,* ed 5, Baltimore, 1994, Williams and Wilkens.

Trussel V et al: Contraceptive failure in the United States: an update, *Stud Fam Plann* 21:51, 1990.

5

Dysmenorrhea

ELIZABETH A. KENNARD

Most women report that they experience some sort of dysmenorrhea. *Primary dysmenorrhea* occurs when no underlying pathologic condition exists, whereas *secondary dysmenorrhea* is diagnosed when an underlying pelvic condition is thought to cause the pain. Studies to determine the incidence of dysmenorrhea have usually found that 75% of women have some sort of dysmenorrhea, with 15% to 20% complaining of dysmenorrhea severe enough to interfere with school or work. The severity of the pain appears to correlate with early menarche, longer duration, and amount of menstrual bleeding. Dysmenorrhea is decreased by treatment with oral contraceptives and by undergoing childbirth.

PATHOPHYSIOLOGY

Several studies suggest that dysmenorrhea is caused by prostaglandin release from the endometrium. The symptoms of dysmenorrhea are replicated by administering prostaglandins to women. Those women who complain of more severe dysmenorrhea have higher concentrations of prostaglandins in their menstrual fluid and their endometrium seems to have higher prostaglandin production capacity when tested in vitro. The mechanism of the pain appears to be threefold. First, prostaglandins increase painful uterine contractions. Furthermore, these contractions reduce uterine blood flow and the resultant ischemia also causes pain. Lastly, pain fibers within the pelvis seem to be sensitized by high concentrations of prostaglandins and some of the intermediates in their synthetic pathway. The underlying determinants of the amount of prostaglandin produced have not been determined. Why one woman produces an incapacitating amount of prostaglandin and another very little, is unknown.

DIAGNOSIS

An attempt should be made to distinguish primary and secondary dysmenorrhea. The usual presentation of primary dysmenorrhea is crampy suprapubic pain of 2 to 3 days duration during the heaviest menstrual flow. Primary dysmenorrhea has an onset before age 20 and is associated with regular menstrual cycles and a normal pelvic exam. Many of the causes of secondary dysmenorrhea can be ruled out by performing a simple history and physical exam.

DIFFERENTIAL DIAGNOSIS

Secondary dysmenorrhea can be caused by cervical stenosis, endometriosis, uterine anomalies, PID, ovarian cysts, adenomyosis, leiomyoma, and pelvic congestion. Evaluations for these underlying causes is part of the initial history and physical exam of these patients. However, endometriosis can be difficult to diagnose. Often the physical exam is normal in these patients. Therefore if the dysmenorrhea cannot be controlled with the usual treatment regimens, or if there is a strong suspicion of endometriosis, laparoscopy may be considered to aid in diagnosis.

TREATMENT

The mainstay of treatment for dysmenorrhea is prostaglandin synthetase inhibition. The nonsteroidal antiinflammatory drugs (NSAIDs) have repeatedly been shown to decrease dysmenorrhea. They are best used if begun with onset of menses and taken continuously for 48 to 72 hours. Not only do these medications decrease the prostaglandins that cause dysmenorrhea, they also reduce the amount of blood flow and act as systemic analgesics. Different women will respond differently, and two or three types of NSAIDs should be tried for up to 6 months if pain is not initially controlled. Examples of NSAIDs effective in the treatment of dysmenorrhea are listed in Table 5-1.

Another approach to dysmenorrhea is to place the woman on oral contraceptives. These medications will diminish dysmenorrhea by decreasing the amount of blood flow and the amount of prostaglandin produced by the endometrium. The vast majority of women will have complete relief

TABLE 5-1
Prostaglandin Synthetase Inhibitors for Dysmenorrhea

Drug	Dosage
Ibuprofen	400-600 mg tid
Naproxen sodium	550 mg once then 275 mg tid
Mefenamic acid	250-500 mg qid
Indomethacin	25 mg qid

of dysmenorrhea in response to oral contraceptives. If contraception is desired, these should be prescribed first and supplemented with NSAIDs if dysmenorrhea persists.

Severe cases of dysmenorrhea may be approached with transcutaneous electrical nerve stimulation (TENS). This treatment has been shown to be as effective as naproxen in a randomized crossover trial. Since most women will respond to either oral contraceptives or NSAIDs, TENS is a supplemental treatment sometimes added to treatment with NSAIDs.

In rare cases, women may be treated with a surgical procedure. Presacral neurectomy interrupts nerve fibers to the lower uterus and is only effective in centrally located pelvic pain. Uterosacral ligament division is used by some surgeons, although its efficacy has not been tested in a randomized controlled prospective trial. Both procedures are more commonly used for treatment of chronic pelvic pain and should be very sparingly used for dysmenorrhea, if at all.

The treatment of secondary dysmenorrhea is directed toward the underlying cause. Endometriosis can be treated with ablation or medical therapy. Cervical stenosis will usually respond to dilation. Uterine anomalies may require reconstruction or removal. Uterine polyps or myomas may need to be surgically removed. Persistent ovarian cysts that do not respond to hormonal manipulations will also require a surgical approach.

KEY POINTS

1 Most women have some dysmenorrhea, with 15% to 20% reporting severe episodes that interfere with work or school.

2 Dysmenorrhea will decrease after childbirth.

3 Dysmenorrhea is worse in women with early menarche, longer menses, and heavier menses.

4 Primary dysmenorrhea usually begins shortly after menarche and is associated with a normal pelvic exam.

5 Current treatment for primary dysmenorrhea consists of NSAIDs and/or oral contraceptives.

6 Treatment of secondary dysmenorrhea is targeted at the underlying etiology.

SUGGESTED READINGS

Dawood MY: Nonsteroidal antiinflammatory drugs and reproduction, *Am J Obstet Gynecol* 169(5):1255, 1993.
Gomibuchi H et al: Is personality involved in the expression of dysmenorrhea in patients with endometriosis? *Am J Obstet Gynecol* 169:723, 1993.
Heisterberg L: Factors influencing spontaneous abortion, dyspareunia, dysmenorrhea, and pelvic pain, *Obstet Gynecol* 81:594, 1993.
Milsom I, Hedner N, Mannheimer C: A comparative study of the effect of high-intensity transcutaneous nerve stimulation and oral naproxen on intrauterine pressure and menstrual pain in patients with primary dysmenorrhea, *Am J Obstet Gynecol* 170:123, 1994.
Robinson JC et al: Dysmenorrhea and use of oral contraceptives in adolescent women attending a family planning clinic, *Am J Obstet Gynecol* 166:578, 1992.
Stout AL et al: Relationship of laparoscopic findings to self-report of pelvic pain, *Am J Obstet Gynecol* 164:73, 1991.

6

Ectopic Pregnancy

Moon H. Kim

Ectopic pregnancy is defined as the condition where gestational implantation occurs outside of the uterine cavity. The incidence of ectopic pregnancy has risen dramatically over the past two decades. Despite remarkable advances in early diagnosis and management, it remains a leading cause of maternal mortality.

EPIDEMIOLOGY

In the United States, the Centers for Disease Control and Prevention reports that there were 17,800 cases (4.5 per 1000 pregnancies) in 1970, 52,200 (10.5 per 1000 pregnancies) in 1980, and 88,400 cases (16.8 per 1000 pregnancies) in 1989. A similar trend in incidence has been reported worldwide. Early detection of the condition accounts for the remarkable reduction in mortality by 90% despite a more than threefold increase in reported cases in the United States since 1970.

ETIOLOGY

The majority of ectopic pregnancies occur in the fallopian tube. Any impairment, mechanical or hormonal, in the transportation of the fertilized ovum (zygote) from the fallopian tube into the uterine cavity may result in an ectopic implantation. Many risk factors have been well documented.

1. PID: The risk of ectopic pregnancy increases six fold after a documented episode of PID. *Chlamydia trachomatis* is the most common offender.
2. Reconstructive surgery of the fallopian tubes: Although anatomical patency may be restored by surgery, partial luminal occlusion and peritubal adhesions may form, impairing tubal motility. After microsurgical reversal of a previous tubal sterilization, a 2.5% to 4.0% incidence of ectopic pregnancy has been reported. On the other hand, rates up to 25% to 30% are associated with neosalpingostomy.
3. Tubal sterilization: Although the incidence may vary depending on the type of tubal sterilization, more than 50% of conceptions diagnosed after laparoscopic tubal sterilization are ectopic. However, the relative risk of ectopic pregnancy in women undergoing tubal sterilization is lower than that of women using no contraception.
4. IUDs: Approximately 4% and 15% of conceptions that occur in women using copper-containing IUDs and progestin-containing IUDs, respectively, are reported to be ectopic.
5. History of previous ectopic pregnancy: 10% to 20% of pregnancies in women with a history of previous ectopic pregnancy are ectopic. In women whose first pregnancy was ectopic, the repeat ectopic pregnancy rate is as high as 30%.
6. Other risk factors include diethylstilbestrol exposure in utero, pelvic surgery, multiple ovulation induced by HMG and clomiphene citrate, and assisted reproductive technologies.

PATHOPHYSIOLOGY

Following implantation of the trophoblast to the luminal epithelium of the fallopian tube, trophoblast proliferation takes place into the muscularis. The duration of viability of the ectopic pregnancy, the degree of invasion into the muscularis, maternal tissue damage, and clinical manifestation vary depending on implantation site. Many ectopic pregnancies of the distal fallopian tube may end in early tubal abortion. Implantation in the isthmus portion, however, tends to invade maternal tissue and vasculature, resulting in early-tubal rupture and intraabdominal hemorrhage. Common sites of ectopic gestation are the ampulla (80%), the isthmus (15% to 20%), and the cornual or interstitial portion (2%) of the fallopian tube. Extratubal (ovary, cervix, and abdominal) gestations occur in less than 1% of cases.

During an ectopic pregnancy the endometrium becomes decidual and hypersecretory (Arias-Stella reaction). When HCG secretion declines in association with demise of the ectopic gestation, irregular shedding of the decidual endometrium occurs with bleeding and occasional passing of a decidual cast.

The clinical course of an ectopic pregnancy varies widely. At times, there may be no clinical symptoms when spontaneous resorption or tubal abortion occurs at an early stage. At the other extreme, patients may experience acute abdominal pain, intraperitoneal hemorrhage, and shock caused by tubal rupture.

DIFFERENTIAL DIAGNOSIS

Depending on clinical presentation, the following conditions must be excluded: abortion (threatened, incomplete, or complete); corpus luteum cyst, particularly ruptured; PID; endometriosis; appendicitis; ovarian cyst, with or without torsion; and heterotopic pregnancy (coexistence of intrauterine and extrauterine pregnancies).

DIAGNOSIS

Early diagnosis of the ectopic pregnancy is crucial to successful management and minimizes morbidity and mortality. A high index of suspicion is critical in early diagnosis, which is based on clinical findings, measurement of β-hCG titers, ultrasonography, and diagnostic laparoscopy.

A classic clinical triad of symptoms includes abdominal or pelvic pain, adnexal mass, and irregular uterine bleeding. However, a substantial number of patients with an ectopic pregnancy are either asymptomatic or experience only minimal pain or vaginal bleeding when first seen by their physicians. Abdominal or pelvic pain, diffuse or localized, is the most common symptom, and is often a complaint even before tubal rupture. When a significant amount of bleeding occurs intraperitoneally, syncope and referred shoulder pain from diaphragmatic irritation may be noted.

Physical findings are so varied that it is a clinical challenge to make a diagnosis of unruptured ectopic pregnancy. When tubal rupture occurs, patients often experience an acute condition resulting from hemodynamic compromise, shock, and hypovolemia. Often, the physical examination in such a situation is quite restricted because of severe pain, abdominal guarding, and time constraints in managing hemodynamic changes. Abdominal rebound tenderness suggests intraperitoneal bleeding. Orthostatic changes in blood pressure and pulse rate may be present in patients with a greater than 15% total blood loss from hemorrhage. Although it is uncommon, mild fever may be present. The frequency of common symptoms and signs are amenorrhea (75% to 85%), vaginal bleeding or spotting (75% to 85%), abdominal or pelvic pain (90% to 100%), adnexal tenderness (90%), and adnexal mass (40%).

DIAGNOSTIC EVALUATION

Early detection of ectopic pregnancy has become possible through highly sensitive HCG assays, transvaginal ultrasonography, and advanced laparoscopic technique. There are other potentially helpful methods such as the determination of serum progesterone levels and endometrial curettage, but these are not as sensitive and specific. In the past, culdocentesis has been widely used for diagnosis of ectopic pregnancy. However, it is rarely indicated because more specific tests have become available to physicians.

The ultimate goal is to detect and treat early ectopic pregnancies before they rupture.

Every pregnant woman with risk factors for an ectopic pregnancy should be closely monitored with determination of β-HCG levels complemented by transvaginal ultrasonography to detect the presence of intrauterine pregnancy. The most commonly used reference standard is the International Reference Standard (IRP), however some laboratories may still use the Second International Standard (Second IS). One unit of IRP approximately equals one unit of Second IS multiplied by a factor of 1.7. In normal pregnancy, serum concentrations of HCG rise exponentially for the first 5 to 7½ weeks after ovulation by doubling the titers every 2 to 3 days. During the first 7 weeks, a random value of β-HCG is lower for the gestational stage in 60% of cases of ectopic or nonviable pregnancies compared with normal gestation. Furthermore, a slow doubling time of β-HCG titers is highly predictive of abortion or ectopic pregnancy. Serial determinations of the titer are critical when an ectopic pregnancy is suspected.

The primary goal of transvaginal ultrasonography is to exclude an intrauterine gestation. Transvaginal ultrasonography has better resolution than the transabdominal approach in detecting an early gestational sac. An intrauterine gestational sac can be visualized by transvaginal ultrasonography as early as five weeks gestation, at which time the HCG titer is about 1500 mIU/ml (IRP). This discriminatory zone or threshold, along with doubling time of HCG titers, is important in early diagnosis of ectopic pregnancy (Table 6-1).

One should differentiate a pseudosac produced by decidual reaction in an ectopic pregnancy or a leiomyoma from a true intrauterine gestational sac. In such a situation, follow-up sonography is necessary. Although it is not sensitive, the presence of moderate to large amounts of fluid in the cul-de-sac has been shown to correlate with likelihood of ectopic pregnancy.

Diagnostic laparoscopy is the most definitive diagnostic procedure for ectopic pregnancy. Laparoscopy should be performed for suspected

TABLE 6-1
Relationship of Gestational Age, β-HCG Levels, and Vaginal Ultrasonographic Findings

		β-HCG (mIU/ml)	
Sonographic findings	Days from LMP	IRP	2nd IS
Gestational sac	35	1400	900
Fetal pole	42	5100	3800
Fetal heart motion	49	17,200	13,000

Modified from Fossom G, Davajan V, Kletzky O: Early detection of pregnancy with transvaginal ultrasound, *Fertil Steril* 49:788-791, 1988.

symptomatic but hemodynamically stable patients. Because laparoscopy allows visualization of the entire pelvis, definitive surgical treatment for ectopic pregnancy or other coexisting pathologic conditions can be carried out.

Dilation and curettage is frequently done in patients with uterine bleeding when an abortion is suspected. The presence of chorionic villi is highly suggestive of incomplete abortion. However, either ectopic pregnancy or completed abortion must be considered where there is an absence of chorionic villi in curetted tissue.

TREATMENT

When an ectopic pregnancy is suspected, a baseline CBC and blood typing should be done in addition to a pregnancy test (urinary or serum β-HCG titer) (Fig. 6-1). When the patient is completely asymptomatic and in early stage of ectopic pregnancy, conservative management is feasible. However, emergency surgical management should be performed in hemodynamically unstable women in whom ruptured ectopic pregnancy is suspected.

In certain patients, expectant management is an acceptable alternative to more traditional surgical management. Spontaneous resolution of tubal pregnancy has been well documented. A guideline for selection of the patients for expectant management should include hemodynamically stable state with no clinical evidence of rupture, falling HCG titers with an initial titer less than 1500 mIU/ml (IRP), and minimal or no abdominal pain. Expectant management should only be attempted when the patient is compliant with the necessary rigid monitoring. Subsequent fertility rates in this select group of patients managed expectantly are comparable with other methods of treatment.

Methotrexate, a folic acid antagonist, has been a mainstay of chemotherapy for trophoblastic neoplasms. For the past decade, it has been widely used for the treatment of unruptured ectopic pregnancy. Generally recommended selection criteria for methotrexate treatment include ectopic gestation size less than 3 cm in diameter, HCG titer less than 15,000 mIU/ml (IRP), no evidence of tubal rupture, no active bleeding, and desire for future fertility. It is also indicated for treating selected cases of cornual or cervical ectopic pregnancy. Patients with abnormal liver or renal function, active peptic ulcer, poor compliance, and/or leukopenia or thrombocytopenia should not be treated with methotrexate. Excellent resolution of ectopic pregnancy has been observed with a single dose of methotrexate (50 mg/m^2 body surface). If the HCG titer does not fall within a week or two, or if the titer rises, a second dose of methotrexate should be given. Other therapeutic approaches include direct injection of methotrexate, potassium chloride, urea, or prostaglandins into the gestational sac under sonographic or laparoscopic guidance.

The recent advancement in operative laparoscopy along with increased capability of early diagnosis of the ectopic pregnancy has brought the evolution of surgical treatment from laparotomy to less invasive, conservative laparoscopic approaches. Indeed, laparotomy is only indicated when the patient is hemodynamically unstable, the surgeon's skill in laparoscopy

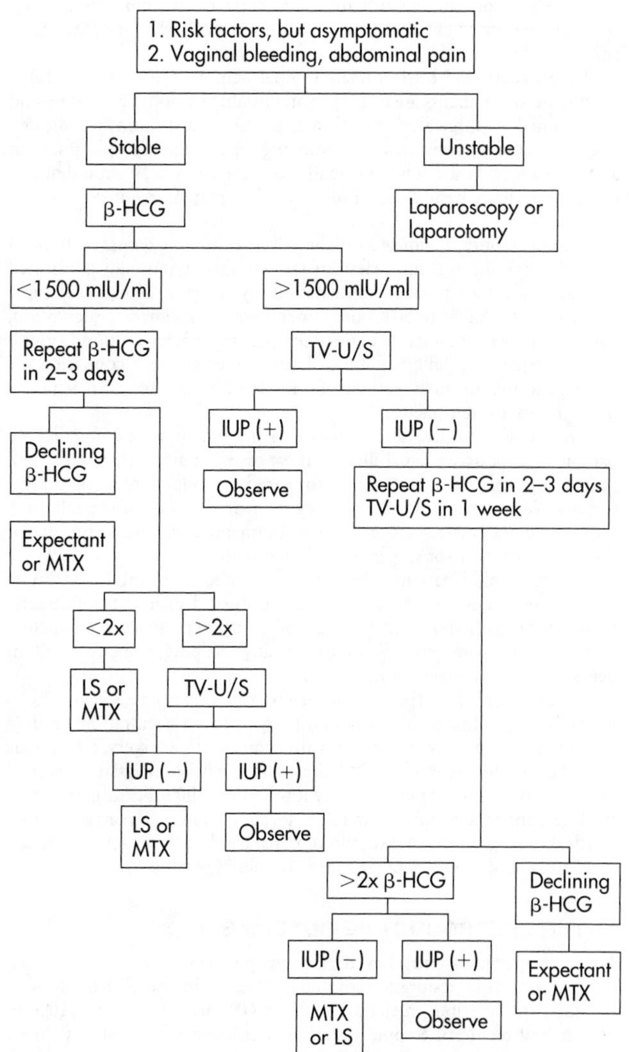

FIG. 6-1 Suspected ectopic pregnancy. *β-HCG,* mIU/ml (IRP); *2x,* doubling titer of β-HCG; *TV-U/S,* transvaginal ultrasound, *MTX,* methotrexate; *LS,* laparoscopy; *IUP,* intrauterine pregnancy.

is limited, a contraindication to laparoscopy exists, and when pelvic conditions are not favorable to laparoscopic approaches (i.e., extensive adhesions and cornual or abdominal pregnancy).

When acute and brisk intraabdominal hemorrhage caused by tubal rupture occurs, patients are usually in an unstable hemodynamic state and need immediate surgical intervention. Exploratory laparotomy is indicated to quickly achieve hemostasis by removing the ruptured ectopic gestation and the damaged tube. Though laparoscopy can be done, it should not be undertaken in a hemodynamically unstable patient by inexperienced surgeons.

Salpingectomy is indicated if the fallopian tube is damaged beyond repairable condition or future fertility is not desired. It is usually performed laparoscopically or through minilaparotomy. In view of higher ectopic pregnancy rates (20% to 50%) and low subsequent pregnancy rates (30%), patients with a history of PID or prior ectopic pregnancies or infertility with a single remaining fallopian tube should be extensively counseled for salpingectomy. In such patients future fertility can be best achieved through in vitro fertilization.

The goal of conservative surgical management is to preserve the patient's reproductive capability. In most cases, laparoscopy is preferred. Linear salpingostomy should be considered for ampullary ectopic pregnancies. When the ectopic pregnancy is in the isthmus of the fallopian tube, segmental resection is generally recommended with reanastomosis of the tube at the time of surgery or at a later date.

Viable trophoblasts may remain in the tube following conservative surgical treatment. Peritoneal reimplantation of displaced trophoblastic tissue has been also reported as a cause of persistent presence of circulating β-HCG. Approximately 5% of conservative salpingostomies result in persistent ectopic pregnancy.

When removal of the ectopic pregnancy is complete, serum HCG levels should decline within 72 hours of surgery to a concentration less than 20% of the preoperative value. Thus after conservative surgery, HCG titers must be monitored weekly until the titers reach nonpregnant levels. If HCG levels decline or persist at very low levels (<100 mIU/ml), expectant management is appropriate. If HCG levels remain at a plateau or rise, medical or surgical therapy should be considered, including methotrexate administration, repeat salpingostomy, or salpingectomy.

FUTURE REPRODUCTIVE OUTCOME

New therapeutic approaches to ectopic pregnancy yield encouraging results, including restoration of tubal patency in more than 80% of patients; intrauterine pregnancy rates of 40% to 60%, with a 10% to 20% risk of recurrent ectopic gestation after linear salpingostomy; lower intrauterine pregnancy rates (40%) after ectopic pregnancy in women with a history of infertility than in women with normal reproductive history (85%); and, higher recurrence risks in patients with a history of two or more ectopic pregnancies (a 30% pregnancy rate with 20% to 50% ectopic pregnancy rate).

NONTUBAL ECTOPIC PREGNANCY

Although ectopic gestations can occur in the ovaries, the uterine cervix, and the abdominal cavity, the incidence is extremely low. Approximate rates for ovarian, cervical, and abdominal pregnancies are 1 in 7000 to 40,000 deliveries, 1 in 50,000 deliveries, and 1 in 8000 deliveries, respectively.

Both ovarian and abdominal pregnancies present a diagnostic challenge because of the tendency to be initially asymptomatic. Diagnosis may be confirmed by ultrasonography. Surgical removal of ectopic gestation is required. In abdominal pregnancy, the placenta may be left in situ to avoid hemorrhage if it is attached to a wide area of peritoneal surface.

Cervical pregnancy carries a high morbidity because of the frequent, profuse accompanying hemorrhage. Diagnosis is made clinically and confirmed by ultrasonography. In most cases surgical treatment is indicated, usually with hysterectomy. Dilation and curettage may be attempted when the diagnosis is made early. Methotrexate treatment should be considered if the patient is stable without acute hemorrhage.

KEY POINTS

1. The incidence of ectopic pregnancy has risen steadily over the past three decades, and ectopic pregnancy is a leading cause of maternal mortality in the United States.
2. Risk factors include a history of PID, reconstructive surgery of the fallopian tubes, previous tubal sterilization, IUD use, previous ectopic pregnancy, and the use of ovulation-inducing agents.
3. Over 95% of ectopic pregnancies occur in the fallopian tube, most frequently in the ampulla.
4. A substantial number of patients with ectopic pregnancy may be asymptomatic or only have minimal pain or irregular vaginal bleeding when first seen by physicians. However, abdominal pain and irregular vaginal bleeding are the two most common complaints.
5. Laparoscopy is the most definitive diagnostic procedure for ectopic pregnancy.

SUGGESTED READINGS

ACOG Technical Bulletin: *Ectopic pregnancy,* No. 150, Dec, 1990.

Centers for Disease Control and Prevention: Ectopic pregnancies–United States, 1990-1992, *MMWR* 44:46-48, 1995.

Fernandez H et al: Spontaneous resolution of ectopic pregnancy, *Obstet Gynecol* 71:171-174, 1990.

Hahlin M et al: Single progesterone assay for early recognition of abnormal pregnancy, *Hum Reprod* 5:622-626, 1990.

Helsa JS, Rock JA: Emergent management of ectopic pregnancy, *Infert Reprod Med Clin North Am,* 3:775-793, 1992.

Pouly JL et al: Multifactorial analysis of fertility after conservative laparoscopic treatment of ectopic pregnancy in a series of 223 patients, *Fertil Steril* 56:453, 1991.

Seifer DB et al: Persistent ectopic pregnancy following laparoscopic linear salpingostomy, *Obstet Gynecol* 76:1121, 1990.
Stovall TG et al: Emergency department diagnosis of ectopic pregnancy, *Ann Emerg Med* 19:1098, 1990.
Stovall T, Ling F: Expectant management of ectopic pregnancy, *Obstet Gynecol Clin North Am* 18:135-144, 1991.
Stovall T, Ling F, Gray LA: Single-dose methotrexate for treatment of ectopic pregnancy, *Am J Obstet Gynecol* 168:1759, 1993.
Yankowitz J et al: Cervical ectopic pregnancy: review of the literature and report of a case treated by single-dose methotrexate therapy, *Obstet Gynecol Surv* 45:405, 1990.

7

Endometriosis

ELIZABETH A. KENNARD

Endometriosis is defined as the presence of the glands and stroma of the lining of the uterus in an aberrant location. The incidence of endometriosis is difficult to estimate because the disease cannot accurately be diagnosed without direct visualization of the pelvic cavity. Endometriosis is found in 5% to 15% of surgeries performed on reproductive-age females and in up to 30% of infertile women.

PATHOPHYSIOLOGY

The etiology of endometriosis has been the subject of much investigation. No theory completely explains all cases of endometriosis. The most common explanation focuses on retrograde menstruation. First suggested in 1920 by Sampson, retrograde menstruation postulates that endometrial tissue flowing out the fallopian tubes implants in the abdominal cavity. A number of animal experiments have demonstrated the development of classic endometriosis when the cervix is sutured, and endometriosis is very common in women with outflow obstruction of the genital tract. However, other investigators have shown that retrograde menstruation is probably a normal occurrence and that some underlying abnormality of the immune system must explain why endometrial tissue is able to implant in the pelvic cavity. A large body of confusing research surrounds the investigation of the immunology of endometriosis. Some authors have shown increased numbers of macrophages and cytokines in the peritoneal fluid from women with endometriosis. Some have found impaired functioning of these intraperitoneal cells. Others have found defects in natural killer cell proliferation in response to exposure to autologous endometrium. It is clear however, that women with endometriosis are not immunocompromised. They do not demonstrate a propensity for infection, and they do not have increased susceptibility to the development of tumors.

There are cases of endometriosis that defy the theory of retrograde menstruation. For example, endometriosis has occurred in women with uterine agenesis. In addition, endometriosis has been found in the lungs, nose, spinal column, and other areas distant from the pelvis. Two theories advanced to explain these types of situations exist. The theory of coelomic metaplasia postulates that epithelium will retain the ability for multipotential development and differentiate into endometrial tissue after some type of induction. Vascular and lymphatic dissemination are advanced as etiologies when endometriosis has been found in locations that do not arise from coelomic epithelium.

DIAGNOSIS

Usually, endometriosis is asymptomatic. Many women will be diagnosed with endometriosis only incidentally during laparoscopy or laparotomy for other reasons. Women can also demonstrate pelvic pain or infertility. On physical exam they may have cul-de-sac nodularity or adnexal masses. The pain of endometriosis does not correlate well with the extent of disease and can include pain with menses, defecation, and/or intercourse.

Diagnosis of endometriosis depends on direct visualization and biopsy if possible. The appearance of endometriosis is varied. Implants may progress from red or clear to blue, then black and powdery or scarred. Endometriomas of the ovary will appear as cloudy cysts on ultrasound and may mimic corpus luteum cysts. During surgery, rupture of an endometrioma will result in spilling chocolate-colored material.

Endometriosis is usually described as being minimal, mild, moderate, or severe. A classification system was devised by the American Fertility Society, however this classification has not been shown to be helpful in predicting resolution of symptoms after treatment.

DIFFERENTIAL DIAGNOSIS

Endometriosis may be suspected when pain or infertility is present. The differential diagnosis consists of other sources of pelvic pain including ovarian cysts, ovarian torsion, irritable bowel syndrome, uterine fibroids, dysmenorrhea, pelvic adhesions, and other causes.

TREATMENT

No controlled study has ever demonstrated a benefit of treating minimal or mild endometriosis to restore fertility. Several studies show the pregnancy rate with expectant management to be approximately 30%. This is no different from the pregnancy rates in groups treated with various methods. Treatment of endometriosis that is painful has been shown to help with resolution of symptoms.

Endometriosis can be treated medically or surgically. The glands and stroma of endometriosis respond to steroid hormones and contain steroid receptors. Surgical treatment seeks to physically destroy implants.

Danazol is a derivative of ethisterone and has androgenic and anabolic side effects. The exact mechanism of action of danazol is controversial. It definitely results in a hypoestrogenic, hypoprogestational state. The standard dose is 400 to 800 mg/day for 6 months. Adverse side effects are experienced by most women using this medication. Danazol is metabolized by the liver and liver function tests should be checked if the medication is prescribed for longer than 6 months.

Kistner popularized the use of continuous oral contraceptives for treatment of endometriosis in an attempt to produce a "pseudopregnancy." The clinical impression was that endometriosis regressed during and after a pregnancy. This method is less commonly prescribed now that comparison studies have shown other methods to be superior in providing symptom relief.

GnRH agonists are peptide analogues of GnRH. They bind the GnRH receptor and induce down-regulation caused by prolonged receptor occupation. These medications result in a dramatic suppression of the pituitary-ovarian axis within 2 weeks of initiating therapy. The drugs are administered either subcutaneously or intranasally and produce pseudomenopause without the androgenic or anabolic side effects of danazol. However, the hypoestrogenic state that is induced does lead to bone loss, and the use of these medications is currently limited to 6 months. Studies have recently been published suggesting that the disease may be successfully treated with GnRH therapy combined with steroid hormone "add-back" therapy. This therapy would allow prolonged treatment with the GnRH agonist, however the data are limited. Multiple comparison trials have shown danazol and GnRH agonists to be comparable in suppressing implants and alleviating symptoms.

Surgical treatment of endometriosis involves ablating all implants. This can be done by excision or by physical destruction using endocoagulation or laser. The surgery may be performed as a laparoscopy or a laparotomy, depending on the extent of disease and experience of the surgeon. Since the definitive diagnosis of endometriosis requires surgical evaluation, the main advantage to surgical treatment is that it can be accomplished at the same time. At times, the only solution to unremitting symptomatic endometriosis is a total abdominal hysterectomy. There is controversy in the literature about whether a bilateral oophrectomy should be performed simultaneously. This would avoid further hormonal stimulation of endometriotic implants that were not removed at the time of the hysterectomy but would subject the woman to increased cardiovascular and osteoporosis risk as a result of hypoestrogenism.

KEY POINTS

1. Endometriosis represents the presence of the glands and stroma of the lining of the endometrium in another location.
2. Theories about the etiology of endometriosis include retrograde menstruation, coelomic metaplasia, and vascular spread.

3 Endometriosis cannot be accurately diagnosed without visualization and/or biopsy.

4 Endometriosis often causes no symptoms.

5 Surgical treatment of the disease can be performed by laparoscopy or laparotomy and may involve excision, laser, or endocoagulation. Surgical treatment has the advantage of occurring at the time of definitive diagnosis.

SUGGESTED READINGS

ACOG Technical Bulletin Number 184, *Endometriosis,* 1993.

Adamson GD, Pasta DJ: Surgical treatment of endometriosis-associated infertility: meta-analysis compared with survival analysis, *Am J Obstet Gynecol* 171:1499, 1994.

Howell R et al: Gonadotropin-releasing hormone analogue (goserelin) plus hormone replacement therapy for the treatment of endometriosis: a randomized controlled trial, *Fertil Steril* 64:474, 1995.

Hughes EG, Fedorkow DKM, Collins JA: A quantitative overview of controlled trials in endometriosis-associated infertility, *Fertil Steril* 59:963, 1993.

Inoue M et al: The impact of endometriosis on the reproductive outcome of infertile patients, *Am J Obstet Gynecol* 167:278, 1992.

Namnoum AB et al: Incidence of symptom recurrence after hysterectomy for endometriosis, *Fertil Steril* 64:898, 1995.

Rock JA, Truglia JA, Caplan RJ, Study Group: Zoladex (goserelin acetate implant) in the treatment of endometriosis: a randomized comparison with danazol, *Obstet Gynecol* 82:198, 1993.

Rock JA, Markham SM: Pathogenesis of endometriosis, *Lancet* 340:1264, 1992.

Wheeler JM, Knittle JD, Miller JD: Depot leuprolide versus danazol in treatment of women with symptomatic endometriosis, *Am J Obstet Gynecol* 167:1367, 1992.

8

Gestational Trophoblastic Disease

LARRY J. COPELAND AND JAMES L. NICKLIN

Gestational trophoblastic diseases are both biologically interesting and therapeutically challenging. Choriocarcinoma, the most malignant spectrum of trophoblastic disease, is one of the few metastatic tumors that is curable. These patients seek treatment from primary care physicians and specialists of many different disciplines with a vast array of symptoms. Unfortunately, delays in diagnosis, usually attributable to the rarity of the disease and the diverse symptomatology, remain a problem and compromise opportunities for cure.

Physicians, usually gynecologic oncologists, who are thoroughly familiar with the multiple nuances of this disease should direct the management of patients with gestational trophoblastic disease.

MORPHOLOGIC DIAGNOSIS

Hydatidiform Mole

Incidence

Hydatidiform mole incidence varies by geography and is as frequent as 1 in 85 pregnancies in Indonesia, to 1 in 150 pregnancies in the Orient and Mexico, to approximately 1 in 1500 pregnancies in the United States. The wide variability in reported incidence may be the result of the bias of reporting hospital-based studies rather than population-based studies. The clinical risk factors for molar pregnancy with approximate relative risks (RR) include the following:

Prior mole	20-40 RR
Young (teens) < 20	1.5 RR
Older > 40	5.2 RR
Prior spontaneous abortion	1.9-3.3 RR
Professional occupation	2.5 RR

Protective factors for molar pregnancy with approximate relative risks (RR) include the following:

Dietary vitamin A	0.6 RR
Parity > 0 and no abortions	0.2-0.6 RR

Clinical presentation and diagnosis

First trimester vaginal bleeding or spotting is often the first symptom. The uterus is large for dates in approximately 50% of patients with moles, 25% are normal, and 25% are small for dates. Hyperemesis or toxemia can be associated with high HCG levels. Fetal heart tones are absent. Theca-lutein cysts are present as an adnexal mass in 15% to 20% of patients. Before the widespread use of sonography to evaluate first trimester bleeding, the vaginal passage of molar tissue was the most common symptom that led to the diagnosis of molar disease.

The characteristic ultrasound finding is a snowstorm pattern and the differential diagnosis for this sonographic finding includes tangential cuts of placenta, fibroids, missed abortion, and multiple gestation. Commonly the β-HCG is 40,000 mIU/ml or greater, but the HCG level is not a reliable basis for the diagnosis of molar disease because multiple gestations and other hyperplacental situations can produce high levels of HCG. In a normal pregnancy, serial HCG values normally decline after 10 weeks gestation. Before the availability of ultrasound, the amniogram was a useful diagnostic procedure. Currently, the amniogram is of only historic interest.

Pathology

Grapelike vesicles fill the uterine cavity. The villi are all hydropic and avascular. There are no normal villi. There is proliferation of trophoblastic tissue (syncytiotrophoblast or cytotrophoblast cells). The usual chromosomal pattern is 46,XX, paternal homologous based on the empty egg theory with 23,X sperm fertilization with reduplication.

Management

Evacuation by suction curettage is the preferred technique because mechanical probing or scraping of a uterus with molar disease places the uterus at risk for perforation should the molar disease invade in an occult fashion into the myometrium (Fig. 8-1). Because perforation leading to hysterectomy is a potential complication, the uterus should be evacuated with the safest possible technique, especially in a patient desirous of future childbearing. If suction equipment is not available, it is reasonably safe to evacuate a small uterus (<13- to 14-week size) by mechanical dilation and curettage. However, if the uterus is significantly enlarged, consideration should be given to transferring the patient to a facility with suction equipment or evacuating the uterus by hysterotomy.

Contractions should be avoided. Active uterine contractions on a molar pregnancy, especially a large molar pregnancy, present an increased risk of trophoblastic embolization, an event similar to amniotic fluid embolism and with similar potential sequelae. Therefore it is contraindicated to start Oxytocin or administer prostaglandins before evacuation. This is sometimes erroneously done in an attempt to either abate bleeding or evacuate the uterus. If bleeding is a problem, then this presents a relative urgency to proceed with evacuation of the uterus and to not enhance uterine contractions by pharmacologic means. Oxytocin can be started concurrent with the suction evacuation.

After evacuation, some recommend the uterine cavity have a sharp curettage performed. There is no evidence that curettage provides meaningful information, and it probably subjects the patient to uterine trauma and serious sequelae, including perforation and Asherman's syndrome.

Theca-lutein cysts are functional ovarian cysts, an exaggerated response to elevated HCG levels. These cysts should be managed conservatively because after HCG stimulation has been eliminated, they will usually regress over an interval of many months.

Hysterectomy is an acceptable form of primary treatment in the patient who also desires sterilization. Hysterectomy is justified on the basis of reducing the risk of requiring chemotherapy for persistent gestational trophoblastic neoplasia (GTN) from the 15% to 20% range down to the 1% to 4% range.

Surveillance after evacuation is necessary to identify patients who demonstrate persistent viable tumor as evidenced by a plateau or increase in HCG levels. Titres should be obtained weekly until three normal titres have been obtained and then monthly for 6 to 12 months. Factors favoring abnormal regression include high HCG levels, large uterus, theca-lutein cysts, age over 40, and prior GTN. Effective contraception during the surveillance period is important. If the patient conceives before complete resolution of the prior GTN, the new pregnancy will demonstrate increasing HCG levels and assessment of the status of the prior GTN is severely handicapped. In these rare situations, evidence of progressive GTN is limited to sonographic imaging studies of the pelvis and chest radiography.

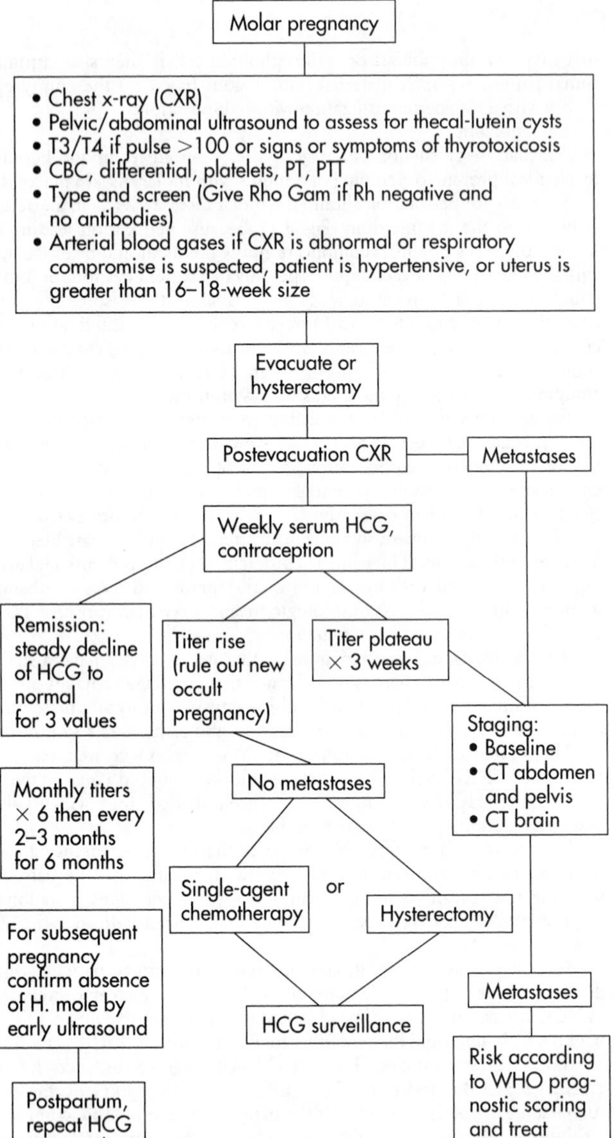

FIG. 8-1 Molar pregnancy management. (From Copeland LJ: Gestational trophoblastic neoplasia. In *Textbook of gynecology,* Philadelphia, 1993, WB Saunders, pp 1137.)

Beyond 10 to 12 weeks, the HCG in a normal pregnancy is expected to decline and a sustained increase would raise the level of concern for the possibility of coexisting progressive GTN. Oral contraceptives are recommended for birth control during the surveillance interval.

Chemotherapy is required for the 15% to 20% of patients who can be expected to demonstrate a plateau or an increase in HCG levels. Patients with either nonmetastatic molar disease or metastatic low-risk disease are usually treated with single-agent chemotherapy, usually either actinomycin-D or methotrexate. It is estimated that only 3% to 4% of patients with complete hydatidiform mole are at risk of progressing to choriocarcinoma if untreated.

Partial Mole

Incidence

The true incidence of partial hydatidiform mole is difficult to assess. It is safe to say that the incidence is probably higher than previously suspected, possibly accounting for 15% to 40% of molar pregnancies.

Clinical presentation and diagnosis

The epidemiology of complete moles is not applicable to partial moles. The average gestational age is 20 weeks, 6 weeks later than the average for a complete mole. The uterus is also more frequently small for dates. The diagnosis is often suspected on ultrasound findings and is supported by specific pathologic features.

Pathology

Normal villi are intermingled or adjacent to hydropic villi. Villi contain vessels, best documented by the presence of nucleated RBCs within the vessel. Hyperplasia is usually minimal. Portions of fetus, cord, or membranes are often identified. The karyotype is usually triploidy or trisomy and rarely diploid. Metastases are rare.

Management

Management principles for partial mole are similar to those for a complete mole. The timing and method of uterine evacuation may be influenced by the fetal karyotype and gestational age of the fetus. Depending on the size of the accompanying fetus and experience of the clinician, evacuation is performed by either hysterotomy or mechanical evacuation. Only 2% to 7% of patients with partial mole may require chemotherapy treatment. Postevacuation surveillance is necessary to identify patients with persistent molar disease, as evidenced by a plateau of increased HCG levels. Titres should be obtained weekly until three normal titres have been obtained and then monthly for 6 to 12 months.

Chorioadenoma Destruens (Invasive Mole)

Incidence

The true incidence of invasive mole is difficult to assess because the diagnosis usually requires a hysterectomy to demonstrate the invasive element. Probably about 10% to 20% of moles have an invasive focus.

Clinical presentation and diagnosis

The classic clinical symptom of invasive mole is bleeding, most commonly vaginal. However, bleeding from metastatic sites (i.e., hemoptysis from lung metastasis) or intraperitoneal bleeding from direct uterine extension may be the initial symptom.

Diagnosis is based on demonstrating invasive trophoblastic tissue with persistent villi and is most commonly done at the time of hysterectomy.

Pathology

Proliferation of trophoblastic tissue is usually limited to the uterus but may be metastatic. Most commonly the invasion is into the myometrium. The pathologic feature that sets chorioadenoma destruens apart from choriocarcinoma is the presence of persistent hydropic villi.

Management

The greatest management problem is the detection and treatment of bleeding. This may require surgical intervention, most commonly a hysterectomy for uterine bleeding. Although the disease may be self-limiting, all patients should receive chemotherapy.

Placental Site Trophoblastic Tumor

Incidence

Placental site trophoblastic tumor (PSTT) is a rare entity, but the diagnosis has been made more frequently in recent years. PSTT can follow any type of gestation.

Clinical presentation

The most common symptom of PSTT is persistent postpartum bleeding and low elevated levels of HCG. Characteristically this tumor produces small amounts of HCG, <3000 mIU/ml, and tends to metastasize later than choriocarcinoma. PSTT can be associated with toxemia and nephrotic syndrome. Human placental lactogen (HPL) may be a better tumor marker than HCG.

Pathology

The origin of PSTT tumors appears to be the placental bed trophoblast. In contrast, choriocarcinoma arises from the villous trophoblast. The cells are predominantly cytotrophoblasts and intermediate-type cells and syncytial trophoblasts are rare. Hemorrhage and necrosis are absent or focal. The tumor cells stain poorly for HCG and stain better for HPL by immunoflourescence.

Management

Since the response to chemotherapy may be poor, management considerations include early hysterectomy and resection of solitary resistant foci.

Choriocarcinoma

Incidence

Choriocarcinoma following term pregnancy is rare, occurring as a sequela in 1 of 20,000 to 40,000 term pregnancies. There is little data to extrapolate the frequency after abortion. The frequency of choriocarcinoma following therapeutic or ectopic abortion is probably similar to the frequency after term pregnancy. Choriocarcinoma frequency may be slightly higher after an apparent spontaneous abortion. Choriocarcinoma occurs as a sequela to complete mole in 3% to 4% of patients.

Clinical presentation

The clinical progression of choriocarcinoma can be very rapid, with death (usually hemorrhage-related) often occurring within 3 to 12 months of disease onset. Choriocarcinoma develops after any form of previous pregnancy. The precursor gestation in 50% of patients with choriocarcinoma is hydatidiform mole. Term pregnancy and aborted pregnancies are the precursor pregnancies in about a fourth of the cases.

The clinical presentation of choriocarcinoma may be quite variable and often masquerades as other diseases. Although vaginal bleeding from uterine, cervical, or vaginal disease often results in a timely diagnosis, other sites of bleeding such as hemoptysis, hematuria, and hematochezia are frequently associated with a delay of diagnosis. Other presentations include focal neurologic symptoms secondary to spinal or intracranial metastasis, upper or lower gastrointestinal bleeding, abdominal pain secondary to liver metastasis or intraperitoneal bleeding, hematuria from renal tract metastasis, and pulmonary complaints including respiratory failure, hemoptysis, or asthmalike symptoms secondary to extensive pulmonary metastasis.

Since the tumor is characterized by extensive necrosis and hemorrhage, tissue obtained from either the uterus or metastatic sites may not yield the histologic diagnosis. Even uterine curettings in a patient with postpartum bleeding may reveal only necrosis and hemorrhage. Also, tissue-sampling techniques such as fine-needle aspiration or needle biopsy are at risk of being misdiagnosed as another primary.

Diagnosis

Diagnosis is based on history, clinical suspicion, and a serum β-HCG. Tissue sampling is not necessary and if attempted could initiate serious bleeding. Choriocarcinoma is noted for early widespread metastasis and a complete metastatic survey should be performed before initiating treatment. The metastatic survey should include a chest x-ray and CT of the abdomen, pelvis, and brain. Metastases are predominantly arteriovenous rather than lymphatic. Table 8-1 provides an approximation of the frequency of metastasis to the various anatomic sites.

Pathology

Choriocarcinoma is characterized by sheets of proliferative trophoblasts, hemorrhage, and necrosis. No villi are present.

Management

Chemotherapy recommendations vary with the risk level of the clinical situation (Table 8-2). Radiotherapy is employed for prevention of hemorrhage from brain metastasis. Surgery has a role in the management of hemorrhagic complications and may also be indicated for resistant foci.

Chemotherapy for nonmetastatic or low-risk metastatic disease is usually single-agent chemotherapy with methotrexate, actinomycin-D, or 5-fluorouracil. Repeat cycles are given with recovery of blood counts and clearance of stomatitis. Treatments are usually given at about two-week intervals. Chemotherapy is usually administered to at least one treatment beyond a normal titre for low-risk disease and two or three cycles beyond a normal titre for high-risk disease. High-risk metastatic disease is usually treated by combination chemotherapy, and treatment should be per-

TABLE 8-1
Common Sites for Metastatic Choriocarcinoma

Site	Percent
Lung	60-95
Vagina	40-50
Vulva/cervix	10-15
Brain	5-15
Liver	0-5
Kidney	0-5
Spleen	0-5
Gastrointestinal	0-5

NOTE: Frequency varies, depending on whether data are based on autopsy studies or are obtained from pretreatment imaging.

From Copeland LJ: Gestational trophoblastic neoplasia. In *Textbook of gynecology,* Philadelphia, 1993, WB Saunders, pp 1141.

TABLE 8-2
WHO Prognostic Scoring

	Score			
Prognostic factor	0	1	2	4
Age (years)	<39	>39	—	—
Antecedent pregnancy	Mole	Abortion, ectopic	Term pregnancy	—
Time interval (mos)	<4	4-6	7-12	>12
Initial HCG	$<10^3$	10^3-10^4	10^4-10^5	$>10^5$
Blood group	—	OxA	B or AB	—
Largest tumor (cm)	<3	3-5	>5	—
Sites of mets	Lung, pelvis	Spleen, kidney	GI tract, kidney	Brain, liver
Number of mets	—	1-4	4-8	>8
Previous chemo	—	—	Single drug	2 or more

From Copeland LJ: Gestational trophoblastic neoplasia. In *Textbook of gynecology,* Philadelphia, 1993, WB Saunders, pp 1146.
Low risk, 4 or lower; medium risk, 5-7; high risk, 8 or higher; *HCG,* human chorionic gonadotropin; *GI,* gastrointestinal.

formed in a treatment center specializing in the management of gestational trophoblastic disease.

RECURRENT GTN

Recurrences after three negative titres occur in 2.5% of patients with nonmetastatic GTN, in 3.7% of patients with good prognostic metastatic GTN, and in 12% of patients with poor prognostic disease. Before 1978, the salvage rate for recurrent GTN was only about 40%. However, with the introduction of additional chemotherapy agents such as cisplatin, etoposide, carboplatin, and ifosfamide the salvage rate for recurrent disease now exceeds 80%.

SPECIAL SITUATIONS

Special treatment situations such as CNS or liver metastases and extensive pulmonary disease may require innovative and complex treatment plans and should be managed by a gynecologic oncologist.

KEY POINTS

1 Choriocarcinoma is one of the few metastatic tumors that is curable.

2 Delays in diagnosis are attributed to the rarity of the disease, the diverse symptomatology, and compromised opportunities for cure.

3 Hysterectomy is an acceptable form of primary treatment in patients with gestational trophoblastic disease who also desire sterilization.

4 The clinical presentation of choriocarcinoma can be very rapid, with death often occurring within 3 to 12 months from disease onset.

5 Recurrences after three negative titres occur in 2.5% of patients with nonmetastatic GTN, in 3.7% with good prognostic metastatic GTN, and 12% of patients with poor GTN.

SUGGESTED READINGS

ACOG: *Management of gestational trophoblastic disease:* Technical Bulletin, No. 178, March 1993.

Copeland LJ: Gestational trophoblastic neoplasia. In *Textbook of gynecology,* Philadelphia, 1993, WB Saunders, pp 1133-1151.

DeiCas RE et al: The role of contraception in the development of postmolar gestational trophoblastic tumor, *Obstet Gynecol* 87:221-226, 1991.

Kelly MP et al: Respiratory failure due to choriocarcinoma: a study of 103 dyspneic patients, *Gynecol Oncol* 38:149-154, 1990.

Mutch DG, et al: Recurrent gestational trophoblastic disease: experience of the Southeastern Regional Trophoblastic Disease Center, *Cancer* 66:978-982, 1990.

Rice LW et al: Persistent gestational trophoblastic tumor after partial hydatidiform mole, *Gynecol Oncol* 36:358-362, 1990.

Schlaerth JB: Tumors of the placental trophoblast. In *Synopsis of gynecologic oncology,* ed 4, New York, 1993, Churchill Livingstone, pp 311-350.

9

Hirsutism

Chad I. Friedman

Hirsutism is a sign of hyperandrogenemia and as such is the sentinel of many underlying causes of ovulatory dysfunction. Androgens in the female are produced either by the adrenal gland or the ovary. Testosterone (T), dehydroepiandrosterone (DHEA), and androstenedione are significant secretory components of both the adrenal gland and ovary, whereas dehydroepiandrosterone sulfate (DHEA-S) is secreted almost exclusively by the adrenal gland. Peripheral conversion of androgens and androgen precursors is responsible for a major portion of circulating potent androgens and their clinical manifestation. In fact, expression of hirsutism is primarily dependent on peripheral conversion of androgens to dihydrotestosterone.

Approximately 98% of testosterone, the "classic" androgen in circulation, is bound to albumin and a carrier protein called *steroid hormone binding globulin* (SHBG). Biologic activity of testosterone depends on the free and albumin-bound testosterone concentrations, testosterone's intracellular conversion to dihydrotestosterone, and its interaction with the androgen receptor.

The most common pathophysiologic causes for hirsutism include polycystic ovarian disease (PCOD) (also termed *hyperandrogenic chronic anovulation*), enzyme defects (21 hydroxylase, 11β-hydroxylase, 3β-hydroxysteroid dehydrogenase), hyperthecosis, adrenal hyperplasia, androgen-producing tumors, and utilization of anabolic steroids. For most of these entities, ovulatory function is also disturbed. By definition, idiopathic hirsutism is not associated with ovulatory dysfunction. In PCOD and most cases of subtle enzyme defects, hirsutism is slowly progressive, with its onset shortly after menarche. Rapid progression of hirsutism and the presence of virilization are the hallmarks of androgen-producing tumors.

Fig. 9-1 highlights the proposed pathophysiology of PCOD. There are many potential etiologies leading to the clinical syndrome of PCOD. Women with mild adrenal enzyme defects, hyperprolactinemia, and acromegaly could also manifest PCOD. The key for PCOD is excessive stimulation of the theca by LH and insulin to secrete excessive androgens. The low SHBG amplifies the androgenic action, whereas peripheral aromatase activity maintains a chronic estrogenic state.

Hirsutism is a frustrating disorder to treat. Telogen, the phase of active hair growth, can last for 6 to 24 months. Thus actual clinical improvement

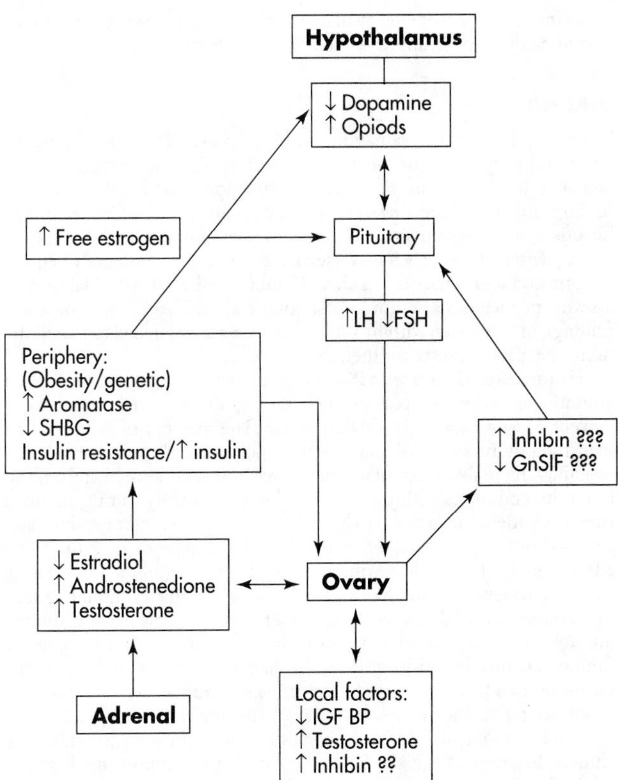

FIG. 9-1 PCOD may have many potential etiologies. Shown are some of the observed and hypothetical findings associated with PCOD. *LH,* luteinizing hormone; *FSH,* follicle stimulating hormone; *GnSIF,* gonadotropin surge inhibiting factor; *IGF-BP,* insulinlike growth factor binding protein; *SHBG,* steroid hormone binding globulin.

requires a prolonged course of therapy. Admittedly, with a reduction in circulating androgens, a reduction in the rate of hair growth and hair shaft thickness may be observed within several months of therapy, though this has little effect on the patient's perception of efficacy. The physician's obligations in the management of hirsutism are to (1) ensure the absence of an underlying neoplastic process, (2) establish a therapeutic intervention to limit future hair growth, (3) establish ovulatory function or cyclic endometrial withdrawal bleeding if anovulation is present, (4) counsel the patient regarding cosmetic therapies available, and (5) educate the patient as to the overall medical implications related to the cause of hirsutism.

DIAGNOSIS

Pertinent points in the evaluation of hirsutism include characterizing the onset and progression of hirsutism, excluding virilizing symptoms, and assessing for symptoms of ovulatory function. Specific key physical findings include blood pressure, striae, documentation of the extent of hirsutism, and assessment of the ovaries. Determination of the clitoral index (sagittal diameter × transverse diameter in mm) is extremely helpful. A normal clitoral index is less than 35 mm. Finally, the basic laboratory assessment includes a serum testosterone and DHEA-S. Based on these findings, most women with hirsutism can be readily assigned to neoplastic or nonneoplastic causes for their hirsutism.

Historically, patients with PCOD typically have the onset of hirsutism around menarche or occasionally after significant weight gain. Sixty percent of women with PCOD are obese. The majority of subjects have menstrual dysfunction (oligomenorrhea, polymenorrhea, or anovulatory bleeding). A family history of females with irregular periods, hirsutism, and infertility and males with premature balding frequently can be obtained from the patient. In addition to hirsutism, a normal-size clitoris, abundant cervical mucus that ferns when dried, and the absence of a unilateral adnexal mass should all be observed on physical examination. During vaginal ultrasound, more than 10 small (4-9 mm) follicles should be seen in a given section of the ovary along with a hyperechogenic stroma. Routine ultrasounds to establish the diagnosis should be discouraged because the findings are merely consistent with the diagnosis, neither establishing the diagnosis of PCOD nor excluding it. Many woman with ultrasound-diagnosed polycystic ovaries are ovulatory and nonhirsuit, and many obese women commonly do not have polycystic ovaries on scans, yet fulfill the clinical diagnosis of PCOD. Laboratory studies to support the diagnosis of PCOD include an elevated LH/FSH ratio, a serum testosterone of <2 ng/ml, DHEA-S value <700 μg/dl, and 17 hydroxyprogesterone (17OH P_4) value <2.5 ng/ml.

One variant of PCOD is the HAIR-AN syndrome (hyperandrogenism, insulin resistance, acanthosis nigricans). In addition to the previously described history for PCOD, these women typically manifest hyperpigmentation of the intertriginous regions commencing at or before menarche. Obesity is more prevalent, and the hyperandrogenic signs are commonly more severe. Clitoromegaly, defined as a clitoral diameter of 1 cm at the base, may in fact be present. When it is, a thorough hormonal and ultrasonographic evaluation is required. The hallmark of the HAIR-AN syndrome is insulin resistance. A fasting insulin is typically elevated (>25 uU/ml), though the glucose response to a GTT may be normal. 17OH P_4 and DHEA-S concentrations are typical of PCOD. Testosterone values may exceed 2 ng/ml and the LH/FSH ratio is seldom elevated. Vaginal ultrasound reveals symmetrical ovaries with hyperechogenic stroma. The number of follicles may or may not be increased.

Androgen-producing ovarian tumors, at least by the time of diagnosis, have a distinctly different presentation. Acute disruption of previously regular menses is noted and a rapid progression of hirsutism often distant from menarche is observed. Virilization (increased muscle mass, clitoromegaly, deepening voice, and temporal balding) is accompanied by defeminization (decreasing breast size and often absent cervical mucus). Pelvic examination in 75% of the cases reveals a unilateral adnexal mass. Testosterone serum concentrations are elevated, commonly exceeding 2 ng/ml. DHEA-S is normal or slightly elevated with 17OH P_4 serum concentrations being variable. Ultrasound of the pelvis is helpful in confirming a unilateral, solid ovarian tumor.

Regrettably, the ovarian tumor cannot always be identified on pelvic examination or even with the aid of ultrasound. In these cases an adrenal source must be excluded either with the use of an iodomethylnorcholesterol scan or ovarian and adrenal catheterization studies. A proposed evaluation for androgen-producing tumors is shown in Fig. 9-2.

Several exceptions to the classic presentation of an androgen-producing tumor must be born in mind. Patients with PCOD may also develop an androgen-producing tumor, blurring the acute onset. Although Sertoli-Leydig cell tumors are the most common androgen-producing tumors in reproductive-age women, adrenal rest and hilus cell tumors are more prevalent in postmenopausal women. In these patients, an acute onset of hirsutism and virilization is still observed though actual total serum testosterone levels are often only moderately elevated (i.e., <2 ng/ml). Adnexal masses are also not necessarily readily apparent on pelvic examination or ultrasound. Diagnosis relies on the exclusion of an adrenal tumor and surgical exploration.

Sertoli-Leydig cell tumors and adrenal androgen-producing tumors have been reported in association with pregnancy. However, the luteoma of pregnancy is the most common cause for acute hirsutism and virilization noted during pregnancy. In 50% of the cases the tumor is unilateral. Although many luteomas are asymptomatic, tumor range testosterone levels may be present. With the exception of a prior history of a luteoma, there is no effective way of differentiating a newly symptomatic androgen-producing ovarian neoplasm from a luteoma of pregnancy. Differentiation after delivery is easy, however, as luteomas readily regress and androgen levels fall.

Several enzyme inefficiencies (i.e., 21 hydroxylase, 11β-hydroxylase, 3β-hydroxysteroid dehydrogenase) have the potential to mimic PCOD. In contrast to classic congenital adrenal hyperplasia with genital ambiguity, adult-onset adrenal hyperplasia may manifest as hirsutism, oligovulation, or acne. The most common cause, 21 hydroxylase deficiency, is relatively prevalent in Jewish subjects of Eastern European descent (disease frequency ≈ 1 in 30). The hallmark for 21 hydroxylase deficiency is an elevated early morning follicular phase 17 hydroxyprogesterone >2.5 ng/ml. Diagnosis is confirmed by an abnormal rise in 17OH P_4 30 to 60 minutes after the administration of 250 μg of Cortrosyn and symptomatic improvement following glucocorticoid therapy. As previously mentioned, physical findings, time of onset, and ultrasound appearance may all

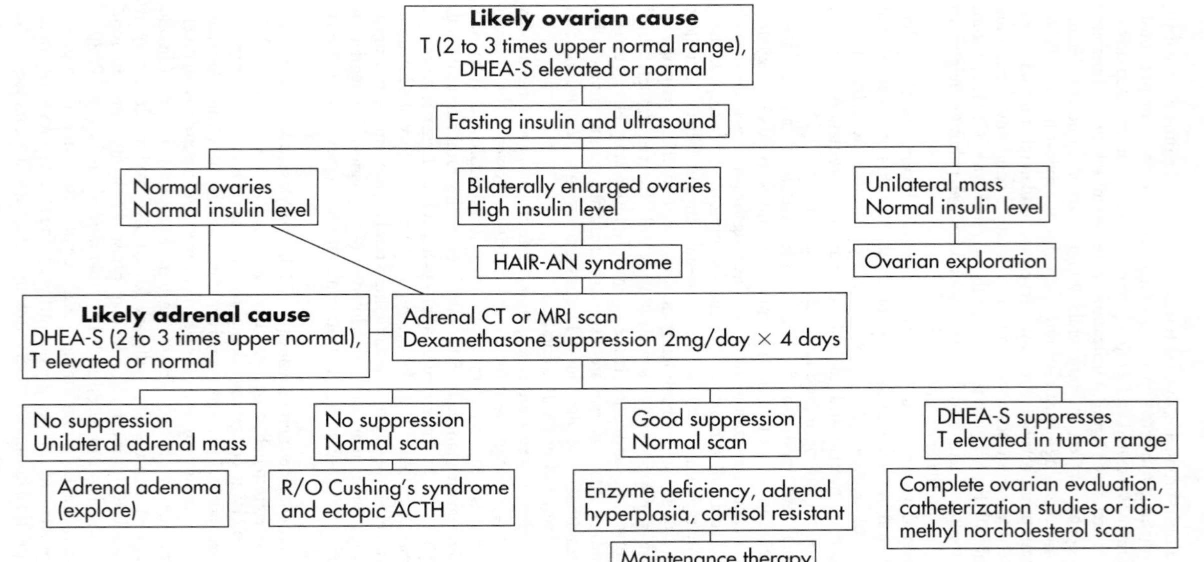

FIG. 9-2 Proposed evaluation of markedly elevated androgens to rule out an androgen-producing tumor. *T*, testosterone.

be consistent with PCOD. Excluding Jewish individuals of Eastern European descent, adrenal enzyme deficiencies will be present in <5% of hirsute women. Testing is frequently restricted to high-risk populations, women not responding to standard treatments for PCOD, women with hirsutism and acne but regular menstrual cycles, and women with elevated DHEA-S but normal testosterone serum concentrations.

Virulizing adrenal adenomas have a similar presentation to ovarian androgen-producing tumors. Markedly elevated DHEA-S serum concentrations are almost always observed. Rare adrenal testosterone-secreting tumors without an elevation in DHEA-S have been reported. In most cases, a dexamethasone suppression test, 2 mg/day × 4 days, fails to suppress the DHEA-S concentration into the low normal range. CT or MRI is highly sensitive in detecting adrenal adenomas. However, nonfunctional adrenal adenomas are relatively common, limiting specificity. Adrenal and ovarian catheterization studies may be required before surgical evaluation.

Cushing's syndrome causes hirsutism and menstrual dysfunction in up to 80% of affected females, though this is rarely the primary complaint. Facial plethora, hypetension, striae, and obesity are commonly seen with Cushing's syndrome. When the syndrome is suspected, a 24-hour free urinary cortisol and 1 mg overnight dexamethasone suppression test should be performed. A subsequent 2-day, 2 mg/day dexamethasone suppression test should be obtained if either of the screening tests are abnormal.

Idiopathic hirsutism, by definition, is a diagnosis of exclusion. In these individuals menstrual cyclicity should be normal. Present and past history for medications known to cause hirsutism (i.e., minoxidil, danocrine, oxandrolone, Dilantin, and cyclosporine) should be negative. Free or biologically active testosterone, DHEA-S, 17OH P_4, and androstenedione should all be normal. Perhaps the greatest importance, hirsutism (coarse hair) excluding the extremities needs to be carefully demonstrated. In heterogeneous societies it is difficult to establish norms of hirsutism. Table 9-1 summarizes the likely hormonal and clinical finding for the various causes of hirsutism.

With the exception of excluding idiopathic hirsutism, measuring free testosterone, SHBG, or androestanediol glucuride has very limited clinical utility.

THERAPY

Given the prolonged duration required to observe clinical improvement, therapy is aggressive initially. Medications to inhibit hair growth and suppress hyperandrogenemia are started concurrently. Once androgens are adequately suppressed, cosmetic interventions are initiated. Following clinical improvement, suppression of the androgen source often suffices for long-term management.

Ovarian Hyperandrogenemia

Despite an associated elevation in DHEA-S, the vast majority of women with PCOD show significant improvement in their androgen profile after

TABLE 9-1
Findings Associated With Various Causes of Hirsutism

	T	DHEA-S	17OH P_4	Clitoral index	Insulin	Ovarian ultrasound
PCOD	nl-↑	nl-↑	nl-↑	nl	nl-↑	Symmetric
Hyperthecosis	↑↑	nl-↑	nl-↑	↑-↑↑	↑↑	Symmetric
Adult 21 hydroxylase deficiency	nl-↑	nl-↑	↑-↑↑	nl	nl	Symmetric
Congenital 21 hydroxylase deficiency	↑-↑↑	↑	↑↑↑	↑↑	nl	Symmetric
Sertoli-Leydig cell tumor	↑↑↑	nl-↑	nl-↑	↑-↑↑	nl	Unilateral (80%)
Adrenal adenoma	nl-↑↑	↑↑(rare-nl)	↑	nl-↑↑	nl-↑	Symmetric
Cushing's syndrome	nl-↑	nl-↑↑	↑	nl-↑	nl-↑↑	Symmetric
Idiopathic hirsutism	nl	nl	nl	nl	nl	Symmetric
Iatrogenic	nl-↑	nl	nl	nl-↑↑	nl-↑	Symmetric

ovarian suppression alone. Clinically, oral contraceptives represent the primary means for obtaining ovarian suppression. Although there is little data to support one formulation over another in terms of suppressing androgen production, the use of less andorgenic progestins (e.g., norgestimate, desonorgesteryl, and cyproterone acetate) is strongly encouraged. Oral contraception, in addition to suppressing androgen production, increases circulatory SHBG, possibly inhibits androgenic manifestations at the hair follicle, and of equal importance provides cyclic menstrual bleeding in women at risk for endometrial carcinoma and anovulatory bleeding. Improvement in HDL cholesterol levels may also be appreciated with the use of oral contraceptives, a potential benefit in a population at increased risk for cardiovascular disease. Because many women with PCOD demonstrate abnormal lipid profiles, a fasting cholesterol and triglycerides test should be considered before initiating treatment with oral contraceptives. Severe hypertriglyceridemia with potential pancreatitis may be a relative contraindication to oral contraceptives. After 3 to 6 months of treatment, evaluation of the previously abnormal androgen values may be indicated in cases where clinical improvement is not readily apparent or when baseline androgens approached the "tumor range." Failure to normalize the androgens of concern should prompt a reassessment of the diagnosis and consideration given for a combined ovarian and adrenal source for the hyperandrogenemia. Yearly androgen profiles are of limited value unless an inadequate therapeutic response is observed.

Exercise and weight loss should also be strongly encouraged. This is especially true in the women with obesity and the HAIR-AN syndrome. Weight loss in obese, anovulatory women lowers circulating androgen levels while increasing SHBG. Exercise, by improving insulin sensitivity, should reduce androgen production and at the same time lower cardiac risk factors. Women with PCOD or HAIR-AN are at increased risk for the development of hypertension, diabetes, and atherosclerosis.

Secondary treatment regimens for ovarian hyperandrogenism have included GnRH agonists, oophorectomy, ovarian wedge resections or drilling, enzyme blockers, and oral hypoglycemics. Only limited benefit of the GnRH agonist regimens over standard oral contraceptive-antiandrogen therapy has been demonstrated to date. Treatment of hirsutism with the GnRH agonist requires concurrent administration of estrogen and cyclic progestens to avoid the consequence of long-term estrogen deficiency. Because this form of therapy must extend over years, the cost involved severely limits its clinical potential.

Ovarian wedge resection and laparoscopic ovarian ablative techniques (i.e., drilling) are effective in inducing ovulation in PCOD subjects. Reductions in circulating androgens and LH are also observed. Whether such therapy is effective for hirsutism has not been adequately evaluated. In the absence of clear infertility indications, such procedures should not be performed for the treatment of hirsutism until more is known regarding the duration of androgen suppression and cost/benefit ratio.

Oophorectomies are unquestionably effective in reducing hyperandrogenemia when the source of excess androgen production has been clearly localized to the ovary. Such treatment should be restricted to women having completed their reproductive desires and who have failed medical therapy or in whom oral contraceptives are contraindicated. The women must clearly believe that the potential cosmetic benefits justify the risks and expense. Hormonal replacement therapy is indicated postoperatively. Despite studies suggesting that ovulation-inducing agents may increase the risk of ovarian cancer, prophylactic oophorectomy cannot be justified simply for women who have utilized clomiphene citrate and have troublesome hirsutism.

Androgen-producing ovarian neoplasms (i.e., Sertoli-Leydig cell tumors, hilus cell tumors) should be managed surgically. For most reproductive-age women, this entails a unilateral oophorectomy and surgical staging. The overall survival rate exceeds 90%. More aggressive surgical management and possible chemotherapy is appropriate for women who have fulfilled their reproductive desires and women with aggressive tumors (extraovarian spread or high mitotic counts). In contrast, luteomas of pregnancy should be managed expectantly because regression after delivery is common.

Adrenal Hyperandrogenemia

Hyperandrogenemia resulting from inefficient cortisol production (21 hydroxylase deficiency, 11 β-hydroxylase deficiency, 3 β-hydroxysteroid dehydrogenase deficiency) may be treated effectively with glucocorticoid replacement therapy (i.e., dexamethasone 0.25-0.5 mg/day or prednisone 5-7.5 mg/day). After 2 weeks of therapy, DHEA-S and testosterone levels are repeated. DHEA-S should suppress to the low normal range. Failure to achieve this implies an inadequate dose of glucocorticoids, noncompliance, possible adenoma, Cushing's syndrome, depression, or drug interactions enhancing glucocorticoid metabolism. Failure to suppress the testosterone into the low normal range despite good suppression of DHEA-S implies an ovarian contribution to the hyperandrogenemia or a very rare testosterone-secreting adrenal adenoma. In most cases, good suppression of both androgens is observed. For maintenance therapy, further reduction of the glucocorticoid dose or the use of alternate-day therapy should be the goal. The assumption should always be that the pituitary-adrenal response to stress is also depressed, thus these individuals should have a medic alert identification. During medical or surgical emergencies, high-dose glucorticoids should be administered to cover the stress response. Commonly, in the absence of classic congenital adrenal hyperplasia (CAH) treatment is restricted to approximately 1 year, followed by reassessment of clinical complaints after establishing a regimen of cosmetic intervention and cycle regulation. Regrettably, long-term glucocorticord therapy is generally necessary to maintain normal androgens.

Management of adrenal adenomas and Cushing's disease are beyond the scope of the text.

Follicular Therapy

Multiple drugs have been shown to inhibit hirsutism, typically by reducing 5-α-reductase activity or competing at the androgen receptor. These drugs are useful in combination with regimens to suppress the cause of hyperandrogenemia and are the mainstay for treating idiopathic hirsutism. Such drugs include cyproterone acetate (not available in the United States), finasteride (contraindicated in women who may become pregnant, the drug is also expensive and occasionally liver toxic), and spironolactone (not an FDA-approved indication). In the United States, spironolactone at a dose of 50 to 200 mg/day is commonly used for the treatment of hirsutism. Doses exceeding 100 mg/day are associated with abnormal uterine bleeding. To avoid the risk of pregnancy as well as maintain regular menstrual bleeding, combined use of oral contraceptions and spironolactone is encouraged. Women should not become pregnant while utilizing any of these antiandrogenic compounds to avoid concerns of antagonizing virilization of male infants. Spironolactone should not be utilized with other potassium-sparing agents or in women with renal disease without careful monitoring of potassium. The need for spironolactone or follicular-unit inhibitors should be reassessed after 1 to 2 years of therapy.

Cosmetic Therapy

Hormonal treatment of hirsutism should be viewed as long-term preventive therapy. Once major pathologic conditions have been ruled out, aggressive cosmetic intervention should be initiated. Although this is beyond the arena of physician expertise, inclusion of such therapy in the overall management is often necessary for the patient's psychological well-being and overall satisfaction. In fair-skinned individuals, bleaching and trimming may be highly efficacious. For darker-complexioned women, waxing, depilatories, and plucking may be beneficial provided folliculitis is not a problem. Shaving of the face, abdomen, or extremities does not increase the number of growing hairs nor does it make them thicker. Admittedly, shaving may result in a "stubblelike" sensation within a few days of the procedure. Electrolysis is the one means available for permanently eliminating the follicle producing terminal hair. Electrolysis needs to be performed by a licensed technician, as severe folliculitis and scarring are possible complications. The process is uncomfortable, protracted, and not inexpensive. Despite these problems, incorporation of electrolysis into the treatment of facial hirsutism should be encouraged once suppression of androgens has been achieved.

KEY POINTS

1. Androgen-producing tumors, in contrast to nonneoplastic processes, are characterized by rapidly progressive hirsutism, virilization, and testosterone serum concentration exceeding 2ng/ml or DHEA-S levels exceeding 700 μg/dl.
2. Treatment of hirsutism is accomplished by first establishing the cause.
3. The chronic unopposed estrogen state frequently found with hyperandrogenism should be treated either by establishing ovulatory cycles or administering a progestational agent in cyclic or continuous regimen.
4. Suppression of hyperandrogenemia inhibits but does not eliminate

hirsutism. Cosmetic measures are often necessary to improve the patient's self-image.

5 Women with PCOD, the most common cause of hirsutism, are at increased risk for hypertension, diabetes, and coronary heart disease.

SUGGESTED READINGS

Azziz R, Dewailly D, Owerbach D: Clinical review 56: nonclassic adrenal hyperplasia: current concepts, *J Clin Endocrinol Metab* 78:810-815, 1994.

Barnes R, Rosenfeld RL: The polycystic ovary syndrome, *Ann Intern Med* 110:386-99, 1989.

Burkman RT: The role of oral contraceptives in the treatment of hyperandrogenic disorders, *Am J Med* 98(1A):1305-1365, 1995.

Cusan L et al: Comparison of flutamide and spironolactone in the treatment of hirsutism: a randomized trial, *Fertil Steril* 61:281-7, 1994.

Dahlgren E et al: Women with polycystic ovary syndrome resected in 1956 to 1965: a long-term followup focusing on the natural history and circulating hormones, *Fertil Steril* 57:505-13, 1992.

Donesky BW, Adashi EY: Surgically induced ovulation in the polycystic ovary syndrome: wedge resection revisited in the age of laparoscopy, *Fertil Steril* 63:439-463, 1995.

Ehrmann DA et al: Detection of functional ovarian hyperandrogenism in women with androgen excess, *N Engl J Med* 327:157-162, 1992.

Poretsky L, Piper B: Insulin resistance, hypersecretion of LH, and a dual defect hypothesis for the pathogenesis of polycystic ovary syndrome, *Obstet Gynecol* 84:613-21, 1994.

Rittmaster RS: Clinical review 73: Medical treatment of androgen-dependent hirsutism, *J Clin Endocrinol Metab* 80:2559-63, 1995.

10

Infertility

Moon H. Kim

The diagnosis of infertility is made when conception does not occur after a year without contraception. It is a relative term when applied to a couple, and in some situations it merely means reduced fertility or subfertility. The term *primary infertility* means that the couple has never conceived, and *secondary infertility* is the term used when a couple experiences an infertility problem after having had at least one previous conception.

In managing the infertile couple, the physician's awareness of the importance of treating the couple as a unit is essential in helping them through the often frustrating and stressful experience of various tests and treatment. Periodic counseling and compassionate understanding will inspire the couple to cooperate and accept the outcome of treatment more readily, even if conception fails to occur.

INCIDENCE

The incidence of infertility has been estimated to be 10% to 15% of all married couples in the United States. Human fertility is affected by many factors, such as the ages of the couple, frequency of sexual intercourse, and emotional factors. It has been well demonstrated that fertility declines as age advances. Women not using any contraception have an expected pregnancy rate in 12 months of 86%, 78%, 63%, and 52% for age groups of 20 to 24 years, 25 to 29 years, 30 to 34 years, and 35 to 39 years, respectively.

FACTORS AFFECTING THE INFERTILE COUPLE

In addition to biologic factors such as age and the sexual life of the couple, various physical factors that cause infertility must be considered. Although the exact incidence of each factor affecting infertility cannot be determined, Table 10-1 shows the approximate incidence of various factors. Many couples have more than one factor contributing to their infertility. Therefore it is important to thoroughly evaluate the couple.

DIAGNOSIS

The workup of the infertile couple is aimed at determining the factors contributing to infertility so that appropriate counseling and therapeutic options can be provided. Various factors must be taken into consideration while organizing the evaluation. The evaluation may need to be reassessed periodically when a new contributing factor is discovered.

TABLE 10-1
Incidence of Infertility Factors

Factors	Incidence (%)
Male factor	35-40
Female factors	
Tubal	25-30
Ovulatory	10-15
Cervical	10-15
Other	5
Unexplained	5-10

History and Examination of the Couple

General information should be obtained during history taking. This includes present illness, ages of the couple, duration of infertility, history of contraceptive use, and results of previous studies. Menstrual and obstetric history details irregular menses and obstetric complications. History of pelvic infection, pelvic surgery, intestinal surgery (e.g., ruptured appendix), and endocrine disease is noted. Other information, such as sexual history (e.g., frequency, ejaculatory difficulty, and use of any lubricant), exercise, and weight loss or gain is also included.

At the conclusion of the initial interview and examination the couple should be assured that all necessary tests will be done as rapidly and thoroughly as possible. It is also important to explain the basics of human reproduction, monthly fecundity, and the prognosis of various infertility factors.

Basic Diagnostic Evaluation

Basic tests should include evaluation of the (1) male factor, (2) cervical factor, (3) tubal and uterine factors, (4) ovulatory factors, and (5) others if indicated. In addition, a CBC, blood typing, Pap smear, and rubella antibody titer should be ordered. The couple should be informed that these tests must be scheduled at appropriate times in relation to the woman's ovulation.

Male factor

Semen analysis is the single most important test in evaluating male factor infertility. Because of the well-known fluctuation in sperm counts in an individual, two semen samples collected at least 2 weeks apart should be evaluated. The commonly used criteria of "normality" for a semen analysis are shown in Table 10-2. Oligospermia refers to a sperm count of less than 20×10^6 per ml, and asthenospermia is present when fewer than 50% of spermatozoa show forward motility.

TABLE 10-2
Normal Semen Analysis

Factor	Normal value
Volume	2.0 ml
pH	7.2-7.8
Sperm concentration	20×10^6/ml
Total sperm count	40×10^6
Motility	At least 50% of spermatozoa with forward progression within 60 minutes after collection
Fructose	+

Modified from the WHO Laboratory Manual, 1987.

Cervical factor

The cervical canal is the first path in the female reproductive tract that spermatozoa must pass through to achieve fertilization. The endocervical epithelium secretes mucus, and is stimulated by the rising level of estrogens near ovulation. Evaluating sperm survival in the cervix following coitus (postcoital test [PCT], also called the *Sims-Huhner test*) is an important test. Although its prognostic value is controversial, this test evaluates sperm-mucus interaction in vivo. The test is best scheduled as close as possible to the presumed day of ovulation (i.e., days 12 to 14 in women having a 28-day menstrual cycle). The mucus is collected from the endocervical canal and examined under a coverslip with high-power microscopy. A common cause of poor mucus quality is inappropriate timing. An abnormal test must be confirmed by repeating the test.

Tubal and uterine factors

The fallopian tubes provide a channel for the transport of sperm and for the ovum picked up by the fimbria. The ciliary motion and muscular contractions of the tubes promote gamete transport, and their secretions provide nourishment for the fertilized gamete in transit to the uterus. Pelvic adhesions and tubal occlusion, frequently sequelae of PID, are common pathology causing infertility. The uterus must be anatomically normal to allow for growth of the fetus. Any pathologic condition compromising normal uterine cavity (e.g., septate uterus, intrauterine synechia, or submucous fibroid) should be evaluated.

Hysterosalpingography (HSG) is the basic radiographic technique for evaluating tubal patency and the contour of the uterus. It is best scheduled during the mid-follicular phase after menstrual bleeding ceases. Several studies have shown that the incidence of pregnancy increases after HSG, suggesting some therapeutic benefit. Therefore it should be performed in all infertile patients unless it is contraindicated by any known allergy to iodine, active pelvic infection, or severe cervicitis or vaginitis.

Laparoscopy is the most definitive technique for evaluating peritoneal factors (e.g., tubal adhesions and endometriosis), fimbrial status, and tube patency (Box 10-1). Tubal patency is evaluated by chromopertubation using a marker dye (i.e., indigo carmine or methylene blue). Although laparoscopy is essential for evaluating the pathologic condition of the

BOX 10-1
Indications for Diagnostic Laparoscopy

Unexplained infertility after complete basic evaluation
Abnormal hysterosalpingogram
Anovulatory patients not conceiving after six ovulatory cycles after induction of ovulation
History of PID, use of IUDs, or clinical evidence of endometriosis
Preoperative evaluation for tubal surgery
Before treatment with HMG

BOX 10-2
Hysteroscopy

INDICATIONS

Abnormal HSG findings of uterine cavity (e.g., synechiae, submucous fibroid, polyp, or septate uterus)
Allergy to iodine
Technical inability to do HSG (e.g., cervical stenosis or unable to tolerate HSG)

CONTRAINDICATIONS

Active pelvic infection
Profuse bleeding

pelvis, it should be performed after weighing the advantages against potential complications. Such complications, although rare, include bowel perforation, bleeding, retroperitoneal hematoma, infection, problems resulting from pneumoperitoneum, and anesthesia-related complications. In general, it should be deferred until all other basic evaluations are completed. HSG and laparoscopy each fulfill a unique role and thus are complementary.

Hysteroscopy is an endoscopic examination of the uterine cavity. It is usually performed to confirm the findings of the HSG or to therapeutically correct an intrauterine pathologic condition. Also, hysteroscopy is indicated as a method of evaluating the uterine cavity in patients who have contraindications to HSG (Box 10-2).

Ovulatory factor

Ovulation and the quality of luteal function must be carefully evaluated. Three methods commonly used are (1) BBT recordings, (2) determination of serum progesterone levels, and (3) endometrial biopsy. In addition, other hormonal evaluations (i.e., prolactin, TSH, and androgens) may be necessary. However, these tests offer only presumptive evidence of ovulation.

Although daily BBT recordings cannot determine the exact time of ovulation, one can estimate an approximate time of ovulation and length of luteal phase when a biphasic pattern is evident after the entire cycle is completed. The rise in BBT usually lasts for 13 to 15 days in an ovulatory cycle. A shorter luteal phase (rise in BBT lasting less than 12 days) suggests luteal phase deficiency (LPD), in which ovulation occurs with a deficiency of progesterone secretion and/or of the development of secretory endometrium. Because both progesterone and a normal endometrial environment are important in maintaining early conception, LPD must be confirmed by endometrial biopsy and/or midluteal progesterone levels.

A serum progesterone level greater than 3 ng/ml is presumptive evidence of luteal function, and a level greater than 15 ng/ml suggests normal function of the corpus luteum.

TABLE 10-3
Evaluation of Ovulatory Factor

	BBT	Serum progesterone	Endometrial biopsy
Time for the test	Daily throughout the cycle	Midluteal phase (days 20 to 22)	Late luteal phase (days 25 to 27)
Normal luteal phase	BBT rise for >12 days	>15 ng/ml (days 20 to 22)	In-phase secretory endometrium (within ±2 days)
Evidence suggestive of LPD	BBT rise for <12 days	<10 ng/ml (days 20 to 22)	Out-of-phase endometrium >3 days)

The endometrium is a target tissue for ovarian hormones. It develops a secretory pattern when progesterone stimulation occurs after ovulation. Histologic evaluation of the endometrium correlates well with days of the ovulatory cycle. Therefore a successful endometrial biopsy gives valuable information regarding ovulation, corpus luteum function, and the normalcy of the endometrium (Table 10-3). Because the objective of the biopsy is to evaluate the condition of endometrium in relation to luteal function and implantation of the conceptus, it is best performed during the late luteal phase. The risk of disturbing a pregnancy is apparently minimal, but the patient may be advised to avoid conception in the study cycle.

Further evaluation of unexplained infertility

Usually the basic evaluation will reveal etiologic factors for infertility. However, frequently some of the evaluations may have to be repeated. Additional tests also may be necessary when infertility is unexplained after the initial evaluation. Although the role of mycoplasma and ureaplasma as a cause of infertility is not well established, sexually transmitted diseases (i.e., gonorrhea or chlamydia) are often responsible for causing infection in the upper reproductive tract. Sperm immunologic tests can determine if antisperm antibodies are present. Such antibodies can interfere with sperm migration in the reproductive tract and also with sperm penetration into an oocyte. The hamster zona-free egg penetration test also has been advocated. However, because their clinical correlation is questionable, such tests are generally not helpful. A more direct approach is to perform an in vitro fertilization, which offers diagnostic and therapeutic benefits to the patients.

THERAPEUTIC CONSIDERATIONS

Male Factor Infertility

Treatment of male factor infertility often requires a urologist's consultation. The etiologic factors will guide the selection of therapeutic options, which include donor sperm insemination (DSI), intrauterine insemination

(IUI) with washed sperm, and in vitro fertilization (IVF), gamete intrafallopian transfer (GIFT), or intracytoplasmic sperm injection (ICSI). Other options are antibiotic treatment for infection in the male genital tract, gonadotropin treatment for hypogonadotropic hypogonadism, and, other hormonal treatments, including thyroid medications, bromocriptine for hyperprolactinemia, and corticosteroids for sperm antibodies.

Female Factor Infertility

Lack of cervical mucus can be caused by inadequate mucus secretion or inappropriate timing of PCT. In the latter situation, more accurate timing can be achieved with the use of urinary LH-detection kits. If inadequate mucus is responsible, low-dose estrogen or stimulation with HMG can be used to improve the mucus secretion. IUI should be considered and is often effective because it bypasses the cervix.

Tubal occlusions and pelvic adhesions causing infertility are managed by surgical therapy. The type of surgical therapy used and its outcome depend on the extent of diseases. Success rates vary for lysis of adhesions and neosalpingostomy. In reversal of prior tubal ligation, microsurgical anastomosis results in 70% to 80% pregnancy rates when the tubal length is greater than 5 cm. Transcervical catheterization (luminoplasty) and cornua-to-isthmus anastomosis for proximal tubal occlusion are additional surgical options. When surgical therapy fails or is not feasible, ultimately IVF should be considered.

Intrauterine synechiae or selected cases of submucous fibroids can be treated with hysteroscopy. Although the role of fibroid tumors causing infertility is controversial, myomectomy may be considered if the tumors distort the uterine cavity or occlude the tube. Likewise, when pregnancy loss occurs in association with a uterine septum, hysteroscopic resection is warranted.

Anovulation is treated with various ovulation-inducing agents (Tables 10-4 and 10-5). In patients who respond to clomiphene, most pregnancies occur during the first four treatment cycles. Hypoestrogenic patients rarely respond to clomiphene alone. In hyperandrogenic patients, dexamethasone (0.5 mg/day) may help in suppressing androgen production as an adjuvant therapy to clomiphene. In women with hypogonadotropic hypogonadism or with failed clomiphene therapy, HMG or urofollitropin treatment is most effective. Because of risks of hyperstimulation of the ovaries and a high incidence of multiple gestation, the patients must be monitored carefully. Severe hyperstimulation occurs in less than 1% of cases and requires hospitalized care. Fortunately, most patients with mild and moderate hyperstimulation can be managed conservatively without hospitalization.

Assisted Reproductive Procedures

Approximately 10% of infertile couples have no definitive cause of their infertility, thus called *unexplained infertility*. They are often empirically treated with IUI using washed sperm in cycles stimulated with either clomiphene or HMG. Ultimately, most of these patients who do not conceive and those with irreparably damaged tubes will be offered one of

TABLE 10-4
Induction of Ovulation

Methods	Indications	Mechanism
Clomiphene citrate (CC)	Anovulation Eustogenic Normal FSH and LH Intact H-P-O axis	*Antiestrogenic *Blocking estrogen receptors in the hypothalamus
HMG OR Urofollitropin (Menotropin)	Hypogonadotropic state CC failure Intact ovary	*Replacing FSH, LH *Direct stimulation of ovary
GnRH	Hypothalamic dysfunction Intact P-O axis	*Stimulation on gonadotrophs *Pulsatile stimulation
Bromocriptine	Hyperprolactinemia Intact P-O axis	*Dopamine agonist *Decreased PRL secretion
Surgical therapy (ovarian drilling)	Polycystic ovary not responding to medical therapy	*Decreased androgen-producing tissue

*Hypogonadotropic group

TABLE 10-5
Therapeutic Outcome of Ovulation Induction

Drugs	Ovulation rates (%)	Pregnancy rates (%)	Multiple gestation (%)
Clomiphene	80	35-40	6-8
HMG	90	70-80* 20-30†	15-20
GnRH	80	50-80	5
Bromocriptine	90	70-80	0
Ovarian drilling	70-80‡	45-65	0

*Hypogonadotropic group
†Euestrogenic/eugonadotropic
‡Immediate response (recurrence rate: 50%)

the following assisted reproductive procedures: IVF, GIFT, zygote intrafallopian transfer (ZIFT), or ICSI. Donor oocyte IVF is offered to women with no functioning ovaries.

These new techniques require four major steps; stimulation of multiple follicles, retrieval of mature preovulatory oocytes, IVF and embryo culture, and embryo transfer to the endometrial cavity. In GIFT the latter two steps are not needed because oocytes and sperm are transferred into the tubal ampulla for fertilization in vivo. Those with severe oligospermia or IVF failure may be candidates for ICSI, where a sperm is directly injected into the ooplasm. Pregnancy rates of 10% to 20% for IVF, 20% to 30% for GIFT, and 25% to 35% for ICSI can be expected.

KEY POINTS

1 Infertility is defined as the inability to conceive for at least 12 months without the use of contraception.

2 The incidence of infertility varies depending on age. Monthly fecundity declines sharply after the age of 35 years in women.

3 A thorough review of the couple's history and a physical examination should be done.

4 The male factor is responsible for 35% to 40% of infertility causes.

5 Various therapeutic options, including assisted reproductive procedures, are directed at each etiologic factor of infertility.

SUGGESTED READINGS

American Fertility Society Registry: 1991 results for assisted reproductive technologies, *Fertil Steril* 59:956, 1993.

Fluke MR et al: Exogenous gonadotropin therapy in WHO Groups I and II ovulatory disorders, *Obstet Gynecol* 83:189, 1994.

Karlstrom PO et al: A prospective randomized trial of artificial insemination versus intercourse in cycles stimulated with human menopausal gonadotropin or clomiphene citrate, *Fertil Steril* 59:554, 1993.

Mosher WD, Pratt WF: Fecundity and infertility in the United States: incidence and trends, *Fertil Steril* 56:192, 1991.

Rasmussen F et al: Therapeutic effect of hysterosalpingography: oil versus water-soluble contrast media: a randomized prospective study, *Radiology* 179:75, 1991.

Sauer MV et al: Reversing the natural decline in human fertility: an extended clinical trial of oocyte donation to women of advanced reproductive age, *JAMA* 268:1275, 1992.

Schlaff WD et al: Neosalpingostomy for distal tubal obstruction: prognostic factors and impact of surgical technique, *Fertil Steril* 54:984, 1990.

Speroff L, Glass RH, Kase NG: Female infertility. In *Clinical gynecologic endocrinology and infertility,* ed 5, Baltimore, 1994, Williams and Wilkins.

Wentz AC et al: The impact of luteal phase inadequacy in an infertile population, *Am J Obstet Gynecol* 162:937, 1990.

11

Lower Genital Tract Infections

WAYNE C. TROUT

ULCERATIVE INFECTIONS OF THE VULVA

Chancroid

Haemophilus ducreyi is a short, nonmotile, gram-negative rod that grows in chains often called a *school of fish* pattern. *H. ducreyi* infection results in a "soft," painful, ulcerative vulvar lesion. These lesions typically occur 7 days after infection. The ulcers begin as small papules and progress to pustules that ulcerate and have an irregular, scallop-shaped border. Unilateral adenopathy usually develops 1 week after ulcer onset. Suppurative inguinal adenopathy with a genital ulcerative lesion is the classic presentation, but tender inguinal lymphadenopathy is present in only 30% of cases.

Diagnosis

H. ducreyi is a facultative anaerobe that has fastidious growth requirements. Specimens for direct microscopic examination should be prepared by swabbing the bed of the ulcer.

Treatment

Treatment consists of azithromycin 1 g orally as single dose, ceftriaxone 250 mg intramuscularly as single dose, or erythromycin base 500 mg orally 4 times daily for 1 week.

Herpes

Herpes simplex virus (HSV) causes recurrent, painful genital ulcerations. HSV is a double-stranded DNA virus that has two identified serotypes: HSV-1 and HSV-2. Recurrent infections are three to four times more common with HSV-2 and 85% of all genital herpes infections are caused by HSV-2. Serologic studies indicate 4% to 6% of the U.S. population has been infected. Barrier contraception may prevent spread.

Primary HSV infections can be asymptomatic or highly symptomatic and result from the first exposure to either serotype of the virus. Primary outbreaks are associated with higher levels of viral shedding, high infectivity, and a prolonged (14-day) course.

Nonprimary first-episode genital HSV infections result when previous exposure to HSV-1 becomes infected with HSV-2. The course of these infections typically is shorter (5 to 7 days). Recurrences are typically shorter than primary infections (7 to 10 days), are less symptomatic, and have fewer lesions.

Diagnosis

Diagnosis of HSV is made by cell culture.

Treatment

There is no cure for HSV infection. Symptomatic relief and shortening of the primary infection can be provided with the antiviral medication acyclovir. For primary infection, acyclovir 200 mg is given orally 5 times daily for 7 to 10 days. For recurrent infection, acyclovir can be prescribed at 200 mg 5 times daily, 400 mg 3 times daily, or 800 mg 2 times daily, all for 5 days of therapy. Alternatively, valcyclovir 500 mg twice daily or famcyclovir 125 mg twice daily for 5 days may be given.

Women who have six or more episodes per year will benefit from prophylactic/suppressive acyclovir therapy (400 mg 2 times daily or 800 mg/day) with a 75% decrease in the frequency of symptomatic episodes. Suppressive therapy should be stopped after 1 year to determine the frequency of recurrence.

Syphilis

Syphilis is caused by the spirochete *Treponema pallidum* and if untreated progresses through three clinical stages and a latent period.

Primary. A painless ulceration (chancre) at the site of infection occurs after an incubation period of 10 to 90 days. The lesions begin as small, painless macules that rapidly ulcerate, forming a sharply demarcated, erythematous border with a "hard," indurated base. Spontaneous healing will occur over 3 to 6 weeks.

Secondary. This bacteremic phase is marked by the formation of mucocutaneous lesions, rash, and adenopathy. These are seen from 6 weeks to 6 months after the primary lesion. The rash is pale red, macular, nonirritative, and symmetric and typically will involve the soles and palms.

Latent. By definition, the patient is asymptomatic during this phase. Diagnosis is made based on serologic evidence of infection and is divided into two groups: early (<1 year) and late (>1 year).

Tertiary. Left untreated, one third of patients will manifest the CNS, cardiovascular, and musculoskeletal defects seen with tertiary infection.

Diagnosis

Primary. Serologic testing is usually negative while the primary lesion is present, but darkfield examination of the ulcer bed is diagnostic for *T. pallidum*.

Secondary. Darkfield examination of the condyloma lata may demonstrate treponemas, but serologic testing is more reliable. The cutaneous lesions are infectious and yield spirochetes that can be detected by darkfield examination or direct fluorescent antibody testing.

Latent. Serologic testing is the only means of diagnosing women during this asymptomatic period. The Rapid Plasma Reagin (RPR) and Venereal Diseases Reference Laboratory (VDRL) tests are the two tests used for syphilis screening. A positive tests requires confirmation with a specific treponemal test such as the Fluorescent Treponemal Antibody-Absorbed

(FTA-ABS) or the Microhemagglutination assay for *T. pallidum* (MHA-TP), because false positive RPRs and VDRLs can occur. A significant change in the nontreponemal tests is a fourfold change in titers.

Neurosyphilis. CSF results will show elevated leukocyte counts (>5 WBC) and the VDRL-CSF test will be positive.

Treatment

The mainstay of treatment is parenteral penicillin. Duration and route depend on the severity and site of the infection (Box 11-1).

Posttreatment monitoring of patients for clinical symptoms and serologic testing should be done at 1, 3, 6, and 12 months after completing therapy. A failure for the titer to decrease by fourfold is indicative of treatment failure or reinfection. Lumbar puncture should be done to exclude neurosyphilis and, if negative, the patient should be retreated. The Jarisch-Herxheimer reaction (manifestation of fever, headache, myalgias, and the rash of secondary syphilis) may become more prominent after treatment with penicillin.

Lymphogranuloma Venereum

Lymphogranuloma venereum (LGV) is caused by infection with the L_1, L_2, and L_3 serotypes of *Chlamydia trachomatis* and is uncommon in the United States. The first symptom is a painless genital ulcer that will often go unnoticed after an incubation of 1 to 3 weeks and will heal within days. Typically, patients will have tender adenopathy, occurring 1 to 4 weeks after the ulcer. Fevers, myalgia, malaise, and headache may also be present. Later, the adenopathy may coalesce, adhere to the overlying skin, and

BOX 11-1

Treatment of Syphilis

Primary

Benzathine penicillin 2.4 million units IM in single dose

Secondary

Benzathine penicillin 2.4 million units IM in a single dose,

alternative therapy for PCN allergy:

doxycycline 100 mg orally 2 times daily for 14 days or

tetracycline 500 mg orally 4 times daily for 14 days

Early latent

Benzathine penicillin 2.4 million units IM in single dose

Late latent or unknown duration

Benzathine penicillin 2.4 million units IM weekly for 3 weeks

Neurosyphilis

Penicillin G aqueous 2-4 million units IV every 4 hours for 10-14 days become very painful. Eventually these matted lymph nodes will suppurate and form fistulas.

Diagnosis

Chlamydia can be recovered from aspiration of lymph nodes in 50% of cases. Identification of the serotypes can then be done. More commonly, complement fixation titers for chlamydia are diagnostic.

Treatment

Treatment consists of doxycycline 100 mg orally 2 times daily for 21 days, erythromycin 500 mg orally 4 times daily for 21 days, or sulfisoxazole 500 mg orally 4 times daily for 21 days.

VAGINAL INFECTIONS

The normal, healthy vagina is a complex microbiologic system. The predominant organism is *Lactobacillus acidophilus.* This bacterium is able to produce H_2O_2, which inhibits the growth of other potentially pathogenic bacteria. One of the metabolic byproducts of the lactobacilli is lactic acid, which lowers the pH of the normal vagina. The pH of vaginal secretions is >4.5. Antibiotic use can also upset the balance of the microbiologic system, predisposing women to symptomatic infections.

Trichomoniasis

Trichomonas vaginalis is a motile, flagellated, protozoan parasite, and is sexually transmitted. Women with trichomonas infections typically complain of a watery, yellow-green vaginal discharge that may have a slightly foul odor. Urinary complaints can also result from urethral infections.

Diagnosis

The best means of diagnosis is observation of the motile trichomonads by microscopic examination of the vaginal secretions (saline wet prep). Both DNA and antigen detection kits are available, but it is unlikely that they will replace direct microscopic examination.

Treatment

Treatment consists of metronidazole 2 g orally in one dose, or 500 mg orally 2 times daily for 7 days.

Bacterial Vaginosis

Bacterial vaginosis (BV) represents an alteration in the normal flora of the vagina with a predominance of anaerobic bacteria. Women with bacterial vaginosis complain of a foul-smelling vaginal odor with gray, homogeneous discharge. Vaginal pH is >5.0. Diagnosis requires the presence of "clue cells" in vaginal secretions and an amine odor released with potassium hydroxide (whiff test).

Treatment

Either systemic or topical therapy may be utilized. Systemic therapy is less expensive, but can have side effects. Topical treatments deliver high concentrations of antibiotics directly to where the infection is, but are more expensive, messy, and inconvenient.

Oral therapy consists of metronidazole 500 mg orally 2 times daily for 7 days, metronidazole 2 orally in a single dose, or clindamycin 300 mg orally 2 times daily for 7 days. Topical therapy consists of metronidazole gel 0.75%, 5 g vaginally twice daily for 5 days, or clindamycin cream 2%, 5 g vaginally each night for 7 days.

Candida

Vulvovaginal candidiasis can cause vaginal and perineal pruritus and vaginal discharge. *Candida albicans* is the most common cause of these infections. Women with a candidal infection will complain of a white, clumpy (cottage cheese-like) discharge, vaginal itching with erythema, and edema of the epithelium.

Diagnosis

Examination of vaginal secretions will usually reveal an acidic pH (<4.5), and mycelial forms (pseudohyphae) observed on microscopic examination. Yeast will appear as large, gram-positive organisms if a gram stain is performed. Culture is performed on Sabouraud's or Nickerson's media. Nonalbicans strains are becoming increasingly important in vulvovaginal candidiasis.

Treatment

Antifungal medications can be either topical or oral preparations. The duration of treatment can be from 1 to 7 days depending on the drug and dosage used. Recurrent vulvovaginal candidiasis occurs in 5% of women and is commonly treated prophylactically with one of the oral medications (fluconazole or ketoconazole).

CERVICAL INFECTIONS

Gonorrhea

N. gonorrhea (GC) is a sexually transmitted, gram-negative diplococcus. GC can cause symptomatic infections of the cervix, the columnar epithelium of the urethra, pharynx, rectum, and vestibular glands (i.e., Bartholin's gland). There are an estimated 1 million new cases of gonorrhea each year. Infection with GC causes inflammation and a mucopurulent discharge, although women can be asymptomatic. Spread of the organism to adjacent pelvic organs can result in PID or it can also spread to the bloodstream as a disseminated gonococcal infection.

Diagnosis

Culture of *N. gonorrhea* is difficult because it is a fastidious organism. Specimens should be plated immediately on a special medium such as Thayer-Martin or Gembec, which suppress the growth of yeast and other bacteria, and placed in a CO_2-rich (3% to 10%) environment. Alternative diagnostic tests for GC are available that use ELISA. DNA probe techniques are also available and are useful because one can avoid the difficulties of culturing GC and provide results more quickly.

Treatment

Fortunately, GC is very sensitive to many of the antibiotics used; however, in some areas, resistant, plasma-mediated, penicillinase-producing strains have emerged. Therapy effective against *Chlamydia trachomatis* should also be given because of the high rate of coinfection (Table 11-1).

TABLE 11-1
Therapy Choices for GC

Drug	Dose
Ceftriaxone	125 mg IM, single dose
Cefixime	400 mg orally, single dose
Ciprofloxacin	500 mg orally, single dose
Ofloxacin	400 mg orally, single dose
Spectinomycin	2 gm IM, single dose
ALTERNATIVE THERAPIES	
Injectable cephalosporins	
Ceftizoxine	500 mg
Cefotaxime	500 mg
Cefotetan	1 g
Cefoxitin	2 g
Oral cephalosporins	
Cefuroxime axetil	1 g
Cefpodoxime proxetil	200 mg
Quinalones	
Enoxacin	400 mg
Lomefloxacin	400 mg
Norfloxacin	800 mg

Chlamydia

Since its recognition in 1959, *C. trachomatis* has been increasingly recognized as a significant sexually transmitted pathogen. Infection is frequently asymptomatic, yet has significant effects on the reproductive system. Chlamydia is the most frequently encountered STD with over 4 million new infections annually. Chlamydia is an obligate intracellular organism and detection must be with a cell culture system.

Urethritis and cervicitis can occur frequently, but asymptomatic infection is most common. Chlamydial infection can lead to acute salpingitis, peritonitis with periappendicitis or perihepatitis, pelvic pain, infertility, and ectopic pregnancy.

Diagnosis

Cell culture on McCoy cell lines is the gold standard for detection but is a labor-intensive, time-consuming test. Alternate detection techniques are available. Direct fluorescent antibody (DFA) staining has aided the identification of the intracellular particles in cell culture and this technology can also be applied directly to clinical samples. Enzyme immunoassay (EIA) techniques are used in most labs, but DNA hybridization testing is also available as is PCR (polymerase chain reaction) technology. The

TABLE 11-2
Treatment for Chlamydial Infection

Drug	Dose
Doxycycline	100 mg orally, 2 times daily for 7 days
Azithromycin	1 g orally, single dose
	OR
Ofloxacin	300 mg orally, 2 times daily for 7 days
Erythromycin base	500 mg orally for 7 days

TABLE 11-3
Treatment Options for Condyloma

Treatment	Description
CHEMICAL THERAPY	
Podophyllin resin	Keratolytic agent; destroys infected tissues. Should not be used on mucous membranes or during pregnancy.
Condylox	Commercial product similar to podophyllin, self-administered. 0.5% solution, applied directly to wart twice daily for 3 days. Repeat treatment weekly.
Trichloracetic acid (TCA) 85%	Applied directly to warts, can be used on cervix and in vagina. Repeated application by trained health care provider at 1- to 2-week intervals.
5-Fluorouracil (5-FU)	Chemotherapeutic agent in cream applied to vulvar lesions or into vagina. Applied weekly for 1-3 months. Sloughing of tissue occurs, can be uncomfortable.
PHYSICAL AGENTS	
Cryotherapy	Liquid nitrogen, limited to cervix. Can be used on vulva with local anesthesia. Probe coated with lubricant, freeze-thaw-freeze cycle (3-5-3 min) preferred by most physicians.
Laser ablation	Very effective for cervical and vulvar condyloma. Ability to control depth, lateral spread, and provide hemostasis.
Electrotherapy	Either loop electrode or direct to condyloma advocated as effective outpatient therapy. Local anesthetic must be used on vulva, scarring more pronounced.
IMMUNOTHERAPY	
Interferon	Injections given systemically, 2.5-3 million units 3 times weekly for 6-10 weeks. Or, injections of 250,000-1 million units can be given into base of each lesion 3 times weekly for 3-6 weeks. Intralesional injections—no more than 5 lesions at a time. Side effects: fatigue, headache, myalgias, fever.

specificities of these tests are not 100% (actually closer to 97% to 99%), so in low-prevalence populations the false positives may outnumber the true positives.

Treatment

Empiric treatment for chlamydia for patients being treated for gonorrhea is appropriate (Table 11-2). Pregnant women should be treated with erythromycin or amoxicillin 500 mg orally 3 times daily for 7 to 10 days.

Condyloma

Genital warts caused by HPV can be found anywhere in the lower genital tract. Evidence of HPV infection can be found with cervical cytology. Cervical HPV infection is currently believed to be a cause of dysplasia and to increase the risk of cancer. HPV infection is asymptomatic in 70% of people. Symptomatic infection will result in a raised pink or white lesion that may be flat or have fingerlike projections. Genital warts can be found around the anus, vulva, vagina, or cervix.

Diagnosis

There are currently no culture systems for HPV. Diagnosis requires an observable tissue effect to be present. Techniques such as PCR and hybrid capture may be useful in the future for HPV diagnosis and typing.

Treatment

HPV treatment options fall into three groups: chemical therapy, physical agents, and immunotherapy (Table 11-3).

KEY POINTS

1. Genital ulcerative infections of the vulva include chancroid, herpes, syphilis, and lymphogranuloma venereum.
2. Vaginal infections include trichomoniasis, bacterial vaginosis, and candidiasis.
3. Cervical infections include gonorrhea, chlamydia, and HPV, which can be found anywhere in the lower genital tract.

SUGGESTED READINGS

Centers for Disease Control and Prevention: 1993 sexually transmitted diseases treatment guidelines, *MMWR* 42(No-RR14); 1993.

Centers for Disease Control and Prevention: Recommendations for the prevention and management for *Chlamydia trachomatis* infections, *MMWR* 42(No. RR12); 1993.

Csonka GW, Oates JK, eds: *Sexually transmitted disease: a textbook of genitourinary medicine,* 1990, Bailliere Tindall.

Mead PB, Hager WD, eds: *Infection protocols for obstetrics and gynecology,* 1992, Medical Economics Publishing.

Sweet RL, Gibbs RS: *Infectious diseases of the female genital tract,* ed 3, 1995, Williams & Wilkins.

12

Menopause

Cynthia B. Evans

The mean age of menopause in the United States is 51.4 years. With a current female life expectancy of 78 years, a woman spends almost one third of her life in menopause. Currently, there are 36 million women in the United States over age 50. The timing of menopause is genetically determined and is not related to race, socioeconomic level, education, height, weight, use of oral contraceptives, or number of pregnancies. Smokers, however, have an earlier menopause than nonsmokers.

ENDOCRINOLOGY

The perimenopausal period typically begins approximately 5 years before menopause. Regular menses can persist, or the patient may begin to have irregular menses. Intermittent episodes of hot flashes, insomnia, and vaginal dryness typically occur. Estradiol levels are normal or slightly low, and FSH levels are frequently elevated. LH levels are normal or elevated.

Menopause is defined as a single point in time when no further menses occur as a result of insufficient follicular maturation and inadequate estrogen production. Postmenopausally, therefore, the patient is amenorrheic, FSH and LH levels are elevated (>40 mIU/ml), and estradiol levels are low (<20 to 30 pg/ml). The ovarian theca cells degenerate, fail to respond to gonadotropins, and produce less estrogen. Symptoms include hot flashes, vaginal dryness, insomnia, and possibly mood changes and memory loss.

Postmenopausal women continue to produce some estrogen. The elevated LH stimulates the ovarian stromal cells to produce androgens. Both the adrenal glands and the ovaries produce androstenedione, which is converted to estrone and then estradiol in the adipose tissue. It is because of this peripheral production of estrogens that obese women, in general, have fewer menopausal symptoms than thin women. It is also this continued production of adrenal and ovarian androgens that causes some menopausal women to complain of androgenic side effects. Many women will complain of acne, mild temporal balding, and some increased hair growth on their arms and face.

DIAGNOSIS

Diagnosis of menopause is usually clear in a patient with hot flashes who is 50 years of age and amenorrheic. The difficulty arises in evaluating

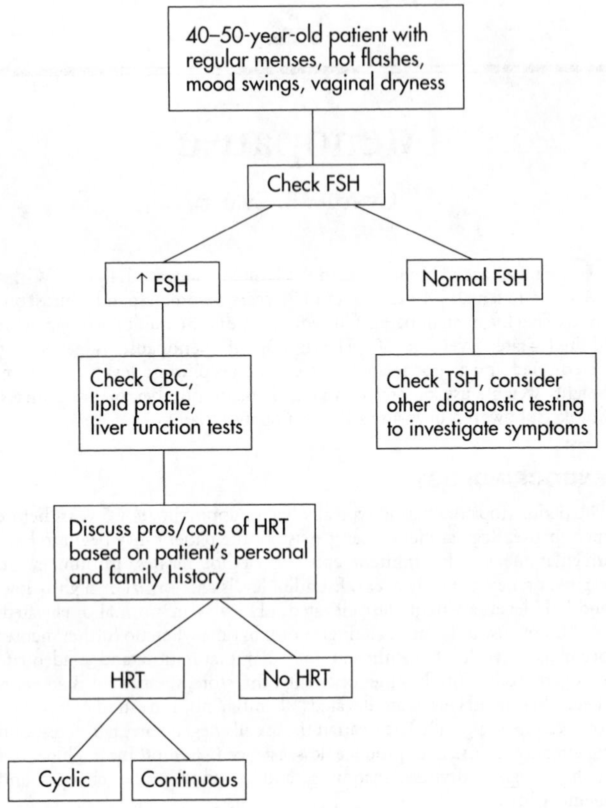

FIG. 12-1 Menopause management.

women ages 40 to 50 with regular or mildly irregular menses, insomnia, mood changes, and an occasional hot flash or night sweat (Fig. 12-1). The differential diagnosis would include perimenopause, PMS, thyroid disease, stress, psychiatric diseases (depression, anxiety disorder, or bipolar disorder), collagen vascular disease, or alcoholism. A complete history and physical examination should be completed and should include a thorough social history. Symptom and menstrual charting can be a significant aid in diagnosing PMS. Thyroid function tests and/or a collagen vascular battery can aid in evaluating for these diseases, and obtaining FSH levels can help to evaluate for the perimenopausal state. Usually, an FSH level is borderline or elevated in the perimenopausal patient.

TREATMENT

Hormone Replacement Therapy

Indications

Vasomotor symptoms such as hot flashes occur in approximately 75% of menopausal women and are often extremely disruptive to daily life and result in insomnia. They are most pronounced in thin women and in women with an abrupt decrease in their endogenous estrogen levels. Hot flashes typically last 30 seconds to 5 minutes and are characterized by increases in digital perfusion, peripheral skin temperature, and heart rate.

The cause of hot flashes is unclear. They seem to coincide with an LH surge, but are not directly related to LH release. They are associated with an elevation in norepinephrine, LH, ACTH, and cortisol, but are not associated with elevated FSH or decreased estradiol. Typically, hot flashes spontaneously improve or disappear 1 to 5 years after menopause and are effectively treated with estrogen replacement therapy (ERT).

Currently, an estimated 1 to 2 million fractures per year are the result of osteoporosis. Vertebral compression fractures occur in 25% of white and Asian women over 60 years of age, and femoral neck fractures occur in 20% of white women over age 80. After experiencing femoral neck fractures, 10% to 20% of women will die within 6 months, and the survivors are frequently invalids. Risk factors include women who are white or Asian, short, thin, lead a sedentary lifestyle, smoke, and have a family history of the disease. Dietary factors, including a low calcium intake, excessive caffeine use, excessive alcohol consumption, and a high protein intake increase a woman's risk.

Osteoporosis is defined as a loss of the structural material in trabecular bone. Women lose bone at a rate of approximately 3% per year during the 7 years before menopause. After menopause, there is a steady 1% to 1.5% per year loss of bone. ERT reduces the amount of postmenopausal bone loss and reduces the incidence of fracture. The etiology is not completely clear, but it is thought that sex steroids block the action of parathyroid hormone on bones, increasing calcitonin levels and resulting in less resorption. Estrogen also increases the gastrointestinal absorption of calcium. It does not, however, stimulate new bone growth. Its use is therefore preventative.

The literature supports the following as minimal doses to prevent osteoporosis: Premarin 0.625 mg, Estraderm 0.05 mg, and Estrace 0.5-1 mg. Calcium supplementation at 1000 mg/day and weight-bearing exercise are also important.

Cardiovascular disease is the leading cause of death in the United States. Normal ovarian function is cardioprotective. Premenopausal women (ages 40 to 44) have a cardiovascular disease risk of 1.3 per 1000 compared with 5.7 per 1000 for similarly aged men. After menopause, women ages 65 to 69 have a risk of 22.1 per 1000 and men have a risk of 26.7 per 1000. Many large epidemiologic studies have shown a 50% reduction in cardiovascular disease risk with ERT.

The reasons behind this beneficial effect are not entirely clear. Estrogen has been shown to decrease total cholesterol by 4% and low-density lipoprotein (LDL) by 11%, and increase high-density lipoprotein (HDL) by 10%. Triglycerides are also increased by 26%. This beneficial effect on lipids seems to be maintained despite the therapeutic addition of progestins to the hormone regimen. Estrogen may also have a direct vasodilatory effect on arterial walls, it may affect the prostaglandin-thromboxene system, and it may have control over the release of nonepinephrine and epinephrine. Estrogen may also be an antioxidant.

Regardless of the mechanism, the epidemiologic studies seem to unanimously support a 50% reduction in cardiovascular disease with ERT. Prospective placebo-controlled studies of ERT and HRT and their effect on cardiovascular disease are currently underway.

Many postmenopausal women complain of symptoms of atrophic vaginitis, including itching, burning, vaginal bleeding, and dyspareunia. Urinary symptoms are also common and include frequency, nocturia, and stress incontinence. Uterine descensus, cystocele, and rectocele can occur with estrogen deprivation. Estrogen can maintain the integrity of these tissues and prevent or delay many of these symptoms.

Many women describe symptoms of moodiness, headache, anxiety, memory loss, or irritability at the time of menopause. It is difficult to assess how often these there symptoms are directly related to a decline in estrogen levels and how often they are related to insomnia from vasomotor symptoms, stress, or depression. Some recent randomized, placebo-controlled, double-blind, crossover studies have shown improvement in memory, insomnia, anxiety, and irritability with estrogen use. Estrogen is not a panacea, however.

Significant skin changes occur postmenopausally. Estrogen users maintain premenopausal skin thickness and collagen content. Wrinkling is minimized.

Complications

ERT alone increases the risk of adenocarcinoma of the endometrium by a factor of four to eight. Typically, these are lower-grade, well-differentiated carcinomas and the incidence correlates with the amount and duration of estrogen used.

Progestins inhibit the growth of the endometrium, thereby lowering the risk of cancer. They prevent receptor synthesis and further growth and division of cells despite the continued presence of estrogen. Studies suggest that the duration of exposure to a progestin is more important than the dose used. Continuous ERT is associated with a 40% risk of endometrial hyperplasia. The addition of 7 days of progestin use lowers this risk to 3%. Ten days of progestin use lowers the risk to 2%, and after 13 days of progestin use the risk of endometrial hyperplasia approaches zero.

Because of this increased risk of adenocarcinoma of the endometrium on estrogen alone, this therapy is primarily indicated for women who have had a hysterectomy. Combination therapy, estrogen and progestins, is the more appropriate replacement regimen for most women.

The effect of ERT and/or HRT on breast cancer remains the most controversial topic related to menopause. Despite the many studies completed, this issue remains unclear. This is a difficult topic to study because breast cancer can be in a preclinical state for up to 8 years before it becomes palpable. Drug studies also can lead to an increased detection rate as a result of increased awareness by patients, regular physical examinations, and scheduled mammography.

Most studies published to date do not support an increased risk of breast cancer secondary to ERT. There is some concern of a possible 30% increased risk after 5 or more years of use, but most studies do not support this. The effect of estrogen and progestin replacement therapy (HRT) is even less clear.

Although the potent, high-dose, synthetic estrogens found in oral contraceptive pills have been associated with an increase in blood pressure, postmenopausal estrogens in general result in a stable or even slightly decreased blood pressure. This is probably caused by the vasodilatory effect of these low-dose natural estrogens. A rare idiosyncratic reaction can result in increased blood pressure.

High-dose, synthetic oral contraceptive pills are also associated with increased risk of thromboembolic disease. Postmenopausal estrogens are not associated with an increased risk because of their lowered potency and therefore a different effect on liver globulins.

Because all estrogens increase the cholesterol content of bile, an increase in cholesterol stones occurs. Both oral contraceptive pills and postmenopausal estrogens are associated with an increase in gallbladder disease.

Contraindications

Contraindications to hormone replacement therapy include uterine bleeding of unknown origin, liver disease (acute and chronic), acute vascular thrombosis, and possibly a history of breast cancer and recent history of endometrial cancer. Many oncologists and gynecologists are currently treating endometrial cancer survivors with ERT or HRT because of the multiple documented benefits of the therapy and the low risk of recurrence of well-differentiated, low-stage cancers of the endometrium.

Conditions requiring close monitoring include familial hyperlipidemia, in which unopposed estrogens significantly increase the circulating triglyceride levels of patients, possibly leading to pancreatitis, and migraines, for which the effect of ERT and/or HRT is highly variable. In seizure disorders, progestins raise the seizure threshold and estrogens lower it. In addition, there are a few published case reports of an endometrial adenocarcinoma arising in implants of endometriosis in patients treated with estrogen alone after a hysterectomy for endometriosis. The presence of uterine leiomyomata should also be monitored. These should continue to regress in size postmenopausally despite the presence of HRT. Growth of these tumors should cause concern.

Regimens

In general, it is best to begin with the lowest effective dose that relieves clinical symptoms and maintains bone mineral content. Oral contraceptives should never be used for HRT because of their high-dose, high-potency synthetic estrogens.

The two most commonly used regimens are cyclic (conjugated equine estrogens–0.625 mg daily *or* days 1 to 25 of a month and medroxyprogesterone acetate–5-10 mg for 10 to 14 days each month), with up to 80% of patients having regular withdrawal bleeding, and continuous (conjugated equine estrogen–0.625 mg daily and medroxyprogesterone acetate–2.5-5 mg daily).

In the continuous regimen, this combination can also be given days Monday through Friday for patients with significant breast tenderness on HRT. Despite irregular bleeding initially, 80% of patients will be amenorrheic after 12 months on this regimen. Without a uterus, only daily estrogen therapy is needed. There is no consistent evidence at this time that the addition of a progestin lowers the risk of breast disease.

Equivalent doses (approximately) are as follows:

Estrogens
- Conjugated equine (Premarin) 0.625 mg
- Conjugated estrogen sulfate (Ogen) 0.625 mg
- Micronized estradiol (Estrace) 1.0 mg
- Transdermal estradiol (Estraderm, Climara) 0.05 mg

Progestins
- Norethindrone acetate (Aygestin, Norlutate) 1.0-5 mg
- Medroxyprogesterone acetate (Amen, Cycrin, Provera) 2.5-10 mg
- Micronized progesterone 200-300 mg

KEY POINTS

1 The mean age of menopause in the United States is 51.4 years.

2 Indications for HRT include vasomotor symptoms, prevention of cardiovascular disease and osteoporosis, genitourinary symptoms, psychologic symptoms, and dermatologic symptoms.

3 Contraindications to HRT include uterine bleeding of unknown origin, presence of liver disease, or acute vascular thrombosis. The use of ERT and/or HRT is currently being studied in breast cancer survivors.

SUGGESTED READINGS

Archer DF et al: Bleeding patterns in postmenopausal women taking continuous combined or sequential regimens of conjugated estrogens with medroxyprogesterone acetate, *Obstet Gynecol* 83(5):686, 1994.

Christiansen C et al: Five years with continuous combined oestrogen/progestogen therapy: effects on calcium metabolism, lipoproteins, and bleeding patterns, *Br J Obstet Gynaecol* 97:1087, 1990.

Colditz GA et al: Prospective study of estrogen replacement therapy and risk of breast cancer in postmenopausal women, *JAMA* 264:2648, 1990.

Colditz GA et al: The use of estrogens and progestins and the risk of breast cancer in postmenopausal women, *N Engl J Med* 332(24):1589, 1995.

Creasman WT: Estrogen replacement therapy: is previously treated cancer a contraindication? *Obstet Gynecol* 77:308, 1991.

Felson DT et al: The effect of postmenopausal estrogen therapy on bone density in elderly women, *N Engl J Med* 329(16):1141, 1993.

Nachtigall MS: Incidence of breast cancer in a 22-year study of women receiving estrogen-progestin replacement therapy, *Obstet Gynecol* 80(5):827, 1992.
Stanford JL et al: Combined estrogen and progestin hormone replacement therapy in relation to risk of breast cancer in middle-aged women, *JAMA* 274(2), 1995.
Steinberg KK et al: A meta-analysis of the effect of estrogen replacement therapy on the risk of breast cancer, *JAMA* 265:1985, 1991.
Woodruff JD: Incidence of endometrial hyperplasia in postmenopausal women taking conjugated estrogens (Premarin) with medroxyprogesterone acetate or conjugated estrogens alone, *Am J Obstet Gynecol* 170(5):1213, 1994.
The Writing Group for the PEPI Trial: Effects of estrogen or estrogen/progestin regimens on heart disease risk factors in postmenopausal women: the Postmenopausal Estrogen/Progestin Interventions (PEPI) trial, *JAMA* 273(3):199, 1995.

13

Mood Disorders

Stephen L. Stern and Stephen F. Pariser*

Mood disorders affect nearly one of every four women. They are divided into the depressive and bipolar disorders. The principal depressive disorders are major depressive disorder (MDD), dysthymic disorder, and depressive disorder not otherwise specified (DDNOS). The chief bipolar disorders are bipolar I, bipolar II, and cyclothymic disorder.

The diagnosis of MDD is used for patients who have had at least one major depressive episode but never a manic or hypomanic (mild manic) episode. Dysthymic disorder refers to a less severe but chronic form of depression. DDNOS is used to describe patients whose symptoms do not meet criteria for any other depressive diagnosis and do not occur within 3 months of a psychosocial stressor. It includes premenstrual dysphoric disorder.

Patients who have had at least one manic episode have bipolar I disorder. Those who have had at least one hypomanic and major depressive episode but never a manic episode are diagnosed with bipolar II disorder. Cyclothymic disorder refers to patients who have multiple hypomanic and mild depressive mood swings without major depressive episodes. Patients with bipolar I disorder who concurrently meet full criteria for both a major depressive and a manic episode are diagnosed as having a mixed episode.

* We gratefully appreciate the helpful comments of Nicholas A. Votolato, RPh, and the secretarial assistance of Ms. Sheri Temple.

Bipolar patients with at least four episodes of mood disorder per year have rapid cycling. Women comprise 70% to 90% of patients with rapid cycling bipolar disorder.

During a manic or hypomanic episode, patients typically have significantly impaired judgment (e.g., they may drive too fast, go on spending sprees, or be hypersexual without control or discretion, which can put them at risk for STDs, including HIV). Drug and alcohol problems, bankruptcy, and divorce are common in bipolar patients. Mood disorders are associated with reduced quality of life, increased disability from comorbid physical illnesses, elevated risk of suicide, and increased mortality from cardiovascular disease.

EPIDEMIOLOGY

Mood disorders are among the most common illnesses seen in general medical practice, with 6% to 10% of patients meeting criteria for MDD, compared with 8% for URIs and 7% for hypertension. Mood disorders can affect persons of any age. In a recent national survey, 21.3% of women and 12.7% of men experienced a major depressive episode at some point during their lifetimes. Dysthymic disorder (8.0% versus 4.8%) was also more common in women, but bipolar I disorder was not (1.7% versus 1.6%). Young women had the highest lifetime rates of MDD and dysthymic disorder, which is consistent with other evidence that the likelihood of experiencing an episode of mood disorder is greater in persons born since 1940. Rates for bipolar II disorder were not assessed, though other investigators report that this disorder is more common in women. Premenstrual dysphoric disorder affects approximately 3% to 8% of women (see Chapter 22). Often women with other forms of mood disorder will have increased symptoms during the luteal phase of their cycle, in which case the additional diagnosis of premenstrual dysphoric disorder is not given.

Approximately 10% of women experience a postpartum depressive episode, with a higher risk in those with a history of postpartum blues, premenstrual dysphoric disorder, or another mood disorder. The risk of a postpartum manic or hypomanic episode is less than 2% overall but greater than 25% in women with bipolar disorder. Though postpartum psychosis occurs in only 1 of 1000 births, it is more common in women with histories of mood disorder, especially bipolar illness.

PATHOGENESIS

Genetic, other biological, and psychosocial factors can all contribute to the development of mood disorders. First-degree relatives of patients with MDD have an increased lifetime risk of MDD. First-degree relatives of bipolar patients have an increased risk of both bipolar disorder and MDD. A family history of alcoholism is associated with an increased risk of MDD.

Mood syndromes can be caused by a neurologic, endocrine, infectious, or other general medical disorder or be a side effect of medications or other substances. Alcohol, narcotic analgesics, sedative-hypnotics, hormonal preparations (such as depot progestins), and antihypertensives, among others, can cause depressive syndromes. Antidepressants, steroids, and stimulants may trigger a manic or hypomanic syndrome.

Hormonal factors appear to play a role in women's greater vulnerability to depression as suggested by the fact that the incidence in females does not exceed that in males until age 11 (the approximate time of menarche), women with a past history of major mood disorder are more likely to experience premenstrual dysphoric disorder and vice versa, and the 4 to 6 months after childbirth is a time of increased risk for major mood disorders. The perimenopause also appears to be a period of increased risk for depressive symptomatology, and women with early menopause are at increased risk for subsequent depression.

Stressful life events and lack of social support both increase the vulnerability to mood disorder and likely contribute to the greater incidence of depression in women (e.g., women are more likely than men to live in poverty and to experience bereavement). Certain psychological traits such as perfectionism and lack of assertiveness may be associated with an increased risk of depressive disorders.

Some patients experience a major depressive episode each fall and winter as a result of the decreased amount of sunlight. This pattern, often referred to as *seasonal affective disorder,* is more common in women.

Recent evidence suggests that each major mood episode may cause permanent neurochemical changes in the brain that increase the patient's vulnerability to recurrence.

COURSE

An untreated major depressive episode lasts 5 or 6 months on average, with 80% of patients recovering within a year. Most, however, go on to experience recurrences and many have residual interepisode symptoms. Patients with dysthymic disorder often have episodes of MDD as well. Manic episodes last from a few weeks to a few months. Untreated bipolar disorder is recurrent in over 90% of cases, with interepisode symptoms frequent.

Alcohol and drugs, though often used by patients in an effort to modify their mood symptoms, tend to make the symptoms worse. Approximately two thirds of female alcoholics suffer from a mood disorder before the onset of their alcoholism. In patients with both a mood disorder and substance abuse, it is essential to treat both disorders.

The lifetime risk of suicide is approximately 15% in patients with MDD (a figure 30 times that of the general population) and 19% in bipolar disorder. The suicide rate is higher in men than women, though women make more attempts. It is also greater in older women than in younger ones.

DIAGNOSIS

To meet criteria for a major depressive episode a patient needs to have five of the following nine signs or symptoms for most of the day nearly every day for 2 weeks or more: depressed mood, decreased interest in usual activities (patients must have one of the preceding two symptoms), decreased or increased sleep, feelings of guilt or worthlessness, low energy, poor concentration, appetite or weight change, psychomotor agitation (motor restlessness) or retardation (slowed speech and movements), and thoughts of death or suicide. (Refer to the American Psychiatric Association's DSM-IV for complete diagnostic criteria.) Other common symptoms of depression include physical pain, decreased libido, menstrual disturbance, and gastrointestinal complaints, as well as anxiety, worry, irritability, hopelessness, indecisiveness, and social withdrawal. Psychotic symptoms (i.e., hallucinations or delusions) may also occur as part of a major depressive episode. Some older patients may demonstrate a dementialike syndrome as a feature of their depression.

The criteria for a hypomanic episode require a 4-day period marked by elevated or irritable mood and three of the following seven symptoms (four if the mood is irritable): increased energy and activity, poor judgment, decreased need for sleep, marked talkativeness, racing thoughts, inflated self-esteem, and distractibility. Diagnosis of a manic episode requires marked impairment in social or occupational functioning plus either hospitalization or a duration of at least 7 days. Psychotic symptoms are common during a manic episode.

In addition to being depressed most of the time for 2 years or more, patients with dysthymic disorder need to have at least two of the following six symptoms: appetite disturbance, sleep disturbance, decreased energy, low self-esteem, poor concentration or indecisiveness, and feelings of hopelessness. Patients must not be without the above symptoms for more than 2 months at a time and must not meet criteria for MDD within the first 2 years of their mood disturbance.

Patients whose mood disorder is believed to be physiologically caused by a physical illness are given the diagnosis of mood disorder due to a general medical condition. If the mood disorder is believed to be caused by a prescribed or nonprescribed drug, the diagnosis is substance-induced mood disorder.

To meet criteria for premenstrual dysthmyic disorder, patients need to have 5 of the following 11 symptoms: markedly depressed mood, marked anxiety or tension, marked affective lability, persistent and marked irritability (one of the preceding four symptoms is required), decreased interest in usual activities, decreased concentration, low energy, appetite change, insomnia or hypersomnia, feeling out of control, and other physical symptoms (e.g., breast tenderness or swelling). Symptoms must be present most of the time during the last week of the luteal phase, remit within a few days of the onset of menses, and be completely absent for more than 1 week postmenses. In addition to being present during most menstrual cycles in the preceding year, this disorder must be confirmed by prospective daily ratings during two or more symptomatic cycles.

DIFFERENTIAL DIAGNOSIS

Depressive symptoms following the loss of a loved one should be considered to represent bereavement rather than a depressive disorder unless they persist for 2 or more months, cause marked impairment of functioning, or are accompanied by suicidal thoughts, psychotic symptoms, psychomotor retardation, or marked feelings of worthlessness.

In older patients with memory complaints and depressive symptoms, a prior mood disorder history increases the probability that the patient is suffering from a mood disorder rather than dementia, as does a cognitive decline that coincided with or followed the onset of depressive symptoms.

TREATMENT

There are a variety of treatments available for patients with mood disorders. The great majority of patients can be helped. Patients who do not respond to one treatment often will respond to another.

Pretreatment Assessment

Most depressed and manic or hypomanic patients seen by an OB/GYN or primary care physician have a complaint unrelated to mood. It is useful to screen all new patients and any others in whom depression is suspected with a self-rating scale such as the Beck Depression Inventory. A score ≥10 on the Beck scale alerts the physician to the possibility of clinically significant depressive symptoms, which should be followed up with a clinical interview. Patients with elated or irritable mood, rapid speech, or intrusive behavior should be interviewed to elicit the symptoms of a manic or hypomanic episode. To establish if a depressed patient suffers from bipolar disorder, it is important to specifically question her and, if possible, a family member about a history of manic or hypomanic symptoms. Eliciting a bipolar diagnosis is important because these patients may require a different pharmacotherapeutic approach and also because of their higher rates of postpartum depression and mania. Given high rates of comorbidity, one should inquire in all patients with mood symptoms about current or past symptoms of substance abuse, anxiety, and eating disorders.

All new patients with significant mood symptoms need a thorough medical history and physical examination to evaluate whether any general medical conditions or prescribed or nonprescribed drugs could be contributing to their psychiatric problem. The onset of depressive or manic/hypomanic symptoms within a few weeks of starting or increasing the dosage of a medication suggests the possibility of a causal relationship. A CBC with differential, serum chemistry profile, urinalysis, TSH test, and free T4 or total T4 plus T3 resin uptake should be part of the standard workup.

All patients with mood disorders need to have their suicidal risk evaluated and documented. When a patient acknowledges that she might kill herself, a psychiatric consultation is indicated on an emergent basis.

Antidepressant Medication

Antidepressants are most commonly used in the treatment of depressive disorders but can also be helpful for the depressive phase of bipolar disorder and for anxiety and eating disorders. All patients who meet criteria for a major depressive episode should be considered candidates for

(1) antidepressant pharmacotherapy, though psychotherapy alone can also be appropriate for some patients with mild to moderate depression; (2) phototherapy for patients with winter depression; and (3) electroconvulsive therapy (ECT) for severely depressed patients. Antidepressant medication may also be helpful for some patients with dysthymic disorder and DDNOS. Several new drugs have been approved for the treatment of depression in recent years (Table 13-1).

These new antidepressants, especially the three SSRIs, are preferred as first-line agents because they are safer than both the tricyclic antidepressants, which have a high lethality in overdose and can cause orthostatic hypotension and a slowing of intracardiac conduction, and the monoamine oxidase inhibitors, which can cause hypertensive crises if certain foods or drugs are ingested. The new antidepressants are better tolerated than the tricyclics and are infrequently associated with typical tricyclic side effects such as sedation, anticholinergic effects, and weight gain. However, they can sometimes cause nausea, diarrhea, headaches, nervousness, or insomnia. In addition, nefazodone can cause dizziness, venlafaxine can cause sustained diastolic hypertension in about 5% of patients, and bupropion has an incidence of seizures of 0.4%, approximately twice that of the other new antidepressants.

Except for bupropion and nefazodone, which are less frequently associated with sexual side effects, the new antidepressants can cause anorgasmia or decreased libido in approximately 20% of patients, especially early in treatment. In patients for whom sexual side effects are a persistent problem, options include reducing the dosage, switching to a different drug, skipping a dose before anticipated sexual activity, or adding

TABLE 13-1
New Antidepressants

Generic name	Brand name	Usual total daily dosage*	Dosing schedule
SSRIs			
Fluoxetine	Prozac	10-50 mg	qd
Paroxetine	Paxil	10-50 mg	qd
Sertraline	Zoloft	25-200 mg	qd
NON-SSRIs			
Bupropion	Wellbutrin	225-450 mg	bid or tid†
Nefazodone	Serzone	200-600 mg	bid
Venlafaxine	Effexor	150-375 mg	bid or tid

*In some elderly and medically ill patients the maximum recommended dosage is lower than listed.
†No single dose of bupropion should exceed 150 mg; doses must be given at least 4 hours apart.

another agent, such as amantadine, bupropion, buspirone, cyprohepadine, or yohimbine.

The new antidepressants should not be given in proximity to an MAO inhibitor because of the risk of a potentially fatal reaction characterized by hyperthermia, confusion, and myoclonus. These drugs may also affect bleeding time when used with warfarin. By inhibiting the 2D6 isoenzyme of the cytochrome P450 hepatic microsomal enzyme system, the SSRIs can increase the plasma levels of certain other drugs, such as tricyclics, neuroleptics, beta blockers, and dextromethorphan, and block the analgesic action of codeine and oxycodone. Sertraline has less of an effect on 2D6 than the other SSRIs. Nefazodone inhibits the 3A4 isoenzyme, which can increase plasma levels of the nonsedating antihistamines terfenadine and astemizole, as well as the motility agent and antinausea drug cisapride and the benzodiazepines alprazolam and triazolam. Nefazodone is contraindicated with terfenadine, astemizole, and cisapride because high levels of these three drugs can interfere with intracardiac conduction. Fluoxetine, and to a much lesser extent sertraline, may affect the 3A4 isoenzyme. Fluoxetine may also affect the 2C9 and 2C19 isoenzymes, which metabolize tricyclics and benzodiazepines, among other drugs. Venlafaxine has been reported to have a significant effect on 2D6. There has been little research to date on bupropion's possible effects on the hepatic microsomal enzyme system.

Several of the new antidepressants, including fluoxetine, sertraline, paroxetine, and nefazodone, are effective in the treatment of premenstrual dysphoric disorder. Current evidence supports the use of these drugs on a daily basis rather than simply during the luteal phase of the cycle.

The tricyclic antidepressants are still widely used, primarily for patients who do not respond to the newer agents. They may be particularly effective for patients with more severe depressions. Nortriptyline (Pamelor) and desipramine (Norpramin) are usually preferred because they have fewer side effects than the older tricyclics such as imipramine (Tofranil) and amitriptyline (Elavil). The MAO inhibitors phenelzine (Nardil) and tranylcypromine (Parnate) can be very helpful for certain patients, especially those with symptoms such as increased sleep and appetite, even though they can cause orthostatic hypotension, sexual dysfunction, weight gain, and sleep disturbance, as well as the food and drug interactions noted.

Mood-Stabilizing Medication

Lithium carbonate, divalproex sodium (Depakote), and carbamazepine (Tegretal) are the treatments of choice for the bipolar disorders. (Divalproex sodium is an enteric-coated coordination compound consisting of equal proportions of valproic acid and sodium valproate. It is much better tolerated gastrointestinally than valproic acid [Depakene], which is not recommended.) All three drugs are effective for the acute treatment of manic episodes; lithium and divalproex have been approved by the FDA for this indication. The overall acute antimanic efficacy of divalproex is approximately equal to that of lithium, but it may have a more rapid onset of action and be more effective for patients with rapid-cycling bipolar disorder, a mixed episode, or comorbid substance abuse. Lithium is effective for the prophylaxis of recurrent manic and depressive episodes in bipolar patients. There have been few studies reported of the prophylactic efficacy of divalproex and carbamazepine, though they are widely used for this indication. Lithium has acute antidepressant efficacy in some bipolar patients, though it generally works slower than the antidepressant drugs. Carbamazepine has also some efficacy in this regard.

The most common side effects of lithium are nausea, diarrhea, polyuria (a result of decreased renal concentrating ability), and polydipsia, as well as a fine tremor, muscle weakness, mild sedation, and weight gain. Patients whose serum lithium level 12 hours after their last dose exceeds the therapeutic range of 0.5 to 1.3 mEq/L can develop lithium toxicity, symptoms of which include nausea and vomiting, coarse tremor, oliguria, seizures, and lethargy, which may progress to coma and death. Occasionally, older or medically ill patients can develop lithium toxicity at levels within the therapeutic range. Lithium causes hypothyroidism in 5% to 35% of patients, with women more commonly affected; this is easily treated with levothyroxine. In the absence of episodes of lithium toxicity, which can adversely affect renal function, long-term lithium treatment appears to have little or no clinically significant effect on the glomerular filtration rate. Lithium may occasionally interfere with cardiac sinus node function, leading to bradycardia, and can also cause T wave flattening and inverted T waves. Nonsteroidal antiinflammatory drugs should be used very cautiously in patients taking lithium, since these drugs can increase the lithium level into the toxic range; sulindac may be less likely to cause a problem than other NSAIDs. Since lithium's antimanic effect usually does not take effect for 5 to 7 days, high-potency benzodiazepines or neuroleptics are often needed as adjuncts early in treatment.

The most common side effects of divalproex are nausea, diarrhea, weight gain, sedation, tremor, and loss of hair (which generally will grow back with continued treatment). Thrombocytopenia, elevated hepatic enzymes, pancreatitis, and menstrual irregularities can also occur. Divalproex can increase the plasma levels of certain other drugs (e.g., tricyclics, other anticonvulsants, and benzodiazepines) by inhibiting their metabolism in the hepatic microsomal enzyme system. Patients on divalproex should be advised to be cautious about taking aspirin, since it may reduce the plasma protein binding of valproate and thereby cause a possible increase in side effects. The most common side effects of carbamazepine are nausea, sedation, diplopia, and ataxia. By inducing hepatic isoenzymes, carbamazepine can lower the plasma levels of a number of coadministered drugs, including estrogen compounds. Since pregnancies have been reported in women taking carbamazepine and oral contraceptives (presumably caused by this interaction), the carbamazepine-oral contraceptive combination should be used very cautiously. Carbamazepine can also induce its own metabolism, which means that the dosage may need to be increased early in treatment to maintain therapeutic plasma levels. Carbamazepine can also rarely cause aplastic anemia (1 case in 200,000 treatment-years). It is more commonly associated with benign leukopenia (approximately 10% of patients in the first 4 months of treatment). Like the tricyclics, carbamazepine can cause a slowing of intracardiac conduction. It is the least likely of the mood stabilizers to cause weight gain.

Before starting lithium, patients should have the standard laboratory workup for new patients, plus an ECG if they are over 50 or have a history of syncope or risk factors for cardiac disease. These tests should be repeated yearly, with serum creatinine levels monitored every 6 months. Patients starting carbamazepine or divalproex need a baseline CBC with differential and quantitative platelets, LFTs, and (for carbamazepine) an ECG. The CBC and LFTs should be obtained every 2 to 4 weeks for the first 3 months, then repeated 3 months after that and every 6 months thereafter. Patients should be told to let the physician know right away about any signs of infection or abnormal bleeding. Frequent serum level monitoring is necessary early in treatment for patients on any of the mood stabilizers. This is especially true for carbamazepine because of its capacity for inducing its own metabolism. Once the patient is stabilized on a maintenance dosage, lithium levels should be measured approximately every 3 months and valproate and carbamazepine levels every 6 months, more often if clinical problems or side effects emerge.

Psychotherapy

The key elements of supportive psychotherapy, an essential part of the treatment of all patients with mood disorders, consist of establishing and maintaining a positive, accepting relationship and providing education and reassurance. Patients and family need to be told that mood disorders are very treatable. Pamphlets or books about mood disorders and support groups are often quite helpful. Patients should be cautioned against making major life decisions, because they are usually unable to view matters objectively while they are experiencing an episode of mood disorder.

Although supportive therapy is best provided by the patient's own physician, it can also be provided by a psychiatrist or other mental health professional who can provide other forms of psychotherapy if needed. Both cognitive and interpersonal therapy are effective treatments in their own right for major depressive episodes of mild to moderate severity, though most clinicians feel that symptom relief is more rapid when psychotherapy is combined with medication. Psychotherapy can enhance treatment compliance and psychosocial adjustment in patients with bipolar disorder. It should not, however, be used as the sole treatment for bipolar patients. It is often helpful to see the patient with her spouse or significant other to educate and offer suggestions for support.

Electroconvulsive Therapy

Electroconvulsive therapy (ECT) remains the most rapid and effective acute treatment for severe depression and is also very effective for manic episodes. It is not commonly used as the initial treatment, however, in part because of the amnesia it can cause for events that occur around the time of the ECT. Patients need to be started on medication after a course of ECT to reduce the risk of a recurrence.

Phototherapy

Treatment with bright artificial light is effective for patients who suffer from winter depressions. Antidepressant drugs may also be helpful.

Pregnancy and Mood Disorders

The lifetime risk of a mood disorder in the offspring is 27% if one parent has bipolar disorder or MDD and 50% to 74% if both parents are affected. In general, the presence of a mood disorder in the patient and/or her spouse should not be a contraindication to having a child.

It is usually desirable to avoid use of psychotropic medication during pregnancy, especially the first trimester, because of possible risks to the embryo and fetus. In view of this consideration, shorter half-life antidepressants such as paroxetine and sertraline may be preferable in general for women of child-bearing potential because they can be rapidly cleared in case of an unanticipated pregnancy.

Fluoxetine, sertraline, paroxetine, and bupropion are classified as Class B agents in pregnancy, whereas venlafaxine and nefazodone are classified as Class C. Lithium, carbamazepine, and divalproex are teratogens. Lithium is associated with an increase in the relative risk for all congenital malformations of 1.5 to 3 and for fetal cardiac malformations of 1.2 to 7.7. Both carbamazepine and divalproex have an increased overall risk of congenital malformations, with carbamazepine associated in particular with spina bifida and divalproex with neural tube defect and IUGR. Both drugs may have the potential for causing an adverse effect on the child's later cognitive development.

In those depressed patients for whom the severity of their illness makes medication use during pregnancy advisable, the SSRIs and the tricyclics nortriptyline and desipramine may be associated with the fewest risks. For bipolar patients, lithium is the mood stabilizer of choice during pregnancy. To minimize withdrawal symptoms in the neonate, it may be advisable to reduce lithium dosage in the week before delivery. If mood-stabilizing medication is discontinued during pregnancy, it should be restarted immediately after delivery, given the high risk of a postpartum recurrence. The American Academy of Pediatrics has rated divalproex and carbamazepine as compatible with breastfeeding, but lithium as contraindicated. More data is needed with regard to the SSRIs and other agents.

Guidelines for Treating Mood Disorders

Before starting treatment, it is helpful to review therapeutic options with patients and encourage them to participate in the decision-making process (Fig. 13-1). In so doing, you are implicitly telling them that you value what they have to say, as well as increasing the likelihood that they will follow through with treatment. During a manic or hypomanic episode patients typically have little insight that anything is wrong with them; the family can play a crucial role in persuading them of the need for treatment. Patients should be advised about potential side effects, including the possibility that they might feel worse psychologically. If possible, family members should be informed as well. Patients should also be informed about possible drug

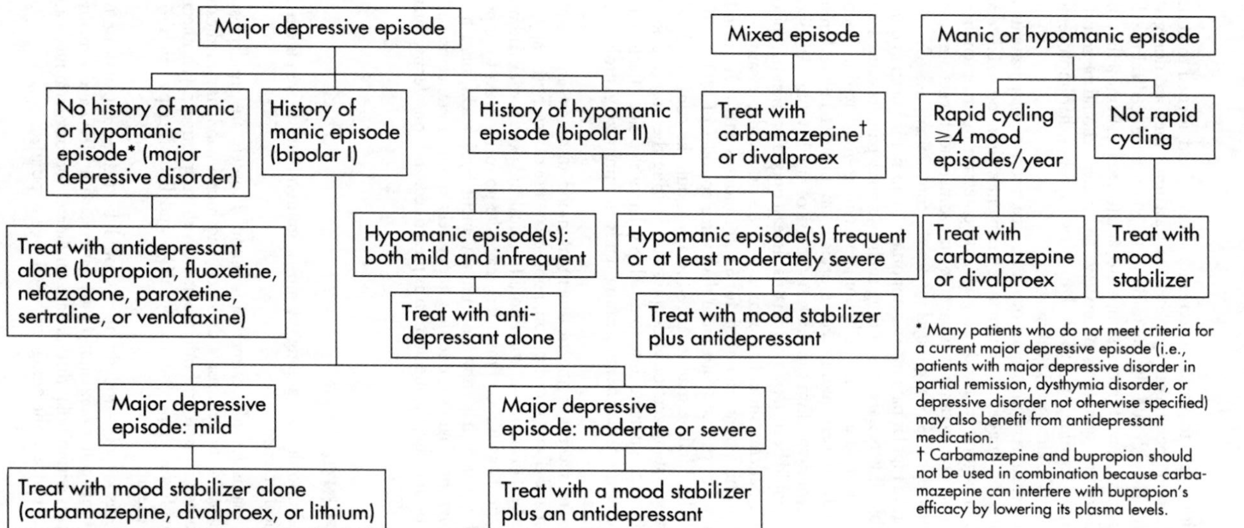

FIG. 13-1 Initial pharmacologic approach to an episode of mood disorder.

interactions, told to avoid all recreational drugs, and advised to abstain from alcoholic beverages completely at least until they are doing well clinically. They should also be told not to go on a reduced-calorie diet, since this can aggravate mood symptoms, and to avoid caffeine if they have insomnia or any symptoms of anxiety. The patient should be told that treatments sometimes start to work in a few days, but that improvement also could take a few weeks or longer.

Given their very high rates of recurrence, most bipolar patients are candidates for long-term maintenance treatment with mood stabilizers. If possible, it is good to avoid using an antidepressant for maintenance in bipolar I patients because these agents may sometimes trigger a manic or hypomanic episode or rapid cycling despite concomitant use of a mood stabilizer. In bipolar patients it is important to normalize sleep as quickly as possible, if necessary with a drug such as clonazepam, because lack of sleep can aggravate manic or hypomanic symptoms. Thyroid function needs to be closely monitored, especially in patients taking lithium, because hypothyroidism can increase the risk of rapid cycling. All bipolar patients should be seen by a psychiatrist at least once. For an initial episode of MDD, patients should be maintained on an antidepressant, at the dosage to which they responded, for 6 to 12 months after they are in full remission. For patients with more than three episodes of MDD and for older adults, lifetime maintenance therapy should be considered. With either mood stabilizers or antidepressants, raising the dosage gradually often allows the patient time to develop tolerance to side effects; taking medication immediately after eating tends to minimize gastrointestinal symptoms.

Keys to success in the treatment of mood disorders are adequate duration and dose of medication, appropriate use of psychotherapy, and management of comorbid conditions (medical and psychiatric). Although some patients with mood disorders may take up to 12 weeks to respond fully, if a patient has shown no improvement by 6 weeks, one should reconsider the diagnosis, question her closely about substance use, ask if she has been taking the medication as prescribed, and consider psychiatric consultation.

KEY POINTS

1 Mood disorders are among the most common illnesses seen in general medical practice.

2 The mainstays of treatment for mood disorders are antidepressant medication for depressive disorders and mood-stabilizing medication for bipolar disorder, both provided with supportive psychotherapy. Other forms of psychotherapy, ECT, and light therapy can also be very useful.

3 An episode of mood disorder should be treated for at least 6 to 12 months after remission. Many patients with MDD and virtually all patients with bipolar disorder are candidates for long-term medication maintenance at the dosage to which they responded.

SUGGESTED READINGS

American Psychiatric Association: *Diagnostic and statistical manual of mental disorders, ed 4 (DSM-IV),* Washington, DC, 1994, American Psychiatric Press.

American Psychiatric Association: Practice guidelines for major depressive disorder in adults, *Am J Psychiatry* 150(supp.):1-26, 1993.

American Psychiatric Association: Practice guideline for the treatment of patients with bipolar disorder, *Am J Psychiatry* (supp.) 151:1-36, 1994.

Briggs GG, Freedman RK, Yaffee SJ: Reference guide to fetal and neonatal risk, drugs in pregnancy and lactation, ed 4, Baltimore, 1994, Williams & Wilkins.

Depression Guideline Panel: *Depression in primary care: quick reference guide for clinicians,* U.S. Dept. of Health and Human Services, Agency for Health Care Policy and Research, 1993.

Frank E et al: Three-year outcomes for maintenance therapies in recurrent depression, *Arch Gen Psychiatry* 47:1093-99, 1990.

Goodwin FK, Jamison KR: *Manic-depressive illness,* New York, 1990, Oxford.

Hekkinen ME, Isometsa ET, Aro HM: Age-related variation in recent life events preceding suicide, *J Nerv Ment Dis* 183:325-31, 1995.

Kessler RC et al: Lifetime and 12-month prevalence of DSM-III-R psychiatric disorders in the United States: results from the National Comorbidity Survey, *Arch Gen Psychiatry* 51:8-19, 1994.

Pariser SF: Women and mood disorders: menarche to menopause, *Ann Clin Psychiatr* 5:249-54, 1993.

Pearlstein TC: Hormones and depression: what are the facts about premenstrual syndrome, menopause, and hormone replacement therapy? *Am J Obstet Gynecol* 173:646-53, 1995.

Post RN: Transduction of psychosocial stress into the neurobiology of recurrent affective disorder, *Am J Psychiatry* 149:999-1010, 1992.

Steiner M et al: Fluoxetine in the treatment of premenstrual dysphoria, *N Engl J Med* 332:1529-34, 1995.

Stowe ZN, Nemeroff CB: Psychopharmacology during pregnancy and lactation. In Schatzberg AF and Nemeroff CB, eds: *The American Psychiatric Press textbook of Psychopharmacology,* Washington, DC, 1995, American Psychiatric Press, Inc.

Stowe ZN, Nemeroff CB: Women at risk for postpartum-onset major depression, *Am J Obstet Gynecol* 173:639-45, 1995.

Yonkers KA, Halbreich U, Freeman E: Efficacy of sertraline for treatment of premenstrual dysphoric disorder, *Psychopharmacol Bull* (in press).

Reading material for patients and families

National Institute of Mental Health: Pamphlets on depression and bipolar disorder, 1-800-421-4211.

Papolos DF, Papolos J: *Overcoming depression,* ed 2, New York, 1993, Harper & Row.

Support groups for patients and families

National Depressive and Manic Depressive Association, 1-800-82-NDMDA

National Alliance for the Mentally Ill, 1-800-950-NAMI

14

Nutrition and Menopause

MAUREEN O'BRIEN PLATT

Educating patients about nutritional concerns and exercise during perimenopause will enable these women to enhance their quality of life during the sometimes difficult transition into menopause.

BALANCED DIET

To maintain a healthy lifestyle during the menopause transition, following a balanced, nutrient-rich diet should be a primary goal. Good nutritional habits before, during, and after menopause can help decrease the risk of complications of menopause and maintain a healthy body.

During midlife, a woman's dietary focus should be on following a diet higher in nutrients and lower in calories. A balanced diet should consist of the following:

Food group	Number of servings/day
Milk	3-4
Meat	5 (1 oz = 1 serving)
Vegetables/fruit	5+
Bread	6-11
Fats	In moderation
Water	6-8 glasses

Calories can be divided among three meals plus two snacks daily for optimal utilization by the body.

Calcium

Calcium is probably the most important nutrient concern during menopause. Women need calcium to help prevent osteoporosis. If a woman is not eating at least three dietary sources of calcium or taking calcium supplements daily, she may be at risk for osteoporosis. To help maintain a greater bone mass and to reduce the chances of developing osteoporosis, it is recommended that women have an intake of 1000 to 1500 mg of calcium daily. A menopausal woman who is receiving HRT should consume 1000 mg of calcium. The woman not using HRT should consume 1500 mg of calcium daily.

The best source of calcium is food. However, women who do not like dairy products or who are lactose intolerant can meet the calcium requirements with a calcium supplement. Calcium carbonate, which is

40% elemental calcium, provides a significant amount of calcium per tablet and is economical. Elemental calcium is the amount of calcium available for absorption. Calcium carbonate should be taken in divided doses. For women with low stomach acid, calcium citrate malate, taken with meals, is recommended.

A woman who is relying solely on supplements for calcium should be advised to also take a multivitamin/mineral supplement. The large amount of calcium required can interfere with zinc absorption. Also, additional vitamin D and magnesium help to increase calcium absorption and bone mineralization. Women should avoid excessive amounts of caffeine, protein, alcohol, and tobacco, which alter the body's absorption of calcium.

Cholesterol

From approximately 2 years before to 6 years after menopause, cholesterol levels increase. The LDL cholesterol increases and the HDL decreases. The rise in cholesterol is found to be significantly lower in women who choose their dietary fats from the monounsaturated fat group rather than from those fats that are saturated; monounsaturated fats include olive oil, canola oil, and peanut oil. Monounsaturated fats and exercise increase HDL levels. Estrogen therapy decreases total cholesterol levels by 8% to 10%.

Cholesterol is found in animal foods such as egg yolks, meat, fish, poultry, and whole milk products. Foods from the vegetable group do not contain cholesterol. However, saturated oils such as coconut oil and palm oil, ingredients found in chocolate candy, commercial baked goods, and nondairy creamers, increase cholesterol levels.

The current recommendation is to reduce dietary cholesterol to 300 mg/day. Fat in the diet should be approximately 25% of the total dietary calories.

Fiber

Getting adequate amounts of fiber in the diet is difficult. The fiber intake for many women falls below the recommended amount of 20 to 35 g/day.

Both classes of fiber, soluble and insoluble, are especially beneficial to menopausal women. Soluble fiber reduces cholesterol levels and helps to regulate blood sugar. Foods that contain insoluble fiber help to add bulk to the digestive system. As women age, the GI tract functions more slowly. Insoluble fiber is effective in relieving constipation.

High-fiber foods also help with weight maintenance. High-fiber foods are generally low in fat and calories, high in vitamins and minerals, and are filling. Sources of high-fiber foods include whole grains, fruits, vegetables, legumes, and brans.

Antioxidants

Antioxidants are believed to interfere with certain disease processes by preventing free radical formations. Free radical damage to the body has been associated with the risk of developing cancer, heart disease, cataracts, weakened immune systems, and aging.

Dietary antioxidants are vitamins and minerals such as beta carotene, vitamins C and E, zinc, and selenium. Antioxidants are found primarily in fruits and vegetables. Fortified breakfast cereals and nuts also contain significant amounts of antioxidants.

Data from studies have linked high dietary intakes of fruits and vegetables to a reduction of breast cancer in women when compared with women with low intakes of these foods. Additional information from studies has shown similar results with antioxidants, women, and heart disease. Until an optimal intake of dietary antioxidants can be determined from more studies, women should be encouraged to consume a minimum of five servings of fruits and vegetables daily. Servings should include a dark green vegetable, an orange or yellow vegetable, and a source of vitamin C such as strawberries, broccoli, or citrus fruits.

MAINTAINING APPROPRIATE BODY WEIGHT

The majority of women experiencing perimenopause will usually gain weight. The metabolic rate drops significantly during perimenopause and women's activity levels usually begin to decline. As a result, the percent of body fat increases. The weight that is gained tends to be around the stomach area. Women's figures change from a pear shape to an apple shape. It is the extra fat in the abdomen that is considered to cause a greater risk of heart disease, hypertension, and diabetes.

For some women, weight gain is the most frustrating "side-effect" of menopause. Maintaining an appropriate body weight often seems impossible to accomplish. Women need continuing support for successful weight maintenance.

The 1995 edition of the *Dietary Guidelines for Americans* has changed since the guidelines were last introduced in 1990. This change reflects the importance of maintaining appropriate body weight during the aging process. The new guidelines no longer allow for additional weight gain after the age of 35. There is one weight range for all adults.

Exercise can be a significant component of a weight-maintenance program. An exercise routine should include both aerobic exercise and resistance training or weight-bearing exercise. The aerobic exercise will increase the metabolic rate, burn calories, improve cardiovascular health, and relieve stress. Examples of aerobic exercise are jogging, walking, swimming, and bicycling. Weight-bearing exercise, such as weight lifting, improves muscle mass and bone strength to help prevent osteoporosis.

A healthy weight-loss plan should incorporate both a balanced, low-fat diet and an appropriate exercise program. The diet needs to be individualized to meet the food preferences, ethnic practices, and schedules of the patient.

ALTERNATIVE THERAPIES

The use of alternative therapies for HRT is attracting the interest of perimenopausal women. These women are appearing to find relief from hot flashes, vaginal dryness, irritability, and other complaints from nontraditional therapies. Health professionals are not always told of this alternate approach by their patients. The use of phytoestrogens, herbs, homeopathy, and acupressure are among the alternative therapies being used for the treatment of menopausal symptoms. Although these nontraditional treatments may offer relief for some, women need to be cautioned about possible side effects, "too-good-to-be-true" claims, and the expense of these therapies.

Whichever therapy a woman chooses, a healthy lifestyle of a nutrient-rich diet and adequate exercise will help improve her quality of life during perimenopause and menopause.

Phytoestrogens

Phytoestrogens, or plant hormones, are primarily found in soy foods, which contain a very high content of isoflavonoids, a phytoestrogen compound. These isoflavonoids have estrogenlike effects on the body. In Asian countries where high soy diets are popular, the women have fewer complaints of menopausal symptoms and fewer hip fractures. In the Japanese culture, the phrase *hot flash* does not exist.

There are many foods that contain phytoestrogens, but traditional soy foods appear to contain the most potent amount. Sources of traditional soy foods are tofu, tempeh, and miso. The role of phytoestrogens in reducing the incidence of cardiovascular disease and breast cancer is also being studied.

Herbs

The use of herbs for relief of menopausal symptoms is a very popular alternative therapy. Bookstores and health food stores offer a wide range of information regarding medicinal uses of herbal treatments.

Among perimenopausal patients, ginseng and dong quai are often used for menopausal complaints. These herbs act as estrogen precursors. The herbs are used as teas, infusions, or in the most concentrated form, tinctures. Side effects can occur because of the inability to regulate a specific dosage of these herbs. The effects of unopposed estrogen on the body is a concern.

Other herbal remedies that are used include black cohash, chasteberry, horsetail, Lady's slipper, nettles, and motherwort.

Homeopathy

Homeopathy has also been used as an alternative treatment for HRT. Examples of remedies and their claims prescribed by homeopaths include nux vomica for insomnia or constipation, lycopodium for poor memory, lachesis for anxiety, sepia for vaginal dryness, ignatia for hot flashes, and pulsatilla for insomnia.

Acupressure

Acupressure is an alternative therapy used to release stress by putting pressure on designated points of the body. Acupressure points that are thought to increase hormone production are located on the palm of the hand, lower ankle, and on the sole of the foot. Results occur if the acupressure is performed for 5 to 10 minutes, twice daily.

KEY POINTS

1 The calcium requirement for women receiving HRT is 1000 mg daily; without HRT the requirement is 1500 mg of calcium daily.

2 Women who are lactose intolerant can meet calcium requirements with calcium carbonate, a supplement that provides a significant amount of calcium per tablet and is readily absorbed by the body.

3 Using monounsaturated fats in the diet helps to lower the risks associated with increasing cholesterol levels during menopause.

4 Because of a decrease in metabolic rates and physical activity, women in midlife need to reduce caloric intake and increase exercise to achieve and maintain an appropriate body weight.

5 The use of alternative therapies for HRT may be unreported by the patient, can lead to increased health risks, and may cause significant expense for the patient.

SUGGESTED READINGS

Aldercreutz H et al: Dietary phyto-estrogens and menopause in Japan, *Lancet* 339:1233, 1992.

Eisenberg DM et al: Unconventional medicine in the United States, *N Engl J Med* 328:246, 1993.

Foreyt JP, Goodrick GK: Weight management without dieting, *Nutr Today* 28:4-10, 1993.

Hankin JH: Role of nutrition in women's health: diet and breast cancer, *JADA* 93(9):994-999, 1015-1016, 1993.

Jacobs MM: Diet, nutrition and cancer research: an overview, *Nutr Today* 28:19-23, 1993.

Kris-Etherton PM, Krummel D: Role of nutrition in the prevention and treatment of coronary heart disease, *JADA* 39:987-993, 1993.

Ojeda L: *Menopause without medicine,* Alameda, Calif, 1992, Hunter House, Inc.

Pike MC et al: Re: Dietary fat and postmenopausal breast cancer, *J Natl Cancer Inst* 84(21):1666-1669, 1994.

Reid IK et al: Effect of calcium supplementation on bone loss in postmenopausal women, *N Engl J Med* 328:460-464, 1993.

Shangold M: Exercise in menopausal women, *Obstet Gynecol* 75:535-555, 1990.

St. Jean S: The role of weight maintenance in the health of women, *JADA* 93:1007-1012, 1993.

Stein D: *The natural remedy book for women,* Freedom, Calif, 1992, Crossing Press.

Wardlaw GM: Putting osteoporosis in perspective, *JADA* 93:1000-1006, 1993.

Zhang J et al: Moderate physical activity and bone density among perimenopausal women, *A J Public Health* 82:736-738, 1992.

15

Osteoporosis

Rebecca D. Jackson

As a result of health care advances in recent decades, society is aging. It is estimated that a 50-year-old woman will now spend more than one third of her life in her postmenopausal years. Thus medical conditions such as osteoporosis that are influenced by menopause and aging have important public health ramifications.

Osteoporosis is defined as a disease characterized by a decrease in bone mass with impairments in architectural arrangement leading to an increased risk for nontraumatic fractures. It can be assessed indirectly by measurement of bone mineral density (BMD) because BMD accounts for more than 75% of the variance in bone strength. Using the WHO operational definition, osteoporosis is defined as a bone density value more than 2.5 standard deviations below the young normal mean.

The incidence of osteoporosis in the United States exceeds 20 million persons. The clinical manifestations of this disease are directly related to the increased incidence of fractures, with resultant pain, deformity, and loss of physical function contributing to its morbidity. More than 1.3 million fractures are attributable to osteoporosis annually. These fractures predominantly occur at the vertebrae (538,000 fractures/year), the distal radius (172,000 fractures/year), and the hip (more than 250,000 fractures/year). From 12% to 20% of patients with a hip fracture die within 1 year of the injury. These fractures lead to substantial economic burden to both the individual and society.

PATHOPHYSIOLOGY

Bone is a dynamic tissue that constantly undergoes a process of formation and resorption in a coupled process of remodeling. In the young adult, where bone mass is stable, bone formation is equal to the amount of bone resorbed. However, as estrogen levels fall with menopause there is inadequate estrogen to suppress release of local cytokines, leading to an increased number of active remodeling sites, increased osteoclastic resorption, and net loss of bone. These changes can result in bone loss as high as 5% to 7%/year in the first few years of menopause.

There are also changes associated with aging that can result in gradual losses (1% to 2%/year) of bone in the elderly. There is evidence that the extent and depth of the resorption cavity increases with age, leading to cortical thinning and increased porosity of bone. There is also decreased osteoblast recruitment with a reduction in the amount of total bone formed per remodeling cycle, leading to a reduction in bone mass.

DIAGNOSIS

Osteoporosis is a silent disease, and bone loss may occur for years before manifestation. The classic signs and symptoms of osteoporosis relate to its associated fractures and include back pain, kyphosis, and loss of height. Late clinical features of osteoporosis include restrictive lung disease, constipation, reflux esophagitis, and abdominal bloating. Because physical findings will not define the women with early bone loss who would benefit most from aggressive intervention, additional studies to establish the presence and extent of reduced bone mass are critical.

History and Physical Examination

The history should be structured to look at factors that might influence the acquisition of peak bone mass or accelerate bone loss that would affect overall bone mass. It should include a review of risk factors (Box 15-1) and a careful gynecologic history. Late menarche and prolonged secondary amenorrhea are associated with lower bone mass, whereas oral contraceptive use may result in slightly higher than normal bone density. Premature menopause results in earlier-than-normal losses of bone. Parity and lactation seem to have no clear-cut adverse effect on bone mass. This history should also focus on potential secondary causes for osteoporosis

BOX 15-1
Risk Factors for Involutional Osteoporosis

Nonmodifiable	Modifiable
Advancing age	Decreased estrogen exposure
Female gender	Early menarche
Asian or Caucasian ethnicity	Secondary amenorrhea
Small body habitus	Lifestyle
Genetics	Smoking
	Alcohol intake
	Inactivity
	Nutritional intake
	Low calcium
	High protein (>120 g/day)
	High phosphate

that might indicate a need for more aggressive testing and intervention. This should also include a history of medication use to assess the potential effect of pharmacologic strategies that contribute to a negative calcium balance (loop diuretics), increase vitamin D degradation (anticonvulsants), increase bone resorption (thyroid hormone and cyclosporine among others), or decrease bone formation (glucocorticoids). Risk factor analysis should be a critical part of preventive health care and can be utilized to tailor specific recommendations for lifestyle modifications such as nutrition and exercise. However, only a history of a prior fracture after age 50; history of fracture of the hip, wrist, or vertebra in a first-degree relative; current cigarette smoking; or a physical finding of low body weight have been shown to be important clinical determinants of hip fracture risk (in addition to the BMD).

The physical examination is focused on excluding secondary causes of osteoporosis and defining the extent of disease that is already present. Classic physical findings of osteoporosis include a loss of height, the presence of fixed dorsal kyphosis, and an arm span that exceeds height. This latter finding is a result of the presence of multiple compression fractures that decrease axial height, but have no effect on appendicular length. The presence of proximal muscle weakness or diffuse skeletal tenderness may indicate concurrent osteomalacia.

Radiologic Studies

The diagnosis of osteoporosis by radiograph is suggested by the presence of increased skeletal lucency, a loss of horizontal trabeculation, and a decrease in cortical endplate thickness. As a qualitative image, the primary role for radiographs is in the identification of fractures or other skeletal disease. Radiographs may help to stratify risk for fracture because the presence of at least one vertebral fracture increases the relative risk for a second fracture by fourfold to fivefold, independent of the underlying BMD.

The most important determinant of fracture risk is BMD. For every one standard deviation that BMD is decreased there is an approximate doubling of the fracture rate. Although several absorptiometric techniques are available, dual energy x-ray absorptiometry (DEXA) is the technique of choice. DEXA allows for measurement of BMD in the axial skeleton (lumbar spine), peripheral skeleton (forearm or hip), or the total body. The results are expressed in bone mineral content (BMC) or areal BMD (g/cm^2). DEXA has excellent measurement precision (<1% error) and an accuracy error of <3%, which allows for serial follow-up of bone mass at approximate 2-year intervals. The radiation exposure is low (1 to 3 mrads), thus ensuring patient safety.

Clinical indications for bone mass measurement include (1) confirmation of the diagnosis of osteoporosis when osteoporosis is suspected; (2) definition of the extent of bone loss when an alteration can be made to therapy to change an outcome; (3) assessment of bone mass to expedite a decision for therapy; (4) evaluation of the degree of bone loss and effect of treatment in other metabolic diseases such as renal osteodystrophy and parathyroid bone disease; and (5) monitoring efficacy of therapeutic intervention. DEXA is a diagnostic test and at present should not be utilized for mass screening.

Biochemical Testing

Biochemical testing may be used to exclude secondary causes of osteoporosis. At a minimum, when osteoporosis is noted a woman should have serum calcium, phosphorus, and alkaline phosphatase tests performed. These tests are usually normal in involutional osteoporosis. If the history and physical examination suggests an underlying disorder or if there is evidence of accelerated bone loss, additional laboratory testing should be pursued.

In some individuals, it may also be useful to determine the rate of bone turnover. Markers of resorption reflect degradation products of collagen and include the urinary deoxypyridinoline and N-telopeptide. Markers of bone formation include the bone-specific alkaline phosphatase and osteocalcin. Although bone turnover markers cannot quantify bone mass, they may be especially useful in either stratifying the rates of bone loss in a woman with osteopenia in whom the choice to begin treatment is not clear or for early follow-up of therapeutic efficacy with an antiresorptive treatment.

DIFFERENTIAL DIAGNOSIS

Although more than 85% of women with osteoporosis will have bone loss caused by either menopause or age-related reasons, there are also a number of diseases that may cause secondary osteoporosis. These can be divided into several major categories such as endocrinopathies, connective tissue diseases, deficiency states, and hematologic malignancies (Box 15-2). Most

BOX 15-2
Differential Diagnosis of Secondary Osteoporosis

- Endocrinopathies
  - Type I diabetes
  - Cushing's syndrome
  - Hyperparathyroidism
  - Thyrotoxicosis
  - Hyperprolactinemia
- Connective tissue disease
  - Rheumatoid arthritis
  - Osteogenesis imperfecta
- Nutritional disorders
  - Anorexia nervosa
  - Parenteral nutrition
- Hepatobiliary disease
- Hypoxemia
- Hematologic malignancies
- Medications
  - Thyroid hormone
  - Glucocorticoids
  - GnRH agonist/antagonist
  - Chronic lithium
  - Chemotherapy
  - Anticonvulsants
  - Cyclosporine
  - Loop diuretics

secondary causes of osteoporosis increase the rate or amount of bone resorption, although several diseases, most notably Cushing's syndrome, can also diminish bone formation.

TREATMENT

Primary Prevention

The goal of primary prevention is to maximize attainment of peak bone mass during adolescence and young adulthood and to minimize rates of bone loss with menopause and aging. Prevention strategies should include avoiding cigarettes and alcohol, minimizing the use of medications that could contribute to accelerated bone loss, ensuring adequate calcium intake, and getting regular exercise. These recommendations are appropriate for all individuals irrespective of risk for osteoporosis.

Adequate calcium intake is necessary for attainment of peak bone mass and to decrease calcium deficiency–related accelerated bone loss. The recommended daily calcium allowance is 800 to 1000 mg/day for the premenopausal female (or postmenopausal woman on ERT), 1200 mg/day for the pregnant female, and 1500 mg/day for the postmenopausal woman not on ERT. Because calcium is a threshold nutrient, intake beyond an adequate level will not result in additional skeletal benefit. If the recommended amounts of calcium cannot be obtained by dietary modification, calcium supplements can be used. Calcium carbonate is the most commonly prescribed calcium salt because it is inexpensive and 40% of its total content is elemental calcium. However, calcium carbonate is not effectively absorbed in individuals who are achlorhydric. In this situation, calcium citrate or lactate should be prescribed. If supplements are used, they should be taken in divided doses (<600 mg at any one time). Adequate vitamin D is necessary for optimal absorption.

A regular exercise regimen is also an important component of a primary prevention regimen. In addition to increasing bone mass, exercise can improve muscle strength and coordination, thereby decreasing the risk for falls. To date, the most effective exercise regimen has been high-load resistance training with the regimen targeted to stimulate areas at risk for osteoporotic fracture. Other effective strategies for decreasing bone loss include high-impact aerobics, walk/jog/dance regimens, and stationary cycling. Although the most common recommendation is walking, there are no conclusive data that walking is sufficient to prevent bone loss. Exercise must be performed for approximately 30 to 60 minutes/day at least 3 times/week. When exercise is discontinued, any gains in bone mass achieved are quickly lost.

Secondary Prevention

The goal of secondary prevention is to prevent additional bone loss in an individual who already has evidence of some decrement in bone mass. Treatment can be based on either the severity of osteoporosis or on bone turnover markers (Box 15-3).

The standard treatment for postmenopausal osteoporosis is ERT, which can prevent bone loss and reduce the incidence of vertebral and hip

BOX 15-3
Pharmacologic Options for Osteoporosis

+Calcium balance	Antiresorptive	Stimulate formation
Calcium supplements	Estrogen	$1,25(OH)_2$ vitamin D (?)
Vitamin D analogues	Calcitonin	Fluoride
Thiazides	Etidronate	Anabolic steroids
	Alendronate	PTH

fractures by 50% to 75% after 10 or more years of use. It appears to be most effective when started within the first several years of menopause, but studies have shown that it is able to prevent additional bone loss even when started after the age of 65. Estrogen is an antiresorptive agent and decreases bone loss by inhibiting local cytokine release. It also improves menopause-induced changes in calcium balance by increasing GI calcium absorption and decreasing renal calcium loss.

ERT may be utilized for prevention of either primary or secondary osteoporosis. Other potential benefits of ERT include a decrease in vasomotor symptoms, a reduction in coronary heart disease incidence and mortality, and prevention of genitourinary atrophy. In an individual whose only indication to begin ERT is to prevent or treat osteoporosis, an initial bone mass measurement may help to facilitate a treatment decision. If the BMD T score is greater than −1, it is reasonable for a woman to begin a primary prevention strategy, withhold initiation of estrogen, and repeat the bone mass measurement. This conservative approach is safe because these individuals are at low risk for osteoporotic fracture. In contrast, if a woman already has evidence of significant osteopenia (BMD T score <-2), initiation of ERT may be more appropriate (Fig. 15-1).

A daily dose of 0.625 mg of a conjugated equine estrogen or equivalent will reduce vertebral bone loss and hip bone loss to less than 1% in 98% and 95% of women, respectively. Progestin, with either a cyclic or continuous regimen, may be utilized to reduce the incidence of endometrial cancer. Therapy should be lifelong. Within 10 years after ERT is discontinued, the risk for hip fracture is nearly identical to that of a woman who never used ERT.

For women who cannot or will not take ERT, there are several other antiresorptive options. Synthetic calcitonin, as either a subcutaneous injection or nasal spray, is an FDA-approved treatment for osteoporosis. Calcitonin inhibits osteoclastic bone resorption, thus retarding the rate of bone loss. There are no definitive data regarding the effect of long-term calcitonin use on fracture incidence. Calcitonin is most effective in individuals with high bone turnover, and its beneficial effect is observed as long as the medication is used. Its greatest therapeutic benefit, however, is based on evidence that calcitonin has inherent analgesic properties.

The recommended dose of calcitonin is 50 to 100 U of subcutaneous salmon calcitonin taken on an alternate or daily basis or 200 U of calcitonin

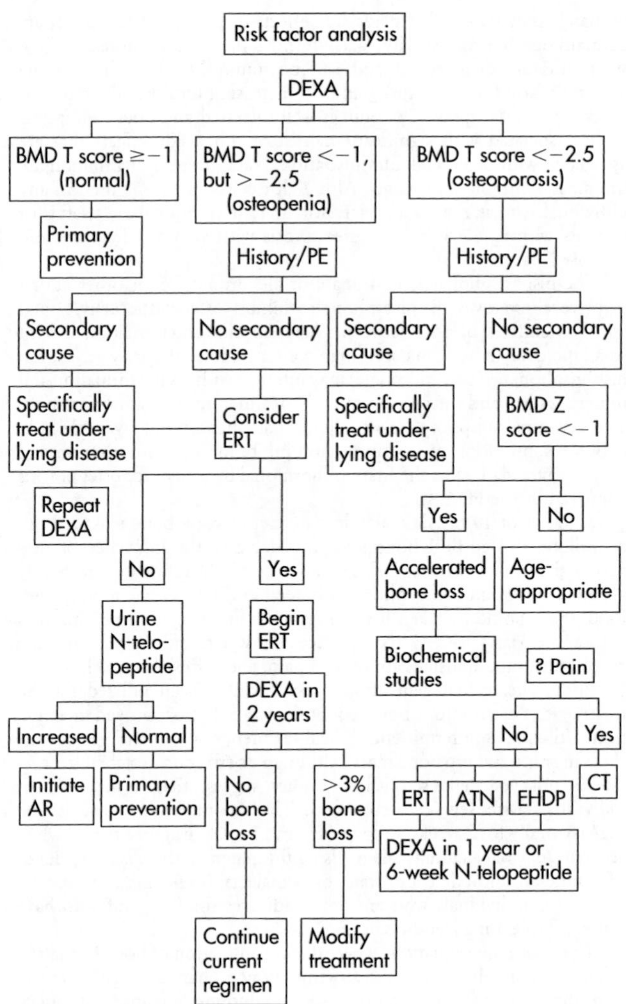

FIG. 15-1 Suggested diagnosis and treatment plan for suspected osteoporosis. *AR*, antiresponsive.

by nasal spray daily. The major side effects of parenteral calcitonin are dermatologic hypersensitivity, facial flushing, nausea, and anorexia. These symptoms are dose-related and can be diminished by initiating the calcitonin at a low dose and gradually increasing until the desired dose is reached. Nasal spray calcitonin is well tolerated and does not appear to be associated with significant nausea or other side effects that are associated with parenteral administration. Nasal dryness or irritation are the most common complaints. Although calcitonin can be used in any individual who is not a candidate for ERT, it is particularly useful for patients with severe vertebral osteoporosis with vertebral fractures and increased pain.

The bisphosphonates, etidronate or alendronate, offer other antiresorptive alternatives. Bisphosphonates inhibit osteoclastic activity and appear to shift the balance between bone resorption and formation to favor small increases in bone mass. At high concentrations, the early generation bisphosphonates (e.g., etidronate) may interfere with crystal formation and mineralization and thus require a cyclic regimen for safe administration. The new aminobisphosphonate, alendronate, has a more favorable ratio between suppression of resorption and inhibition of mineralization and may be given daily. It is the first nonhormonal treatment for osteoporosis approved by the FDA.

At doses of 10 mg/day, alendronate can increase bone mass at both cancellous and cortical bone sites and decrease the incidence of new vertebral and hip fractures by 50%. Because bisphosphonates are poorly absorbed orally and absorption is obliterated if taken concurrently with food, they should be taken first thing in the morning (30 to 60 minutes before breakfast) with 6 to 8 ounces of water. Side effects include esophagitis, mild transient abdominal pain, and diffuse bony aching.

Etidronate, a first generation drug, has also been utilized for the treatment of osteoporosis but is currently not an FDA-approved intervention. Utilizing an intermittent cyclical regimen, one can anticipate small gains in spine and hip bone mass. Although its effect on vertebral fracture rate is not yet well established, studies suggest that it may benefit individuals with severe osteoporosis. The recommended dose is 400 mg/day orally for 2 weeks, followed by an 11-week drug-free period when 1500 mg/day of calcium is taken. Using this regimen, there is no evidence of a mineralization defect or frank osteomalacia. It remains a therapeutic option for individuals who are not candidates for ERT and who have difficulty tolerating alendronate.

There are some situations where direct stimulation of bone formation might be desirable. Unlike the aforementioned pharmacologic interventions that decrease bone resorption, sodium fluoride can directly stimulate osteoblast proliferation and bone formation. Initial studies utilizing 50 to 75 mg of sodium fluoride (NaFl) daily show significant increases in bone mass. However, there is little evidence that this increase in bone mass is associated with a significant reduction in vertebral fractures but there is the suggestion of a higher incidence of appendicular fractures. Recent studies focus on a slow-release NaFl with more promising effects. Slow-release

NaFl limits conversion of fluoride to hydrofluoric acid, thus maintaining fluoride concentrations within the therapeutic window. Utilizing cycles of slow-release NaFL (25 mg twice daily) for 12 months followed by 2 months off therapy, there is evidence of substantial increases in bone mass at the spine and proximal femur and decreases in both loss of height and fracture incidence. Slow-release NaFL appears to be most beneficial in women who have an initial BMD that is >65% of the average BMD seen in young normal adults. This intervention is still investigational.

There are two additional treatment options for osteoporosis that work through maximizing calcium balance. Calcitriol can increase GI calcium and phosphate absorption and increase renal tubular calcium and phosphate reabsorption. Its effect on bone directly is not clear. Doses of 0.5 μg/day or higher prevent cancellous and cortical bone loss and potentially reduce the incidence of new fractures. The primary side effect of calcitriol is a 20% incidence of hypercalciuria and hypercalcemia. Thiazide diuretics may also be useful in decreasing fracture risk. They can influence a positive calcium balance by increasing renal calcium reabsorption. Epidemiologic studies show a reduction in the incidence of hip fractures in populations using thiazides for more than 5 years. Although thiazides are not recommended as a single agent for osteoporosis, they may have a role as the diuretic of choice in individuals with osteoporosis in whom a diuretic is indicated.

Monitoring Therapeutic Efficacy

After therapy is initiated, appropriate follow-up of therapeutic efficacy is warranted. In individuals in whom rapid assessment of the efficacy of an antiresorptive regimen is desired, a baseline followed by a repeat N-telopeptide 6 weeks later may be helpful. If the N-telopeptide has not declined by at least 25% to 30%, an adjustment in dose or a change in medication may be warranted. To help determine that the pharmacologic agent has prevented additional bone loss, however, repeat DEXA is necessary in 2 years. DEXA at shorter intervals may be appropriate in specific situations where more rapid losses of bone mass are anticipated (e.g., in women taking glucocorticoids or in the first few years of menopause). For the young menopausal woman, follow-up studies of the spine BMD should be selected for close monitoring. For individuals with severe hip osteoporosis or with degenerative changes or scoliosis in the spine, only the hip should be monitored serially.

KEY POINTS

1. Osteoporosis is a common disease characterized by a decrease in bone mass leading to an increased incidence of fractures. Bone loss occurs for years before the clinical manifestations of osteoporosis are evident. Early primary prevention may decrease the risk of osteoporosis.
2. Risk factor analysis is useful for designing preventive health strategies, but it has insufficient ability to discriminate who is likely to have osteoporosis.

3 The diagnosis of osteoporosis is made by DEXA (or other absorptiometric technique). For every one standard deviation that BMD declines, there is a doubling of the fracture risk.

4 ERT can prevent bone loss and reduce the incidence of fractures in most women. Although it is most effective when started early in menopause, it has some benefit in women with established disease. Newer FDA-approved antiresorptive agents, alendronate and the nasal spray calcitonin, offer treatment alternatives to women who cannot or will not take ERT.

SUGGESTED READINGS

Consensus Development Conference: Diagnosis, prophylaxis and treatment of osteoporosis, *Am J Med* 94:646-650, 1993.

Grady D et al: Hormone replacement therapy to prevent disease and prolong life in postmenopausal women, *Ann Intern Med* 117:1016-1037, 1992.

Kanis JA et al: Diagnosis of osteoporosis, *J Bone Miner Res* 9:1137-1141, 1994.

Liberman UA et al: Effect of oral alendronate on bone mineral density and the incidence of fractures in postmenopausal osteoporosis, *N Engl J Med* 333:1437-1443, 1995.

Lindsey R: Prevention and treatment of osteoporosis, *Lancet* 341:801-805, 1993.

New drugs for osteoporosis, *The Medical Letter* 38:1-3, 1996.

16

Ovarian Cancer

JAMES L. NICKLIN AND LARRY J. COPELAND

In the United States and most of the Western world, ovarian cancer is the fifth most common cancer among women and the second most common genital tract malignancy. Of note, the mortality rate from ovarian cancer exceeds those of all other genital tract malignancies combined. This largely reflects the propensity for this malignancy to present in advanced stage. Because the ovaries are anatomically free intraabdominal organs, the development of considerable tumor burden and metastatic dissemination to the upper abdomen and retroperitoneal nodes are frequently found at the onset of clinical symptoms.

Malignancies can arise from any of the cell types normally found in the ovary, and the ovary is a common site for metastasis of nonovarian malignancies. A histogenic classification of ovarian cancers is included in

BOX 16-1
Modified 1993 WHO Classification of Ovarian Cancer

Epithelial tumors
- Serous
- Mucinous
- Endometrioid
- Clear cell
- Brenner
- Mixed
- Undifferentiated
- Unclassified
- Mixed mesodermal tumors

Germ cell tumors
- Dysgerminoma
- Endodermal sinus tumor
- Embryonal carcinoma
- Polyembryoma
- Choriocarcinoma
  - Teratoma
  - Mature cystic
  - Immature
  - Monodermal
- Mixed
- Gonadoblastoma

Sex cord–stromal tumors
- Granulosa-theca
- Sertoli-Leydig
- Gynandroblastoma
- Lipoid cell
- Unclassified
- Mixed

Soft tissue tumors not specific to the ovary

Unclassified tumors

Secondary (metastatic) tumors

Box 16-1. Epithelial ovarian carcinomas are the most common type of ovarian malignancy, constituting 80% to 85% of all ovarian cancers. These occur predominantly in the perimenopausal and postmenopausal groups, with a mean age of 59. Germ cell tumors constitute 10% to 15% of ovarian cancers and occur mainly in the second and third decades. Sex cord–stromal cell tumors account for 3% to 5% of ovarian cancers and can occur at any age. All remaining malignancies combined total 1% to 5% of ovarian cancers.

EPITHELIAL OVARIAN CANCER

Epidemiology

Although the etiology of epithelial ovarian cancer (EOC) is not known, epidemiologic risk factors have been increasingly appreciated. EOC is more common in Western, industrialized countries and in Caucasian races, partly a result of dietary and other environmental factors, and partly caused by differing racial susceptibility. This has been demonstrated by the changing patterns of incidence experienced by emigrant populations. The total number of ovulatory menstrual cycles has been found to positively correlate with the incidence of this disease. Consequently, increasing parity, oral contraceptive use, lactation, and early menopause are associated with decreased relative risk. Other factors associated with increased risk include high socioeconomic class, high dietary fat consumption, perineal talc usage, previous mumps infection, and a history of breast, colon, or endometrial cancer. The risk associated with ovulation-induction agents is contentious because these agents are utilized in a population demonstrably at risk because of infertility. Tubal ligation is associated with a decreased incidence of the disease.

Family history is a reliable marker of risk in a small population of women. In 5% to 7% of women with EOC there is a positive family history of ovarian cancer, of which greater than 90% of these persons have a single first-degree relative with the disease. Approximately 1% of EOC presents as part of a familial ovarian cancer syndrome as defined by two or more first-degree relatives with the disease. Although this represents a small percentage of the overall population, members of these families have a risk of developing disease of 30% to 50% by virtue of an autosomal dominant transmission and incomplete penetration of oncogenes. There are three familial ovarian cancer syndromes: site-specific ovarian cancer syndrome, hereditary breast-ovarian cancer syndrome, and Lynch Syndrome II. The latter syndrome is characterized by pedigrees with an autosomal dominant risk of nonpolyposis colorectal cancer in association with adenocarcinomas of the breast, endometrium, upper GI tract, and other sites.

Staging

Ovarian cancer has four primary modes of spread. It can spread by local extension, transperitoneal seeding, lymphatic embolization, and less commonly by hematogenous embolization. Iatrogenic tumor implantation has also been described. Recognizing these biologic features and correlating them with survival, the International Federation of Gynecology and Obstetrics (FIGO) has published a staging schema for ovarian cancer that is based on the surgicopathologically proved extent of disease (Box 16-2).

Clinical Features

Early ovarian cancer is often asymptomatic and only detected during routine clinical examination. Symptoms are often mild, vague, and inconsistent, and include abdominal discomfort or pain, pressure sensation in the bladder or rectum, pelvic fullness or bloating, and sometimes dyspareunia. Occasionally patients have acute pain as a consequence of intralesional hemorrhage, rupture, or torsion. Patients with advanced disease often have abdominal swelling and pain, and sometimes a palpable mass. GI symptoms such as nausea, early satiety, anorexia, dyspepsia, and constipation are common. Because of the lateness of symptomatology and the biology of this cancer, approximately 75% of ovarian cancers are in an advanced stage when detected. An important aspect of the history is to exclude the likelihood of primary pathology from other anatomic sites,

BOX 16-2
FIGO Staging for Primary Carcinoma of the Ovary

Stage I	Growth limited to the ovaries.
IA	Growth limited to one ovary; no ascites. No tumor on the external surface; capsule intact.
IB	Growth limited to both ovaries; no ascites. No tumor on the external surfaces; capsules intact.
IC	Tumor either stage 1A or 1B but with tumor on the surface of one or both ovaries; or with capsule ruptured; or with ascites present containing malignant cells or with positive peritoneal washings.
Stage II	Growth involving one or both ovaries with pelvic extension.
IIA	Extension and/or metastases to the uterus and/or tubes.
IIB	Extension to other pelvic tissues.
IIC	Tumor either stage IIA or IIB but with tumor on the surface of one or both ovaries; or with capsule(s) ruptured; or with ascites present containing malignant cells; or with positive peritoneal washings.
Stage III	Tumor involving one or both ovaries with peritoneal implants outside the pelvis and/or positive retroperitoneal or inguinal nodes. Superficial liver metastasis equals stage III. Tumor is limited to the true pelvis, but with histologically proved malignant extension to small bowel or omentum.
IIIA	Tumor grossly limited to the true pelvis with negative nodes but with histologically confirmed microscopic seeding of abdominal peritoneal surfaces.
IIIB	Tumor of one or both ovaries with histologically confirmed implants of abdominal peritoneal surfaces, none exceeding 2 cm in diameter. Nodes negative.
IIIC	Abdominal implants >2 cm in diameter and/or positive retroperitoneal or inguinal nodes.
Stage IV	Growth involving one or both ovaries with distant metastasis. If pleural effusion is present, there must be positive cytologic test results to allot a case to stage IV. Parenchymal liver metastasis equals stage IV.

especially the breasts, the GI tract, and the remainder of the genital tract. A full systems review is mandatory for all patients as an indicator of fitness for surgery and other treatment.

Comprehensive physical examination is critical to the diagnosis because the symptoms described will often be attributed to lesser pathologies by both patient and physician alike.

Pertinent features of the physical examination include evaluation of general nutritional status, the supraclavicular lymph nodes, the breasts, and the lungs, as well as abdominal and pelvic examinations. Patients with advanced disease may have supraclavicular lymphadenopathy (rarely), pleural effusions, ascites, and palpable abdominal masses. Examination of the pelvis should begin by excluding disease in the external genitalia, vagina, and cervix. Although the Pap smear has a limited capacity to detect malignant ovarian cells shed through the fallopian tubes and uterus, it does not play a significant part in the workup of these patients and should only be performed as a screen for cervical dysplasia as indicated. Similarly, endometrial biopsy should be reserved for workup of suspected intrauterine pathology. Bimanual pelvic examination, including rectovaginal examination, is of fundamental importance in the clinical evaluation of this condition. Pelvic masses should have their size, consistency, position, and the extent of fixation to surrounding structures determined. The cul-de-sac should be carefully examined for nodularity that is highly suspicious for intraperitoneal malignancy.

The minimum investigation of patients in whom ovarian cancer is suspected should include routine preoperative hematologic and biochemical parameters (including renal and hepatic function tests), ECG, and chest x-ray. Ultrasonography or abdominopelvic CT scanning is useful in refining the preoperative clinical diagnosis and evaluating sites difficult to palpate intraoperatively. All other investigations should be employed only where clinically indicated to exclude extraovarian primary disease, for example, upper and lower GI tract endoscopy or imaging, mammography, and intravenous urography. Although a number of tumor markers have been evaluated in the management of EOC, serum CA 125 has the greatest utility in evaluating the response of disease to treatment and is of some value in distinguishing benign from malignant disease. Approximately 85% of nonmucinous EOC will be associated with an elevated serum CA 125 level. Mucinous EOC has a lower incidence of raised CA 125 levels and may be associated with raised levels of CA 19-9, CEA, or NB 70/K.

Differential Diagnosis

Differential diagnoses can be separated into genital tract pathology and extragenital tract pathology. With genital tract pathology, the most important lesions to consider include functional and benign neoplasms of the ovary, endometriosis, neoplasms of other genital tract sites, and pelvic inflammatory masses. With extragenital tract pathology, consider neoplasms of the bowel and other intraperitoneal structures; inflammatory masses secondary to appendicitis, inflammatory bowel disease, or diverticular disease; metastatic cancer from any site; and other rare conditions associated with a pelvic mass.

Treatment

In all but the earliest stage and lowest grade of EOC, management is a combination of both surgery and chemotherapy. Neither modality works optimally in isolation. Indeed, the most favorable results can only be reliably achieved with the optimal deployment of both components of treatment. Treatment of EOC can be considered in terms of early and advanced disease.

Early disease

When the possibility of EOC exists, surgery is of fundamental importance. Although the laparoscopic approach to early EOC has been described, this concept is unproved compared with conventional open surgery. Until sophisticated laparoscopic techniques are widely mastered and comparative trials can demonstrate the safety and utility of this approach, laparoscopic surgery should be restricted to specialized centers as part of investigational protocols. Surgery for early EOC must be undertaken with three objectives in mind: (1) the presence of malignancy must be confirmed, (2) the true extent or stage of surgery must be determined, and (3) consideration must be given to reproductive requirements of younger women. Figure 16-1 suggests options for surgical management of EOC.

Unless comprehensive staging is performed during surgery, 11% to 24% of apparent stage I disease will be understaged as will up to 50% of apparent stage II. This has significant prognostic and therapeutic ramifications.

Normally, stage IA, grade 1 EOC is treated with surgery alone, provided that the patient has been adequately staged. The prognosis for this group is approximately 90% 5-year survival. No randomized study has demonstrated a survival advantage for any adjuvant therapies compared with close observation in this group. The use of adjuvant treatment for stage IA, grade 2 is contentious. Most physicians, however, would recommend adjuvant treatment to all patients with grade 3 lesions and any lesion of stage IC or greater. The adjuvant treatment most popularly utilized is cisplatin (or carboplatin) and Taxol for three to six cycles. Other adjuvant regimens that have been successfully employed include intraperitoneal chemotherapy, intraperitoneal ^{32}P, whole abdominal radiotherapy, and other chemotherapy regimens.

Advanced disease

For advanced disease the extent or stage of disease is usually evident, and the surgical objectives are different. The primary goal of surgery becomes optimal removal of tumor, or *cytoreduction*. Survival from advanced EOC is inversely correlated with the amount of residual disease at completion of surgery. Every effort should be made to remove as much tumor as possible, within the bounds of acceptable postoperative morbidity. Consequently, it is not uncommon for radical pelvic surgery, resection of segments of bowel and bladder, and sometimes even splenectomy and partial phrenectomy to be performed to facilitate optimal cytoreduction.

The current standard for adjuvant therapy after maximal cytoreductive effort is six cycles of cisplatin and Taxol chemotherapy. Carboplatin is frequently used interchangeably with cisplatin. Other adjuvant chemotherapies have been utilized, as well as whole abdominal radiotherapy, intraperitoneal ^{32}P, and intraperitoneal chemotherapy. Patients treated with platinum-containing combination regimens perform consistently better than those treated with alternative regimens. There are several

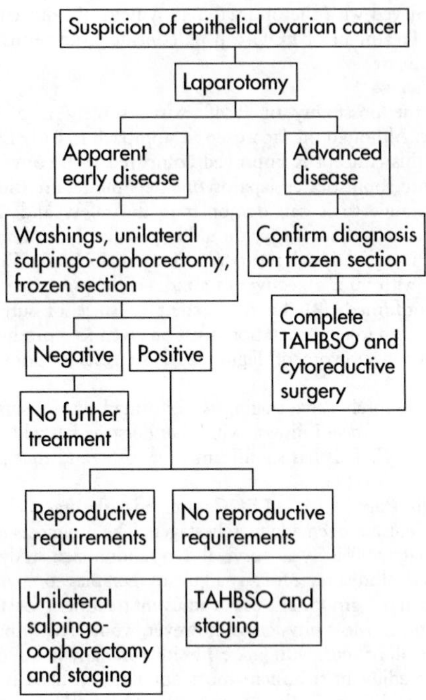

FIG. 16-1 Primary surgical management of ovarian cancer. *TAHBSO,* Total abdominal hysterectomy and bilateral salpingo-oophorectomy; *staging,* pelvic and paraaortic lymph node sampling, multiple peritoneal biopsies, infracolic omentectomy, inspect all peritoneal surfaces and biopsy suspicious lesions.

multicenter randomized trials currently being conducted to evaluate new and promising regimens.

Response to treatment is evaluated by sequential clinical evaluation and tumor marker analysis as well as periodic imaging studies. Response to debulking surgery and optimal first-line chemotherapy approximates 85%. Despite this high response rate, recurrence is common. Furthermore, in patients with an apparent complete clinical response, persistent disease can be demonstrated in up to 50% to 70% of patients. The practice of using second-look laparotomy (SLL) to more accurately evaluate disease status at the completion of primary therapy has been debated. SLL is, by definition, a laparotomy to evaluate disease status in a patient with no clinical, tumor marker, or imaging evidence of disease. This is a controversial aspect of management because no large, quality, prospective randomized trials have been conducted to evaluate the effect of this practice on survival. In patients undergoing SLL after therapy for advanced EOC, approximately 50% will have macroscopically positive disease, 20% will have microscopically positive disease, and 30% will have no histologic evidence of disease. The results of this operation have both prognostic and therapeutic implications. Patients with persistent disease have a very poor prognosis and can be offered second-line therapies at an earlier time instead of waiting for clinical evidence of disease. For those with negative disease, 50% will recur with time. This subgroup can be closely followed clinically or offered consolidation therapies.

Recurrent or persistent ovarian cancer has a poor prognosis and has been treated with second-line chemotherapy and radiotherapy. Response rates tend to be lower and of shorter duration than those with primary therapy. For patients with refractory EOC, the terminal course is usually the complication of bowel obstruction. Substantial palliative measures can be provided for these patients, using both surgical and nonsurgical measures. Although cure becomes unrealistic, quality of life and patient dignity become of primary importance.

Screening

The rationale behind screening for EOC is that with the large difference in survival between early and advanced disease, the detection and treatment of disease at the earliest possible stage may improve overall survival rates. The current screening modalities of clinical examination, serum CA 125, and transvaginal sonography have insufficient predictive value in distinguishing benign from malignant disease to be cost-effective in the general community. There may be a greater role for screening relatives of patients with EOC, in whom the prevalence of disease is greater. The NIH is considering a large, prospective, randomized trial comparing a screened with a nonscreened population. With the recent advances in molecular biology of EOC, it is possible that this may have a role in the preventive management of this disease.

GERM CELL TUMORS

Germ cell tumors characteristically arise in children and young women. These tumors typically grow very quickly, become symptomatic early, and consequently are detected most often in stage I. They commonly present in pregnancy. Whenever a rapidly growing pelvic mass, particularly with significant solid areas, is detected in a woman under 30, it should be considered a germ cell tumor until proved otherwise and treated expeditiously. There is an association between testicular feminization and other types of dysgenetic gonads and germ cell tumors, particularly dysgerminoma.

In addition to the workup discussed for EOC, there are several additional relevant tumor markers that can assist in the management of this condition such as β-HCG, alphafetoprotein (AFP), and LDH. Disgerminoma is associated with raised β-HCG in 8% of cases and frequently is associated with elevated LDH. Endodermal sinus tumor is associated with raised AFP. Immature teratoma is rarely associated with elevated tumor markers, whereas choriocarcinoma, embryonal carcinoma, and polyembryoma are all consistently associated with raised β-HCG. It should be noted that germ cell tumors are often of mixed type and the tumor marker status will reflect this.

Similar to the management of EOC, the initial treatment of germ cell tumors is surgical, and its goal is to establish histologic diagnosis, determine extent of disease, and cytoreduce the tumor load. All germ cell types have a better prognosis than EOC and are potentially curable, so in the young population in which they occur it is of paramount importance to maintain reproductive potential whenever possible. These lesions also have a greater propensity for lymphatic spread, so this aspect of staging requires particular attention. Dysgerminomas are bilateral approximately 15% of the time, whereas nondysgerminomatous germ cell tumors are rarely bilateral.

Most germ cell malignancies require adjuvant treatment after surgery. The exceptions are stage IA dysgerminomas and stage IA, grade 1 immature teratomas that have been comprehensively staged. Chemotherapy has become the mainstay of adjuvant therapy. The most commonly used regimen includes bleomycin, etoposide, and cisplatin (BEP), with vincristine, actinomycin-D, and cyclophosphamide (VAC) used as a second-line regimen. Dysgerminoma is an exquisitely radiosensitive malignancy, but this approach is rarely used as first-line adjuvant therapy because of the success of the surgicochemotherapeutic approach in curing disease and maintaining fertility. Radiotherapy does have a limited role in patients in whom reproductive potential is not required and in patients with metastatic disease unresponsive to chemotherapy.

SEX CORD–STROMAL TUMORS

These uncommon tumors can occur at any age, with a peak incidence in the postmenopausal age group. The primitive gonadal stroma has a potentially bisexual capacity. Therefore neoplasms can develop along a male pattern (Sertoli-Leydig cell tumors), along a female pattern (granulosa cell tumors), in a mixed pattern (gynandroblastoma), or in a general stromal pattern such as fibroma. Up to 30% are hormonally active, synthesizing any of the gonadal or adrenal steroid hormones. The type of hormone secreted and the patient's age at presentation will often determine the mode of presentation, for example precocious puberty, menstrual irregularity, virilization, postmenopausal bleeding, or even Cushing's syndrome. The hormonal production can be used as a tumor marker. Serum inhibin has also been used as a tumor marker for granulosa cell tumors.

The principles of treatment remain the same in management of patients with these tumors; however, because of the low incidence, the place for chemotherapy not yet been clearly defined. In younger patients with early stage, well-differentiated lesions, consideration can be given to conservative, fertility-preserving surgery. Chemotherapy regimens that have been used include BEP, VAC, VBP (vincristine, bleomycin, and cisplatin), and PAC (cisplatin, doxorubicin, and cyclophosphamide).

OTHER MALIGNANCIES

Of the remaining malignant subtypes, metastatic cancers are the most common, usually arising from the breast and GI tract. The Krukenberg tumor is a specific type of metastatic ovarian tumor characterized by the presence of signet ring cells. These are usually solid, lobulated lesions that are metastatic from the stomach or less commonly the colon. On rare occasions, no primary site can be identified.

Management of all malignancies must be individualized, based on the nature of the malignant primary cell type. Generally speaking, metastatic ovarian cancers have a poor prognosis. This may influence the radicality of surgery to the extent that a more palliative approach may be considered.

KEY POINTS

1. Ovarian cancer is a moderately common malignancy with a high fatality rate. For each malignant cell type there are distinct epidemiologic characteristics and biologic behavior patterns.
2. Treatment strategies must make allowance for these characteristics and patterns, especially with regard to the age and reproductive requirements of the patient.
3. Most ovarian malignancies are optimally managed by a combination of both surgery and chemotherapy.

SUGGESTED READINGS

Copeland LJ: *Textbook of gynecology*, Philadelphia, 1993, WB Saunders, pp 1083-1095.

Gershman DM: Epithelial ovarian cancer. In Copeland LJ, ed: *Textbook of gynecology*, Philadelphia, 1993, WB Saunders, pp 1046-1082.

McGuire WP et al: Cyclophosphamide and cisplatin compared with paclitaxel and cisplatin in patients with Stage III and Stage IV ovarian cancer, *N Engl J Med* 334:1-6, 1996.

Nicklin JL, Copeland LJ: Second-look laparotomy and secondary tumor reduction in epithelial ovarian cancer, *Adv Obstet Gynecol*, 3:439-455, 1996.

17

Papillomavirus Infections and the Abnormal Pap Smear

George S. Lewandowski

The appropriate treatment and counseling of patients with condyloma acuminata (genital warts) relies on a familiarity with pertinent issues in infectious disease, virology, epidemiology, and preventive medicine. Condyloma acuminata are visible manifestations of infection with the human papillomavirus (HPV). Research into the behavior of HPV has been hampered by an inability to grow the virus in culture. Therefore HPV may be suggested by cytology but is identified only through histologic appearance or molecular biologic testing. At present, over 70 different types of HPV have been identified.

Data obtained in the early 1980s suggests that at that time approximately 2 million women in the United States had sought treatment for HPV infection. More recent information obtained using the sensitive polymerase chain reaction (PCR) molecular biologic technique suggests that more than 30% of sexually active women may carry evidence of viral infection. The insidious nature of HPV infection in both men and women makes disease prevalence very difficult to estimate. Equally distressing is the fact that although condyloma acuminata can be treated by a number of methods, the virus *cannot* be eliminated from the genital tract by these treatments.

PATIENT PRESENTATION

Some patients ultimately found to have evidence of HPV infection will have symptoms of persistent vaginal burning or irritation unresponsive to patient-directed attempts at therapy, such as douches and nonprescription antifungal medications. Other patients will describe the intermittent appearance of genital warts or report a history of another sexually-transmitted disease or involvement with a symptomatic partner. Dyspareunia is another common symptom in HPV-exposed women.

In contrast, many women are without symptoms. The sole indication of disease may be an abnormal cervical cytologic specimen. Cytologic or molecular biologic evidence of HPV infection is found to coexist with many dysplastic lesions and cancer. Yet most women with abnormal Pap smears will have neither high-grade dysplasia nor cancer. An epidemiologic profile has been drawn that identifies women who have an increased risk for squamous cervical cancer. Some of these features include first intercourse at an early age, multiple sexual partners, a history of other sexually-transmitted diseases, low socioeconomic status, and women who have inadequate opportunities for screening.

MANAGEMENT OF THE ABNORMAL PAP SMEAR

Pap smears are for screening, and biopsy is required for diagnosis. Any visible gross lesion suspicious for cancer should be biopsied immediately, even if colposcopy is not available. Most patients with abnormal Pap smears should be considered for colposcopic evaluation with biopsy of the identified lesions. An adequate colposcopic examination of the cervix requires that the entire squamocolumnar junction is visualized, each lesion is seen in its entirety, a nondysplastic endocervical curretage is obtained (in nonpregnant patients), and the biopsy results correlate with the Pap findings.

Once the criteria for adequate colposcopy have been satisfied, appropriate therapy may be instituted with little risk of "missing" an invasive lesion. In the event of an inadequate colposcopic exam, the clinician should consider repeating the exam, perhaps focusing additional attention on the vulva and vagina. If dysplastic areas are still not identified, a cone biopsy or a loop electrical excision procedure (LEEP) should be considered. LEEP, an in-office procedure, can often replace operative cone biopsy. LEEP is performed by passing an ultrafine wire that is vibrating at radio frequency through the cervix to excise a cone or wedge of tissue; specific lesions and/or the entire transition zone may be removed. Ideally, LEEP has the potential to provide diagnostic material and complete therapy with a single procedure. It appears that in experienced hands colposcopy followed by LEEP is a safe, effective, and cost-effective means to diagnose and treat high-grade dysplastic lesions (HGSIL) and carries little risk of missing an invasive lesion. Laser vaporization and cryotherapy of the cervix are other appropriate management options for high-grade cervical dysplasia. A surgically-obtained cone biopsy with clear margins would be considered a curative procedure for squamous dysplasia. The use of hysterectomy to treat HGSIL would ordinarily constitute overtreatment in the absence of other confounding gynecologic indications.

Low-grade squamous intraepithelial lesion (LSIL) occupies a category within the Bethesda classification, which encompasses changes of viral infection as well as those formerly classified as mild dysplasia. Other cytologic descriptions refer to atypical cells, metaplasia, inflammation, or atypical squamous cells of uncertain significance (ASCUS). In the absence of a clinically obvious bacterial or fungal source of cervicitis, viral infection will often be the cause. Several authors suggest that greater than half of low-grade lesions will regress to normal without therapy. Consideration should be given to merely following a reliable LGSIL patient without therapy and reserving treatment to those who develop high-grade lesions or

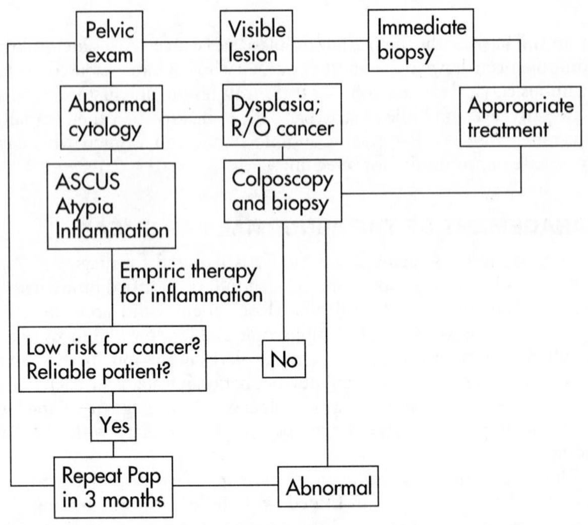

FIG. 17-1 Managing an abnormal Pap smear or a visible lesion.

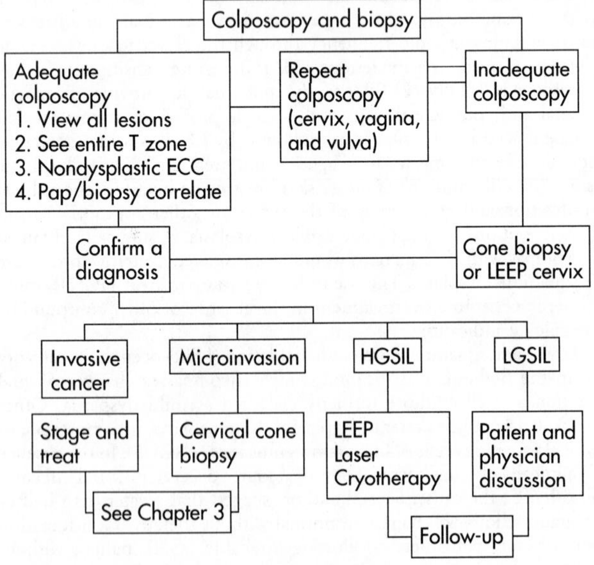

FIG. 17-2 Colposcopy and biopsy and the management of genital dysplasia.

those who are poor follow-up candidates. One proposed approach to management is shown in Figs. 17-1 and 17-2.

ADDITIONAL HPV EVALUATION

Although certain viral types (HPV 16, 18, 31, 33, 35, 45, 51, 52, and 56) are more frequently associated with higher grade dysplasias and cancer, experts disagree on the clinical utility of HPV typing. In addition to cost and individual assay sensitivity and specificity, questions exist concerning the proper management of patients who carry one of the so-called *high-risk* types. Although many patients with high-grade dysplasia or cancer are found to carry HPV 16 or 18, the majority of patients with these HPV types have *not* developed high-grade changes and may never do so. Infection with a high-risk HPV type seems to be necessary for developing high-grade genital dysplasia in most cases, but alone it is not sufficient.

TREATMENT

Goals of Therapy

Before treating HPV-related disease, the goals of the planned intervention should be clearly identified. Partners may infect one another even when both are asymptomatic. In addition, control of symptoms guarantees neither a cure nor freedom from recurrence. Three potentially achievable goals can be defined: the elimination of currently dysplastic lesions, control of distressing symptoms, and directing limited therapy at small-volume indolent and benign disease in a theoretical attempt at preventing disease intensification.

Modalities of Therapy

Treatment plans for nondysplastic HPV-related disease should address the intensity of symptoms, the modification of factors such as tobacco abuse, and the evaluation for immune suppression that may increase the risk for malignant progression. The cost of therapy, along with the patient's ability to comply with a follow-up regimen, should also be considered.

Patients with extensive involvement of the vulva, vagina, and perineum present a distinct management challenge. Systemic conditions such as pregnancy and diabetes mellitus should be ruled out. A social and sexual history should be obtained that addresses the patient's risk for AIDS. Confirmatory testing may be appropriate. Colposcopically-directed biopsies should be performed at the initial visit if needed to rule out the presence of high-grade dysplasia. Empiric antibiotic therapy with ampicillin or metronidazole for 5 to 7 days followed by a short course of antifungal medication can facilitate both symptomatic relief and shrinkage of visible virus-related lesions.

At a second visit, topical therapies can often be introduced. Podophyllin compounds (10% to 25%) have historically been used for external genital condylomas. Because of potential systemic neurotoxicity, treated areas should be rinsed in 4 to 6 hours. Podofilox (Condylox) is a 0.5% solution that is applied twice daily for 3 consecutive days followed by 4 days without treatment. Up to four weekly cycles may be used. With Podofilox, no rinsing is required; however, no more than 10 cm^2 should be treated each day. Burning, pain, inflammation, erosion, and itching have been reported in 63% to 78% of female patients.

Therapy with 85% trichloroacetic acid (TCA) is another option for topical therapy. Although it is widely used, little literature describes its efficacy. Its caustic effect is immediate, and no rinsing is required. Discomfort is also immediate, but of short duration. Unlike podophyllin, TCA has only minimal systemic absorption so it can be used on the vulva, cervix, and vagina. With either topical treatment modality, repeated treatments over several visits may be required before evaluating the success of treatment. Patients with an immediate complete response should be examined periodically and return if they develop symptoms of pain or discharge that might suggest an early recurrence.

If initial local therapy is unsuccessful, several management options should be discussed with the patient. Residual small-volume disease can be managed with outpatient excisional biopsies. Vulvar and vaginal LEEP has been proposed in this setting, and laser vaporization can be considered, but with extensive vulvovaginal or perirectal disease a regional anesthetic may be required.

A salve of 5% 5-fluorouracil (Efudex, 5-FU) can be used intravaginally to manage widespread or recurrent disease. One applicator full (10 g) may be placed into the vagina at night after application of petroleum jelly or silver sulfadiazine cream to nonaffected vulvar areas. The following morning a gentle tap water douche is used to remove additional medication from the treated areas. One to two treatments per week can generally be tolerated and a 2-to 3-month course of therapy is common. Patients should be cautioned to refrain from therapy if severe discomfort is encountered. Patients should be examined at regular intervals while on treatment to assess response and to survey for toxicity. The development of chronic ulcers that heal poorly represents a significant potential side effect. These ulcers respond poorly to medical or hormonal management; surgical excision is usually required. Using this regimen of 5-FU to treat vulvar dysplasia is not as well tolerated as vaginal treatment.

A final modality that may be successful in certain patients is the use of interferon compounds. Common side effects of interferon therapy include fever, myalgia, and malaise. The significant recurrence rate and the cost of this modality prohibit its widescale use.

ATYPICAL CYTOLOGY AND HPV INFECTION

Both the American College of Obstetricians and Gynecologists and the Centers for Disease Control and Prevention state that HPV typing is not indicated for routine clinical use. HPV testing may lack the specificity to unequivocally predict behavior. The relatively high cost of colposcopy with biopsy or LEEP provides the driving force behind a search for more efficient triage methods.

KEY POINTS

1. HPV infection is ubiquitous and often indolent and is often found in association with genital dysplasia and cancer.
2. HPV infection can be controlled by therapy, but the virus is not eliminated from the genital tract by therapy.
3. Evaluation of a patient with an abnormal Pap smear includes a pertinent history and examination followed by colposcopy and biopsy.
4. Since the virus is not eliminated by therapy, goals of treatment include elimination of dysplasia and control of symptoms.
5. Relatively few HPV-related lesions have a high malignant potential; all require careful follow-up.

SUGGESTED READINGS

Bigrigg MA et al: Colposcopic diagnosis and treatment of cervical dysplasia at a single clinic visit, *Lancet* 336:229-231, 1990.

Cecchini S et al: Follow-up Papanicolaou smear for cervical atypia: a method for identifying cases with false negative smears, *Acta Cytol* 34:778-780, 1990.

Cox JT et al: Human papillomavirus testing by hybrid capture appears to be useful in triaging women with a cytologic diagnosis of atypical squamous cells of undetermined significance, *Am J Obstet Gynecol* 172:946-954, 1995.

Cuzick J et al: Human papillomavirus testing in primary cervical screening, *Lancet* 345:1533-1536, 1995.

Gordon P, Hatch K: Survey of colposcopy practices by obstetricians/gynecologists, *J Reprod Med* 37:861-863, 1992.

Hines JF, Jenson AB, Barnes WA: Human papillomaviruses: their clinical significance in the management of cervical carcinoma, *Oncology* 9(4):279-291, 1995.

Kataya S et al: Prospective follow-up of genital HPV infections: survival analysis of the HPV typing data, *Eur J Epidemiol* 6:9, 1990.

Lorincz AT et al: Human papillomavirus infection of the cervix: relative risk associations of 15 common anogenital types, *Am J Obstet Gynecol* 79:328, 1992.

Miller BE et al: The presentation of adenocarcinoma of the uterine cervix, *Cancer* 72:1281-1285, 1993.

Sherman ME et al: Correlation of cytopathologic diagnoses with detection of high-risk human papillomavirus types, *Am J Clin Pathol* 102:182-187, 1994.

Schiffman MH: Recent progress in defining the epidemiology of human papillomavirus infection and cervical neoplasia, *J Natl Cancer Inst* 84:394, 1992.

Schiffman MH et al: Epidemiologic evidence showing that human papillomavirus infection causes most cervical intraepithelial neoplasia, *J Natl Cancer Inst* 85:958-964, 1993.

18

Pelvic Inflammatory Disease and Its Sequelae

WAYNE C. TROUT

The female genital tract is unique among organ systems in that a direct connection exists from the microbiologically diverse vagina to the sterile protected space of the peritoneal cavity. Bacteria that enter these normally sterile spaces can result in symptomatic infections of the endometrium, fallopian tube, ovary, and adjacent peritoneum; these upper tract infections (endometritis, salpingitis, tuboovarian abscess, and peritonitis) are collectively termed *pelvic inflammatory disease (PID).* The body's response to pelvic infection often results in damage to the mucosal surfaces of the fallopian tubes, which may have long-term medical consequences.

EPIDEMIOLOGY

Sexually transmitted infections have been epidemic since the sexual revolution of the 1960s. PID is typically the result of infection with sexually transmitted organisms that have bypassed the protective barriers of the cervix and gained access to the upper genital tract.

An estimated 1 million women are treated for PID annually; 250,000 to 300,000 of these women require hospitalization. Approximately 150,000 surgical procedures are performed each year because of complications of pelvic infections. Treatment of PID and its sequelae cost over $4 billion in 1990; this number is expected to surpass $10 billion by 2000.

Age is inversely proportional to the risk of having PID. Hospitalization rates are highest among sexually active females from ages 15 to 19 (three times higher than from ages 25 to 29). Race has been a risk factor for PID. Twice as many nonwhites than whites have PID (23% versus 13%). Women with multiple sexual partners are at higher risk of PID. IUDs are associated with upper genital tract infections. Barrier contraceptives and oral contraceptives are protective.

The symptomatic onset of PID often corresponds with the menstrual cycle. Two thirds of patients will become symptomatic during or within days after ending their menstrual cycle when there are breaks in the natural protective barriers of the genital tract. One of the protective host defenses is the cervical mucous plug; the endometrium may provide some additional protection. During the menstrual phase the mucous plug is lost and the endometrium is sloughed; the sloughed endometrium is an exceptional culture medium. Most cases of PID occur as an ascending infection (possibly aided by spermatozoa or the motile *Trichomonas vaginalis*), though hematogenous or lymphatic spread may also occur.

Iatrogenic causes of PID include hysterosalpingography, IUD insertion, and cervical dilation for pregnancy termination.

DIAGNOSIS

Laparoscopic visualization of the fallopian tubes is the ideal procedure for diagnosis of PID, however the surgical risks and costs of laparoscopy have prevented its widespread use. In acute salpingitis the tubes appear erythematous, with capillary injections; they may appear edematous. In advanced infection the surface will have a sticky exudative covering and frank pus may be seen coming from within the lumen. Only two thirds of women suspected of having PID will have laparoscopic confirmation of the disease, reflecting the shortcomings of the clinical criteria.

Diagnosis of PID cannot be made in the absence of abdominal, uterine, and adnexal tenderness; other systemic signs of infection should be identified. The most commonly used diagnostic criteria are shown in Box 18-1.

Endometrial biopsy has recently been described as a means to demonstrate inflammation of the uterus and can be utilized when the diagnosis is unclear. The identification of neutrophils and plasma cells in the endometrial stroma has correlated well with the laparoscopic diagnosis of PID. A contemporary approach to PID is depicted in Fig. 18-1. The rationale is to have broad defining criteria when the clinical presentation is mild (high sensitivity, low specificity) but to demand exact criteria when the patient is clinically ill (high specificity).

BOX 18-1
PID: Clinical Diagnostic Criteria

Major criteria: all should be present
Abdominal tenderness
Cervical motion tenderness
Adnexal tenderness
Minor criteria: one of the following should be present
Temperature $\geq$ 38° C
WBC $\geq 10.5 \times 10^3$/cc
ESR > 15mm/hr
Evidence of *N. gonorrhoeae* or *C. trachomatis* in the endocervix
Culdocentesis positive for bacteria and WBC in peritoneal fluid
Presence of inflammatory mass noted on pelvic exam or sonography

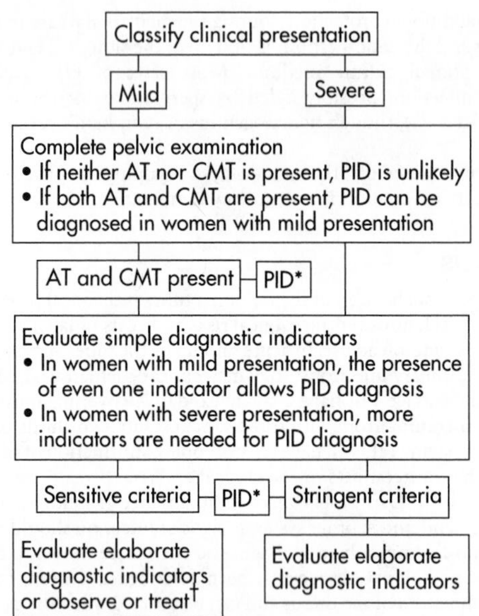

FIG. 18-1 PID diagnostic model. *PID was diagnosed in the absence of strong evidence for a competing diagnosis. †Management depends on available tests, compliance, and patient preference. *AT,* adnexal tenderness; *CMT,* cervical motion tenderness. (From Kahn JG et al: *JAMA* 266(18):2594, 1991.)

MICROBIOLOGY

Gonorrhea is recovered from the cervix in 25% to 50% of patients with PID. The infection is able to ascend through the genital tract. Production of endotoxin can cause tubal mucosal damage. Marked elevations in temperature are frequently seen in women with PID caused by gonorrhea, which is also endotoxin mediated.

Chlamydia is similarly recovered from the cervix in 25% to 50% of women with acute PID. The clinical course of chlamydial PID is typically milder than that of gonorrhea. Women with chlamydial infections are more likely to be afebrile and have a more indolent course. Chlamydia is playing a greater role as a causative agent for PID, and as a result *silent PID* has become increasingly more common. Chlamydia replicates intracellularly, causing destruction of the tubal mucosa. Some of the tubal damage and peritoneal scarring are believed to be caused by an autoimmune phenomenon. In some women an immunologic response to the chlamydial heat shock protein can elicit a delayed hypersensitivity reaction that has been correlated with the degree of tubal scarring. The Fitz-Hugh–

Curtis syndrome refers to the observation of adhesions between the diaphragm and the liver seen frequently with PID.

C. trachomatis and *N. gonorrhoeae* are recovered from the cul-de-sac or the fallopian tubes at a much lower rate than from the cervix. The bacteria most commonly encountered are mixed anaerobic (peptostreptococcus and bacteroides) and aerobic (*E. coli,* streptococcus). The most likely reason for this discrepancy is that after the initial tubal infection bacterial superinfection is more likely to occur in the damaged mucosa. Subsequently alterations of the local environment (i.e., pH, oxygen tension, and redox potential) favor the growth of these mixed infections. Overgrowth with these bacteria may alter the environment such that the original sexually transmitted organism can no longer be recovered. Histologically diagnosed endometritis has recently been associated with bacterial vaginosis. This may represent another cause (or risk factor) for the development of PID because the abnormal vaginal flora may ascend into the upper genital tract.

TREATMENT

Outpatient

Successful outpatient management of uncomplicated cases of acute salpingitis requires patient compliance. Approximately 70% to 75% of patients with acute PID are initially managed on an ambulatory basis. To be eligible for outpatient treatment, a patient must reliably take the prescribed antibiotics and be able to return for a follow-up visit in 48 to 72 hours. Patients who fail these criteria should be treated on an inpatient basis (Box 18-2). Those patients in whom an adnexal abscess is suspected or who fail to improve after initial outpatient treatment should be hospitalized. The consensus is that the outpatient treatment failure rate is high. Because PID is most common in younger women and is associated with serious, long-term reproductive sequelae, many practitioners advocate hospitalization of all adolescents suspected of having acute salpingitis.

Treatment of acute salpingitis should be effective against the sexually transmitted bacteria that initiated the infection as well as cover the mixed aerobic and anaerobic bacteria that are present in later stages of the

BOX 18-2
Indications for Hospitalization for PID

Diagnosis is uncertain (appendicitis, ectopic pregnancy)
Pelvic abscess is suspected
Patient is pregnant
Patient is an adolescent (noncompliant)
Severe symptoms prevent outpatient management
Patient is unable to follow or tolerate outpatient treatment
Failure of outpatient treatment
Unable to have patient follow up in 72 hours for evaluation

BOX 18-3

Outpatient Treatment of PID

REGIMEN A

Single dose of one of the following:

Ceftriaxone 250 mg IM

Cefoxitin 2 g IM with probenecid 1 g orally

Other third generation cephalosporin (e.g., ceftizoxime or cefotaxime)

PLUS

Doxycycline 100 mg orally 2 times daily for 2 weeks

REGIMEN B

Ofloxacin 400 mg orally 2 times daily for 2 weeks

PLUS

Clindamycin 450 mg orally 4 times daily for 2 weeks

OR

Metronidazole 500 mg orally 2 times daily for 2 weeks

BOX 18-4

Inpatient Treatment of PID

REGIMEN A

Cefoxitin 2 g IV every 6 hours, or

Cefotetan 2 g IV every 12 hours

PLUS

Doxycycline 100 mg IV/orally every 12 hours

REGIMEN B

Clindamycin 900 mg IV every 8 hours

PLUS

Gentamicin 2 mg/kg load followed by 1.5 mg/kg IV every 8 hours

infection. The CDC has recommended several antibiotics as first-line agents for outpatient therapy and also recommend treatment with a second agent to cover for chlamydia (Box 18-3). Alternative antibiotic therapies have also been used. Their success depends on their ability to cover mixed aerobic/anaerobic infections and chlamydia.

Inpatient

Patients who do not meet criteria for outpatient management should be admitted for observation and treated with parenteral antibiotics (Box 18-4). Treatment should be continued until the patient is afebrile and the abdominal and pelvic tenderness resolves. Usually a clinical response is seen within 48 hours of treatment. If the patient fails to improve, the clinician should suspect either pelvic abscess or incorrect diagnosis.

SEQUELAE

Tuboovarian Abscess

In advanced disease, an inflammatory complex of the ovary and fallopian tubes, a tuboovarian abscess (TOA), will form. The host defenses will attempt to isolate this infection, and the resulting abscess may be confined to the ovary and tube or may extend to the adjacent peritoneum and bowel.

Diagnosis

Because of the limitations of the pelvic exam in women with PID, the tender, fluctuant mass suggestive of a TOA is difficult to diagnose. The clinician must rely on radiologic studies to diagnose many of these abscesses. Ultrasound is the most useful diagnostic radiologic test because of its familiarity to the gynecologist, and it is the study of choice for most gynecologic disorders. With TOA, the typically sharp ovarian border seen with ultrasound will be obscured, and the ovary may be replaced by a heterogenic echodense mass. CT can also be used; its advantage is the ability to identify nongynecologic pathology. Abscesses on CT scan have a typical appearance, and small gas bubbles can be observed. Nuclear medicine imaging techniques are limited and provide little help in differentiating an abscess from inflammation.

Treatment

Surgical. A ruptured TOA is a surgical emergency; delayed diagnosis and treatment will result in significant mortality. Broad spectrum antibiotics, if not already being used, should be administered while the patient is prepared for surgery. Cardiovascular and respiratory support may be required. Peripheral vasodilation should be treated with fluid administration. Typically, a vertical skin incision is required to perform thorough abdominal exploration because purulent fluid may be located between loops of bowel. The subdiaphragmatic spaces should be explored and copiously irrigated. There is no evidence that antibiotics in the irrigation fluid are of any benefit.

The classic treatment for abscesses has been incision and drainage. Extension of the inflammatory mass into the cul-de-sac can allow transvaginal drainage through a colpotomy incision. The requirements for this procedure are that the mass be felt dissecting (pointing) into the rectovaginal space, be midline, and be fixed. Mobile, lateral masses are likely to be pushed up away from the incision and cause intraperitoneal leaking. Drainage of the abscess can also be performed radiologically with a CT-guided aspiration. Other surgical approaches include laparoscopy, with or without drain placement, and laparotomy. Therapeutic removal of the uterus and both adnexa has been advocated in the past, but it is now recognized that more conservative treatments are equally effective.

Medical therapy. Improvements in the antibiotic armamentarium have allowed for successful nonsurgical therapy in two thirds of patients with a TOA. The contemporary approach to the patient with a TOA is a trial of broad spectrum antibiotics effective against the mixed aerobic/anaerobic flora present in the abscess cavity. *E. coli,* anaerobic streptococci, *B. fragilis,* and other *Bacteroides* species are the most commonly recovered organisms in these abscesses, and coverage against these organisms is the mainstay of modern antibiotic therapy.

Infertility

Approximately 20% of women with PID will become involuntarily infertile. An estimated 255,500 new cases of infertility occur each year as a result of PID. Tubal factor infertility is seen in 37% of women in developed countries where antibiotics are readily available (versus 85% in developing countries). Serologic studies have shown antibodies to chlamydia in a large number of women with infertility, and infertility is more common in those women who have had nongonococcal PID than those with gonococcal PID. The increasingly young age of sexual experience coupled with the recent trend of postponed childbearing has created a window of opportunity for chlamydia to cause tubal scarring. Some studies show that early (before 2 days after the onset of symptoms) treatment of chlamydia correlates with a lower rate of infertility. Many practitioners advocate hospitalization of *all* women with PID to ensure adequate compliance and prevent future infertility. The rate of infertility increases with each episode of PID (first episode, 11%; second, 34%; three or more, 54%).

Ectopic Pregnancy

Tubal scarring may allow the relatively small spermatozoa to traverse the fallopian tube but prevent the migration of the fertilized ovum into the uterus. The zygote will therefore implant in the tube as an ectopic pregnancy. Approximately 44,000 ectopic pregnancies each year result from the sequelae of PID. A single episode of PID will increase the risk of subsequent ectopic pregnancy sixfold.

Pelvic Pain

Chronic pelvic pain will be a long-term sequela in an estimated 15% to 20% of women with PID. Pelvic pain can be incapacitating for these women and may result in inability to work, multiple physician visits, and surgical intervention. Pelvic adhesions are one of the etiologic factors of pelvic pain, and minimal scarring can be seen in women with significant discomfort.

KEY POINTS

1 PID is typically the result of infection with sexually transmitted organisms that have bypassed the protective barriers of the cervix and gained access to the upper genital tract.

2 Age is inversely proportional to the risk of having PID. Hospitalization rates are highest among sexually active females from ages 15 to 19.

3 Diagnosis of PID cannot be made in the absence of abdominal, uterine, and adnexal tenderness.

4 Sequelae of PID include tuboovarian abscess, ectopic pregnancy, chronic pelvic pain, and infertility. Approximately 20% of women with PID will become involuntarily infertile.

SUGGESTED READINGS

Centers for Disease Control and Prevention: 1993 sexually transmitted diseases treatment guidelines, *MMWR* 42 (No-RR14).

Kahn JG et al: Diagnosing pelvic inflammatory disease: a comprehensive analysis and considerations for developing a new model, *JAMA* 266(18):2594-2604, 1991.

Mead PB, Hager WD, eds: *Infection protocols for obstetrics and gynecology*, Montvale, NJ, 1992, Medical Economics Publishing.

Soper DE: Pelvic inflammatory disease, *Infect Dis Clin North Am* 8(4):821-840, 1994.

Sweet RL, Gibbs RS: Mixed anaerobic-aerobic infections and pelvic abscess. In *Infectious diseases of the female genital tract*, ed 2, Baltimore, 1990, Williams & Wilkins, pp 75-108.

Sweet RL, Gibbs RS: Pelvic inflammatory disease. In *Infectious diseases of the female genital tract*, ed 2, Baltimore, 1990, Williams & Wilkins, pp 241-266.

19

Pelvic Masses—Benign

MICHAEL L. BLUMENFELD

Many pelvic masses are totally asymptomatic and may be incidentally diagnosed during a routine pelvic examination, an x-ray examination, or an ultrasound scan. A concise patient history, careful physical examination, and appropriate evaluation and diagnostic imaging can help to narrow the diagnosis and determine further medical or surgical options.

The differential diagnosis of a pelvic mass should be initially organized with respect to three stages during a woman's life: premenarchal, reproductive, and postmenopausal. Generally, malignant masses are more often found in older women, whereas functional cysts, benign neoplasms, and complex masses caused by infection are predominant in younger patients.

DIAGNOSIS

A careful review of the patient's history and a physical examination that includes a pelvic examination will focus the evaluation. The patient's age and menstrual history are also important.

Serum qualitative and quantitative β-HCG levels should be checked to rule out pregnancy when evaluating a woman in her reproductive years with a pelvic mass. A blood profile should include a CBC with a differential and ESR to evaluate the possibility of infectious cause (Fig. 19-1).

Cultures of the cervix for sexually transmitted diseases such as chlamydia and gonorrhea should be performed in selected patients. The Pap smear may also provide information for hormonal evaluation and microbiology. Other endocrine tests should be done when certain types of hormone-secreting ovarian tumors are suspected. The measurement of tumor markers such as CA 125 should also be performed on a selective

History
- Premenarchal
- Reproductive
- Postmenopausal

Physical examination

Laboratory tests
- β-HCG
- CBC
- ESR

Imaging studies
- Flat plate abdominal x-ray
- Ultrasonography
- MRI

Differential diagnoses

Congenital

Functional
- Follicular
- Hemorrhagic corpus luteum
- Theca-lutein

Endometrioma

Mature teratoma

Leiomyomas
- Pedunculated/subserosal

Infections
- Hydrosalpinx
- Pyosalpinx
- Tuboovarian abscess

Management/treatment

Observation

Pharmacologic
- combination

Surgical

FIG. 19-1 Evaluation of benign pelvic masses.

basis. However, it is not recommended as a routine screening test for ovarian epithelial tumors. HIV status may be evaluated in selected patients. Grossly reactive lymphadenopathy has been seen in the pelvis and resembles a large pelvic mass.

Ancillary diagnostic procedures such as culdocentesis, sigmoidoscopy, cystoscopy, imaging procedures, and laparoscopy should be performed when indicated.

Imaging procedures that are frequently used in the assessment of pelvic masses include a flat plate x-ray of the abdomen, pelvic ultrasonography, CT, and MRI. The flat plate of the abdomen may show evidence of calcification or dental structure in the pelvis, findings highly suggestive of a benign ovarian teratoma. A CT scan is an excellent way to look at detailed anatomy of the pelvis, particularly in the obese patient where an ultrasound scan may be compromised. CT can also be used to guide biopsies into pelvic tissue to avoid major surgery. MRI is a good method for evaluating uterine anomalies and adenomyosis of the uterus. Ultrasonography of the pelvis is the most important, practical imaging technique used to evaluate pelvic disorders. Assessment should include both abdominal and transvaginal techniques, and in certain patients the use of transperineal or transrectal scanning may be necessary. Occasionally, color Doppler flow will add significant information.

DIFFERENTIAL DIAGNOSIS

Premenarche

Before menarche, it is rare to have a physiologic cause of the enlargement of an organ or the development of a mass in the pelvis and thus careful and complete assessment is required. Investigation and treatment should not be delayed because most occurrences will be related to pathology, such as a germ cell tumor of the ovary. The young child has a small pelvis, thus a moderate-sized mass will move out of the pelvis and into the abdomen.

The following conditions can cause a pelvic mass in the premenarchal female:

1. Neoplasms (ovarian): Germ cell tumor (mature or immature teratoma, dysgerminoma, endodermal sinus tumor, choriocarcinoma, embryonal cell carcinoma, polyembryoma, and mixed tumors), gonadoblastoma (rare in this group), epithelial ovarian tumor (rare), gonadal stromal tumor (granulosa cell tumor), and others (sarcoma botryoid, presacral teratoma, lymphoma, and neuroblastoma).
2. Congenital abnormalities: Pelvic kidneys (incidence 1 in 600), uterine anomalies (bicornuate or didelphic uterus), and vaginal septum.
3. Functional ovarian cyst: Follicular cyst, germinal inclusion cyst, and paraovarian cyst (all rare in this age group).

Reproductive Phase

Follicular or corpus luteum cysts and pathologic complications of these account for the majority of etiology. Pregnancy and pregnancy-related complications must *always* be considered in the initial evaluation of patients in this age group. Infectious exposure may result in PID and subsequent hydrosalpinx, pyosalpinx, or TOA. Uterine leiomyomas and benign ovarian teratomas are also quite common.

Masses that occur during the reproductive years include congenital anomalies of the uterus and, functional cysts (Fig. 19-2). Follicular cysts account for 20% to 50% of ovarian cysts, can reach in size from 6 to 8 cm in diameter, are usually incidentally found on pelvic examination, and usually regress after two to three menstrual cycles but may cause acute pain secondary to torsion or rupture. Hemorrhagic corpus luteum cysts result

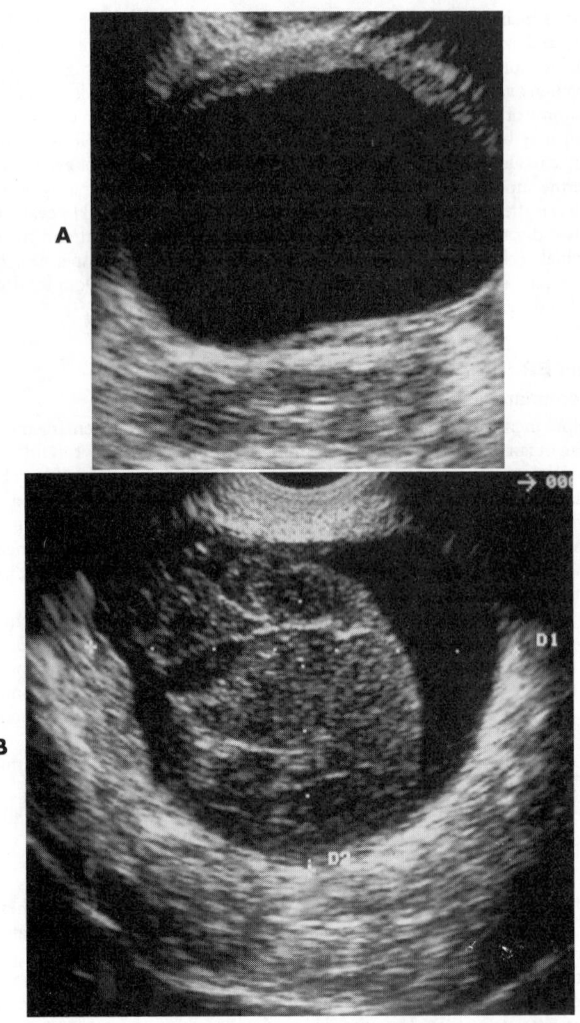

FIG. 19-2 A, Functional ovarian cyst. **B,** Hemorrhagic corpus luteum cyst with clot retraction.

Continued

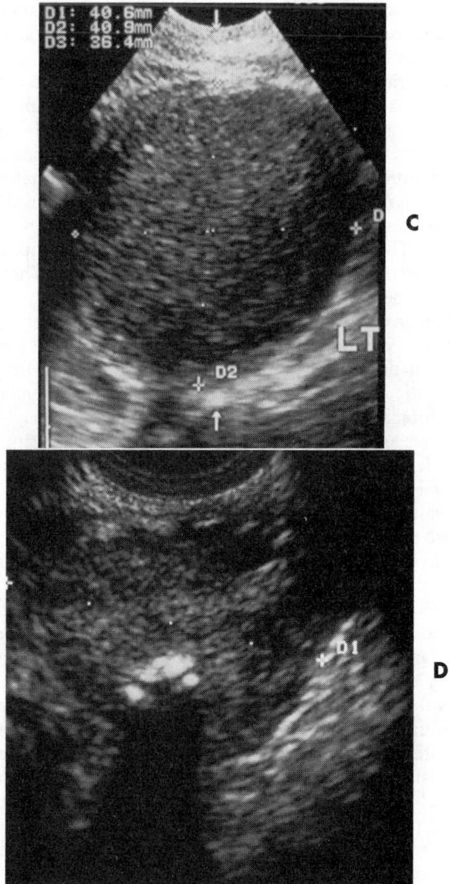

FIG. 19-2, cont'd C, Endometrioma–a typical ultrasound appearance. **D,** Benign teratoma with calcified structure.

after ovulation and subsequent hemorrhage into the cystic cavity; these cysts are usually smaller than 8 cm in size, and generally regress after two to three menstrual cycles. Theca-lutein cysts are occasionally seen in normal pregnancies; often accompany trophoblastic disease or hyperplacentosis in patients with diabetes or multiple gestations; show rapid growth (up to 15 cm), with widespread luteinization of the ovary and multiloculation; usually spontaneously regress when HCG stimulation is discontinued; and can rupture under torsion, causing subsequent acute abdominal pain.

Endometriomas ("chocolate cysts") occur secondary to cyclic bleeding into the cyst, are usually smaller than 10 to 12 cm in diameter, often are immobile because of ovarian adhesions, and occasionally are associated with increased pelvic pain, peritonitis, and pelvic adhesions.

The mature cystic teratoma, often inappropriately referred to as a *dermoid cyst,* is one of the most common ovarian neoplasms (10% to 20%). Teratomas constitute 20% to 40% of all pelvic tumors that complicate pregnancy. These ovarian neoplasms are actually composed of well-differentiated tissue arising from all three germ cell layers. These neoplasms have three types:

1. The benign cystic teratoma contains derivatives of two or more germ cell layers with differentiation and maturity of those tissue elements.
2. A malignant teratoma, a predominantly solid tumor, frequently contains cystic structures that are malignant and lack differentiation.
3. A carcinoma-sarcoma arising in a benign cystic teratoma. Mature cystic teratomas are believed to originate from primordial germ cells. Also, multiple studies have demonstrated that these benign ovarian teratomas have karyotypes of 46,XX origin.

The vast majority of these tumors occur during the reproductive years. About two thirds of the mature cystic teratomas are incidentally discovered during physical examination, imaging procedures, or abdominal surgery. These tumors usually measure 5 to 10 cm in diameter and are bilateral in 10% to 15% of the cases. On pelvic examination, the ovary often palpates as enlarged and cystic in nature and is often anterior to the uterus. Within the cystic areas may be a solid mass projecting from the wall, referred to as *Rokitansky's protuberance.* It is a common sign of malignant transformation and thus should be appropriately examined in the pathology laboratory.

On ultrasound scan, a benign teratoma will usually be a well-defined, encapsulated, complex, solid, cystic mass with heteroechogenic components. Characteristic sonographic images of the contents, including teeth, bone, and hair, as well as sebaceous or fatty material, may allow for a precise narrowing of the differential diagnosis.

Although most teratomas are asymptomatic, torsion of the adnexa is the most common complication, with the torsion rate at around 3.2%. Mature cystic teratomas have been reported to undergo spontaneous rupture, although this is a rare event. When a teratoma ruptures, the patient may experience acute peritonitis. On a more chronic basis, the development of granulomatous peritonitis may be found.

Two other areas of interest regarding teratomas are the development of thyroid tissue and malignancies associated with mature cystic teratomas. Thyroid tissue is a relatively frequent component of a mature cystic teratoma and is found in up to 20% of the cases. Called *struma ovarii,* these tumors can cause clinical hyperthyroidism. Malignant association occurs in less than 2% of teratomas, with invasive squamous cell carcinoma being the most common.

Uterine leiomyomas are also common and are found in 20% of all females over 35 years of age. They are twice as frequent in black females (one in two) as in white females. They vary in size from microscopic to large, multinodular masses. Myomas are rarely noted to occur before puberty and usually undergo various degrees of atrophy after menopause. This suggests that myoma growth is probably hormonally stimulated. Myomas are classified based on growth. The vast majority are intramural. Subserosal myomas are commonly pedunculated and rarely become parasitic to the omentum or peritoneal structures. Approximately 5% to 10% of myomas are submucosal, and 1% to 5% are cervical. Myomas are frequently multiple. The incidence of malignant degeneration, leiomyosarcoma, is less than .5% of all leiomyomas. It should be remembered, however, that the peak incidence of leiomyosarcoma is actually in the 30 to 40 years of age group. Most leiomyomas are asymptomatic. However, 30% of women with leiomyomas may have pelvic pain and abnormal uterine bleeding. Clinical symptoms depend on size and location of the lesions.

Other clinical and pathologic concerns include degenerative changes such as carneous (red degeneration), hyaline, cystic, fatty, myxomatous, calcification, or malignant degeneration; urological problems; obstetric complications; and intravenous leiomatosis.

Infection of related structures in the pelvis may produce an acute pelvic mass during an active episode of PID. The mass may be a pelvic abscess or TOA involving the fallopian tube, ovary, broad ligament, uterus, and nearby omentum or bowel. These masses may require surgical excision and drainage, but often can be successfully treated with aggressive antibiotic therapy. Inflammatory masses may include hydrosalpinx, pyosalpinx, or TOAs.

Paraovarian cysts and hydatid of Morgagni account for 10% of adnexal masses; are remnants of the wolffian duct; are benign and usually unilocular; can reach very large sizes up to 20 cm, but usually do not torse; have a mass effect that displaces the uterus; and necessitate surgical removal to differentiate them from other neoplasms.

Miscellaneous pelvic masses in the reproductive-age woman include a distended bladder, usually caused by a neurogenic disorder or entrapped uterus; appendiceal abscess; epiploic appendagitis (torsion or infarction of the epiploic appendage); lymphatic hemangioma of the pelvis; and lymphadenopathy. With the alarming increase of heterosexual spread of the HIV virus, more and more women are being seen with immune suppression and lymphadenopathy. A conglomerate of enlarged pelvic lymph nodes may present as an adnexal mass.

Postmenopausal Women

During menopause and postmenopause, any mass or abnormal bleeding must be considered a neoplastic process until proved otherwise. Aggressive investigation is needed for these patients. Nongynecologic pathologic processes may also present during these years as an apparent pelvic mass. It is important to note that small ovarian cysts (less than 3 cm) are more common than was once thought. The following conditions must be considered in the differential diagnosis of a pelvic mass in postmenopausal women:

1. Ovarian: Epithelial, germ cell, and stromal tumors and functional cysts, usually small–less than 3 cm
2. Uterus: Endometrial carcinomas or sarcomas
3. Fallopian tube: Rare carcinomas
4. Urogenital: Diverticulum or carcinoma of the bladder, neuropathies
5. Gastrointestinal mass from diverticula, appendiceal abscess, or Crohn's disease
6. Abdominal aneurysms and pelvic hemangiomas
7. Metastatic disease (Krukenberg's tumor): primary lesion sites most common in the breast or colon

MANAGEMENT

Management should ultimately be based on observation, pharmacologic therapy, surgical therapy, radiation therapy, and combinations of these. Based on these options, a final management plan can be established in a sequential manner. Some important considerations to keep in mind include the following:

1. It is rare to have a functional cyst before menarche or after menopause.
2. Any mass or abnormal bleeding after menopause should be considered a malignancy until proved otherwise.
3. One must rule out the possibility of pregnancy in a woman in the reproductive years before an extensive workup is ordered.
4. Any mass in excess of 8 cm in any age group and any solid mass should be considered for surgical evaluation by laparoscopy or laparotomy.

THERAPY

Therapy will vary based on the patient's age, parity, and plans for childbearing, as well as symptoms. For follicular luteal cysts, if an incidental finding is a cyst less than 6 to 8 cm, follow conservatively and observe for spontaneous regression over two to three menstrual cycles. If a cyst is symptomatic or persists or enlarges, proceed with a laparoscopy for aspiration or excision of the cyst. Ovarian suppression with oral contraceptives may be tried with the functional cyst, although the therapeutic effect has not been well studied. Endometriomas are primarily managed surgically with or without medical suppressive therapy. All teratomas are surgically treated via laparoscopy or laparotomy, oophorectomy, or conservative cystectomy.

For leiomyomas, the physician should treat anemia, if present, with iron supplementation and/or transfusion, if needed. With the administration of a GnRH analogue, pituitary suppression can be temporarily achieved, allowing for cessation of the bleeding and subsequent restoration of normal hemoglobin.

Conservative therapy with close observation and follow-up every 4 to 6 months is appropriate for those with minimal symptoms, small tumors in pregnancy, or postmenopausal women.

Indications for myomectomy include repetitive miscarriages, long-standing infertility, persistent abnormal bleeding, pain or pressure, and a rapidly expanding mass or enlargement of an asymptomatic myoma to more than 8 to 10 cm in a woman who has not completed her childbearing. Recurrence after myomectomy has been reported to be 5% to 25%.

Hysterectomy indications include severe symptoms (i.e., pain and pressure), considerable size (greater than 12 weeks gestation) uterus in a patient who has completed childbearing who desires definitive treatment, and rapid growth of the myoma. For paraovarian cysts, surgical excision is usually indicated if cysts are large. Hydatid of Morgagni do not need to be removed.

TORSION

All pelvic masses can potentially undergo torsion, causing acute intermittent or persistent pain. With torsion of the pedicle there may be a compromise in the venous return and secondary vascular congestion with subsequent edema. In mild cases of vascular compromise, there may be no significant findings. In severe cases, the adnexa will significantly enlarge. There may be an increase in the surrounding peritoneal fluid. If untreated in an early stage, necrosis may be seen. Sonographic examination will show an enlarged ovary with midlevel echoes throughout in a very homogenous pattern suggestive of a very edematous ovary secondary to significant vascular congestion.

KEY POINTS

1. The differential diagnosis of a pelvic mass should be initially organized with respect to three stages during a woman's life: premenarchal, reproductive, and postmenopausal.
2. Ultrasonography is an excellent adjunct to history and physical examination in the assessment and diagnosis of pelvic masses.

SUGGESTED READINGS

Droegemueller W et al: *Comprehensive gynecology,* St. Louis, 1987, Mosby.

Gabbe SG, Neibyl JR, Simpson JL: *Obstetrics: normal and problem pregnancies,* ed 2, New York, 1991, Churchill-Livingstone.

Copeland LJ, Jarrell JR, McGregor J: *Textbook of gynecology,* Philadelphia, 1993, WB Saunders.

Sweet RL, Gibbs RS: *Infectious diseases of the female genital tract,* ed 2, Baltimore, 1990, Williams & Wilkins.

Reich H: New techniques in advanced laparoscopic surgery. In Sutton C, ed: *Valeries clinical obstet gynecol,* Philadelphia, 1989, WB Saunders.

20

Pelvic Pain—Chronic

John S. McDonald

The workup, diagnosis, and management of the female patient with lower abdominal pain or pelvic pain are often frustrating processes for the clinician. Careful review of the history and a thorough physical examination by an experienced physician are essential.

DIAGNOSIS

The workup begins with the history and physical. Pertinent information obtained in chronologic order includes the names of physicians consulted, tests and procedures they used in diagnosis and therapy, and medications used. A unisex diagram can be used to quickly pinpoint the location of the pain and as a reference for later visits. The effect of the pain on the patient's functioning also is evaluated. This determination can be used to measure the effectiveness of treatment regimens. Follow-up and outcome studies of all patients treated are essential.

In the physical exam the practitioner thoroughly evaluates noticeable sensory, motor, reflex, and visual changes. This process includes identifying areas of pain and types of stimulation that cause the pain. For example, the exam for a patient with pain in her right pelvic area begins with the abdomen and includes the lower extremities and a pelvic examination. The physician attempts to elicit pain by superficial and deep pressure applied by the examining finger, an elongated "Q" tip in the pelvis, or the blunt end of a pen or pencil on the abdomen. During this process the physician carefully notes the anatomic relationships of pelvic organs and other tissues with nearby nerves and pain areas.

Psychologic Interview

The psychologic interview is performed during the first visit and often before the physical examination, confirming to the patient the importance of this aspect of her health. Ideally, the examiner is experienced in the area of sexual function and aware of causes of gynecologic pain problems, which may include childhood abuse. If childhood abuse is the cause for sexual and psychologic dysfunction, the patient may not disclose this information immediately because a trusting relationship has not been established or the experience has been repressed. Significant psychologic impairment can negatively affect a treatment's success. A "dyssexualis" history helps identify patients with significant sexual dysfunction early in treatment (Fig. 20-1).

Have you been treated by any other health care professionals for your pelvic pain? Yes No

If yes, what was done? ______________________________

____

How would you rate the pelvic pain you are experiencing?

|-------|-------|-------|-------|-------|-------|-------|-------|-------|

1 2 3 4 5 6 7 8 9 10

least pain ever experienced in life — worst pain ever experienced in life

Over the last 2 years, about how often have you had sex with a partner?

1+/day 3–4/week 1/week 1–2/month <6/year

Are you comfortable with your current sexual frequency? Yes No

If no, why are you uncomfortable? ______________________________

Do you ever experience pain/discomfort during sexual intercourse?

Yes No

If yes, how frequently do you have pain?

always most times sometimes rarely

How would you rate the intercourse pain you have most often?

|-------|-------|-------|-------|-------|-------|-------|-------|-------|

1 2 3 4 5 6 7 8 9 10

least pain ever experienced in life — worst pain ever experienced in life

What is the worst the intercourse pain has ever been?

|-------|-------|-------|-------|-------|-------|-------|-------|-------|

1 2 3 4 5 6 7 8 9 10

least pain ever experienced in life — worst pain ever experienced in life

About how long ago did the pain begin? ________

Which of the following best describes the location of your pain during intercourse?

___ closer to the opening of the vagina

___ deeper in the vagina

___ both close to the opening of the vagina and deep in the vagina

___ other (rectum, stomach, etc.), please specify____________

Is the intercourse pain worse with thrusting? Yes No

Is your pain worse with different intercourse positions (e.g., male on top, female on top, rear entry, etc.)? Yes No

If yes, what position(s) feels more painful?______________________________

FIG. 20-1 An example of the "dyssexualis" history.

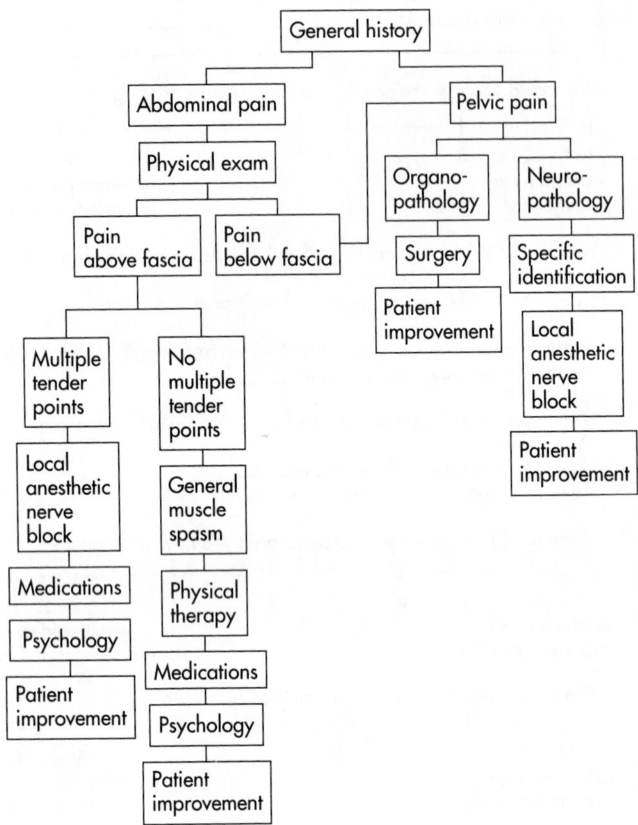

FIG. 20-2 Management of pelvic pain.

DIFFERENTIAL DIAGNOSIS

Differentiation of gynecologic disease processes is difficult because pelvic and abdominal pain are interchangeable. The pelvic examination is essential because it identifies locations of maximum pain that will direct diagnosis and treatment (Fig. 20-2). Adhesions from past surgeries are sometimes cited as the reason for pelvic pain but are rarely the cause. The clinician also performs diagnostic blocks to rule out neuropathic processes.

The neuropathic aspect of pain must be considered. Abdominal nerve entrapment is an important associated problem in lower abdominal pain.

Ilioinguinal and Iliohypogastric Nerve Disturbances

The histories of patients with ilioinguinal and iliohypogastric nerve disturbances often include surgery or trauma involving the lower abdominal wall. The pain is thought to result from overstretch or avulsive neural injuries incurred when nerves near or at the lower corners of the incision were retracted during surgery. The onset of pain varies depending on the intensity of the injury and possibly the nerve fiber size. For example, the Pfannenstiel-type incision crosscuts the ilioinguinal and iliohypogastric nerves and is found in many gynecologic patients. Many patients have had repeated abdominal explorations because their physicians attributed the cause of abdominal pain to adhesions or undefined "organ-related pathology," necessitating more surgery. Laparoscopy has decreased the incidence of repeat surgery, but may cause abdominal neuropathy from placement of a scope or obturator or from an ancillary site being made percutaneous.

Some patients initially have eight or more pain points identified and undergo repeated spaced local anesthetic nerve blocks. Most patients respond in 4 to 6 weeks. Those who do not may benefit from abdominal catheter placement with continuous local anesthetic irrigation of the nerves between the transversalis and oblique muscle groups. The next method is cryotherapy for destruction of refractory nerves. When multiple nests of neuromas are active after the previous techniques have been tried, surgical removal of the local nests is the next option.

Genitofemoral Nerve Disorders

Patients with genitofemoral nerve disorders initially complain of low abdominal pain or back pain that has migrated to the front of their bodies and now descends into the vulvar area. The pain is often incapacitating when it occurs in sharp, repeated attacks. For almost all patients, a significant reduction in pain occurs after individual nerve blocks and maximum tender point injections, often within minutes of office therapy. If this treatment is unsuccessful, search for a pathologic condition should resume.

Hymenal Syndrome

In hymenal syndrome the affected area is the vaginal outlet bordered by the hymen. Pelvic examination may be difficult because of patient complaints of pain, and no evidence of pain may be found in the vagina, cervix, uterus, fallopian tubes, and ovaries. The patient history often reveals repeated infections with *Candida albicans,* which may cause irritation of the superficial nerves in the area of the hymenal ring. Patients usually have a history of normal sexual patterns before the onset of their vaginal pain, but develop significant sexual dysfunction secondary to the disease process, often manifest as severe dyspareunia near the vaginal outlet. Two or three successful hymenal blocks can be performed before surgery is considered.

Endometriosis

Endometriosis is one of the most common causes of chronic pelvic pain (see Chapter 7). Timing, location, and duration of pain vary depending on location of the implanted tissue. The presence of endometrial tissue in or around nerve fibers can result in compression neuropathy over time. Laparoscopy confirms the diagnosis, and treatment involves drugs and/or surgery.

Sympathetic Pelvis Syndrome

Innervation of the pelvis includes the vagina and cervix from the pudendal nerves with derivation from S2 to S4 and the uterus, tubes, and ovaries from the sympathetic pelvic branches of T10 to T12. Many patients with gynecologic pain have a deep pain in the pelvis not associated with physically detectable abdominal wall tenderness or myofascial disease of the abdominal musculature. This disease entity has been classified as *sympathetic pelvis syndrome* and results from pain transmitted to cutaneous areas (referred pain). Some patients obtain relief from repeated local anesthetic nerve blocks if the origin of pain is identified. Laparoscopy can be used for lateral uterosacral nerve ablation or superior hypogastric ganglion resection. Patients unresponsive to local anesthetic block therapy are usually rendered pain free after the surgical resection.

Pelvic Joint Instability

Persistent pelvic pain and pelvic joint instability have been associated with precocious puberty and use of oral contraceptives before reproduction. This diagnosis should be considered in patients with this history in whom diagnostic processes have not identified a cause.

Pyramidal Muscle Hematoma

Hematoma of the pyramidal muscle is a rare complication that may cause impingement of the sciatic, inferior gluteal, and pudendal nerves resulting from compression between the muscle and the iliac spine. A CT scan helps confirm the diagnosis.

Osteitis Pubis

Osteitis pubis should be considered in active females involved in competitive sports who are seen with pubic and adductor pain. Recovery may take as long as 7 months. Pelvic malalignment and sacroiliac dysfunction are associated findings.

Adductor Tendonitis

Adductor tendonitis is usually seen in marathon walkers or runners who suffer from acute injury to the adductor muscle of the anterior thigh, which attaches directly to the pubic ramus. This condition is often misdiagnosed as pelvic pain because of the diffuse ache that radiates into the involved pelvic area laterally. Diagnosis is made by running the examining finger along the medial margin of the adductor muscle to the point of insertion on the pubic ramus. The patient will experience exquisite pain and identify the point of insertion as the location. A local anesthetic injection completely eradicates the pain within minutes of injection. Treatment may need to be repeated for complete eradication.

Osteoporotic Sacral Fractures

According to research, osteoporotic sacral fractures are associated with pelvic pain complaints in which other pathologic causes are excluded.

Focal Vulvitis

Focal vulvitis involves superficial dyspareunia and focal areas of inflammation and/or ulceration of the mucosa. Patients may disclose a history of treatment failures. The typical symptom is extreme pain with intercourse. The characteristic signs are 3- to 10-mm areas of inflammation focused in the area of the vestibule that may not be detected as superficial ulcers. Most lesions are located in and around Bartholin's ducts. Treatment includes creams that may contain antibiotics, cryotherapy to destroy the local ulcerative lesions, and surgical removal of the hymenal ring with a surgical perineoplasty.

TREATMENT

Physical causes of chronic pelvic pain are difficult to identify. Special physical examination techniques are needed, and the physician must consider neuropathic conditions such as nerve compression and neuropraxsis resulting in hyperalgesia and allodynia, myofascial pain syndrome, or pressure neuropathy of the pudendal nerve, obturator nerve, and inferior hypogastric ganglia.

Therapeutic Procedures

Laparoscopy can detect endometriosis and adhesions. The laser beam or electrosurgery can be used to lyse or ablate abnormalities.

Laparotomy is used when multiple and thick adhesions obscure peritoneal anatomy or a substantial mass must be removed.

Treatment Trials

Therapy in the form of medication or rest or exercise programs should begin on the first visit after careful analysis of current medications and treatment history. A low-dose antidepressant medication such as amitriptyline can be prescribed if sleep habits are a problem. This decreases the reception of pain centrally and improves sleep. Another approach is to outline to the patient the conditions, causes, and therapies that may be involved and assure continued support.

The first treatment step is use of over-the-counter drugs such as salicylates. The next step is often over-the-counter nonsteroidal antiinflammatory drugs. The use of tricyclic antidepressants, which are thought to block the uptake of serotonin and norepinephrine in the CNS, is the next phase. Anticonvulsant drugs are effective in certain pain syndromes such as trigeminal neuralgia and are the next treatment option. Last is administration of opioid-type drugs. Normally, this class of drug is not the first line of therapy, but if the patient is currently taking these agents or if their use results in fewer side effects than tricyclic antidepressants and some anticonvulsant drugs, the patient can continue using these drugs for a short time. The incidence of side effects among opioids such as morphine sulfate, codeine, and pentazocine is approximately 20%, whereas oxycodone has an incidence of 10%. Adverse effects include pruritus, drowsiness, nausea, vomiting, dizziness, headache, euphoria, dry mouth, and swelling.

Assessment by Medical Log

The medical log consists of the patient making daily notes of medications and subsequent effects. It is used to adjust dosages and measure progress, with the goal being to reduce the level of medication.

Assessment by Activity Log

This component of the medical log should note the patient's functioning level before onset of the disorder. The goal is to encourage continued activity and function, regardless of the state of the pain disorder, and also measures progress of therapeutic regimens.

Special Studies

MRI is a cross-sectional, high-resolution image of the body. The advantage of using MRI for pelvic evaluation is that the contrasting images of the tissues are superior to the images found on CT and ultrasound scans and are more effective in distinguishing normal and abnormal tissues.

Ultrasound scan is the best image method currently available for abdominal and vaginal views of the pelvis. It is less expensive and more readily available than MRI. It can detect abnormalities of pelvic organs and displacement resulting from pathologic entities.

The CT scan is also valuable as a diagnostic tool in determining pelvic abnormality, especially in relation to bony anatomy. Tumor growth, tumor invasion, and distortion of pelvic anatomy can be detected.

Laparoscopy is the most widely applied diagnostic technique used today in gynecology, and its application obviates many operative exploratory procedures performed in the past. Experience and expertise are required, but laparoscopy is an invaluable diagnostic tool.

KEY POINTS

1. Integrated workup includes detailed history and physical examination as well as diagnostic techniques.
2. Local anesthetic techniques, over-the-counter medicines, and psychotherapy are used in treatment of chronic pelvic pain.

SUGGESTED READINGS

Baskin LS, Tanagho EA: Pelvic pain without pelvic organs, *J Urol* 147:683-686, 1992.

Drossman DA et al: Sexual and physical abuse in women with functional or organic gastrointestinal disorders, *Ann Intern Med* 113:828-833, 1990.

Fricker PA, Taunton JE, Ammann W: Osteitis pubis in athletes, *Sports Med* 12(4):266-279, 1991.

Ghia JN, Blank JW, McAdams CG: A new interabdominis approach to inguinal region block for the management of chronic pain, *Reg Anesth* 16:72-78, 1991.
Miyazaki F, Shook G: Ilioinguinal nerve entrapment during needle suspension for stress incontinence, *Obstet Gynecol* 80(2):246-248, 1992.
Peters AAW et al: A randomized clinical trial to compare two different approaches in women with chronic pelvic pain, *Obstet Gynecol* 77(5):740-744, 1991.
Reiter RC: A profile of women with chronic pelvic pain, *Clin Obstet Gynecol* 33(1):130-136, 1990.
Slocumb JC: Chronic somatic, myofascial, and neurogenic abdominal pelvic pain, *Clin Obstet Gynecol* 33(1):145, 1990.
Spitzer M, Krumholz BA: Human papillomavirus-related diseases in the female patient, *Urol Clin North Am* 19(1):71, 1992.
Walker EA et al: An open trial of nortriptyline in women with chronic pelvic pain, *Int J Psychiatry Med* 21(3):245-252, 1991.
Whitehead: Researchers delineate scope of visceral pain syndromes, *Pain Topics* 5(4):2-3, 1992.

21

Pelvic Floor Support

Renee M. Caputo

Vaginal prolapse is a disorder of pelvic floor support. It is estimated to be present in 50% of all parous women and is a significant problem in 10% to 20% of all women.

It is defined as a herniation of either the anterior, posterior, or apical vagina into the lumen of the vagina, which may extend outside of the introitus in the severest of cases. The type of vaginal prolapse present depends on which part of the vagina has lost its support. There are five types of prolapse: cystocele, rectocele, uterine prolapse, vaginal vault prolapse, and enterocele.

PATHOPHYSIOLOGY

Prolapse is the result of either a functional or structural defect of one or more of the components of the pelvic floor supporting structures. Denervation injury of the pelvic floor musculature is the major pathophysiologic mechanism behind the development of female pelvic floor disorders, including vaginal prolapse. Significant nerve damage has been documented in women with these disorders compared with controls. The most common cause of denervation injury is vaginal delivery. During a vaginal delivery the pelvic floor and its nerve supply are stretched beyond their normal limits. Although nerve function is restored in most patients within several months, in some patients denervation persists. Obstetric risk factors that increase a woman's chance for denervation injury include a large baby, prolonged second stage labor, forceps delivery, and multiple vaginal deliveries.

Other causes of vaginal prolapse include conditions that chronically increase intraabdominal pressure, such as obesity, chronic constipation with heavy straining, chronic lung disease, and possibly postural changes. Other diseases that affect nerve function and tissue strength can also contribute to vaginal prolapse, such as neurologic diseases, diabetes, pelvic surgery, aging, collagen disorders, and hypoestrogenism.

DIAGNOSIS

Symptoms associated with vaginal prolapse depend on the type and severity of prolapse. Patients can be asymptomatic. The more severe the prolapse, the more likely that symptoms will be present that may include vaginal pressure or heaviness, vaginal or perineal pain, sensation of tissue protrusion from the vagina, abdominal pain or pressure, low back pain, and observation or palpation of a mass at or protruding from the introitus. If the vaginal mucosa is exposed, it will become dry and thus more susceptible to ulceration, bleeding, vaginal discharge, and infection if abrasion of the mucosa occurs. Intercourse may be uncomfortable and women will often avoid it because of discomfort and the fear that they will seriously injure themselves.

Any type of vaginal prolapse is best diagnosed by a pelvic examination with the patient in an upright position and bearing down so that the full extent of the prolapse can be appreciated. Each part of the vagina, anterior and posterior walls as well as the apex, should be examined separately in a systematic fashion so that all defects are appreciated. Grading systems, such as the one developed by the International Continence Society (ICS), are used to assess the severity of the different types of prolapse and define location. This system defines six points whose position with reference to the hymen should be measured and recorded (Fig. 21-1). Positions are expressed as centimeters above or proximal to the hymen (negative number) or centimeters below or distal to the hymen (positive number) with the plane of the hymen being defined as zero. Once the quantitative description is complete, a stage can be assigned to an individual subject according to the most severe portion of the prolapse when the full extent of the protrusion has been demonstrated.

TREATMENT

Symptomatic vaginal prolapse can be treated nonsurgically with a vaginal pessary or with surgical correction. The surgical procedures performed depend on the specific defects present. Because pelvic floor disorders often occur concomitantly, the patient may need multiple procedures to correct each defect appropriately. The goals of surgical repair of vaginal prolapse

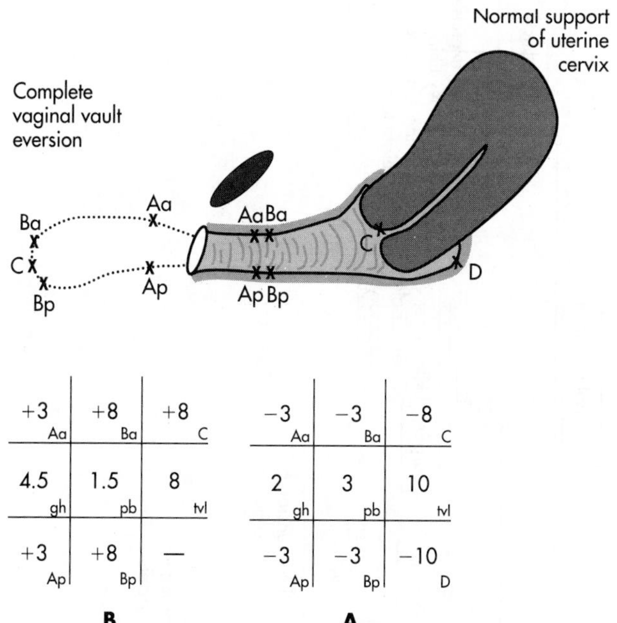

B

+3 Aa	+8 Ba	+8 C
4.5 gh	1.5 pb	8 tvl
+3 Ap	+8 Bp	—

A

−3 Aa	−3 Ba	−8 C
2 gh	3 pb	10 tvl
−3 Ap	−3 Bp	−10 D

FIG. 21-1 International Continence Society Committee on Standardization of Terminology classification of vaginal prolapse. (From Bump R et al: Standardization of terminology of female pelvic organ prolapse and pelvic floor dysfunction, *Am J Obstet Gynecol* 175:10-17, 1996.)

are the restoration of normal vaginal anatomy and the preservation of function (Fig. 21-2).

Cystocele, Urethrocele, and Cystourethrocele

Cystocele can be defined as a herniation of the bladder into the vaginal lumen because of the loss of support to the anterior vaginal wall. If that portion of the anterior vaginal wall closest to the symphysis that supports the urethra is involved, it is sometimes referred to as a *urethrocele.* The term *cystourethrocele* is also used when both the urethra and bladder are herniated.

Symptoms associated with cystocele depend on its severity. The larger the cystocele, the more likely the patient will have symptoms. Patients with cystocele can be asymptomatic. If the bladder descends significantly, a mechanical obstruction can occur at the bladder neck, causing difficulty emptying the bladder, urgency, frequency, frequent UTIs, and urinary incontinence. In rare cases, severe anterior vaginal wall prolapse can lead to ureteral obstruction. In these patients, incontinence can be hidden by the

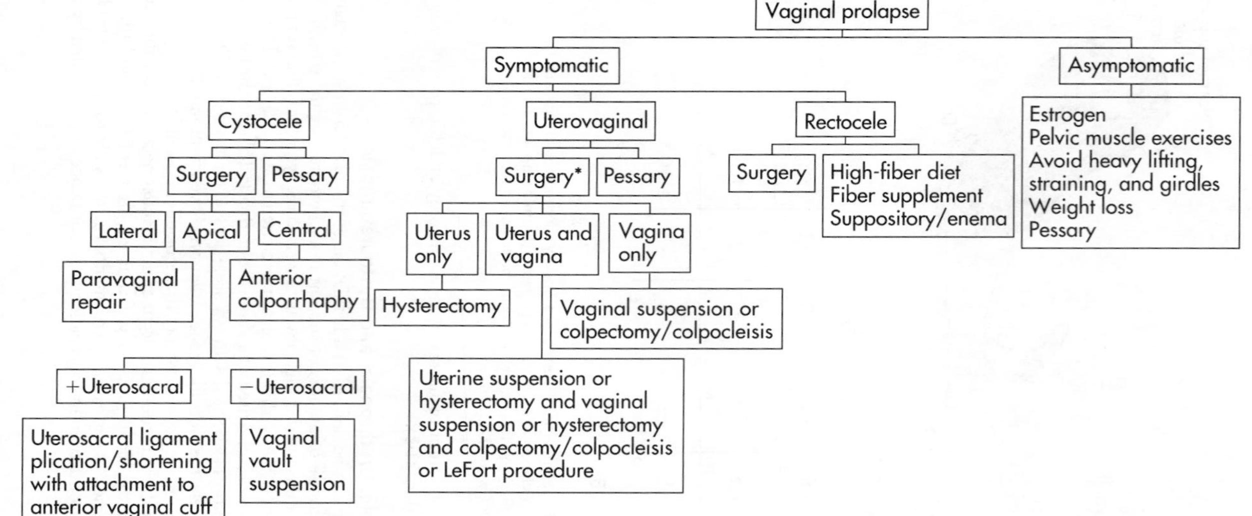

FIG. 21-2 Management of vaginal prolapse. *All procedures should include culdoplasty.

mechanical obstruction of the urethrovesical junction. These patients will deny the presence of incontinence or have a history of incontinence that improved over time as the prolapse worsened.

For diagnosis of a cystocele, the bottom half of a Graves' speculum or a Sims' speculum is placed into the vagina and depresses the posterior vaginal wall out of the way. The anterior vaginal wall is then observed for descensus while the patient performs the Valsalva maneuver. To ensure that the full extent of the defect is observed, the patient should be examined in the upright position. Points Aa and Ba of the ICS system are used to quantitate anterior vaginal wall prolapse. For diagnosis of hidden incontinence, the patient should have a urodynamic evaluation with the anterior vaginal wall reduced.

Different types of cystoceles have been described, and diagnosis depends on what part of the anterior vaginal wall has lost support. If the lateral anterior vaginal wall loses its attachment to the obturator fascia along the lateral pelvic side wall from the pubis to the ischial spine, it is referred to as a *lateral* or *displacement cystocele*. A lateral cystocele is diagnosed by observing loss of one or both of the lateral sulci and preservation of the rugae of the anterior vaginal wall. If the anterior vaginal wall loses its attachment at the cervix, an apical cystocele will be present. This type of cystocele will also be present if the vaginal apex has lost support. The anterior vaginal wall defect of an apical cystocele will be observed superiorly at the cervix or vaginal apex. Many times this cystocele can be diagnosed by elevating the apex of the vagina with a speculum. If the cystocele reduces, an apical cystocele is most likely present. If the anterior vaginal wall loses support in the midline, a central or distention cystocele will occur. A central cystocele is most often diagnosed by observing the absence of anterior vaginal wall rugal folds. More than one type of cystocele can be present simultaneously, making diagnosis more difficult.

The differential diagnosis of a cystocele would include anterior vaginal wall masses, such as a Gartner's duct cyst or urethral diverticulum, and other types of vaginal prolapse such as vaginal vault eversion and enterocele.

The surgical procedures commonly performed for cystocele are anterior colporrhaphy for a central defect, paravaginal repair for a lateral defect, and vaginal vault (apical) suspension procedures for an apical defect. The goal of cystocele repair is the restoration of normal anterior vaginal anatomy.

Rectocele

A rectocele is the herniation of the anterior rectal wall and posterior vaginal wall into the vaginal lumen. Rectoceles occur when the barrier between the vagina and rectum, the rectovaginal septum, becomes attenuated. The rectum is a relatively high-pressure organ, especially during defecation. Over time, the anterior rectal wall dissects through the defect in the rectovaginal septum, pushing the posterior vaginal wall into the vaginal lumen.

The symptom commonly associated with rectocele is difficult evacuation of stool. Classically, patients will have to use heavy Valsalva maneuver, apply pressure manually on the perineum or posterior vagina to complete a bowel movement, and will feel as if they have not completely evacuated. Rectal pressure may be present, especially after a bowel movement and during sexual intercourse. A large proportion of women with rectoceles are asymptomatic.

A rectocele is diagnosed by pelvic and rectal examinations. During the pelvic examination, the speculum is used to hold the anterior vaginal wall out of the way and the posterior vaginal wall is observed for descensus while the patient performs the Valsalva maneuver, preferably in the upright position. Because a rectocele by definition must involve the anterior rectal wall as well, a rectal examination is necessary to confirm the diagnosis. During the rectal examination, attenuation of the rectovaginal septum and herniation of the anterior rectal and posterior vaginal walls are easily appreciated. Rectoceles are classified as either high, mid, or low based on where the defect in the rectovaginal septum occurs. Points Ap and Bp in the ICS system are used to quantitate posterior vaginal wall prolapse.

The differential diagnosis of a rectocele would include any anatomic or functional disorder of the anorectal canal that would interfere with normal defecation. Rectoceles are often cited as the cause for constipation when they are more often the result of it and chronic heavy straining by the patient. Correction of a rectocele in this instance would not improve the patient's symptoms. An enterocele may be confused with a rectocele because it will often present as a bulge in the rectovaginal space. A rectovaginal examination would be needed to confirm its presence.

Rectoceles are treated both nonsurgically and surgically. In all patients with a symptomatic rectocele, increasing fiber in the diet or adding a fiber supplement is recommended before proceeding to surgical therapy. Patients should be encouraged not to strain with defecation and to use suppositories and enemas as needed to avoid progression of the rectocele and other pelvic floor disorders. Pessaries, for the most part, are not helpful. Most surgical repairs involve plication of the posterior vaginal wall in an attempt to reconstruct and strengthen the attenuated rectovaginal septum.

Uterine Prolapse

Uterine prolapse is the descensus of the uterus or cervix into the vaginal canal toward the introitus. It is caused by lengthening of the cervix or loss of support to the cervix by the cardinal/uterosacral ligament complex. Because the vaginal apex is supported by this same complex, it is not uncommon for the patient to have simultaneous vaginal vault eversion. This point becomes important when surgical correction is considered.

Uterine prolapse is diagnosed by a vaginal examination with the patient in the upright position and performing the Valsalva maneuver at maximum effort. The extent of uterine prolapse would be described using points C and D from the ICS system.

Treatment can be accomplished with a pessary or surgery. If surgery is chosen, the type of procedure used depends on whether the patient wants to maintain childbearing potential and whether vaginal vault prolapse is present. If the patient is no longer planning to have children and there is no vaginal vault prolapse present, a hysterectomy would be the treatment of choice. If the patient wants more children, a uterine-sparing procedure, such as a uterine suspension, is indicated. If childbearing is not a concern and vaginal vault prolapse is present, a hysterectomy with a vaginal vault suspension or vaginal ablative procedure should be performed.

Vaginal Vault/Apical Prolapse

Vaginal vault prolapse is the loss of support of the vagina beginning at the apex, the most proximal location of the normally positioned lower reproductive tract. When the vaginal apex loses support, it will evert in the direction of the hymen. This phenomenon is caused by loss of support of the cardinal/uterosacral ligament complex, which is responsible for apical support. With progression of vaginal apical eversion, lateral support to the obturator fascia is also lost bilaterally.

The vaginal apex is represented by the anterior and posterior fornices in a patient who has a cervix (Fig. 21-1, points C and D), and by the vaginal cuff scar in a patient who has had a hysterectomy (point C).

It is important to identify the presence of vaginal vault prolapse if surgical correction is being considered. This defect is corrected with a vaginal vault suspension (sacrospinous suspension, colposacral suspension) in patients who desire sexual function, or a vaginal ablative procedure in those patients who do not (LeFort, colpectomy/colpocleisis). There will be a less than adequate result and increased risk for recurrence of prolapse if vaginal vault eversion goes undiagnosed and uncorrected. This is a common error in the surgical treatment of patients with uterine prolapse, many of whom have a significant degree of concomitant vaginal apical eversion. A hysterectomy alone is not appropriate in these patients. With complete loss of vaginal vault support, loss of anterior and posterior wall support is also present. If sexual function is being preserved, separate procedures to correct these defects will often need to be performed for a satisfactory anatomic result.

Enterocele

Enterocele occurs when a portion of the small or large bowel protrudes into the upper vagina or dissects into the rectovaginal space. It is preceded by and contained within the peritoneum of Douglas' cul-de-sac.

An enterocele can be difficult to diagnose clinically, especially if small. The most accurate way to make the diagnosis in the office is by rectovaginal examination on a patient who is in the upright position and performing at maximum Valsalva effort. If an enterocele is present, the physician will feel a mass come between the rectal and vaginal fingers. In patients with a significant degree of vaginal vault prolapse, an enterocele is almost always present.

An enterocele can be confused with a rectocele because each may cause a protrusion of the posterior vaginal wall. A rectovaginal examination is needed to distinguish between the two.

The surgical treatment for enterocele is the obliteration of Douglas' cul-de-sac, called a *culdoplasty*. Simple uterosacral plication is generally not enough and should be accompanied by the plication of the peritoneum between the uterosacral ligaments, sigmoid colon, and vagina. A culdoplasty should routinely be performed in patients with vaginal vault eversion who are receiving surgical therapy. This will correct the enterocele that most of these patients have and protect the vaginal apex.

NONSURGICAL MANAGEMENT OF VAGINAL PROLAPSE

The only effective nonsurgical therapy for vaginal prolapse is use of the vaginal pessary. A pessary is a device that comes in different shapes and sizes and is placed in the vagina to occupy its lumen and support the vaginal walls. It is most effective for anterior and apical defects.

The pessary has been classically used for the elderly woman who is not a surgical candidate because of her medical condition. However, a pessary can and should be offered as a viable treatment option to any woman with symptomatic prolapse. A pessary is especially helpful with patients who want to delay surgery but would like symptomatic relief. Theoretically, a pessary may act prophylactically to delay prolapse progression by counteracting the forces of intraabdominal pressure and gravity.

A properly fitted pessary cannot be felt by the patient when in place, yet provides adequate support to relieve the patient of her symptoms. It should fill as much of the vagina as possible without undue stretch or tension on the vaginal walls. Although not possible in all patients, the patient should be instructed in pessary insertion and removal so that she can remove the pessary at night or before intercourse and replace it during times when she is active. This will protect the patient from excessive vaginal discharge, ulceration or erosion of the vaginal mucosa, and infection. If a patient is unable to perform this task, a family member or visiting nurse can be trained to do this once per week. The last resort is to remove the pessary and examine the vaginal mucosa one to two times per month in the office. Lubrication should be used for insertion. In those patients who are wearing a pessary long-term, regular use of an antibiotic cream is appropriate. Patients who use a pessary, especially those who cannot remove them on a regular basis, should use ERT if possible to protect the vaginal mucosa.

PREVENTION

For women who have normal support or asymtomatic prolapse, prophylactic measures should be recommended to prevent progression and subsequent symptoms. ERT, either systemic or vaginal, should be offered to the postmenopausal woman who has no contraindications. Regularly performed pelvic floor muscle exercises (Kegel exercises) can strengthen pelvic floor skeletal muscle, reinforcing the mechanisms of support provided by the levator ani. Patients should be instructed to avoid behaviors that will increase intraabdominal pressure, such as heavy lifting, weight gain, smoking, chronic cough, wearing girdles, and straining with defecation.

KEY POINTS

1 Disorders of female pelvic floor support, called *vaginal prolapse,* are caused by denervation injury of the pelvic floor skeletal muscle with subsequent attenuation of secondary supporting structures.

2 Causes of vaginal prolapse include vaginal delivery, activities that increase intraabdominal pressure, neurologic injury or disease, aging, hypoestrogenism, postural changes, and genetic factors.

3 The examination of a woman for vaginal prolapse should include the anterior and posterior vaginal walls as well as the vaginal apex.

4 Treatment of vaginal prolapse includes use of a vaginal pessary, surgical therapy, and preventive measures.

5 The goal of surgical therapy is to correct all defects present simultaneously and restore normal vaginal anatomy and function.

SUGGESTED READINGS

Benson JT: Vaginal approach to cystocele repair. In *Female pelvic floor disorders,* New York, 1992, WW Norton.

Cruikshank SH: Sacrospinous fixation: should this be performed at the time of vaginal hysterectomy? *Am J Obstet Gynecol* 164:1072-1076, 1991.

DeLancey JOL: Anatomic aspects of vaginal eversion after hysterectomy, *Am J Obstet Gynecol* 166: 1717-1728, 1992.

Nichols DH: Fertility retention in the patient with genital prolapse, *Am J Obstet Gynecol* 164:1155-1158, 1991.

Nichols DH: Posterior colporrhaphy and pernineorrhaphy. In *Vaginal surgery,* Baltimore, 1995, Williams & Wilkins.

Nichols DH: Enterocele. In *Vaginal surgery,* Baltimore, 1995, Williams & Wilkins.

Richardson AC: Paravaginal repair. In *Urogynecologic surgery,* New York, 1992, Raven.

Wall LL, DeLancey JOL: The politics of prolapse: a revisionist approach to disorders of the pelvic floor in women, *Perspect Biol Med* 34:486-496, 1991.

Wall LL, Norton PA, DeLancey JOL: Prolapse and the lower urinary tract. In *Practical urogynecology,* Baltimore, 1993, Williams & Wilkins.

Wall LL, Norton PA, DeLancey JOL: Pelvic anatomy and the physiology of the lower urinary tract. In *Practical urogynecology,* Baltimore, 1993, Williams & Wilkins.

22

Premenstrual Syndrome

Cynthia B. Evans

Premenstrual syndrome (PMS) is usually defined as a syndrome during which the patient experiences at least one behavioral and one physical symptom within the 5 days before onset of menses in two consecutive cycles, with relief of those symptoms within 4 days after onset of menses. There should not be a recurrence of symptoms until at least cycle day 12. The definition also requires that there be an identifiable dysfunction in the social or economic performance of the patient (marital discord, poor work or school performance, legal difficulties, or suicidal ideation). Behavioral symptoms include but are not limited to fatigue, irritability, depression, angry outbursts, poor concentration, labile mood, episodes of crying, and anxiety. Physical symptoms include but are not limited to breast tenderness, abdominal bloating, headache, swollen extremities, appetite changes, and pelvic pain. This definition implies that there must be a temporal relationship of the symptomatology to menses in that the symptoms occur only during the luteal phase. This implies as well that ovulation must occur. Symptoms must be repetitive on a monthly basis and should be severe enough to interfere with a normal lifestyle.

Approximately 70% to 90% of reproductive-age women are aware of some physical or behavioral changes in relationship to their cycles. In addition, 20% to 40% have some temporary disability, but it is estimated that only 2% to 5% of women experience true PMS with symptoms severe enough to cause lifestyle disruptions.

Risk factors for PMS include high parity, history of preeclampsia, alcoholism, postpartum depression, and working outside of the home. Interestingly, the risk of PMS does not correlate with marital status, education level, or culture. Monozygous twin and mother-daughter studies, however, do suggest a genetic element.

PATHOGENESIS

Although PMS has been recognized for centuries, its etiology and therefore its ideal treatment remain a mystery. Multiple theories regarding its etiology exist, but data are limited and poorly controlled.

Various dietary factors have been examined, but there are no controlled studies looking at the relationship between diet and PMS. Studies show no change in insulin or glucose metabolism with PMS, but carbohydrate intake may affect mood by increasing serotonin activity. The placebo effect for any therapy used to treat PMS is quite high. A study among college students in Oregon correlated an increase in PMS with an increased intake of chocolate, alcoholic beverages, fruit juice, and caffeine-free soda.

The benefit of calcium supplementation is somewhat unclear. Excessive consumption of dairy products results in a chronic magnesium deficiency and PMS. In fact, aggressive behavior has been observed in girls consuming excessive dairy products. However, calcium supplementation of 1000 mg/day has been shown to improve negative mood, fluid retention, and pain.

Studies have also examined the roles of fluid retention, hyperprolactinemia, prostaglandins, and hormone levels, but results are unclear and inconsistent.

A common aspect of many theories is the involvement of various neurotransmitters. β-Endorphins seem to play a role in PMS, and the effect of the GABA system remains to be proved.

The serotonin system seems to be a promising area of research. Patients with various abnormal behavioral states characterized by depression, anxiety, and aggression have decreased whole-blood serotonin, platelet uptake of serotonin, CSF serotonin metabolites, and brain serotonin content. Whole-blood serotonin and platelet uptake of serotonin are also decreased in the luteal phase of PMS patients. This suggests a possible central deficiency of serotonin. Fluoxetine (Prozac) is a serotonin-reuptake inhibitor and was effective in treating PMS patients in multiple double-blind, placebo-controlled, randomized studies. A greater improvement was noted in behavioral than physical scores, but the difference in symptoms between the luteal and follicular phases was abolished. Buspirone (Buspar) initially suppresses the serotonin system, but later potentiates it through autoreceptor desensitization. It is effective for symptoms of irritability, fatigue, pain, and poor social functioning.

DIAGNOSIS

Because PMS occurs only in the luteal phase, a history consistent with ovulation is important. Sometimes basal body temperature charts are necessary to document ovulation. It is also important to look for sources of stress and to ask about physical or sexual abuse. Do the patient's symptoms suggest another disorder, psychiatric or medical? Are there concurrent psychiatric or medical diseases? Is the patient on any medications? Finally, it is essential to determine the extent to which the symptoms affect her life.

There are no characteristic physical findings consistent with PMS. The role of the examination is to rule out other disorders potentially causing the patient's symptoms. No specific laboratory findings are consistent with PMS. Various laboratory tests can, however, identify other disorders.

Prospective charting is the key to making and confirming the diagnosis of PMS. Patients must chart their symptoms on a daily basis for at least two consecutive menstrual cycles. Retrospective recall of symptoms has been shown to be inaccurate by multiple investigators.

DIFFERENTIAL DIAGNOSIS*

The differential diagnosis is derived from the prospective symptom charting performed by the patient. Emphasis is placed on the timing of symptoms. By definition, PMS occurs only in the luteal phase, so this charting allows clarification of patients' symptomatology.

Other disorders can cause effects throughout the cycle or worsen during the luteal phase. These include psychiatric and medical illnesses such as depression, anxiety disorders, bipolar affective disorders, personality disorders, substance abuse, idiopathic cyclic edema, chronic fatigue syndrome, and fibromyalgia. Other medical illnesses with symptoms similar to PMS include hyperprolactinemia, panhypopituitarism, adrenal disorders, pheochromocytoma, irritable bowel syndrome, and thyroid diseases. The premenstrual dysphoric disorder is considered a subset of PMS and is characterized predominantly by psychologic manifestations of the disease. There are very strict guidelines for the diagnosis as outlined in the *DSM-IV.*

TREATMENT

Because the precise etiology of PMS is unknown, treatments are primarily directed at symptom relief (Fig. 22-1). Long-term therapy is frequently necessary. Each therapy should be in place at least three cycles to assess effectiveness. The goals of treatment should be to reduce but not necessarily eliminate symptoms and to improve the patient's ability to function and her overall sense of well-being. Consultants can be of tremendous assistance when indicated (i.e., psychiatrists, neurologists, and internists).

Self-Help Strategies

Although there is very little scientific data supporting self-help therapies for PMS, they are essentially without adverse side effects and lead to an overall healthier lifestyle. Therefore they are usually recommended as first-line therapy. Education about PMS can be of considerable benefit to patients. Simply reassuring them that there is no serious underlying medical illness helps a significant number of patients. Helping patients to understand our limited knowledge of the etiology of PMS can help them to understand that a "quick fix" is rarely possible, and that it will be a team effort to find the best therapy for the symptoms.

Stress does not cause PMS, but reducing external and internal stressors can reduce the intensity of PMS symptoms. Support groups, relaxation techniques, hypnosis, and counseling can all be of benefit.

Although it has not been proved in placebo-controlled studies, improved nutritional habits may alleviate some PMS symptoms and will lead to an overall healthier lifestyle. Nutritional supplements can be considered. Magnesium supplementation is of some benefit at a dose of

---

*Modified from Johnson SR: Clinician's approach to the diagnosis and management of the premenstrual syndrome, *Obstet Gynecol* 35(3), 1992.

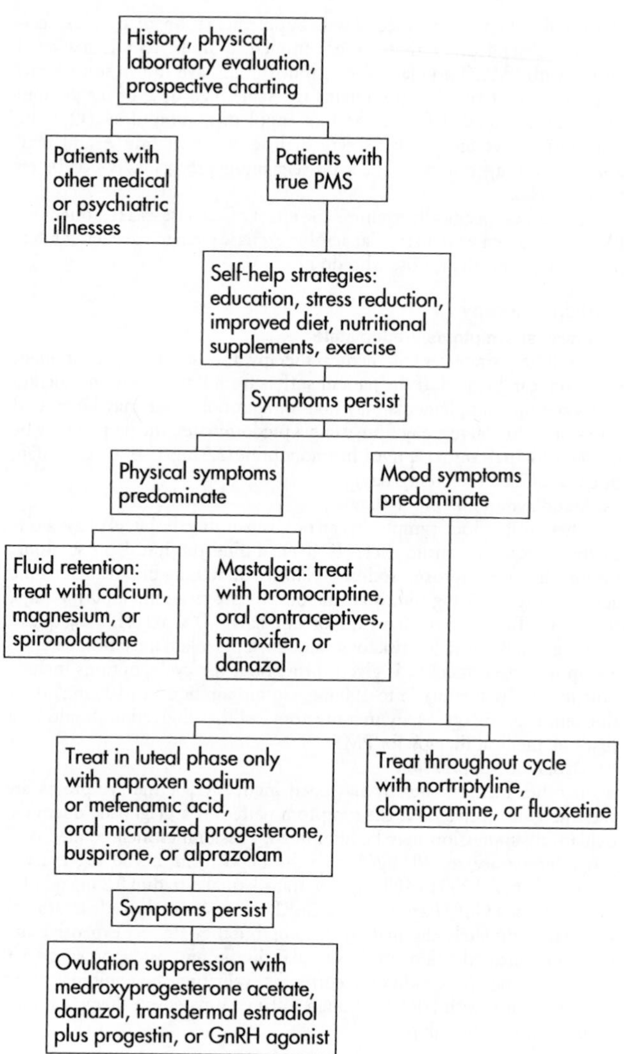

FIG. 22-1 Management of PMS.

360 mg/day in three divided doses. Supplementation of pyridoxine is not recommended. Optivite is a commercial multivitamin marketed for use with PMS. Two placebo-controlled trials have shown some benefit to using Optivite, but it contains the same high dose of magnesium that is recommended for magnesium supplementation alone. Optivite is also expensive and contains very high levels of vitamin A and pyridoxine. Evening primrose oil, a prostaglandin precursor, is not better than placebo.

No studies specifically examine the effect of exercise as a treatment for PMS, but women who do regular aerobic exercise seem to have fewer luteal phase symptoms than those who do not.

Medical Therapy

Physical symptoms predominate

If self-help strategies fail, medical therapy directed at the predominant symptom can be used. If the patient suffers from fluid retention, calcium or magnesium supplements may help or spironolactone may be used at doses of 25 to 200 mg/day. If mastalgia predominates, the patient may be treated with oral contraceptives, bromocriptine (2.5 mg qd-bid), tamoxifen, or danazol (200 to 400 mg/day).

Mood symptoms predominate

Therapy for mood symptoms can be given during the luteal phase alone or throughout the entire cycle. If given during the luteal phase alone, options include naproxen sodium (Naprosyn) 500 mg bid or mefenamic acid (Ponstel) 500 mg bid, oral micronized progesterone (300 mg/day), buspirone (Buspar) 5 to 10 mg tid, or alprazolam (Xanax) 0.125 mg qhs to 0.25 mg qid. Because of a risk for addiction, alprazolam must be tapered to a stop with each menses. If given throughout the cycle, options include nortriptyline (Pamelor) 25 to 100 mg, clomipramine 25 to 100 mg qd, or fluoxetine 20 mg qd. Many investigators feel that fluoxetine should be a first-line medical therapy for PMS.

Ovulation suppression

If other medical therapy has been ineffective, if the symptoms are extremely disruptive, or if the symptom pattern is a diagnostic dilemma, ovulation suppression may be attempted. Possibilities include medroxyprogesterone acetate 30 mg/day or the depo form at 150 mg every 3 months, danazol 200 to 400 mg/day, transdermal estradiol 0.2 mg qd plus progestin, or a GnRH agonist. The GnRH agonists are the only treatment found to completely eliminate symptoms, but they are very expensive and carry an increased risk of cardiovascular disease and osteoporosis after 6 months of therapy. Studies are currently evaluating the combination of GnRH agonists with HRT. Although still a very expensive therapy, it may help minimize the risk profile.

Surgical Therapy

Oophorectomy is almost never an indicated treatment for PMS. If it is to be used as a treatment, all of the following conditions must be met: no response to any other treatment except danazol or a GnRH agonist, complete resolution of symptoms while using danazol or a GnRH agonist for 4 to 6 months, childbearing has been completed, and the patient is believed to have at least 5 years of menstrual function remaining.

KEY POINTS

1 By definition, PMS is a recurrent cyclic disorder with symptoms occurring only in the luteal phase of ovulatory women.

2 The etiology of PMS remains unclear but probably involves neurotransmitters.

3 Self-help strategies including education, stress reduction, improved diet, nutritional supplements, and exercise are usually first-line therapies for PMS.

4 Medical therapy is directed at specific symptoms and can be given during the luteal phase only or throughout the cycle.

5 Surgical therapy is almost never indicated for the treatment of PMS.

SUGGESTED READINGS

ACOG Committee on Gynecologic Practice: *Premenstrual syndrome:* ACOG committee opinion, #155, April 1995, ACOG.

Burnet RB et al: Premenstrual syndrome and spironolactone, *Aust NZ J Obstet Gynaecol* 31(4):366, 1991.

Facchinetti F et al: Oral magnesium successfully relieves premenstrual mood changes, *Obstet Gynecol* 78:177, 1991.

Freeman EW et al: Ineffectiveness of progesterone suppository treatment for premenstrual syndrome, *JAMA* 264:349-353, 1990.

Johnson SR: Clinician's approach to the diagnosis and management of premenstrual syndrome, *Clin Obstet Gynecol* 35(3):637-657, 1992.

Kleijnen J, TerRiet G, Knipschild P: Vitamin B_6 in the treatment of the premenstrual syndrome: a review, *Br J Obstet Gynaecol,* 97:847-852, 1990.

Lurie S, Borenstein R: The premenstrual syndrome, *Obstet Gynecol Surv* 45:220-228, 1990.

Mortola JF, Girton L, Fischer U: Successful treatment of severe premenstrual syndrome by combined use of gonadotropin-releasing hormone agonist and estrogen/progestin, *J Clin Endocrinol Metab* 71(2):252 A-F, 1991.

Plouffe L et al: Diagnostic and treatment results from a Southeastern academic center-based premenstrual syndrome clinic: the first year, *Am J Obstet Gynecol* 169(2):295-307, 1993.

Wood SH et al: Treatment of premenstrual syndrome with fluoxetine: a double-blind, placebo-controlled, crossover study, *Obstet Gynecol* 80(3):339-344, 1992.

23

Sexual Dysfunction

STEPHEN F. PARISER

DIAGNOSIS

The key to assisting patients with sexual dysfunction is a sensitive and nonjudgmental approach by the physician. Professional interviewing regarding sexual concerns should be conducted in a quiet, private setting free from interruptions. Sexual issues should be discussed only when the patient is fully clothed, preferentially in a consultation room. Emphasis should be placed on acknowledging the patient's uneasiness and eliciting feedback.

The history should include the presence or history of psychiatric illness, such as depressive disorders, bipolar disorder, anxiety disorders (including obsessive-compulsive disorder), and eating disorders. A complete gynecologic history is also obtained. Detailed information about medications and drug or alcohol use is also necessary. It is also important to inquire about sexual and child abuse, sexual assault, and spousal abuse. A social history should include questions about family background, sex education, current and past relationships, and religious background.

During the sexual history the physician defines the history of the problem, determines premorbid functioning–lifelong (primary) or after a period of good functioning (secondary)–and clarifies the relationship between symptoms and the sexual response cycle (desire, arousal, orgasm, resolution, or sexual pain). When the patient uses slang or demeaning terms to identify genital anatomy or relate a sexual complaint, it is appropriate to clarify its meaning and redefine it in dignified terms. Educating patients to use anatomic terms and clinical diagnostic labels and definitions can be therapeutic itself.

Initially, members of a dyad are interviewed separately. This gives each partner an opportunity to share information that they may feel is a source of embarrassment or pain. Next, both partners are interviewed to gather more information about their sexual concern and quality of the relationship and to address misunderstandings and myths. Specific questions address onset, circumstances in which the problem occurs, and factors that improve or worsen the situation. Fears, anxieties, avoidance patterns, and the patient's opinion should be explored.

PSYCHOSEXUAL DYSFUNCTIONS AND THEIR DIFFERENTIAL DIAGNOSIS

The possible causes of sexual dysfunction frequently involve combinations of medical, surgical, and psychosexual issues. Careful clinical evaluation is critical to identify all causes. Even when a chronic illness such as diabetes is a source of dysfunction, contributing psychiatric issues should be addressed. Commonly, psychiatric intervention (medical, psychologic, or both) can lead to significant improvement even in the presence of medical, surgical, or gynecologic problems.

The American Psychiatric Association's *DSM-IV* is a valuable resource for physicians. All diagnostic criteria of psychosexual dysfunction in this chapter are directly quoted from the *DSM-IV.*

PHASES OF THE SEXUAL RESPONSE CYCLE

According to the *DSM-IV,* the sexual response cycle can be divided into the following phases:

1. Desire: Sexual fantasies and sexual desire
2. Excitement: Subjective sense of pleasure and associated physiologic changes (e.g., erections in men and vaginal lubrication in women)
3. Orgasm: Peaking of sexual pleasures with release of sexual tension and rhythmic contractions of perineal muscles and reproductive organs
4. Resolution: Muscular relaxation and a sense of comfort or well-being

Men are physiologically unable to experience further erections or to achieve orgasm and ejaculation for some time (refractory period). Women do not appear to have a refractory period.

SUBTYPES OF PSYCHOSEXUAL DYSFUNCTION

The onset of sexual dysfunction can be classified as either *lifelong* or *acquired.* Context can be specified as either *generalized type* or *situational type.* Etiologic subtypes include *psychologic* and *combined factors* (psychologic and general medical). When a general medical condition or substance use (prescribed or otherwise) is sufficient to account for the dysfunction, it should be categorized as either *sexual dysfunction caused by a general medical condition* or *substance-induced sexual dysfunction.*

PSYCHOSEXUAL DYSFUNCTIONS ACCORDING TO PHASE OF SEXUAL RESPONSE CYCLE

Sexual Desire Disorders

Hypoactive sexual desire disorder

Diagnostic criteria for hypoactive sexual desire disorder include persistently or recurrently deficient (or absent) sexual fantasies and desire for sexual activity. The judgment of deficiency or absence is made by the clinician, taking into account factors that affect sexual functioning, such as age and the context of the person's life. Additional criteria are that the disturbance causes marked distress or interpersonal difficulty, the sexual dysfunction is not better accounted for by another axis I disorder (except another sexual dysfunction), and it is not exclusively related to the direct physiologic effects of a substance (e.g., drug abuse or other medication) or general medical condition.

Hypoactive sexual desire is the most common chief complaint among sex therapy clinics. A range of differential diagnoses needs to be considered to determine the cause of low sexual desire (Box 23-1).

When low desire is associated with depression, the patient may benefit from appropriately tailored antidepressant and psychotherapy regimens. This issue is complicated because psychotropic medication, such as antidepressants, can also interfere with sexual desire and function.

Because many patients with low desire have dysfunction secondary to medication, it is important to review all current medication for potential sexual side effects. Approximately 20% to 40% of patients on antidepressants will experience sexual dysfunction. Bupropion is an antidepressant that appears to be relatively free of sexual side effects.

Endocrine causes of low sexual desire (i.e., thyroid and testosterone abnormalities) also need to be explored. Exogenous androgen therapy has no clear role in the treatment of the naturally cycling woman with low levels of desire or any other sexual dysfunction without a clearly defined endocrine syndrome. The role of androgen use in postmenopausal women is controversial.

Sexual desire can wane in an individual or her partner because of changes in body habitus (weight gain, disfigurement from surgery or radiation) or as result of anger. Psychotherapy (often as a couple) can be helpful in resolving these issues or at least clarifying them. The key to

BOX 23-1
Factors Associated With Low Sexual Desire

Endocrine abnormalities (e.g., hypothyroidism, diabetes, hyperprolactinemia)
Drug side effects
Chronic illness (diabetes, inflammatory bowel disease, heart disease, collagen-vascular disease, renal failure, multiple sclerosis)
Mood disorders associated with depressive symptoms
Anxiety (fear of loss of control, pain, death associated with sexual excitement as a result of heart disease or stroke; previous sexual trauma)
Stress
Comorbid sexual dysfunction
History of sexual trauma or abuse
Guilt
Religious prohibitions
Relationship issues
Problems with intimacy

treatment success in these patients is careful delineation of the issues and their contribution to hypoactive sexual desire. Only then can a specifically tailored approach be implemented. Because these patients may have low desire only in the context of their identified partner, clarification of this nature is critical.

Sensate focus is a sex therapy behavioral approach. It can be helpful in the treatment of patients with psychologically mediated low desire and every other sexual dysfunction where psychologic factors play an etiologic role.

Sexual Aversion Disorder

The diagnostic criteria for sexual aversion disorder include persistent or recurrent extreme aversion to and avoidance of all (or almost all) genital sexual contact with a sexual partner, the disturbance causes marked distress or interpersonal difficulty, and the sexual dysfunction is not better accounted for by another axis I disorder (except another sexual dysfunction).

Sexually aversive patients may find themselves repulsed, nauseated, or even panic stricken at the thought of sexual contact in general or one dimension of sexual contact in particular. Obviously, in the event that this response is limited to a specific partner, the implications are quite different. Successful treatment is predicated on the basis of careful identification of the source of aversive feelings (i.e., fear, performance anxiety, religious conflicts, or previous trauma) and employing both behavioral and often dyadic psychotherapeutic techniques to achieve treatment goals. When the aversion is not simply the result of finding a partner unattractive, the approach to treatment involves behavioral desensitization using sensate focus techniques that permit the affected person to begin with the least threatening behaviors, such as touching themselves, and then progress to more threatening behaviors, such as kissing or touching the partner, in a graduated sense.

Sexual Arousal Disorders

Female sexual arousal disorder

The diagnostic criteria for female sexual arousal disorder include persistent or recurrent inability to attain or to maintain until completion of the sexual activity an adequate lubrication and swelling response of sexual excitement, which causes marked distress or interpersonal difficulty. In addition, the sexual dysfunction is not better accounted for by another axis I disorder (except another sexual dysfunction) and is not exclusively related to the direct physiologic effects of a substance (e.g., drug abuse, or other medication) or a general medical condition.

Arousal difficulties can be caused by many of the same issues as those identified in patients with hypoactive sexual desire. In addition, reproductive organ or more generalized somatic pain can contribute. This disorder (when psychogenic) appears to be less common today as a result of more open presentation of sexual information in the media and more open discussion among peers.

Orgasmic Disorders

Female orgasmic disorder

The diagnostic criteria for female orgasmic disorder include persistent or recurrent delay in or absence of orgasm following a normal sexual excitement phase. Women exhibit wide variability in the type or intensity of stimulation that triggers orgasm. The diagnosis of female orgasmic disorder should be based on the clinician's judgment that the woman's orgasmic capacity is less than would be reasonable for her age, sexual experience, and the adequacy of sexual stimulation she receives. Other criteria include marked distress or interpersonal difficulty and the orgasmic dysfunction is not better accounted for by another axis I disorder (except another sexual dysfunction) and is not exclusively related to the direct physiologic effects of a substance (e.g., drug abuse or other medication) or a general medical condition.

Chronic illness, radical surgery, depression, and prescription or nonprescription drugs can all cause orgasmic dysfunction. Psychoactive medication, such as the SSRI antidepressants fluoxetine, sertraline, and paroxetine, can cause either delayed or inhibited orgasm. When psychotropics are thought to be causal, doses may be carefully lowered or in some cases medication changes to other agents will be helpful. When doing so, careful follow-up is absolutely necessary to avert crises.

Performance anxiety is among the common themes for women with orgasmic difficulties. In addition, fear of loss of control, religious guilt, anger with a partner, and lack of attraction to a partner are all considerations. Some women become inhibited by fear that orgasm will lead to vocalization that may lead to discovery by others, including children.

Treatment of psychogenic female orgasmic disorder commences with education, conflict resolution, and then behavioral strategies directed at reduction of performance anxiety and fear. Encouraging the patient to focus on her pleasure while stimulating herself with her own hand or a vibrator can be helpful. Subsequent sensate focus techniques involving her partner can be beneficial. Directed reading is frequently worthwhile. Among the helpful books that provide comfortable education and a strategy the patient can follow for success is Lonnie Barbach's *For Yourself*.

Vaginismus

The diagnostic criteria for vaginismus include recurrent or persistent involuntary spasm of the musculature of the outer third of the vagina that interferes with sexual intercourse, the disturbance causes marked distress or interpersonal difficulty, and the disturbance is not better accounted for by another axis I disorder (e.g., somatization disorder) and is not exclusively related to the direct physiologic effects of a general medical condition.

Vaginismus may develop after an episode of pelvic or vaginal pain associated with dyspareunia. Religious conflict or sexual abuse may contribute. Although it is commonly reported that this diagnosis can be confirmed in the gynecologist's examination room, this is not always the case. For some women, a gentle, communicative gynecologic exam in the presence of an attendant may be far less threatening than intercourse.

Treatment of vaginismus includes appreciation and discussion of potential causative factors, reduction of conflict and guilt, and a behavioral approach based on desensitization. The patient should use her fingers to explore her genitalia as opposed to using a dilator. Once the patient is comfortable touching and exploring her genitals, her partner may be involved in the process with a sensate focus type of approach.

KEY POINTS

1 Initial therapy for sexual dysfunction is aimed at correcting or modifying contributing concurrent medical illness and drug side effects.

2 Concurrent psychiatric illness that may be secondarily contributing to the patient's sexual function needs to be addressed.

3 Therapeutic approaches depend on the specific sexual dysfunction.

4 The goal of treatment is that both partners will be able to share in a mutually satisfying, physically intimate, and loving relationship.

SUGGESTED READINGS

American Psychiatric Association: *Diagnostic and statistical manual of mental disorders, DSM-IV,* ed 4, Washington, DC, 1994, The Association.

Anderson BL: Yes, there are sexual problems: now, what can we do about them? (editorial) *Gynecol Oncol* 52:10-13, 1994.

Balon R et al: Sexual dysfunction during antidepressant treatment, *J Clin Psychiatry* 54:209-212, 1993.

Corney RH et al: Psychosexual dysfunction in women with gynecological cancer following radical pelvic surgery, *Br J Obstet Gynecol* 100:73-78, 1993.

Hutchinson KA: Androgens and sexuality, *Am J Med* 98(suppl 1A):111S-115S, 1995.

Kelstrom L et al: Sexuality after hysterectomy: a factor analysis of women's sexual lives before and after subtotal hysterectomy, *Obstet Gynecol* 81:357-362, 1993.

Rosen RC, Ashton AK: Prosexual drugs: empirical status of the "new aphrodisiacs." *Arch Sex Behav* 22:521-543, 1993.

Rosen RC et al: Prevalence of sexual dysfunction in women: results of a survey study of 329 women in an outpatient gynecological clinic, *J Sex Marital Ther* 19:171-188, 1993.

Webster L: Management of sexual problems in diabetic patients, *Br J Hosp Med* 51:465-468, 1994.

Wilsnack SC et al: Predicting onset and chronicity of women's problem drinking: a five-year longitudinal analysis, *Am J Public Health* 81:305-318, 1991.

24

Sterilization

GERI D. HEWITT

Sterilization is the most common form of contraception in the United States. Because of the growing use of laparoscopy, more women now undergo laparoscopic sterilization than men do vasectomy.

Female sterilization has a typical failure rate of 0.4%, and most failures are caused by technical errors. If a woman conceives after a tubal ligation, she is at increased risk of an ectopic pregnancy, particularly if the pregnancy occurs 2 to 3 years after the procedure. Overall, however, the risk of ectopic pregnancy is less in women who have been sterilized than in noncontraceptors. Female sterilization has a fatality rate of 1.5 per 100,000 procedures.

METHODS OF STERILIZATION

Tubal Occlusion

Female sterilization can be performed by laparoscopy, minilaparotomy, or colpotomy. Laparoscopic tubal occlusion is most common in the United States and has the advantage of being an outpatient procedure with full recovery anticipated within 24 hours. It also leaves minimal scars and gives the surgeon the opportunity to view the abdominal and pelvic organs for any abnormalities. The disadvantages of the laparoscopic approach over the minilaparotomy include the expensive equipment required, the risk of inadvertent bowel or vessel injury, and the laparoscopic training required by the surgeon. Laparoscopic tubal occlusion can be done under general, conduction, or local anesthesia. Although most procedures utilize bipolar electrocoagulation because of the decreased incidence of damage to bowel, unipolar electrocoagulation and mechanical devices such as the Hulka-Clemens clip, Filshie clip, or Falope ring can be used as well. Approximately 2 to 3 cm of the isthmic portion of the fallopian tube should be destroyed.

Minilaparotomy is more commonly used in developing countries to perform female sterilization because it does not require any special surgical equipment or laparoscopic surgical skills. If the patient is not pregnant, a 3 to 5 cm incision can be made suprapubically to perform the procedure. The failure rate is similar to that of the laparoscopic approach. In the United States, the minilaparotomy is often used when performing postpartum tubal ligations. When performed after delivery, a small subumbilical incision can be made to gain access to the fallopian tubes. Postpartum tubal ligations have approximately twice the failure rate as tubal ligations done remote from delivery. Most tubal occlusions done via a minilaparotomy use a Pomeroy type of procedure, although rings or clips could be used. A colpotomy or vaginal approach to tubal occlusion is rarely used in the United States because of a higher rate of failure, infection, and abscess formation.

Patients and their partners should be extensively counseled before undergoing sterilization. They should view the procedure as permanent and also understand that there is a small but significant chance for intrauterine or ectopic pregnancy after the procedure. Alternative contraceptive options should be reviewed, and the risks of surgery and anesthesia should be outlined.

Vasectomy

More vasectomies are performed in the United States than in any other country. Vasectomy is safer and less expensive than female sterilization. The typical failure rate is 0.15%. Unlike female sterilization, vasectomy is not immediately effective and requires 15 ejaculations or 6 weeks before the man is sterile. Vasectomy is performed as an office procedure with local anesthetic and typically takes approximately 15 minutes to complete. There have been no deaths in the United States attributed to vasectomy. Reported minor complications include hematoma formation or infection, which can easily be treated with heat and antibiotics, respectively. Men who have a vasectomy are not at increased risk of cardiovascular or autoimmune disease; however, controversy exists regarding whether vasectomy leads to an increased risk for prostate cancer.

KEY POINTS

1 Sterilization is the most commonly used form of contraception in the United States.

2 Female sterilization has a failure rate of 0.4%, with an increased risk of ectopic pregnancy if conception does occur.

3 All sterilizations should be considered permanent, and the patient should be counseled regarding alternative contraceptive methods, as well as the risks of the procedure and anesthesia used.

4 Vasectomy is safer, less expensive, and more effective than female sterilization.

SUGGESTED READINGS

Mosher WD, Pratt WF: *Contraceptive use in the United States, 1973-1988: advance data from vital and health statistics,* No. 182, Hyattsville, Md, 1990. National Center for Health Statistics.

Peterson HB et al: The risk of pregnancy after tubal sterilization: findings from the U.S. Collaborative Review of Sterilization, *Am J Obstet Gynecol* 174:1161-70, 1996.

Speroff L, Darney P: *A clinical guide for contraception,* Baltimore, 1996, Williams and Wilkins.

25

Urinary Dysfunction

Renee M. Caputo

The bladder and the urethra constitute the lower urinary tract in the female. These structures together perform two functions, the storage and the evacuation of urine. There are two types of urinary dysfunction: urinary incontinence and voiding dysfunction (incomplete bladder emptying). Urinary incontinence is a disorder of the storage phase, and voiding dysfunction is a disorder of the emptying phase.

URINARY INCONTINENCE

Urinary incontinence is the involuntary loss of urine in a patient who has identified it as a social or hygienic problem. Urinary incontinence has enormous social and economic consequences, affecting approximately 10 million Americans at a cost of over 10 billion/year. Women are at least two times more commonly affected than men. Among women in the general community, the prevalence of urinary incontinence has been estimated to be between 10% and 25%. This percentage increases with the age of the patient and has been estimated to be 50% or greater among women in nursing facilities.

Diagnosis

The diagnostic evaluation of a patient with the complaint of urinary incontinence consists of three parts: history, physical examination, and urodynamics (Fig. 25-1). The history of a patient with urinary incontinence should first establish how much of a problem it is for the patient. Second, determine the severity of the incontinence. Third, establish the type of incontinence present by asking the patient for the presence of specific symptoms typically associated with the different types of incontinence. This information can be easily obtained via a questionnaire (Fig. 25-2).

The medical history is essential in the evaluation of a patient with urinary incontinence. Risk factors for development of urinary incontinence can be identified. Surgical history is also important, especially regarding previous pelvic surgery or antiincontinence procedures. Numerous medications can affect lower urinary tract function; therefore a list of the patient's prescription and over-the-counter medications should be obtained.

A bladder diary is valuable in the evaluation of a patient with urinary incontinence. It is a record that the patient keeps (usually in 24-hour

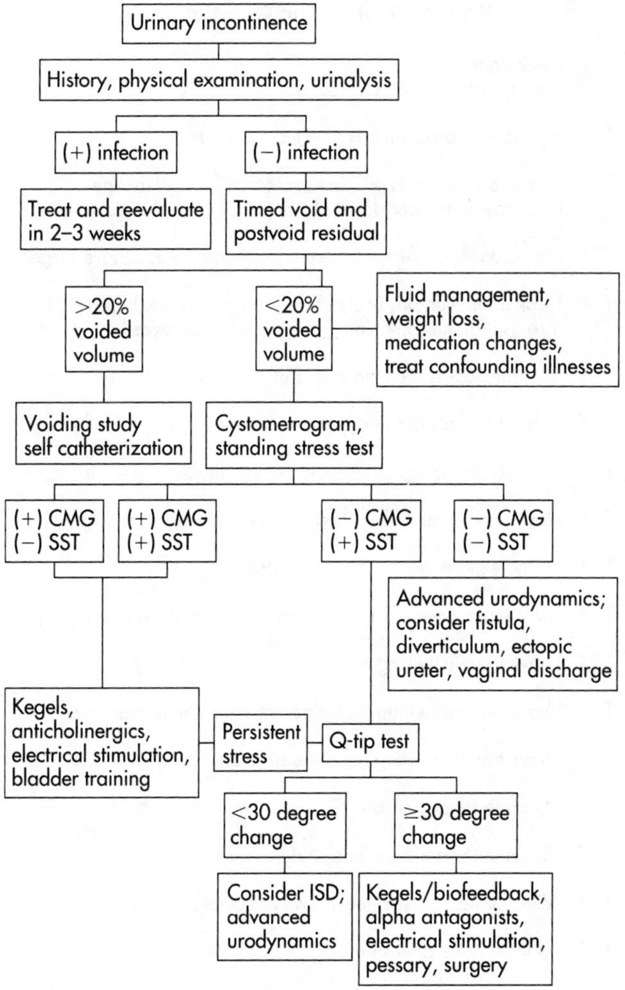

FIG. 25-1 Management of urinary incontinence.

Urinary Dysfunction Questionnaire

T F I leak urine
If so, for how long? ______________________

T F My bladder problem has affected my lifestyle

T F I have to wear pads or other protection for my leakage
If so, how many per day? ______________________

T F My bladder problem is severe enough that I would have surgery

T F I leak urine with physical activity (cough, sneeze, bend, etc.)
If so, is it at the same time_____, or a few seconds later____?

T F My urine loss is a continuous drip

T F I often have a strong urge to urinate even if I am not full

T F I have a strong urge to urinate before I leak

T F I lose urine when I come home and put my key in the lock

T F I urinate more than 10 times per day

T F The need to urinate wakes me up 2 or more times per night

T F I have trouble wetting the bed

T F I have had more than 2 bladder infections in the past year

T F I have trouble starting my urine stream

T F My urine stream is slow

T F My urine stream starts and stops

T F After I urinate, I often feel I have not emptied completely

T F I dribble urine after urinating

FIG. 25-2 Urinary dysfunction questionnaire.

intervals) of her daily voids, voided volumes, incontinence episodes, reasons for the incontinence, and fluid intake. The bladder diary is an objective way to assess the severity of incontinence and response to treatment. It can also be used to determine the type of urinary incontinence present.

The physical examination of a patient with urinary incontinence consists of a general examination to rule out any medical condition that could contribute to incontinence, a neurologic evaluation with particular emphasis on the lumbar and sacral dermatomes, an abdominal examination to rule out a pelvic mass, and pelvic and rectal examinations.

Urodynamics is the term given to the diagnostic tests used to determine the presence, severity, and type of urinary incontinence. The goal of a urodynamic evaluation is to reproduce the patient's symptoms. Urodynamics can be divided into basic, which can be done simply in the office, and advanced, which requires special equipment.

Differential Diagnosis

The differential diagnosis of a patient with urinary incontinence includes the different types of urethral urinary incontinence: stress, urge, mixed, and overflow. Although less common, causes of extraurethral incontinence should be considered, such as a fistula or ectopic ureter. A urethral diverticulum should be suspected, particularly in patients who complain of dribbling of urine following urination, dyspareunia, recurrent UTIs, or who have an anterior vaginal wall mass. Conditions that can be mistaken for urinary incontinence include vaginal discharge and excessive vulvar perspiration.

Urinary incontinence can occur transiently because of treatable medical conditions that can be remembered using the mnemonic *DIAPPERS* (for *d*elirium, *i*nfection, *a*trophic urethritis and vaginitis, *p*harmalogic causes, *p*sychologic causes, *e*xcess fluid excretion, *r*estricted mobility, and *s*tool impaction). These situations are often found in the elderly patient.

STRESS INCONTINENCE

Stress incontinence is the most prevalent type of urinary incontinence in women, occurring in 50% to 70% of cases of urinary incontinence. The classic symptom of a woman with stress incontinence is the loss of urine with physical activity at the same time as the stress event. The urodynamic definition of stress incontinence is the involuntary loss of urine that occurs when the bladder pressure exceeds urethral pressure during times of increased intraabdominal pressure in the absence of a bladder contraction. For continence to be achieved, the urethral pressure must be equal to or greater than bladder pressure.

Pathophysiology

The most common reason for stress incontinence is weakness of the urethral skeletal muscle or muscular supports as a result of a partial denervation injury. The ability of these skeletal muscles to contract in response to increased intraabdominal pressure is compromised and as a result, urethral closure is not maintained.

Denervation injury to the female pelvic floor skeletal muscle is most commonly caused by vaginal delivery. Other risk factors include conditions that chronically increase intraabdominal pressure such as obesity, chronic coughing, heavy lifting, and chronic straining with constipation. Pelvic surgery, neurologic diseases, diabetes, and the effects of aging may also interfere with the pelvic floor nerve supply.

Conditions that interfere with other components of the urethral sphincter or supports may also contribute to the development of stress incontinence. Hypoestrogenism may lead to urethral mucosal thinning and decreased engorgement of the submucosal vascular plexus. Alpha blocking agents commonly used for the treatment of hypertension can decrease urethral smooth muscle tone and are associated with the onset of stress incontinence. Diseases that affect connective tissue may predispose a patient to the loss of urethral support.

Types

There are two types of urinary stress incontinence: stress incontinence with hypermobility and intrinsic urethral sphincter deficiency (ISD). They differ in the degree of urethral sphincter or supports deficiency present. Patients with ISD have very little to no functional sphincter mechanism, little to no mobility of the bladder neck, and severe stress incontinence. It is important to distinguish between the two because they are treated differently.

Diagnosis

The typical history of a patient with stress incontinence will be the loss of urine with physical activity at the same time as the activity, and usually in small amounts. The number of incontinence episodes per day will depend on how severely the urethral sphincter or supports have been compromised and how active the patient is. The voiding diary of a patient with stress incontinence will usually show normal bladder capacity (up to 600 cc), normal frequency (<8 voids/24 hours if fluid intake is <2000 cc), and accidents that occur with physical activity.

The physical examination of a patient with stress incontinence is performed to identify causes for increased intraabdominal pressure (i.e., obesity, a pelvic mass, and lung disease). During the pelvic examination, the vaginal mucosa should be observed for signs of atrophy or prolapse. Many patients with stress incontinence will have vaginal relaxation, especially of the anterior vaginal wall, because stress incontinence and vaginal prolapse have similar pathophysiologic mechanisms.

The urodynamic diagnosis of stress incontinence can be accomplished by basic or advanced testing. The basic evaluation consists of a standing stress test (SST). During this test, the patient is asked to cough while standing with legs shoulder width apart while the examiner observes for the loss of urine. The SST should be performed while the patient has a symptomatically full bladder. A positive SST would be the observation of a small amount of urine loss immediately with the cough. The SST has the highest positive and negative predictive values for the diagnosis of stress incontinence. Advanced urodynamic testing involves placing catheters in the bladder and rectum or vagina to measure bladder, urethral, and abdominal pressure simultaneously.

Once the diagnosis of stress incontinence is made, the type is then determined. Hypermobility of the urethrovesical junction can be confirmed with the cotton swab or "Q-tip" test. A cotton swab is placed into the bladder through the urethra and then pulled back into the urethra until resistance is met. This will place the cotton tip in the proximal urethra. The position of the wooden arm of the swab is then noted with respect to horizontal degrees while the patient is supine and resting. Above the horizontal (0 degrees) is negative, below the horizontal is positive. The patient is then asked to maximally perform the Valsalva maneuver, and the change in the position of the swab is again noted with respect to horizontal degrees. A resting position of negative 30 degrees or more or a change of 30 degrees or more with Valsalva technique is considered by most to be hypermobile. Suspect ISD in patients without hypermobility, with severe stress incontinence, who are elderly, who have a neurologic disease, or who had multiple antiincontinence surgeries. Advanced urodynamics should be performed in patients who are considering surgery in whom the diagnosis is unclear after basic testing or when ISD is suspected.

Treatment

Treatments for stress incontinence either increase urethral resistance or provide urethral support, particularly during increased intraabdominal pressure. This can be accomplished surgically or nonsurgically.

Common sense measures

Common sense measures include restriction of fluid intake to less than 2000 cc/day, eliminating certain foods and drinks that increase urine output, such as caffeinated beverages and alcohol, avoiding large amounts of fluid intake before bed or going out, weight loss, and controlling certain medical illness that can affect lower urinary tract function, such as diabetes and lumbosacral disc disease. Certain medications can also predispose a women to urinary incontinence, including diuretics, alpha antagonists, and sedatives.

Medications

Alpha antagonists promote continence by increasing the smooth muscle tone of the urethral sphincter. The most commonly used medication is phenylpropanolamine in its sustained-release form. Pseudoephedrine and ephedrine are also used.

Estrogen theoretically increases urethral resistance by increasing mucosal thickness, increasing volume within the submucosal vascular plexus, and increasing the concentration of alpha antagonist receptors in the smooth muscle sphincter potentiating the effect of alpha antagonists. Every postmenopausal woman with stress incontinence should be offered ERT if she has no contraindications.

Pelvic floor skeletal muscle exercises

Pelvic floor muscle exercises increase pelvic floor skeletal muscle tone, specifically the urethral skeletal muscle and the levator ani, at rest and reflexively during increased intraabdominal pressure. A Kegel exercise is the voluntary contraction of the pelvic floor skeletal muscle performed by the patient repetitively over time. Patients should be instructed in the correct performance of these exercises and should perform at least 50/day for maximum improvement potential. Biofeedback can be used if necessary to teach the patient how to perform the exercise correctly.

Another way to perform pelvic floor skeletal muscle exercises is to use vaginal cones, tapered weights that the patient holds within the vagina by contracting the pubococcygeal muscle. The heaviest cone a patient can hold is worn 15 minutes twice daily while the patient is in the upright position.

Pelvic floor muscle contraction can also be accomplished using electrical stimulation. Via a rectal or more typically a vaginal surface electrode probe, an electrical current of 5 to 50 Hz is delivered for 15 to 30 minutes daily to weekly. The pelvic floor skeletal muscle is stimulated via the pudendal nerve, causing passive repetitive contractions. Electrical stimulation is ideal for patients who are unable to contract their pelvic floor skeletal muscles voluntarily.

Vaginal pessary

Vaginal pessaries for stress incontinence are devices that when properly placed in the vagina, compress the urethra by placing pressure on the anterior vaginal wall. There are several devices available, all of which come in different sizes that must be fitted.

Surgical therapy

The surgical procedure appropriate for stress incontinence depends on the type present. The procedures used for hypermobility immobilize the hypermobile urethra behind the symphysis using the anterior vaginal wall or periurethral tissues. Continence is achieved during times of increased intraabdominal pressure through two mechanisms, the restoration of the urethral "backstop" and the creation of bladder neck obstruction when the bladder is forced downward. Procedures for stress incontinence with hypermobility can done vaginally or abdominally. The commonly performed vaginal procedure is the needle urethropexy: Pereyra, Raz, Stamey, Gittes. The abdominal procedures are the Marshall-Marchetti-Krantz (MMK) and the Burch colposuspension.

The procedures for hypermobility have a relatively high failure rate when performed in patients with intrinsic urethral sphincter deficiency (ISD). Patients with ISD require a procedure that can affect more complete urethral closure. These procedures include a sling urethropexy, using either autologous or synthetic materials, urethral submucosal collagen injection, or an artificial sphincter.

Unless the patient is going to have surgery for other indications, patients should be offered nonsurgical therapeutic options first. Nonsurgical therapies offer the patient a more than 50% chance of improvement with the advantage of less cost and fewer complications.

URGE INCONTINENCE

Urge incontinence is defined both symptomatically and urodynamically. Patients with urge incontinence will complain of the involuntary loss of urine preceded by a sudden, strong urge to urinate. Urine loss is usually in large amounts and difficult to control once it starts. Urge incontinence occurs spontaneously or on provocation such as physical activity, cold weather, running water, laughing, sexual intercourse, or placing a key in a door lock. Patients with urge incontinence will often complain of frequent voiding, urgency, getting up two or more times at night to urinate (nocturia), or bed wetting (nocturnal enuresis). Urodynamically, urge incontinence is defined as an involuntary bladder contraction that occurs during the storage or filling phase either spontaneously or on provocation. This type of incontinence comprises 10% to 30% of all cases.

Pathophysiology

Urge incontinence is the result of bladder dysfunction during the storage phase. The bladder muscle will contract involuntarily instead of remaining relaxed and accommodating increasing volume. Urethral relaxation occurs simultaneously with the bladder contraction through normal reflex pathways, and a loss of urine will most often occur.

The etiology of involuntary bladder contractions during the storage phase is poorly understood and reflects how little is known about lower urinary tract inhibitory mechanisms. The most common etiology is idiopathic. Neurologic diseases that affect the nerve pathways anywhere from the cortex to the periphery can cause urge incontinence. Conditions that irritate the bladder (i.e., a bladder stone, bladder tumor, infection, or foreign body) can lead to urge incontinence. Smooth muscle disorders or abnormalities of the local conducting system–the pacemaker cells or ganglia–have also been proposed as possible causes of urge incontinence. Medications with cholinergic antagonist activity may also lead to this condition. Patients may develop de novo urge incontinence following antiincontinence surgery for stress incontinence. Urethral outlet obstruction, usually from antiincontinence surgery or anterior vaginal wall prolapse, may cause urge incontinence.

Types

Urge incontinence is the term given to the symptom of loss of urine preceded by a strong urge to urinate. Once uninhibited bladder contractions are confirmed urodynamically, the diagnosis will be one of three types. *Detrusor instability,* the most common type, is the term used for patients who have no identifiable cause. If the urge incontinence can be attributed to a neurologic etiology, such as multiple sclerosis, it is referred to as *detrusor hyperreflexia.* Detrusor hyperactivity with impaired contractions (DHIC) is the term given to those patients who also have an elevated postvoid residual. DHIC is more common in the elderly population.

Diagnosis

Patients should be questioned about the presence of urgency, frequency, nocturia, nocturnal enuresis, and urge incontinence. Many women with urge incontinence as adults were bed wetters as children. Women with urge incontinence will often be given the diagnosis of recurrent UTIs because their symptoms are similar. Documentation of UTIs, either through urinalysis or culture, is imperative. Patients who develop anterior vaginal wall prolapse may develop signs of urge incontinence simultaneously. Previous history of pelvic surgery or radiation should be obtained as well as the patient's estrogen status. Patients with painful bladder syndrome or interstitial cystitis may also have a component of urge incontinence.

A bladder diary would typically reveal more than seven voids in 24 hours given a normal fluid intake of 1500 to 2000 cc, small voided volumes of less than 200 cc consistently, and incontinence episodes caused by "not making it in time," "waiting too long," or preceded by an urge.

Physical examination should include a pelvic examination for signs of atrophy, vaginal infection, urethral or bladder infection, urethral diverticulum, or vaginal prolapse. A neurologic exam, especially of the lower extremities, perineal sensation, and bulbocavernosus reflex, is recommended. Urinalysis is necessary to check for hematuria or infection.

Because urge incontinence is caused by inappropriate bladder contractions during the storage phase, the urodynamic diagnosis is made by observing bladder pressure while the bladder is filling. This urodynamic test is called a *cystometrogram.* A cystometrogram can be performed via a foley catheter, which measures only bladder pressure qualitatively, or using pressure catheters that can quantify bladder pressure as well as measure other parameters simultaneously such as urethral and abdominal pressures. A cystometrogram will give information regarding sensation, bladder capacity, accommodation (compliance), and stability. A positive or unstable cystometrogram will show an elevation of bladder pressure caused by the detrusor muscle, not abdominal pressure, during filling while the patient is attempting to inhibit micturition. The rise in bladder pressure is often associated with a strong urge to void and loss of urine around the catheter, which the patient is unable to control. Most patients with urge incontinence have decreased maximum bladder capacity, less than 400 cc. A postvoid residual should also be obtained from patients with urge incontinence to rule out DHIC.

Treatment

If an identifiable cause for urge incontinence is discovered, such as infection or bladder tumor, then it should be addressed first. In most instances in which the cause is unknown or untreatable, the patient is treated symptomatically. The goal in the treatment of urge incontinence is to increase bladder capacity and decrease frequency, urgency, nocturia, and incontinence. This can be accomplished behaviorally or pharmacologically.

Behavioral therapies include "common sense" measures, bladder training, and pelvic floor muscle exercises. Bladder training is mandatory voiding at increasing intervals. The initial voiding frequency is determined by the patient's voiding diary. Start at her shortest interval and have her void at this interval only during the day, whether she has to void or not. Various relaxation and distraction techniques can be used to get the patient to her next void. This interval is then increased, depending on the severity of the incontinence, by one-half hour every week. The goal is to reach a 3- to 4-hour interval. Bladder training will decrease frequency and incontinence episodes in the majority of patients.

Pelvic floor muscle exercises commonly used for stress incontinence can also be helpful for women with urge incontinence. When the pelvic floor musculature is contracted, a bladder contraction can be inhibited. Electrical stimulation in animal models directly stimulates the sympathetic system and inhibits the parasympathetic system, actions that promote bladder relaxation. All of the pelvic floor muscle exercise techniques described for stress incontinence can be used.

Medications are the most commonly used therapy for urge incontinence. Medications with anticholinergic or antispasmodic activity are the most effective. These agents include oxybutynin chloride (Ditropan), propantheline (Pro-Banthine), imipramine (Tofranil), dicyclomine (Bentyl), and hyoscyamine (Cystospaz, Levsinex). More than 50% of patients with urge incontinence will improve with these medications, but their use is often curtailed by side effects. Common side effects are dry mouth and constipation, which tend to be annoying rather than harmful. More severe side effects include tachycardia, blurred vision, confusion, and urinary retention. Elderly patients are more susceptible to these side effects. Start with the lowest possible dose and increase until the desired effect is achieved or undesirable side effects occur. Estrogen can decrease bladder irritability symptoms in the menopausal patient but does not decrease the number of uninhibited contractions.

Therapies for urge incontinence can be combined to achieve a maximum effect. It is wise to maximize one therapy at a time before adding another.

MIXED URINARY INCONTINENCE

Mixed urinary incontinence is the presence of both stress and urge incontinence and comprises 10% to 20% of all cases of incontinence. It is diagnosed and treated similarly. Treatment should address the component that is believed to be the most predominant. Surgical therapy for the stress component in patients with mixed incontinence has a higher failure rate than in patients with pure stress incontinence. Therefore surgical therapy should only be recommended to patients with mixed incontinence after the urge component is controlled and if the stress component is still present and bothersome to the patient. Pelvic floor muscle exercises, in any form, are ideal for patients with mixed incontinence. Imipramine (Tofranil) is also recommended because it has both anticholinergic and alpha antagonist properties.

VOIDING DYSFUNCTION

Voiding dysfunction is the term given to incomplete bladder emptying. The goal of the emptying phase of the lower urinary tract is the complete evacuation of the bladder when deemed socially acceptable by the patient. This process begins with the voluntary relaxation of the pelvic floor skeletal muscle with subsequent urethral relaxation, followed by a sustained bladder contraction.

Pathophysiology

The etiology of a voiding dysfunction can be attributed to either a functional or anatomic obstruction of the urethra or poor to no bladder contractility. In the female patient, the latter is most common.

Voluntary urethral relaxation and bladder contraction as well as the coordination of the two is neurologically mediated. An insult to any level of this neurologic network may interfere with urethral relaxation or bladder contraction and lead to incomplete bladder emptying.

Urethral obstruction in a woman is uncommon. Urethral stenosis, either congenital or acquired (recurrent UTIs, or urethral surgery), may lead to a voiding dysfunction. Bladder polyps, tumors, or stones could cause urethral obstruction. The most common reason for urethral obstruction in a female is antiincontinence surgery or prolapse of the anterior vaginal wall.

Bladder contractility tends to decrease with age. The elderly patient is more likely to have this problem. Poor to no bladder contractility is also drug related. Many antidepressants, antipsychotics, antispasmodics, antihistamines, and narcotics can decrease the amplitude of a bladder contraction. Diabetes, myesthenia gravis, and fecal impaction may also affect bladder contractility.

A voiding disturbance can be caused by perineal trauma or pain (e.g., following a vaginal delivery, a primary herpes simplex virus infection, or vaginal surgery). Acute cystitis can cause incomplete bladder emptying. Strange surroundings or acute psychologic stress can also interfere with voiding. If a bladder becomes overdistended, such as following an epidural or over time in those patients who void infrequently, its ability to contract can be compromised.

Overflow Incontinence

Overflow incontinence is a symptom of a voiding dysfunction and comprises less than 5% of all incontinence cases. Patients with overflow incontinence will typically complain of a constant dribbling of urine not necessarily associated with increased physical activity or preceded by an urge. They may or may not have other symptoms of a voiding dysfunction. Patients with overflow incontinence generally have very high postvoid residuals of greater than 200 cc.

Diagnosis

The patient with incomplete bladder emptying may be completely asymptomatic. Others will complain of frequency, nocturia, incontinence, hesitancy, slow urine stream, interrupted urine stream, prolonged emptying time, having to use the Valsalva maneuver or change positions to void, feelings of incomplete bladder emptying, recurrent UTIs, or the inability to void. The voiding diary is usually not diagnostic, but may show frequent voids.

It is important to obtain a medical history as well as a list of all medications, both prescription and over-the-counter. The onset of symptoms is important and may correlate with some other event in the patient's history such as the development of prolapse or antiincontinence surgery.

Patients with neurologic disease may experience a voiding dysfunction as their first symptom. Patients with uncontrolled diabetes are more likely to have a voiding dysfunction.

Physical examination should rule out abdominal or pelvic masses that could impinge on the bladder outlet. For example, urinary obstruction has been reported in women with uterine fibroids. A pelvic examination is necessary to confirm the presence of prolapse, especially of the anterior vaginal wall, and to check uterine size and irregularity. A rectal examination should rule out fecal impaction.

Urodynamics evaluate the emptying phase and consist of basic and advanced testing. Basic tests measure the average urine flow rate (voided volume/time [sec] to complete void) and postvoid residual, either by catheterization or ultrasound. Normal average flow rate is ≥10 cc/sec, with a void of 200 cc or more. The amount of postvoid residual considered normal is controversial but generally is believed to be ≤20% of the voided volume. Urinalysis is done to check for infection. In most instances, these tests will identify those patients with a voiding dysfunction as well as patients who are at risk of a voiding dysfunction after antiincontinence surgery. Advanced testing determines whether the bladder or the urethra is responsible for the incomplete emptying. Pressure catheters are placed in the bladder that measure both urethral and bladder pressures while the patient is voiding. Cystoscopy rules out urethral stenosis, bladder tumors, polyps, or stones.

Treatment

The goal of treatment is to affect more complete bladder emptying. Patients with lower urinary tract symptomatology who are found to have an elevated postvoid residual should have the voiding dysfunction treated before addressing any other symptom.

Treatment depends on the etiology of the voiding dysfunction. Reversible conditions such as a bladder infection, bladder tumor, or medication should be addressed. With urethral obstruction, the treatment also depends on the etiology. If anterior vaginal wall prolapse is present, reduction with a pessary or surgical therapy is indicated. Patients who become permanently obstructed after antiincontinence surgery can be taught to intermittently self-catheterize or have the antiincontinence surgery reversed (urethrolysis). Urethral dilation is rarely indicated, but may play a role in those patients with rare urethral stenosis.

If bladder contractility is compromised from reasons other than a medication, many times it cannot be reversed. These patients will need to perform intermittent self-catheterization. For individuals who cannot perform this procedure, a caregiver can be taught to do so. For temporary conditions, a urethral or suprapubic catheter may be used. A chronic indwelling foley catheter is rarely indicated and should be avoided at all cost because of its association with a high rate of morbidity, especially in the elderly. Bethanechol is sometimes used for patients with voiding dysfunction but should be combined with an alpha-antagonist for maximal effectiveness.

KEY POINTS

1 The lower urinary tract (bladder and urethra) serves two purposes: the storage and emptying of urine.

2 Stress and urge incontinence are the result of a storage phase disorder.

3 When dysfunction of the emptying phase occurs, incomplete bladder emptying will result. This condition is called a *voiding dysfunction,* of which overflow incontinence is an example.

4 A thorough history, physical examination, voiding diary, and urodynamics will determine the type of urinary dysfunction present.

5 Treatment of urinary incontinence can be surgical or nonsurgical and depends on the type present. Treatments for stress incontinence increase urethral resistance. Treatments for urge incontinence relax bladder smooth muscle and increase bladder capacity.

6 Treatment of a voiding dysfunction depends on whether it is caused by urethral or bladder dysfunction, and whether the etiology is reversible. The goal is more complete bladder emptying.

SUGGESTED READINGS

Appell RA: Injection therapy for urethral incontinence. In *Female urology,* Philadelphia, 1994, JB Lippincott.

Bergman A, Elia G: Three surgical procedures for genuine stress incontinence: five-year follow-up of a prospective randomized study, *Am J Obstet Gynecol* 173:66-71, 1995.

Fall M, Lindstrom S: Functional electrical stimulation: physiological basis and clinical principles, *Int Urogynecol J* 5:296-304, 1994.

Fantl JA et al: Efficacy of bladder training in older women with urinary incontinence, *JAMA* 265:609-613, 1991.

Farrell SA, Ostergard DR: Choice of surgical procedure for stress incontinence. In *Female pelvic floor disorders,* New York, 1992, WW Norton & Co.

Sand PK et al: Pelvic floor electrical stimulation in the treatment of genuine stress incontinence: a multicenter placebo-controlled trial, *Am J Obstet Gynecol* 173:72-79, 1995.

Summitt RL, Bent AE, Ostergard DR: The pathophysiology of genuine stress incontinence, *Int Urogynecol J* 1:12-18, 1990.

Urinary Incontinence Guideline Panel: *Urinary incontinence in adults: clinical practice guideline,* AHCPR Pub No 92-0038, Rockville, Md, March 1992, Agency for Health Care Policy and Research, Public Health Service, U.S. Dept of Health and Human Services.

Wall LL: Diagnosis and management of urinary incontinence due to detrusor instability, *Obstet Gynecol Surv* 45:1S-47S, 1990.

Wall LL, Norton PA, DeLancey JOL: Conservative management of stress incontinence. In *Practical Urogynecology,* Baltimore, 1993, Williams & Wilkins.

Wheeler JS, Walter JS: Urinary retention in females: a review, *Int Urogynecol J* 3:137-142, 1992.

Wiskind AK, Stanton SL: The Burch colposuspension for genuine stress urinary incontinence. In *TeLinde's operative gynecology* updates, vol 1, no 11, Philadelphia, 1992, JB Lippincott.

26

Uterine Bleeding—Abnormal

Chad I. Friedman

The normal menstrual cycle is characterized by cyclic bleeding every 24 to 36 days, induced by the synchronized withdrawal of both estrogen and progesterone. Duration of menstrual bleeding is typically 3 to 7 days and associated with 20 to 80 ml of blood loss. The fluid loss observed by the individual is actually a combination of blood, transudate, and tissue.

Factors controlling the amount of menstrual bleeding include coagulation factors, platelet aggregation, uterine contractility, local levels of metalloproteinase inhibitors, local levels of tissue plasminogen activator, vascular contractility, and endometrial regenerative capacity.

Although consistency in the amount of blood loss is reported by most women (in the absence of extremes of bleeding), there have been few studies showing a strong correlation between perception of blood loss and actual blood loss. Thus complaints of menorrhagia (heavy menstrual bleeding) must be considered in terms of social acceptability to the patient as well as medical significance (e.g., anemia as documented by hemoglobin or hematocrit levels). The traditional pad count often reflects social acceptability as much or more than actual blood loss.

Although cyclic predictable changes in estrogen and progesterone are instrumental in limiting the amount of menstrual blood loss, they are equally important in controlling the timing of bleeding. After estrogen priming of the uterine endometrium, withdrawal of estrogen will induce endometrial sloughing and bleeding. In the presence of estrogen and progesterone priming, a fall in either hormone will induce uterine bleeding.

There is controversy in the terminology utilized to describe abnormal uterine bleeding. To aid in diagnosis the following working definitions will be used:

Menorrhagia: Excessive or prolonged uterine bleeding occurring at the time of the expected menstrual period.

Metrorrhagia: Bleeding in between the expected menstrual periods. It is assumed that the time of the normal menstrual period can be identified by traditional menstrual characteristics (i.e., premenstrual symptoms or bleeding pattern.)

Polymenorrhea: Menstrual bleeding of normal duration in association with ovulatory cycles occurring more frequently than every 24 days.

Oligomenorrhea: Menstrual bleeding after a presumed ovulatory cycle occurring at intervals less frequent than 36 days. Thus oligomenorrhea is equivalent to oligoovulation.

Anovulatory bleeding: Irregular bleeding in the absence of ovulatory cycles.

Abnormal uterine bleeding is a common gynecologic problem in all age groups. Etiologies vary from those that spontaneously resolve without significant morbidity to those that are life threatening, requiring very active intervention. The diagnosis strongly depends on the patient's stage of reproductive function.

DIAGNOSIS AND TREATMENT

Bleeding In Childhood and Adolescence

Bleeding from the reproductive tract in the prepubertal child is uncommon. With the exception of the newborn who may experience some bleeding following withdrawal of endogenous estrogen, *trauma, sexual abuse, and foreign bodies* always need to considered. Inappropriate parental or child behavior, concurrent vulvitis, or hymenal changes should be evaluated by an individual experienced with the evaluation of sexual abuse. Vulvovaginitis with a bloody discharge is common with a foreign body and frequently requires an examination under anesthesia to adequately inspect the vagina and obtain appropriate cultures.

Malignancies of childhood associated with vaginal bleeding are restricted primarily to sarcoma botryoides (an erythematous polypoid vaginal lesion) and endocrine tumors capable of inducing precocious puberty (i.e., granulosa cell tumors, Sertoli-Leydig cell tumors, and germ cell tumors). Although typically associated with other signs of pubertal development, hormone-producing tumors may have uterine bleeding as the initial symptom. Hormone-producing tumors are typically palpable on abdominal or rectoabdominal examination and are commonly associated with elevated estradiol or testosterone serum concentrations with prepubertal gonadotropin levels. In the absence of a mass, precocious puberty from other causes (i.e., follicular cysts, neurologic lesions, McCune-Albright syndrome, or constitutional) must also be considered. Benign anatomic conditions or lesions, such as prolapsed urethra or lichen sclerosis et atrophicus, are readily apparent and may cause genital bleeding. A careful physical examination is the most important component in the evaluation of abnormal bleeding in prepubertal girls.

Uterine bleeding in adolescents after the onset of puberty is predominantly of endocrine origin rather than anatomic. Although follicular activity is well developed around menarche, positive feedback responses to initiate the preovulatory LH surge often lag in their maturation. Thus a significant percentage of menstrual cycles around menarche are induced by estrogen withdrawal in the absence of a functional corpus luteum. Lacking progesterone, many of the hemostatic measures induced by progesterone (i.e., release of prostaglandins for uterine contractility and increased vascular tortuosity) are absent. Thus menstrual bleeding around menarche is often irregular, prolonged, and occasionally profuse. Anovulation for the first 12 months after menarche does not warrant an evaluation in the absence of physical signs. However, menarchial adolescents with troublesome uterine/vaginal bleeding do require a pelvic examination to exclude anatomic or traumatic lesions. In contrast to adults, endometrial biopsies need not be routinely performed. Heavy bleeding does require performance of a basic coagulation profile (i.e., platelets, PT, PTT, and bleeding time). Menarche is often the first challenge to the coagulation system. Thus in contrast to adults, coagulation defects are a common cause (15% to 20%) of severe menorrhagia during the first 6 months after menarche.

Relatively unique to this age group are müllerian anomalies associated with metrorrhagia. Egress of old menstrual blood may be observed with bicornuate uteri, vaginal septum, and bicollis hemihematocolpos. Although physical examination generally establishes the diagnosis, ultrasound evaluation of the pelvis and kidney may be helpful in confirming the diagnosis.

Treatment of presumed anovulatory bleeding in this age group relies initially on the use of oral estrogen. Conjugated estrogen 2.5 to 10 mg/day should be administered based on the amount of bleeding. Intravenous conjugated estrogen 25 mg every 4 to 6 hours may be used when oral medications can't be tolerated or in cases of profuse bleeding. Bleeding should typically subside within 1 to 3 days. Low-dose oral contraceptives may then be initiated for subsequent regulation of menstruation. Oral contraceptives may be discontinued after a few cycles unless contraception is required. Iron and vitamin supplementation should be added if anemia is present. Adolescents who fail to establish a normal menstrual pattern within 1 year of menarche are likely to persist with anovulatory bleeding and deserve a comprehensive endocrine evaluation.

Reproductive Age

The key decision to make in evaluating a patient in the reproductive age group with abnormal uterine bleeding is whether the patient is anovulatory, ovulatory, or possibly pregnant. Given the multitude of pregnancy tests available, it is imperative that the physician always consider the possibility of pregnancy. Differentiation of ovulatory from anovulatory states cannot always be made with ease based on history or physical examination. Therefore after excluding pregnancy, very liberal use of endometrial biopsies should be made, not only to rule out malignancy, which is rare, but also to confirm the clinical impression of ovulatory or anovulatory bleeding.

Anovulatory bleeding

Women with anovulatory bleeding typically have a history of frequently skipped periods, variable duration and quantity of bleeding, and the absence of premenstrual symptoms. Menstrual cramping is often minimal, but may be severe in the presence of clots. When not actively bleeding, cervical mucus is clear, stretchy, and abundant. The cervical mucus changes when not contaminated with blood are consistent with chronic estrogen stimulation.

Establishing the diagnosis relies on the history and physical findings. In addition, an endometrial biopsy should be performed to evaluate for atypical hyperplasia or endometrial carcinoma and to confirm the diagnosis. Secretory endometrium (luteal phase) on biopsy must make the physician question the diagnosis, though sporadic ovulation and pregnancy do occur in "oligomenorrhic" women.

The laboratory evaluation of a woman with anovulatory bleeding focuses on the cause of anovulation after assessment of hemoglobin and hematocrit levels. Polycystic ovarian disease, Cushing's disease, adrenal hyperplasia, and hypothyroidism may all be associated with anovulatory bleeding. The extent of laboratory evaluation primarily depends on historic and physical findings. Serum TSH and PRL levels should be obtained because hyperprolactinemia and hypothyroidism may be subtle in their presentation as causes of anovulation.

Treatment of anovulatory bleeding relies primarily on providing cyclic progestins with subsequent induction of withdrawal bleeding. In the presence of active bleeding an estrogen is utilized to induce healing of the denuded endometrium and enhance the endometrium's sensitivity to progesterone (e.g., conjugated estrogen–2.5 to 5 mg/day until bleeding stops, then 2.5 mg estrogen and medroxyprogesterone 10 mg for 10 days or oral contraceptives–3 pills/day until bleeding stops, then 2 pills/day until pack completed). For minimal or recent bleeding, medroxyprogesterone (10 mg for 10 days) or megestrol acetate (80 mg for 10 days) may be used. Patients should be informed that after discontinuing the progestin bleeding will return. The bleeding may be heavy, consistent with a lush endometrium. Cramping may also be significant in response to estrogen and progestin withdrawal and release of prostaglandins. After the initial treatment, a plan for correcting the cause of anovulation or for maintaining chronic cyclic withdrawal bleeding (oral contraceptives or medroxyprogesterone 10 mg for 10 days every 4 to 6 weeks) must be established.

In cases where atypical endometrial hyperplasia is detected, hysterectomy or pharmacologic treatment may be considered based on reproductive desires and status. Hysteroscopy and extensive sampling should be performed before commencing progestin therapy in cases of atypical hyperplasia. High-dose progestin therapy (i.e., megestrol 80 mg twice daily, medroxyprogesterone 20 mg/day, or norethindrone acetate 5 mg/day) is utilized continuously for 3 months. Medication is then stopped, and after withdrawal bleeding a repeat endometrial biopsy is performed to confirm restoration of normal endometrium. When successful and normal endometrium is obtained, cyclic progestin therapy must be given. Failure to convert to normal endometrium will require surgical intervention.

Ovulatory bleeding

The diagnostic evaluation of ovulatory abnormal uterine bleeding is quite distinct from anovulatory bleeding. Therefore it is essential to confirm ovulatory function and rule out pregnancy-related complications. Menstrual calendars or preferably a BBT chart with the days of bleeding marked are extremely useful. A progesterone level during the midluteal phase may also be obtained to confirm normal hormonal function.

Pelvic examination, endometrial biopsy, Pap smear, and ultrasound are the initial key elements in the evaluation. In most cases routine ultrasonography should be complemented by hydrodistension of the uterine cavity to enhance detection of fibroids, polyps, and intrauterine neoplasm. Alternatively, in-office hysteroscopy may be utilized in place of the ultrasound evaluation of the uterine cavity. Coagulation studies in most cases can be restricted to women with menorrhagia. (Table 26-1 lists causes, clinical presentation, and suggested management for ovulatory abnormal bleeding.)

Fibroids (leiomyoma) will be present in roughly 20% of all older reproductive-age women; there is a higher incidence in black women than white women. Submucous fibroids are frequently symptomatic (menorrhagia and metrorrhagia), whereas intramural fibroids are less commonly symptomatic and seldom produce metrorrhagia. Subserosal fibroids rarely are a cause of abnormal bleeding. Myomectomy or hysterectomy is the treatment of choice for unacceptably symptomatic women who fail medical management. Oral contraceptives or progestins are the primary treatment for symptomatic bleeding, though both may stimulate growth of fibroids. Antiprostaglandins may also be considered, though their efficacy is significantly less than with adenomyosis. Long-term use of a GnRH agonist to shrink the fibroid followed by low-dose estrogen and progestin therapy has also been utilized to alleviate bleeding problems with fibroids. The high cost of the GnRH agonist limits the utility of this therapy.

Adenomyosis is present in roughly 25% of hysterectomy specimens. Dysmenorrhea frequently accompanies the menorrhagia. Occurrence of both fibroids and adenomyosis is common. Oral contraceptives and progestin are useful in treating the symptoms. Premenstrual and menstrual utilization of antiprostaglandins has been reported to reduce blood loss by 30% while reducing the dysmenorrhea. Endometrial ablation is of limited benefit, and hysterectomy remains the definitive treatment of adenomyosis.

Contraceptive-related bleeding

Irregular bleeding is a common problem with various hormonal contraceptives (oral contraceptives, 5% to 10%; Depo-Provera, 10% to 15%; and Norplant, 10% to 15%). Although reassurance is the primary treatment during the initial few months of therapy, the possibility of underlying pathology should not be ignored. Persistance of complaints will require an evaluation identical to that for ovulatory bleeding. In the case of oral contraceptives, proper daily administration of the medication should be confirmed. Drugs that may alter hormonal absorption or metabolism should also be assessed (i.e., antibiotics, antiepileptics, lipid absorption-inhibiting drugs). Troublesome bleeding in previously asymptomatic women frequently will respond to the use of estrogen supplementation to correct the presumptive progestagen imbalances associated with modern hormonal contraceptives. Conjugated estrogen 0.625 to 1.25 mg/day may be given for 2 to 3 weeks in an attempt to correct the bleeding. Discontinuation of the oral contraceptives, although useful in assessing the cause of bleeding, should be done very reluctantly and only if another reliable means of contraception can be used.

TABLE 26-1
Ovulatory Bleeding

Cause	Signs and symptoms	Treatment
Midcycle bleeding	Recurrent periovulatory bleeding consistent with estrogen fall; use BBT chart to confirm timing	Reassurance or conjugated estrogen 1.25 mg daily for 3-4 days starting the day before bleeding
Endometritis	Metrorrhagia, tender uterus; endometrial biopsy shows plasma cells	Rule out gonorrhea or chlamydia; antibiotic therapy
Polyps	Metrorrhagia; document on hydrohysterosonogram or hysteroscopy	Hysteroscopic polypectomy
Leiomyoma	Metrorrhagia, though more commonly menorrhagia; irregular uterus; diagnosis of submucous fibroid generally confirmed by hysteroscopy, hysterosalpingogram, hydrohysterosonogram	Resection via hysteroscope or laparotomy; gonadotropin-releasing hormone agonist?, hysterectomy
Functional cyst	Irregular bleeding often accompanied by palpable cyst; biopsy-secretory or dyssynchronous endometrium	Generally resolves spontaneously
Cervical carcinoma	Gross cervical lesion, colposcopic lesion, abnormal Pap smear	Biopsy any gross cervical lesion; surgery; radiation
Cervicitis	Postcoital bleeding; metrorrhagia; Inflammatory changes on Pap smear; abnormal colposcopy	Screen and treat for any sexually transmitted disease
Endometriosis	Premenstrual bleeding, dysmenorrhea; abnormal pelvic examination (e.g., nodularity, adnexal mass); confirmed by laparoscopy	Danazol or gonadotropin-releasing hormone agonist: surgical excision or ablation

TABLE 26-1
Ovulatory Bleeding—cont'd

Cause	Signs and symptoms	Treatment
Adenomyosis	Menorrhagia; boggy, tender uterus; dysmenorrhea; ultrasound or MRI may confirm diagnosis	Antiprostaglandins, hysterectomy, endometrial ablation?
Coagulation defects (i.e., von Willebrand's disease, thrombocytopenia, renal failure, anticoagulants)	Menorrhagia, ecchymosis, abnormal PT and PTT, low platelet count, abnormal bleeding time	Hematologic consultation; cyclic oral contraceptives, GnRH agonist for temporary treatment or megestrol 80-160 mg daily, endometrial ablation?, avoidance of antiprostaglandins, iron replacement
Iatrogenic agents		
Spironolactone	Irregular bleeding	Decrease dose to 100 mg daily; add oral contraceptives
Erratic oral contraceptive use	Irregular bleeding	Education
Excessive antiprostaglandin therapy	Menorrhagia	Decrease intake
Depo-Provera or Norplant	Irregular bleeding	Conjugated estrogen 1.25 mg daily until bleeding stops
Tamoxifen	Metrorrhagia	Biopsy endometrium to rule out endometrial cancer
Uterine arteriovenous fistulas	Severe menorrhagia, probably requiring transfusions	Embolization of fistula, hysterectomy
Pregnancy complications	Bleeding and positive pregnancy test; ectopic, threatened, or inevitable abortion; gestational trophoblastic disease	(See Chapter 30)
Vaginal trauma	Acute onset, localized bleeding site	Surgical repair, consider evaluation of foreign body (x-ray or ultrasonography)

Continued

TABLE 26-1
Ovulatory Bleeding—cont'd

Cause	Signs and symptoms	Treatment
Perimenopausal bleeding	Commonly seen in older patients, vasomotor symptoms occasionally, upper range noncastrate FSH	Endometrial biopsy a must; conjugated estrogen 1.25-2.5 mg daily* with cyclic progestin for 14 days (e.g., medroxyprogesterone 5-10 mg daily; later decrease estrogen dose)

*Higher doses of estrogen than the standard menopausal replacement are recommended. This may suppress endogenous ovulatory function, which otherwise might result in unpredictable intermenstrual bleeding. POF and autoimmune oophoritis can present as perimenopausal bleeding in truly reproductive-age females.

POSTMENOPAUSAL BLEEDING

In postmenopausal women the chance of developing endometrial carcinoma is roughly 1:1000 each year. Uterine sarcomas are also more common during the perimenopausal and postmenopausal years. Recognizing the increased prevalence of these disorders, endometrial sampling with visualization of the endometrial cavity (hysteroscopy or ultrasonography) is essential in the evaluation of postmenopausal bleeding. Endometrial sampling for bleeding in the absence of hormonal therapy or in the presence of estrogen-only therapy is associated with a high incidence of malignant or premalignant disorders. Admittedly, given the extensive use of postmenopausal HRT, bleeding secondary to hormonal imbalances, missed pills, malabsorption, and drug interaction, it is likely that the ratio of malignancies detected per endometrial sampling has declined. Regardless, the dictum that unpredictable postmenopausal bleeding requires endometrial sampling remains. Treatment depends on the biopsy and anatomical findings.

MANAGEMENT OF SEVERE UTEROVAGINAL HEMORRHAGE

Although rare, patients may have such severe genital tract bleeding that treatment is required before an appropriate evaluation can be performed. The flow chart in Fig. 26-1 can be used in such situations, though its use should be restricted. Note that only in this setting is parenteral estrogen therapy recommended. Any benefits of parenteral estrogen over oral estrogen are unsubstantiated.

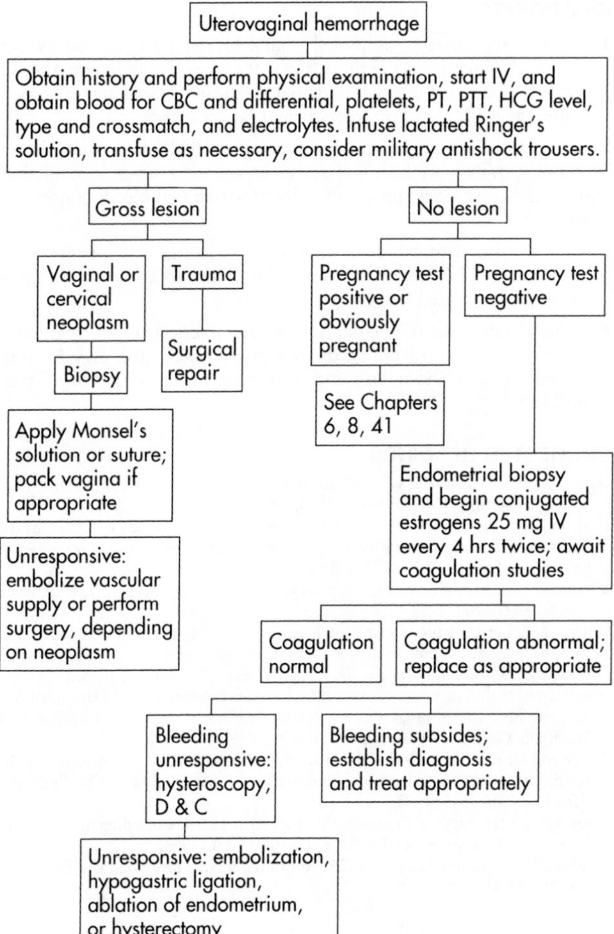

FIG. 26-1 Proposed evaluation and treatment for severe uterovaginal hemorrhage.

KEY POINTS

1 The various causes of abnormal genital bleeding are divided by age groups. Although not the most frequent causes, the following should always be included in the differential diagnosis: premenarcheal sexual abuse, pregnancy, and postmenopausal cancer or sarcoma.

2 Anovulatory bleeding is treated hormonally once the diagnosis is clearly established. Beyond the initial treatment, a plan for restoring ovulation or maintaining cyclic progestin-induced withdrawal bleeding needs to be established.

3 The most frequent causes of metrorrhagia are anatomic or infectious abnormalities. Endometrial biopsy and imaging procedures are essential in planning directed therapy.

4 Menorrhagia is the hallmark for coagulation abnormalities, symptomatic fibroids, and adenomyosis. Antiprostaglandin use may be very helpful with adenomyosis and very detrimental with coagulation problems.

SUGGESTED READINGS

Bayer SR, DeCherney AH: Clinical manifestations and treatment of dysfunctional uterine bleeding, *JAMA* 269:1823-1828, 1993.

Carlson KJ, Miller BA, Fowler FJ: The Maine women's health study II: Outcomes of nonsurgical management of leiomyomas, abnormal bleeding and chronic pelvic pain, *Obstet Gynecol* 83:566-572, 1994.

Chambers JT, Chambers SK: Endometrial sampling: when? where? why? with what? *Clin Obstet Gynecol* 35:28-39, 1992.

Emanuel MH et al: A prospective comparison of transvaginal ultrasonography and diagnostic hysteroscopy in the evaluation of patients with abnormal uterine bleeding: clinical implications, *Am J Obstet Gynecol* 172:547-552, 1995.

Friedman AJ et al: A prospective randomised trial of gonadotropin releasing hormone agonist plus estrogen-progestin or progestin "add-back" regimen for women with leiomyoma uteri, *J Clin Endocrinol Metab* 76:1439-1445, 1993.

Lockwood CJ et al: Steroid-modulated stromal cell tissue factor expression: a model for the regulation of endometrial hemostasis and menstruation, *J Clin Endocrinol Metab* 77:1014-1019, 1993.

Thorneycroft IH: Medical management of abnormal uterine bleeding in the patient in her 40's, *Obstet Gynecol Clin North Am* 20:333-336, 1993.

Wather PI, Henderson MC, Witz CA: Abnormal uterine bleeding, *Med Clin North Am* 79:329-344, 1995.

27

Uterine Cancers

LUIS VACCARELLO

ENDOMETRIAL CARCINOMAS

Endometrial carcinoma comprises 90% to 95% of the malignancies arising from the uterine corpus. It is the most common gynecologic malignancy in the United States; uterine sarcomas comprise the remainder of corpus tumors. Together they rank fourth in incidence behind breast, lung, and colon carcinomas. Estimates for 1996 predicted 34,000 new cases and 6000 deaths from endometrial carcinoma.

The diagnosis of endometrial carcinoma is typically made after the initial symptom of abnormal uterine bleeding. Treatment is mainly surgical, although hormones, radiation, and chemotherapy can also play a significant role. The majority of cases present in early stages, which translates to significant cures and overall survival rates of 80% to 85%.

Epidemiology and Pathophysiology

Endometrial carcinoma is a disease of perimenopausal and postmenopausal women and is uncommon below the age of 40. The mean age at diagnosis and peak incidence is 60. Within the United States the rates are highest among Caucasian and Hawaiian women in contrast to African-American, Asian, or Hispanic women.

Risk factors for the development of endometrial cancer are linked to the exposure to unopposed estrogen of endogenous or exogenous sources. Epidemiologic studies show increased risk with obesity, diabetes, hypertension, nulliparity, early menarche, late menopause, oligoovulation or anovulation, HRT with estrogen alone or the use of tamoxifen, estrogen-secreting tumors such as granulosa cell, and family history. Protective factors are the use of combination oral contraceptives, multiparity, and cigarette smoking.

The stimulatory effect of estrogen on the endometrium is well established; it causes proliferation and cell division during the proliferative phase of the normal ovulatory cycle. The unopposed effect of estrogen is frequently encountered in patients with endometrial hyperplasia as well as carcinoma. Obesity is a major risk factor for endometrial carcinoma, and the pathophysiology is related to unopposed estrogen. Various mechanisms can explain an increased circulating estrogen level in obese women; these include the peripheral conversion of androstenedione to estrone, decreased levels of steroid-binding globulin, and abnormal metabolism of estrogens. Obese women have a higher incidence of anovulation and therefore lack the production of progesterone necessary to counteract the proliferative effect of estrogen. The relative risk of cancer increases proportionally with weight.

HRT for patients with an intact uterus should include cyclic or continuous progestins to protect the endometrium from hyperplasia or carcinoma. Tamoxifen, a drug with estrogen agonist and antagonist properties, is also associated with an increased risk of endometrial pathology. Its use for the treatment and prevention of breast cancer is increasing. These patients should be counseled about the risk of endometrial cancer and undergo an endometrial biopsy for symptoms of abnormal uterine bleeding.

Combination oral contraceptive use is clearly associated with a decrease in the risk of endometrial and ovarian carcinoma. Risk decreases proportionally with length of use and approaches 50% after 5 years of use.

Pathology

Endometrial carcinoma includes a variety of histological subtypes. Endometrioid types comprise approximately 80% of these carcinomas that form glands similar to normal endometrium. The amount of solid components and degree of cellular atypia increases the grade of the tumor. Endometrioid variants can be villoglandular in architecture, contain squamous differentiation, or be secretory.

Less common histologic subtypes are the papillary serous and clear cell carcinomas that resemble their counterparts more frequently seen in the ovaries. These tumors can spread intraperitoneally, as with ovarian carcinoma, and carry a poorer prognosis. Clear cell and squamous carcinomas can be found in conjunction with endometrioid and form a separate group of mixed carcinomas.

Other histologies include mucinous carcinoma, which tends to be well differentiated and has a better prognosis, and pure squamous carcinoma, which is rare and carries a poor prognosis. Undifferentiated and metastatic cancers can also be found in the endometrium.

Presentation and Diagnosis

The most common presenting complaint of women with uterine cancer is abnormal vaginal bleeding, usually postmenopausal. Other common symptoms include mucous or purulent discharge and pain associated with a pyometra or hematometra. In asymptomatic patients, the disease can sometimes be discovered during the evaluation of an abnormal Pap smear. Women who are premenopausal may have menorrhagia or menometrorrhagia.

Not all postmenopausal bleeding can be attributed to uterine cancer. The majority of bleeding is caused by benign conditions such as atrophic endometrium or vagina and cervical or endometrial polyps, benign pathology such as endometrial hyperplasia, or HRT.

The general examination of these patients seldom reveals any signs of pathology. Metastasis can involve the groin nodes or the peritoneum and manifest clinically as lymphadenopathy, ascites, or abdominal masses.

During the pelvic examination, lesions of the vulva, vagina, and cervix must be excluded. With the bimanual and rectovaginal exam, the uterus, adnexa, cul-de-sac, and parametria can be assessed if body habitus permits.

The diagnosis ultimately depends on tissue sampling that can frequently be obtained in the office during the initial visit. A Pap smear, endocervical curettage, and endometrial biopsy should be performed. If cervical stenosis is encountered, a paracervical block and cervical dilation can be attempted before going on to hysteroscopy, dilation, and curettage in the operating room. The role of ultrasound in the evaluation of patients with uterine bleeding is evolving and is currently recommended when tissue diagnosis is unsatisfactory or symptoms persist. The uterus and adnexa can be visualized to evaluate the tubes and ovaries as sources of the bleeding, and the endometrial thickness can be measured. When the endometrial stripe is less than 5 mm, the likelihood of endometrial pathology is *rare.*

Staging and Risk Factors

Clinical staging of endometrial carcinoma results in the understaging of approximately 20% of patients. In 1988, FIGO staging was changed to surgical and pathologic staging (Box 27-1) and requires removal of the uterus, tubes, and ovaries; peritoneal cytology; pelvic and paraaortic lymph node sampling; and biopsy of any suspicious areas. Inoperable patients are still clinically staged. The information obtained from this assessment of risk factors allows an evaluation of risk of recurrence and can be a guide to adjuvant therapy recommendations. Risk factors not included in staging are histologic type, lymph-vascular space involvement, and parametrial extension or metastasis.

Treatment

Surgery is the mainstay of therapy for patients with operable tumors because survival is consistently better than with radiotherapy alone (Fig. 27-1). Patients with gross cervical, vaginal, or parametrial involvement may be best served with initial radiotherapy; all others are candidates for surgical treatment and staging. Surgical staging is carried out through a vertical incision and consists of abdominal exploration, peritoneal cytology, a total abdominal hysterectomy (TAH), bilateral salpingoophorectomy (BSO), and pelvic and paraaortic node sampling. An area of current investigation is the role of a laparoscopic staging approach with vaginal hysterectomy.

The requirement of lymph node sampling is a product of the new FIGO staging system and remains a point of controversy with regards to clinically staged I tumors. The incidence of lymph node involvement varies with the grade of the tumor and the depth of myometrial invasion. It is less than 5% for grades 1 and 2 with superficial myometrial invasion. These patients can probably forgo node sampling, especially if the morbidity and risk outweigh the potential benefits. The final hysterectomy grade will vary from the preoperative grade in 20% of patients. The best estimation

BOX 27-1
FIGO Surgical Staging for Endometrial Cancer (1988)

STAGE I

Stage Ia G123	Tumor limited to the endometrium
Stage Ib G123	Less than 50% myometrial invasion
Stage Ic G123	Greater than 50% myometrial invasion

STAGE II

Stage IIa G123	Endocervical gland involvement only
Stage IIb G123	Cervical stromal invasion

STAGE III

Stage IIIa G123	Tumor in serosa or adnexa, or positive peritoneal cytology
Stage IIIb G123	Vaginal metastases
Stage IIIc G123	Positive pelvic or paraaortic nodes

STAGE IV

Stage IVa G123	Tumor in bladder or bowel mucosa
Stage IVb	Distant spread (inguinal nodes, intraabdominal metastases)

Notes on Grading

G1, 5% or less of a nonsquamous or nonmorular solid growth pattern
G2, 6% - 50% of a nonsquamous or nonmorular solid growth pattern
G3, more than 50% of a nonsquamous or nonmorular solid growth pattern

1. Notable nuclear atypia, inappropriate for the architectural grade, raises the grade of a grade 1 or 2 tumor by 1.
2. In serous adenocarcinomas, clear cell adenocarcinomas, and squamous cell carcinomas, nuclear grading takes precedence.
3. Adenocarcinomas with squamous differentiation are graded according to the nuclear grade of the glandular component.

of myometrial invasion and cervical involvement can be performed by frozen section, and this information can be used in the decision for node sampling.

Adjuvant Therapy

The risk of recurrence is less than 5% for patients adequately staged with grade 1 or 2 tumors and superficial or no myometrial invasion. This low risk group needs no further therapy.

The intermediate-risk group includes those patients with tumors with deep myometrial invasion or endocervical gland involvement with grades 2 and 3. Some clinicians favor the administration of vaginal cuff brachy-

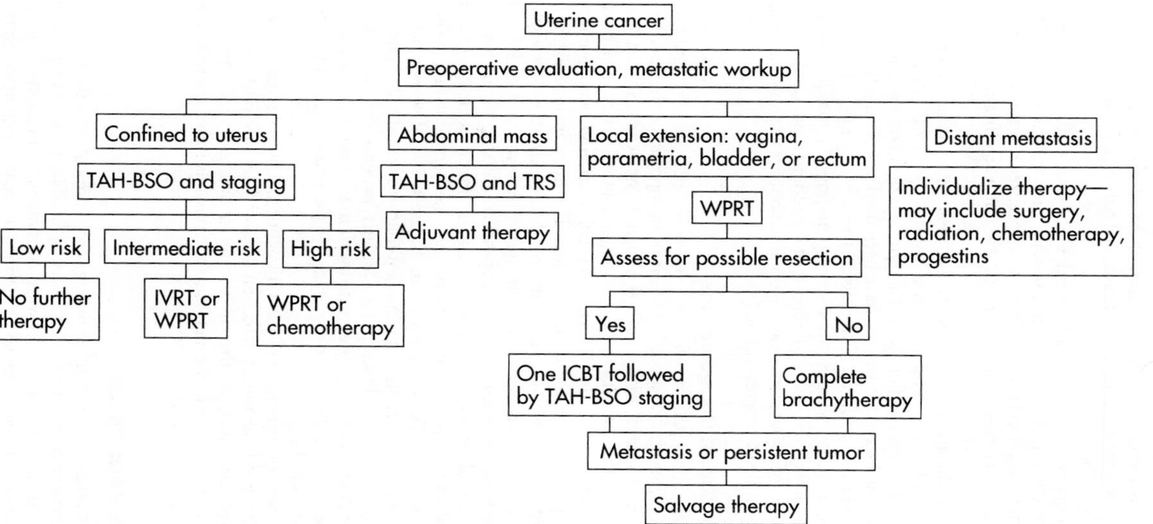

FIG. 27-1 Management of uterine cancers. *BSO,* bilateral salpingo-oophorectomy; *ICBT,* intracavitory brachytherapy; *IVRT,* intravaginal radiation therapy; *TAH,* total abdominal hysterectomy; *TRS,* tumor reductive surgery; and *WPRT,* whole pelvis radiation therapy.

therapy in this group of patients because of the relative ease of administration and low complication rates. Intravaginal radiation can decrease cuff recurrence by 50%.

All other patients comprise a high-risk group that requires additional therapy to prevent recurrence or treat residual disease. The use of pelvic radiation has been a standard for patients with localized disease in the pelvis and appears to decrease local recurrence without a significant effect on survival.

Hormonal therapy of advanced or recurrent endometrial cancer has long been used by many clinicians as a first-line therapy because of the relatively low side effects of progestins and the lack of curative alternatives. Megestrol or medroxyprogesterone have been used in low- and high-dose regimens without significant differences. There is a greater chance of response in patients with hormone receptor–positive tumors, which typically occur in the more differentiated endometrioid carcinomas. Response rates of 15% to 20% can be obtained but are of short duration with average time to progression of 4 months.

Special Treatment Considerations

Endometrial cancer patients who are morbidly obese or have multiple medical problems may dissuade clinicians from appropriate therapy. The challenge is just as great with a vaginal hysterectomy, which also has the disadvantage of the inability to explore the abdominal cavity or remove the ovaries and sample nodes. If surgery is totally contraindicated, primary radiotherapy is planned for potential cure. This may include external radiotherapy and/or brachytherapy with low-dose or high-dose rate applicators. Results are lower than with surgery, but survival rates of 60% to 75% can be achieved when the tumor appears confined to the uterus.

Gross cervical involvement, clinical stage II, imparts a greater risk of paracervical and lymphatic involvement and is associated with a poorer chance of survival. These patients can be treated with whole pelvic irradiation and one brachytherapy implant followed by a simple hysterectomy, BSO, and aortic node sampling. Similarly, patients with parametrial or vaginal extension of tumor are treated with irradiation and assessed for surgical resection based on response. Stage IVA patients are rare and can be managed in a similar fashion.

Most stage IVB patients will have intraabdominal metastasis and are managed by maximal tumor resection followed by adjuvant therapy. Distant metastasis such as that in the lung, brain, or bone requires individualized treatment to the metastasis and possibly surgery or radiation to treat and control the pelvic disease.

UTERINE SARCOMAS

Uterine sarcomas are rare tumors that may also present with the onset of abnormal uterine bleeding or as an enlarging uterine mass. Evaluation of uterine sarcoma is the same as with endometrial carcinoma. Unlike endometrial cancer, the diagnosis of uterine sarcoma is often made on the final hysterectomy specimen. The most common preoperative diagnoses are endometrial carcinoma, poorly differentiated cancer, or abnormal uterine bleeding from leiomyomas.

The three most common types of malignant sarcomas in order of incidence are carcinosarcoma (CS), leiomyosarcoma (LMS), and endometrial stromal sarcoma (ESS). These tumors are very aggressive in growth pattern and behavior and are associated with poor prognosis even if confined to the uterus when diagnosed. Epidemiologic factors that are unique to sarcomas include greater incidence in the black population for CS and LMS, median age of mid-60s for CS and ESS but mid-50s for LMS, and previous pelvic irradiation for CS.

CS is a tumor consisting of mixed elements of epithelial and mesenchymal histology of either homologous or heterologous origin. Most authorities believe that the mesenchymal component represents metaplasia of the carcinoma. The most common epithelial histologies are endometrioid and adenosquamous carcinoma, and the mesenchymal are leiomyosarcoma, rhabdomyosarcoma, and chondrosarcoma. LMS and ESS are pure sarcomas of their respective histologies, and each have low- and high-grade variants.

Management of these tumors is primarily surgical and should include a TAH with BSO and surgical staging. Because the prognosis for these tumors is so poor, these patients are excellent candidates for adjuvant therapy. Pelvic radiotherapy can decrease local recurrence from CS and ESS but does not appear to affect survival. Chemotherapy agents with activity in CS include ifosfamide and cisplatin, and in LMS are ifosfamide and doxorubicin. Low-grade ESS is sensitive to hormonal manipulation and is treated with progestational agents. The high-grade counterpart has been treated with various chemotherapy combinations including cyclophosphamide, doxorubicin, and cisplatin.

KEY POINTS

1. Endometrial cancer is the most common gynecologic malignancy in the United States.
2. The major risk factors for endometrial cancer are obesity and unopposed estrogen of endogenous or exogenous sources.
3. Abnormal uterine bleeding is the most common presenting symptom and should be evaluated with endometrial biopsy.
4. The most common types of uterine sarcomas are carcinosarcoma, leiomyosarcoma, and endometrial stromal sarcoma.

SUGGESTED READINGS

Endometrial cancer

Anderson B et al: Obesity and prognosis in endometrial cancer, *Am J Obstet Gynecol* 174:1171-1179, 1996.

Decensi A et al: Effect of tamoxifen on endometrial proliferation, *J Clin Oncol* 14:434-440, 1996.

Homesley HD: Management of endometrial cancer, *Am J Obstet Gynecol* 174:529-534, 1996.

Kilgore LC et al: Adenocarcinoma of the endometrium: survival comparisons of patients with and without pelvic node sampling, *Gynecol Oncol* 56:29-33, 1995.
Morrow CP et al: Doxorubicin as an adjuvant following surgery and radiation therapy in patients with high-risk endometrial carcinoma, stage I and occult stage II: a Gynecologic Oncology Group study, *Gynecol Oncol* 36:166-171, 1990.
Morrow CP et al: Relationship between surgical-pathological risk factors and outcome in clinical stage I and II carcinoma of the endometrium: a Gynecologic Oncology Group study, *Gynecol Oncol* 40:55, 1991.

Sarcomas

Berchuck A et al: Treatment of endometrial stromal tumors, *Gynecol Oncol* 36:60-65, 1990.
Silverberg SG et al: Carcinosarcomas (malignant mixed mesodermal tumor) of the uterus, *Int J Gynecol Pathol* 9:1, 1990.
Vaccarello L, Curtin JP: Presentation and management of carcinosarcoma of the uterus, *Oncology* 6(5):45-59, 1992.

28

Vulvar and Vaginal Carcinoma

LUIS VACCARELLO AND GEORGE S. LEWANDOWSKI

Vulvar Cancer

Vulvar cancer accounts for 3% to 5% of all gynecologic malignancies and approximately 1% of all female cancer deaths in the United States. The most common histology type encountered is squamous cell carcinoma, accounting for almost 90%, followed by melanoma (5%), Bartholin's gland adenocarcinoma (3%), sarcomas (2%), and others.

EPIDEMIOLOGY AND PATHOPHYSIOLOGY

Vulvar cancer is a disease most commonly encountered in older patients with a mean age at diagnosis of 65, and a range of 30 to 90 years. The etiology of vulvar cancer is not known but appears to be multifactorial. Epidemiologic studies indicate an increased risk in women with genital warts, history of abnormal Pap smear, multiple sexual partners, coffee use, and current smokers. Cervical cancer shares these risk factors and may be seen in these patients as a second primary.

A viral etiology in this disease has long been implicated since the detection of herpes virus antigens in these patients. Vulvar intraepithelial neoplasia (VIN) likewise is associated with HPV infection and carries a 4% to 6% risk of progression to carcinoma.

Vulvar cancer arises from the epithelium, skin appendages, and supporting stroma of the vulva and perineal area. The tumor may extend to involve surrounding organs and structures such as the urethra, vagina, bladder, rectum, or pubic symphysis. Lymphatic spread occurs in roughly 30% of patients and is directly proportional to the size and depth of invasion of the primary lesion. The inguinal and femoral nodes are the primary draining site, with pelvic nodes less frequently affected. This spread seems to be sequential, although direct channels from the clitoris and Bartholin's gland have been demonstrated. Hematogenous spread to the lung, liver, or bone can occur, but is more common with advanced or recurrent tumors.

PRESENTATION AND DIAGNOSIS

Patients may delay their visit to a physician for months and even years despite symptoms of pruritis or the presence of a vulvar mass. Less common symptoms may include bleeding, pain or burning, dysuria, or discharge. Physicians must avoid treatment of vulvar disease based on symptoms described during phone conversations with the patient or on the gross appearance of the lesion. A biopsy is mandatory.

Lesions that may be included in the differential diagnosis are condylomata acuminata, VIN, vulvar dystrophy, and infectious or inflammatory processes. These disorders must be recognized because treatment is significantly different from that for carcinoma.

The labia majora and minora are the most frequent sites of disease. Lesions are commonly 1 to 2 cm in size but may vary from evident only on colposcopy to lesions large enough to replace the vulva and extend to adjacent structures. Lesions may vary in appearance, including color, consistency, and location (i.e., exophytic versus subepithelial). They may be multifocal as well as associated with other lower genital cancers; therefore a careful examination of the vagina, cervix, and rectum should be carried out. Because of the incidence of nodal metastasis, the inguinofemoral area should be inspected for lymphadenopathy.

STAGING

In 1989 FIGO approved a surgical staging classification that relies on the histopathologic examination of the groin nodes rather than clinical impression (Box 28-1). Nodal disease status is clearly a significant prognostic factor that was often unreliably clinically assessed. A further staging modification was implemented by FIGO in 1994 when a microinvasive stage was added to recognize a subset of patients without significant risk of nodal metastasis.

BOX 28-1
FIGO Staging of Vulvar Carcinoma

I*	T1, N0, M0
II	T2, N0, M0
III	T3, N0, M0
	T3, N1, M0
	T2, N1, M0
	T1, N1, M0
IV	T4, N0, M0
	any T, N2, M0
	any T, any N, M1
T1,	Tumor confined to the vulva and/or perineum 2 cm or smaller in greatest dimension.
T2,	Tumor confined to the vulva and/or perineum larger than 2 cm in greatest dimension.
T3,	Tumor of any size with adjacent spread to the lower urethra and/or the vagina and/or the anus.
T4,	Tumor of any size invading the upper urethra, bladder mucosa, rectal mucosa, or pelvic bone.
N0,	No lymph node metastasis.
N1,	Unilateral regional lymph node metastasis.
N2,	Bilateral regional lymph node metastasis.
M0,	No clinical metastasis.
M1,	Distant metastasis (including pelvic lymph node metastasis).

*Stage IA: Lesions 2 cm or less in size confined to the vulva or perineum and with stromal invasion no greater than 1 mm. No nodal metastasis. Stage IB: Lesions 2 cm or less in size confined to the vulva or perineum and with stromal invasion greater than 1 mm. No nodal metastasis.

TREATMENT

The mainstay of therapy for vulvar cancers has been radical surgical resection of the primary tumor and its draining lymphatics in the groin (Fig. 28-1). Current therapy stresses individualization of management of the primary tumor and nodes with integration of radiation and/or chemotherapy when appropriate.

Results from various studies have allowed a more conservative approach without sacrificing treatment efficacy. Unifocal lesions are resected with wide and deep margins (radical wide local excision, modified radical vulvectomy), preserving the unaffected vulva. The inguinal lymphadenectomy is performed through separate groin incisions, only on the ipsilateral groin for lateral vulvar lesions, and is avoided altogether in microinvasive lesions. Pelvic lymphadenectomy is no longer routine. For large primary lesions that may involve adjacent organs, the use of radiation therapy

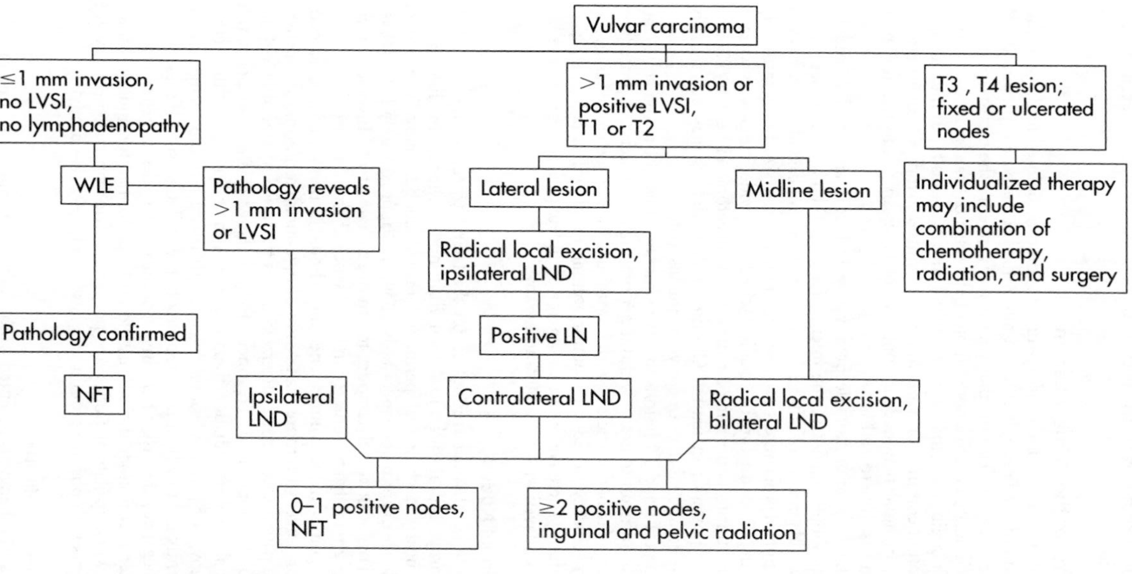

FIG. 28-1 Management of vulvar carcinoma. *LVSI,* Lymph-vascular space invasion; *WLE,* wide local excision; *NFT,* no further treatment; *LND,* lymph node dissection.

and/or chemotherapy has decreased the need for primary exenteration procedures.

Control of the Primary Lesion

Surgery to remove the primary tumor should be tailored to the size and location of the lesion, keeping in mind that the purpose is prevention of local recurrence. Tumors that are microinvasive on the biopsy specimen with clinically negative nodes (potentially stage IA) can be excised with a 1 cm margin of normal epithelium and subcutaneous fat. If microscopic evaluation confirms only microinvasion without lymph-vascular involvement, inguinal lymphadenectomy is not necessary. Cure rate for these patients is close to 100%.

The excision of more deeply invasive T1 lesions and small T2 and T3 lesions should extend to the inferior fascia of the urogenital diaphragm with a wide margin of at least 2 cm. A complete radical vulvectomy is still the standard procedure for tumors larger than 2 cm in size, but occasionally a T2 or T3 lesion can be locally excised with wide margins in what is tantamount to performing a radical hemivulvectomy either lateral, anterior, or posterior in nature. Closure of these defects may occasionally require rotational flaps or a myocutaneous graft.

Large T3 and T4 lesions involve structures adjacent to the vulva and may be difficult to excise without performing an exenterative procedure. The use of radiation therapy with or without concurrent chemotherapy has shown efficacy in reducing tumor volume to allow less radical surgical resections. There are occasions when a complete pathologic response has been achieved with neoadjuvant therapy.

Regional Nodes

Primary lesions that are located on the lateral aspects of the vulva will primarily drain into the ipsilateral groin nodes, whereas midline lesions (i.e., near the clitoris or perineum) may drain bilaterally. The overall incidence of groin node metastasis is 35%, and approximately 20% of these will have positive pelvic nodes for an overall rate of 7%. Involved pelvic nodes are rarely encountered in the absence of groin metastasis.

Inguinofemoral lymphadenectomy should be performed in all cases of vulvar cancer with more than 1 mm of invasion. Exceptions may include those patients with fixed, ulcerated nodes that are not resectable without vascular compromise. Treatment for this latter group of patients will normally require radiation therapy alone or in conjunction with chemotherapy. For primary lesions that are well lateralized, most surgeons are currently limiting lymphadenectomy to the ipsilateral side. If these nodes are negative, the risk of positive contralateral nodes is extremely low. Bilateral groin node dissections should be performed for midline lesions and when ipsilateral nodes are positive. Pelvic lymphadenectomy for patients with positive groin nodes has been largely abandoned.

Adjuvant Therapy

Radiation therapy is accepted in the adjuvant treatment of patients after inguinal lymphadenectomy if two or more nodes are positive. These patients should receive irradiation to the involved groin(s) and pelvis because this decreases recurrence and improves survival. Radiation therapy to the groin for clinical N0/N1 nodes in patients without inguinal lymphadenectomy appears to be associated with a significant failure rate and is not recommended.

The preoperative use of radiotherapy is reserved for advanced lesions that are difficult to resect with clear margins or may require some form of exenteration. This approach has been combined with chemotherapy as a radiosensitizer (usually 5-fluorouracil, mitomycin C, or cisplatin), with good responses in most retrospective series.

Chemotherapy

The use of chemotherapy alone in the treatment of squamous cell cancer of the vulva has been reserved for patients with distant metastatic disease, typically in a salvage situation. The role of chemotherapy in the management of vulvar cancer requires further study.

Treatment Complications

Conservative surgery has been successful in reducing morbidity and mortality rates for vulvar cancer. The most common complications relate to breakdown and infection of the incisions either in the groins or the vulva. Closed system drainage and antibiotics play an important role in the prevention of lymphocysts and infections. Chronic lymphedema of the legs is related to lymphadenectomy and possibly to postoperative infection or chronic lymphangitis. Support stockings and use of intermittent pneumatic compression can alleviate some of this problem. Other complications include thrombophlebitis, femoral neuropathies, vascular injuries, and sexual dysfunction.

Irradiation of the vulvar area and/or the pelvis and groins can be associated with acute and chronic complications such as moist desquamation, nausea, vomiting, diarrhea, bowel obstruction, tissue necrosis, and fistula.

PROGNOSIS

Survival for patients with vulvar cancer can best be related to FIGO clinical stages I through IV with rates of 90%, 80%, 50%, and 20%, respectively. Factors such as tumor size, grade, depth of invasion, vascular space involvement, and lymph node status are of prognostic significance. Of these, the number of positive nodes seems to be most important in determining survival. With negative nodes the 5-year survival rate is greater than 96%, but with three or more positive nodes survival falls to less than 25%.

VULVAR MELANOMA

Malignant melanoma is the second most common cancer of the vulva, accounting for approximately 5% of the cancers. Most patients are postmenopausal and will have symptoms similar to squamous cancers. These tumors may originate de novo or from junctional or compound nevi and are usually pigmented. The three major varieties according to growth pattern are nodular, superficial spreading, and acral lentiginous. These tumors are highly aggressive and have a 5-year survival rate of 30% to 50%.

Thickness of the tumor, the depth of invasion, and lymph node status are important prognostic factors. The survival rate for node-negative patients is ~40% to 50%, whereas node-positive patients rarely survive.

Treatment for vulvar melanoma is mainly surgical and mirrors the conservative approach to squamous cancers. Tumors of <.75 mm thickness or Clark level I-II can be treated with radical wide excision without inguinal lymphadenectomy. The survival rate for these patients is 95%. Larger lesions may require radical vulvectomy to obtain clear margins. Although inguinal lymphadenectomy is usually recommended because of the high incidence of positive nodes in these patients, the therapeutic benefit of the procedure has not been proved and may only be of prognostic value.

Nonsurgical forms of therapy can also be of value in certain circumstances. Melanomas can respond to irradiation. This modality may be useful for palliation of symptoms or to treat inoperable tumors. The use of chemotherapy for melanoma has been disappointing.

Vaginal Cancer

STAGING

Cancers that involve both the vagina and either the cervix or vulva are classified by FIGO convention as if they had arisen from the cervix or vulva. Malignancy seen in the vagina can also be the result of metastatic disease from the endometrium, the GI tract, and other sites. The staging of vaginal cancer is clinical (Box 28-2). Pretherapy evaluation includes radiographic studies and a comprehensive physical assessment, culminating ideally in an examination under anesthesia (with cystoscopy and proctosigmoidoscopy) performed jointly by the radiation oncologist and the gynecologic oncologist or gynecologist.

BOX 28-2
FIGO Staging of Vaginal Cancer

Stage 0	Carcinoma in situ, intraepithelial carcinoma
Stage I	Carcinoma limited to the vaginal wall
Stage II	Carcinoma involves subvaginal tissue, no extension to the pelvic wall
Stage III	Carcinoma extends to the pelvic wall
Stage IV	Carcinoma spread beyond the true pelvis
Stage IV-A	Bladder or rectal mucosa involvement
Stage IV-B	Distant metastasis

Vaginal tissue is highly estrogen-sensitive and has a rich lymphatic supply located within millimeters of the mucosal surface. This suggests that age, menopausal status, and estrogen use can theoretically alter the ability of tumor tissue to enter the lymphatics. Although lesions most frequently occur at the vaginal apex, they can also involve both the middle third or the distal vagina near the vulvovaginal junction. A primary lesion in the proximal two thirds of the vagina would drain into the pelvic nodes, and one in the distal third would find the inguinal nodes at risk for metastatic spread.

TREATMENT

Histologic Review

Histologic review is a critical initial step in developing a treatment plan for vaginal cancer. A large majority of vaginal lesions will have a squamous morphology. There are similarities between vaginal and cervical cancer in the progression from dysplasia and the association of HPV-related disease. Yet 15% to 20% of vaginal cancers will be nonsquamous and represent histologic types including adenocarcinoma, melanoma, sarcomas, and other tumors.

Many women with vaginal cancer will have undergone hysterectomy for benign or preinvasive disease; others will have a remote history of either radiation or radical surgery for cervical malignancy. Most early vaginal cancers will originate at the apex, and are discovered during an investigation of abnormal bleeding or discharge. Patients with an abnormal Pap smear in whom the cervix is normal or surgically absent should be carefully evaluated for vaginal cancer. Unfortunately, many colposcopic changes will be subtle and speculum placement can obscure more distal lesions. At times, an exam with biopsies will require anesthesia because of discomfort. Large areas of dysplasia should be liberally biopsied or excised to rule out invasive disease. Because of these challenges, a lower percentage of vaginal cancers are at stage I than the corresponding staged cervical primary. More advanced lesions that impinge on the bladder, urethra, or rectum may cause expected associated symptoms including urinary frequency, pain, or obstipation.

Should radiation therapy be chosen as the primary treatment modality for a lesion in the proximal two thirds of the vagina, external beam treatments would be delivered to the whole pelvis (see Chapter 3). Disease in the distal third of the vagina increases the risk of involvement of the inguinal lymph nodes. If this is suspected or demonstrated, the teletherapy treatment field should extend to the vulva and include the inguinal nodes.

The brachytherapy techniques used to complete a radiation therapy plan for vaginal cancer may present a greater challenge than those used to treat cervical cancer. A vaginal apex lacking in anterior-posterior depth or that is shallow in width might require the use of smaller ovoids or a Syed template. In a patient whose cervix is surgically absent, the narrower distance between the bladder and rectum increases the risk of fistula formation.

Selected patients with stage I vaginal cancers, most often at the vaginal apex, may be candidates for radical vaginectomy with pelvic lymphadenectomy. This surgery is analogous to the radical hysterectomy done for cervical cancer but must establish a tumor-free vaginal margin several centimeters below the most distal aspect of the disease. Multifocal disease must be ruled out by careful colposcopic examination and biopsy, and vaginal reconstruction will often be required to preserve sexual function.

Identification of nonsquamous pathology is rare. Clinicians encountering patients with these histologies should consider the possibility that the vaginal lesion represents a metastatic site rather than primary disease. Workup, treatment, and outcome could be significantly different in these cases.

KEY POINTS

1 Any vulvar lesion that arises or becomes symptomatic needs to be biopsied.

2 Early stage disease is often curable with surgery alone, whereas patients with advanced primaries or metastatic disease will require adjuvant or combination therapy in the form of radiotherapy and/or chemotherapy.

3 Lymph node status of vulvar cancer is the most important prognostic factor for survival.

4 Most vaginal cancers are squamous in origin, but a variety of other histologies may be encountered that should lead the clinician to consider the vagina as a potential site of metastatic disease.

5 Radiation therapy constitutes the backbone of therapy; however, radical vaginectomy may be appropriate for early lesions.

SUGGESTED READINGS

Vulvar cancer

Burke TW et al: Radical wide excision and selective inguinal node dissection for squamous cell carcinoma of the vulva, *Gynecol Oncol* 38:328-332, 1990.

Homesley HD et al: Assessment of current international federation of gynecology and obstetrics staging of vulvar carcinoma relative to prognostic factors for survival: a Gynecologic Oncology Group study, *Am J Obstet Gynecol* 164:997-1004, 1991.

Rotmensch J et al: Preoperative radiotherapy followed by radical vulvectomy with inguinal lymphadenectomy for advanced vulvar carcinomas, *Gynecol Oncol* 36:181-184, 1990.

Stehman FB et al: Early stage I carcinoma of the vulva treated with ipsilateral superficial inguinal lymphadenectomy and modified radical hemivulvectomy: a prospective study of the Gynecologic Oncology Group, *Obstet Gynecol* 79:490-497, 1992.

Stehman FB et al: Groin dissection versus groin radiation in carcinoma of the vulva: a Gynecologic Oncology Group study, *Int J Radiat Oncol Biol Phys* 24:389-396, 1992.

Thomas GM et al: Changing concepts in the management of vulvar cancer, *Gynecol Oncol* 42, 9-21, 1991.

Vaginal cancer

Eddy GL et al: Primary invasive vaginal carcinoma, *Am J Obstet Gynecol* 165:282, 1991.

Hacker NF, Vaginal cancer. In *Practical gynecologic oncology,* Baltimore, 1994, Williams & Wilkins, pp 441-456.

PART II

Obstetrics

Cynthia B. Evans, Editor

29

Anatomic and Physiologic Changes in Pregnancy

WAYNE C. TROUT

HEMATOLOGIC CHANGES

Uterine perfusion increases by 500 ml/min (which is almost 20% of the total cardiac output near term). The total plasma volume begins to increase by 10 weeks gestation and is typically 30% to 50% higher by 34 weeks gestation. Higher increases are seen in multiple gestations.

The red cell volume increases 25% during pregnancy to provide the oxygen requirements of the fetus and support the respiratory needs of the mother. Expansion of the red cell mass increases iron requirements and depletes iron stores. Serum iron and ferritin levels are decreased and transferrin and total iron binding capacity is increased. Plasma volume increases 30% to 50% with an increase in red cell mass of only 25%, resulting in dilutional anemia. This anemia is physiologic, not pathologic. Elemental iron (1 g), is required during pregnancy to provide for the expansion of maternal blood volume and the requirements of the placenta and developing fetus. The iron requirements are highest in the second half of pregnancy when fetal hematopoiesis is maximal. Daily requirements during this time are 6 to 7 mg/day.

Elevations in white blood cell counts throughout pregnancy range from 5 to 12×10^3/ml and can be as high as 25×10^3/ml after a normal vaginal delivery.

There are also changes in the concentrations of substances responsible for the coagulation of blood, accounting for the "hypercoagulability" of pregnancy. The plasma levels of fibrinogen increase from 250 to 400 mg/dl to 400 to 500 mg/dl during pregnancy as do Factors VII through X, whereas proteins S, C, and antithrombin III decrease.

CARDIAC

An increase in blood volume is associated with a 33% increase in cardiac output (from 4.5 to 6 L/min). The increased perfusion of the uterus, kidneys, and skin surfaces results in a decrease in peripheral vascular resistance so that the mean blood pressure decreases despite the increase in cardiac output. The high levels of progesterone, a smooth muscle relaxant, cause dilation of the vasculature and contribute to a lowering of the mean blood pressure. The right heart and pulmonary artery pressures remain unchanged, so there must be a decrease in the pulmonary resistance. The weight of the gravid uterus on the aorta and vena cava causes positional blood pressure changes; blood pressure is highest when the patient is seated, lower when supine, and lowest when taken with the patient lying on her side. Systolic blood pressure will drop 5 to 10 mmHg and diastolic 10 to 15 mmHg over the first two trimesters and then slowly increase to baseline.

RESPIRATORY

Secretions in the nasopharynx increase during pregnancy, which account for the nasal congestion and stuffiness frequently seen during pregnancy. Epistaxis is also a frequent finding.

Total lung capacity is decreased because of upward pressure on the diaphragm from the enlarging uterus (Table 29-1). Despite this, minute ventilation increases by 30% to 40% based on an increase in tidal volume. A 15% to 20% increase in oxygen consumption also occurs. This results in higher alveolar oxygen concentrations and a higher Pao_2. The effect of increased minute ventilation is a significant decrease in CO_2. Blood gas findings are Pao_2 >100 mmHg and $Paco_2$ 27 to 32 mmHg. The arterial

TABLE 29-1
Pulmonary Changes in Pregnancy

	Function	Change
Respiratory rate	Number of breaths per minute	Unchanged
Vital capacity	Maximum amount of air that can be forcibly expelled after maximal inspiration	Unchanged
Inspiratory capacity	Maximum amount of air that can be inspired from resting expiratory level	Increased 5%
Tidal volume	Amount of air inspired and expired with normal breath	Increased 30%-40%
Inspiratory reserve volume	Maximum amount of air that can be inspired at end of normal inspiration	Unchanged
Functional residual capacity	Amount of air in lungs at resting expiratory level	Decreased 20%
Expiratory reserve volume	Maximum amount of air that can be expired from resting expiratory level	Decreased 20%
Residual volume	Amount of air in lungs after maximal expiration	Decreased 20%
Total lung capacity	Total amount of air in lungs at maximal inspiration	Decreased 5%

pH is slightly increased (a partial compensated respiratory alkalosis) from 7.40 to 7.44. Subjective dyspnea is common in pregnancy, affecting 60% to 70% of women entering their second trimester.

RENAL

With the expanded blood volume of pregnancy, the kidneys must increase their daily workload to remove waste products not only from the mother but also from the fetus. The effective renal plasma flow increases 75% in pregnancy. The glomerular filtration rate (GFR) is increased 50%. Normal ranges for creatinine clearance for pregnancy are 150 to 200 ml/min.

Increases in GFR result in decreases of BUN and creatinine levels by 25% as measured in serum samples. With an increase in GFR of 50%, the sodium delivery to the renal tubules is dramatically increased. The renal tubules must adapt during pregnancy to prevent salt wasting. Sodium reabsorption in the tubules is promoted by aldosterone, deoxycorticosterone (DOC), and estrogen, which are all increased during pregnancy. The hormone most responsible for sodium reabsorption is aldosterone, with increases of serum levels from 100 to 200 ng/L prepregnancy to 200 to 700 ng/L at term. As a result of the increased GFR, the normal values of most of the electrolytes decrease. Serum sodium levels are 3 mEq/L lower, and potassium levels decrease by 0.5 mEq/L.

The lower levels of maternal bicarbonate and P_{CO_2} provide a convenient gradient by which the fetus can eliminate its metabolic byproducts. With a decrease in bicarbonate and sodium, the osmolarity of maternal blood then decreases; the osmoreceptors must therefore be reset to prevent the clearance of free water and diabetes insipidus.

The dramatic increase in GFR coupled with the smooth muscle relaxation of progesterone is combined with the mechanical obstruction of the gravid uterus to cause a physiologic hydronephrosis in the mother. This finding is more pronounced on the right side and can make interpretation of radiologic tests difficult. Dilated ureters promote stasis of urine and make pregnant women particularly prone to pyelonephritis.

GASTROINTESTINAL

During early pregnancy there is a natural increase in appetite that provides the additional caloric intake (300 kcal/day) required for the increased energy demands during pregnancy. The "morning sickness" of pregnancy is usually a self-limited phenomenon of the first trimester. Hyperemesis gravidarum is a severe form of morning sickness that may require parenteral hydration to prevent dehydration.

Occasionally, hypertrophy of the gums and gingival bleeding will occur. Ptyalism is a rare complication of pregnancy in which the patient is unable to swallow her saliva. These women may produce up to 1 to 2 Ls/day. Decreasing the intake of starchy foods may be sufficient to relieve the discomfort.

Much of pregnancy's effect on the remainder of the GI tract is the result of circulating levels of progesterone that, as a smooth muscle relaxant, delays the transit time through the gut. The stomach empties slowly and this effect is exaggerated during labor, which may predispose the laboring woman to aspiration. The tone of the lower esophageal sphincter is also decreased, and when combined with the slower emptying time of the stomach predisposes the pregnant woman to reflux; the subjective complaint of heartburn is extremely common.

Transit time through the small intestine is increased. Constipation is a common complaint in pregnancy; this is caused in part by the effect of progesterone, but also is related to the mechanical obstruction from the gravid uterus and fluid resorption in the colon (probably mediated by aldosterone). Portal venous hypertension is increased in pregnancy and can cause dilation of the hemorrhoidal veins.

There are very few changes that occur in the liver with pregnancy. No changes occur in blood levels of hepatic enzymes (AST, ALT, GGT, and bilirubin), but alkaline phosphatase levels increase as a result of placental production. Total protein and albumin levels decrease, mostly because of expanded blood volume. Albumin levels may reach 3 g/dl at term. Elevated estrogen in pregnancy can increase the hepatic production of some proteins (fibrinogen, sex hormone binding globulin, and thyroid binding globulin are some of the more clinically important). There is little change in the gallbladder during pregnancy with regard to the composition of bile. Although gallbladder contractility is diminished, there is no increase in the rate of gallstone formation during pregnancy.

ENDOCRINE

The thyroid gland increases in size slightly during pregnancy and is easily palpated. TSH is unchanged in pregnancy and remains the best indicator of alterations in thyroid function. Interpretation of the remaining thyroid function test requires an understanding of the changes of pregnancy. Estrogen increases thyroid binding globulin, nearly tripling the concentration near term, so that total T_4 and T_3 are increased. Elevated levels of β-HCG can cross-react with TSH so clinical hyperthyroidism can be seen with molar pregnancy and choriocarcinoma. Parathyroid hormone increases to maintain serum calcium levels despite expanded blood volume and increased urinary excretion.

In the pancreas, hypertrophy of the islet cells occurs, causing higher fasting levels of insulin as the body attempts to compensate for the antiinsulin effects of placentally derived HPL. In addition, the cholesterol levels of pregnancy are twice that of nonpregnant women. Corticosteroid binding globulin increases in response to elevated estrogens during pregnancy. There are also increases in deoxycorticosterone (20 to 100 times normal), cortisol (3 times normal), and aldosterone (2 times normal).

FSH and LH production are suppressed during pregnancy to undetectable levels. Prolactin increases markedly under the influence of elevated estrogens. Oxytocin, vasopressin, and TSH levels are unchanged during pregnancy. Growth hormone is reduced and unresponsive to normal stimuli; ACTH increases slightly.

Estrogen, progesterone, and HCG levels change throughout pregnancy. Estrogens increase throughout gestation, reaching a maximum at term. Progesterone increases rapidly immediately after conception, reaching 25 to 30 ng/ml by 6 weeks and slowly rises from there throughout the remainder of pregnancy. A progesterone value of <15 ng/ml is highly suggestive of an abnormally implanted pregnancy, and levels exceeding 25 ng/ml are usually associated with a normally implanted conceptus. During early gestation, HCG rises exponentially until 38 days after conception. The doubling time ranges from 1.5 days in early pregnancy to 3.5 days at 7 gestational weeks. An HCG level that does not increase by 66% in 48 hours probably represents an abnormal pregnancy.

KEY POINTS

1 Hematologically, plasma volume increases 30% to 50%, RBC volume increases 25%, and WBC counts are higher.

2 Cardiac output increases 33%, and peripheral vascular resistance decreases. Total lung capacity decreases, and minute ventilation increases because of increased tidal volume.

3 Renal blood flow increases because of increased cardiac output. Esophageal reflux increases, and gastric emptying decreases. The thyroid gland increases in size, and estrogen and progesterone are produced in the placenta and are increased during pregnancy.

SUGGESTED READINGS

Cruikshank DP, Hays PM: Maternal physiology in pregnancy. In Gabbe SG, Neibyl JR, Simpson JL, eds: *Obstetrics: normal and problem pregnancies,* ed 2, New York, 1991, Churchill Livingstone, pp 125-146.

Lind T: *Maternal physiology: CREOG basic science monograph,* Washington, DC, 1985, ACOG.

30

Preconceptional, Prenatal, and Postpartum Care

Cynthia B. Evans

PRECONCEPTIONAL CARE

Preconceptional care is an essential aspect of the care of a reproductive-age woman. Intervention at this time can have a great impact on fetal and/or maternal health. First, the patient's medical history needs to be reviewed, focusing on current diseases that may affect a pregnancy. Vaccinations also should be updated, including rubella and hepatitis B. The patient's medication history (prescription and over-the-counter) is next reviewed. Essential medications should be changed to the safest possible alternatives for pregnancy.

A thorough gynecologic and reproductive history, including uterine and lower genital tract anomalies and any endocrinologic abnormalities, should be obtained. A detailed history of any prior pregnancy is also necessary. The next step is a family history. The patient's risk for Tay-Sachs disease, thalassemia, sickle cell disease, cystic fibrosis, muscular dystrophy, and other conditions needs to be determined. The patient's age, relative to an increased risk for chromosomal abnormalities, is also addressed.

The importance of good nutrition is also discussed, including the recommendation of consuming 0.4 mg/day of folic acid to lower the risk of neural tube defects (NTDs). Finally, a complete social history is taken. This covers the patient's use of alcohol and drugs, exercise program, and presence of a support system.

PRENATAL CARE

The initial prenatal visit is probably the most important of all prenatal visits. At this time, a thorough history and physical examination is performed to allow assessment of gestational age and to set a plan of care for the remainder of the pregnancy.

Establishing an estimated date of confinement (EDC) is a critical aspect of early prenatal care. The EDC can be calculated by determining the time of the last menstrual period (LMP) in patients with regular menses or measuring developmental milestones such as the height of the fundus. If the LMP is unreliable or the EDC as established by LMP does not agree with developmental milestones, an ultrasound may be performed to establish an EDC. Ultrasound measurements can establish an EDC for a first trimester pregnancy to within 4 to 5 days, a second trimester pregnancy to within 10 days, and a third trimester pregnancy to within 3 weeks.

The medical history should include any acute or chronic medical problems. A surgical history should also be taken. Teratogenic exposures need to be addressed, including pharmologic, recreational, and occupational. A complete obstetric history should be obtained and verified through previous records. This should include any previous pregnancy losses and problems with a previous pregnancy, labor, or delivery. Infant birth weights and neonatal courses are important, as is any maternal history of congenital anomalies or DES exposure.

A genetic evaluation is made at the first prenatal visit. This should include an assessment of maternal age, family history of anomalies, genetic diseases, or chromosomal problems, and any history of habitual spontaneous abortions. Screening should also be done for Tay-Sachs disease, cystic fibrosis, sickle cell anemia, and thalassemia. In women with a family history of mental retardation, an evaluation should be done for fragile X syndrome. Consultation with a geneticist is appropriate for further evaluation of genetic diseases.

Current problems need to be assessed and treated at the first visit as well. Any symptoms of vulvovaginitis need to be evaluated and treated. Patients should be screened for UTIs. Nausea and/or vomiting needs to be evaluated to ensure adequate hydration and caloric intake. Any symptoms of pelvic or abdominal pain and vaginal bleeding need to be addressed.

Counseling includes information on diet and nutrition. An individual goal for weight gain in pregnancy can then be made, with an optimal weight gain of 20 to 35 lbs for a person who is initially neither underweight nor overweight. Consumption of 0.4 mg/day of folic acid is recommended to lower the risk of NTDs. Women with a history of an NTD are advised to take 4 mg/day of folic acid beginning 1 month before pregnancy and continuing through the first 3 months.

Advice on exercise in pregnancy is also given. Weight-bearing exercise and exercise in the supine position should be avoided. Any exercise with potential abdominal trauma should be avoided. Exercise in pregnancy is contraindicated in some patients with complications such as preeclampsia, premature rupture of membranes, preterm labor, incompetent cervix, second or third trimester bleeding, IUGR, and some maternal medical conditions.

Finally, a background laboratory evaluation should be completed at the first antenatal visit. This should include a CBC; blood type, Rh factor, and indirect Coombs' antibody screen; serology for rubella, syphilis, hepatitis B, and possibly HIV; cervical cytology; urinalysis and urine culture or nitrite sticks; and, gonorrhea, chlamydia, and group B beta streptococcus cultures if appropriate.

In uncomplicated pregnancies, patients are typically seen monthly until 28 weeks, then every 2 to 3 weeks until 36 weeks, then weekly until delivery. The visits entail evaluation of maternal weight, blood pressure, urine, fundal height, and fetal heart tones. Patients are given information about the signs and symptoms of pregnancy complications such as preeclampsia and preterm labor. Counseling should be given regarding prenatal classes available, anesthesia in labor, and breastfeeding versus bottlefeeding. The patient's expectations for labor and delivery should be discussed and clarified.

Routine laboratory evaluation should be performed on subsequent visits. At 15-18 weeks, maternal serum alpha-fetoprotein is assessed. At 24-28 weeks, a 50 g oral glucose load is performed to screen for diabetes, with a possible repeated hemoglobin/hematocrit test and urine culture or nitrite sticks. At 28 weeks, a repeat antibody titer should be obtained for Rhesus (Rh) negative patients, followed by Rhogam administration if the patient remains antibody negative.

POSTPARTUM CARE

Immediate postpartum care should include local cleansing and sitz baths for episiotomy care. Third or fourth-degree episiotomies often require the patient to take stool softeners until the area is healed. Lochia often persists 2 to 3 weeks after a vaginal delivery, and 3 to 4 weeks after a cesarean delivery. Typically, the lochia makes a transition from red to maroon to tan or pink during this time. Tampon use is discouraged. If the patient is breastfeeding, education and support should begin immediately, in the delivery room if possible. If the patient is not breastfeeding, instructions should be given regarding methods of suppressing milk production. Typically, a tight bra or binder worn for 24 hours is recommended when engorgement begins. This is accompanied by oral analgesics and local application of ice packs. Rhogam should be administered if the patient is Rh negative and the infant is Rh positive. The rubella vaccine should be administered if the patient is rubella nonimmune. Extensive education regarding infant care is offered at this time. In addition, the patient is given information about sexual activity, contraception, physical activity, and return to the workplace if applicable. Postpartum examinations are typically scheduled at 4 to 6 weeks after delivery. At this time, the uterus and cervix should have returned to a normal, nonpregnant state. The vaginal vault should be of normal size, but lactating women typically have a very atrophic vagina with minimal elasticity. Vaginal lubricants may be necessary in these patients to achieve comfortable coitus.

Throughout the postpartum period, the patient needs to be evaluated for infections. Endometritis typically presents with fever, tachycardia, abdominal pain, foul-smelling lochia, and a tender uterus. It is usually caused by gram-negative aerobic and anaerobic organisms, so broad-spectrum antibiotics are needed for cure. Risk factors for endometritis include prolonged rupture of membranes, multiple vaginal examinations after rupture of membranes, and cesarean delivery. Endometritis can sometimes be complicated by a pelvic abscess or septic pelvic thrombophlebitis. Wound infections are also fairly common after cesarean deliveries. Obesity, chorioamnionitis, and prolonged rupture of membranes are all risk factors. These are typically caused by endogenous skin flora and respond to local wound care. Occasionally, oral or intravenous antibiotics are necessary. Episiotomy infections do occur, but are uncommon and typically respond to local wound debridement, sitz baths, and antibiotics. Mastitis is a fairly common problem among breastfeeding women. Epidemic mastitis is usually caused by *Staphylococcus aureus* and begins in a hospital nursery. It tends to be more virulent than the more common nonepidemic mastitis. Nonepidemic mastitis is typically caused by endogenous skin flora. Symptoms include fever, malaise, and redness, tenderness, and induration of an area of the breast. Treatment consists of heat to the breast and complete emptying of the breast by nursing and/or pumping the affected breast. Oral antibiotics can help prevent abscess formation. Typically, ampicillin, cephalexin, or dicloxacillin is used. Breastfeeding can be continued unless an abscess is present.

Postpartum hemorrhage usually occurs in the first 24 to 48 hours after delivery, but can occur up to 6 weeks postpartum if caused by endometritis, retained products of conception, or placental subinvolution. For immediate hemorrhage, the patient needs to be evaluated and treated for any obstetric lacerations, uterine atony, or retained products of conception. Uterine inversion is a rare cause of postpartum hemorrhage.

Up to 10% of women can experience postpartum depression. Usually, reassurance and education are sufficient therapy, but sometimes a psychiatric consultation is required. Antidepressant therapy may need to be initiated. Postpartum depression can recur with subsequent pregnancies.

KEY POINTS

1 Preconceptional care involves medical history, medication history, gynecologic and reproductive history, family history, nutrition, and social history.

2 The first prenatal visit should include determination of an EDC, medical and surgical history, medication history, gynecologic and obstetric history, genetic evaluation, nutrition and exercise guidelines, laboratory evaluation, and counseling and education.

3 Subsequent prenatal visits should include measurement of maternal weight and blood pressure; urinalysis for protein, sugar, ketones, and nitrites; fundal height measurements; fetal heart tone assessment; counseling and education; and laboratory evaluation.

SUGGESTED READINGS

American Academy of Pediatrics, American College of Obstetricians and Gynecologists: *Guidelines for perinatal care,* Washington, DC, 1992, APA, ACOG.

American College of Obstetricians and Gynecologists: *Alpha-Fetoprotein,* ACOG Technical Bulletin 154, Washington, DC, 1991, ACOG.

American College of Obstetricians and Gynecologists: *Antepartum fetal surveillance,* ACOG Technical Bulletin 188, Washington, DC, 1994, ACOG.

American College of Obstetricians and Gynecologists: *Current status of cystic fibrosis carrier screening,* ACOG Committee Opinion 101, Washington, DC, 1991, ACOG.

American College of Obstetricians and Gynecologists: *Diethylstilbestrol,* ACOG Committee Opinion 131, Washington, DC, 1993, ACOG.

American College of Obstetricians and Gynecologists: *Down syndrome screening,* ACOG Committee Opinion 141, Washington, DC, 1994, ACOG.

American College of Obstetricians and Gynecologists: *Exercise during pregnancy and the postpartum period,* ACOG Technical Bulletin 189, Washington, DC, 1994, ACOG.
American College of Obstetricians and Gynecologists: *Folic acid for the prevention of recurrent neural tube defects,* ACOG Committee Opinion 120, Washington, DC, 1993, ACOG.
American College of Obstetricians and Gynecologists: *Guidelines for hepatitis B virus screening and vaccination during pregnancy,* ACOG Committee Opinion 111, Washington, DC, 1992, ACOG.
American College of Obstetricians and Gynecologists: *Nutrition during pregnancy,* ACOG Technical Bulletin 179, Washington, DC, 1993, ACOG.
American College of Obstetricians and Gynecologists: *Preconceptual care,* ACOG Technical Bulletin 205, Washington, DC, 1995, ACOG.
American College of Obstetricians and Gynecologists: *Screening for Tay-Sachs disease,* ACOG Committee Opinion 93, Washington, DC, 1991, ACOG.
American College of Obstetricians and Gynecologists: *Vaginal delivery after a previous cesarean birth,* ACOG Committee Opinion 143, Washington, DC, 1994, ACOG.

31

Nutrition and Pregnancy

MAUREEN O'BRIEN PLATT

Nutrition counseling during pregnancy is an integral component of comprehensive prenatal care. A dietitian performs a nutrition assessment early in pregnancy and provides individualized follow-up nutrition education as needed throughout the gestation.

WEIGHT GAIN RECOMMENDATIONS

Prepregnancy weight and pregnancy weight gain are significantly related to the birth weight and subsequent health of the baby. Optimum weight gain for a woman of normal body weight for height is 25 to 35 lbs throughout the pregnancy. Women who are underweight, overweight, or with a multiple gestation should follow other specific recommendations. Teens and black women should strive for gains at the upper limits of the normal weight gain recommendation. Short women (<62 inches) should stay at the lower end of the normal range.

Rate

The rate at which weight is gained during pregnancy is also considered significant. Ideally, a woman should show little weight gain in the first trimester, approximately 2 to 4 lbs. During the second and third trimesters, a woman should have a goal to gain an average of 1 lb/week. Weight gain is sometimes more rapid during the second trimester, with a slowing in weight gain during the third trimester.

Women who begin their pregnancies significantly underweight or overweight are considered to be at risk, and additional nutrition counseling may be indicated. A woman who is underweight before pregnancy (10% or more below her standard weight for height) should be encouraged to gain 28 to 40 lbs during the pregnancy. An overweight woman with a prepregnancy weight of 20% or more above the standard weight for height should limit weight gain to approximately 15 to 25 lbs. The recommended weight gain for an obese woman (30% or more above the standard weight for height) is 15 lbs for the total pregnancy. The recommended weight gain for women with a twin gestation is 35 to 45 lbs.

PRENATAL DIET

The recommended food intake during pregnancy is as follows:

Food group	Daily servings
Milk	3
Meat	5-6
Fruit	2-4
Vegetable (especially dark green leafy and orange choices)	3-5
Bread	6-11
Fats and sweets	Limited (moderate amounts)

Pregnant teens should consume four servings from the milk group and at least six servings from the meat group. An additional 300 kcal/day is recommended during the second and third trimesters to support the demands of pregnancy and fetal growth.

A woman can best meet her caloric and nutrient needs by dividing her daily consumption of food into three meals plus two to three snacks. The evening or bedtime snack is especially important and should include a source of protein. Also, drinking 6 to 8 glasses of water is strongly encouraged. Caffeinated beverages should be limited to 2 cups daily.

Quantities of food should be determined by individual energy requirements to provide an adequate weight gain.

SUPPLEMENTS

Women generally enter pregnancy with minimal iron stores. The amount of iron needed for the fetus during pregnancy, the increase in the maternal blood supply during pregnancy, and the iron lost at delivery also greatly increase the demand for iron. Therefore it is recommended that women take an iron supplement, especially during the second half of pregnancy. A daily intake of 30 mg of elemental ferrous iron is recommended.

Women who become anemic during pregnancy should be given therapeutic doses of iron supplements. A total of 60 to 120 mg/day of iron in divided doses along with 400 μg of folate daily is recommended. Zinc supplementation may also be considered when iron supplements of greater than 60 mg/day are prescribed. Excessive iron supplementation can cause gastrointestinal problems and may also inhibit zinc absorption. The use of folate supplements is particularly advised when the woman is consuming an inadequate diet, pregnant with a multiple gestation, on an anticonvulsant medication, or diagnosed with megaloblastic anemia. The recommended level of folate supplementation is 400 μg to 4 mg daily. Folate supplements are also recommended as preconceptional therapy to help protect against NTDs.

MANAGEMENT OF COMMON PROBLEMS

Nausea/Vomiting

Nausea, or morning sickness, is common during the first trimester of pregnancy and usually subsides by the 14th week. It may be caused by the hormonal changes occurring, and poor dietary habits or strong feelings of anxiety and uncertainty about being pregnant may intensify the nausea. Hospitalization is recommended when the vomiting is severe, urinary ketones are present, and weight loss occurs. IV fluids and electrolyte replacement are usually required to prevent complications of dehydration. Relief measures for the management of nausea/vomiting include eating dry crackers, cereal, or toast before getting out of bed in the morning; eating small, frequent meals throughout the day, never allowing the stomach to be completely empty; separating the intake of fluids and solids by one half to 1 hour; avoiding greasy, fried, and high-fat foods; having good air circulation when cooking; and consumption of vitamin B_6 supplements.

Constipation

Constipation during the latter stages of pregnancy is a common and usually minor problem. Reduced gastrointestinal motility and the pressure of the uterus on the bowel may cause constipation. Dietary remedies for the problem include increasing fluid intake, especially with fruit juices; eating more raw fruits and vegetables with the skin on when possible; adding dried fruits, such as raisins and dates, as snacks; and, choosing high-fiber breakfast cereals. Daily exercise, such as walking, and regular bowel habits also ease elimination problems.

Heartburn

Heartburn is a common problem, often occurring during the third trimester of pregnancy. The pressure of the enlarging uterus on the stomach and the relaxed esophageal sphincter are the usual causes of this complaint. Heartburn can be relieved by eating several small meals throughout the day instead of three large meals; avoiding spicy, fried, greasy, or high-fat foods; limiting caffeine-containing drinks such as coffee, tea, and soda; avoiding laying down for at least 2 hours after eating; wearing loose-fitting clothes; and relaxing during meal times.

Pica

Pica refers to the habit of eating nonfood substances. In the United States, pica during pregnancy most often involves eating dirt or clay (geophagia) or starch (amylophagia), such as laundry starch. Consuming unusual quantities of ice is also common. Other nonfood substances that are eaten are cigarette ashes, coffee grounds, toilet paper, baby powder, mothballs, burnt matches, and coal.

Malnutrition can occur when the mother chooses the nonfood substances in place of nutritious foods. Excessive amounts of starch can lead to obesity. Anemia is common because the substances may contain compounds that interfere with the absorption of minerals, especially iron. Tooth decay, lead poisoning, intestinal obstruction, preeclampsia, and premature births have been observed in women exhibiting pica during pregnancy.

Inadequate Weight Gain

A weight gain of less than 2 lbs/month is usually considered inadequate. Possible causes of inadequate weight gain that need further investigation include nausea, vomiting, or heartburn; improved diet, reducing fats and simple sugars; fear of gaining too much weight and getting fat; depression; eating disorder; and food availability.

Excessive Weight Gain

Weight gains of more than 6.5 lbs per month are considered excessive. Causes for excessive weight gain that may benefit from additional evaluation include poor, calorie-dense food choices; overeating because of stress or depression; errors in measurement; differences in clothing at prenatal visits; fluid retention, especially after week 20; multiple gestation; and, dramatic decrease in physical activity. If a patient is following an inadequate high-fat diet, she should be counseled on specific dietary changes. High-fat foods and cooking techniques to avoid need to be discussed.

BREASTFEEDING

The nutritional requirements of the mother are greater when breastfeeding than during pregnancy. An increased intake of fluids and most nutrients is recommended. Calorie levels should be increased by 500 kcal/day over the prepregnant level.

The quality of the mother's diet can affect the composition and quantity of breast milk. A woman should be encouraged to continue the diet plan she followed throughout pregnancy with emphasis on consuming calcium-rich foods. Fluid intake needs are increased to 10 to 12 glasses/day. Harmful substances such as alcohol, drugs, nicotine, caffeine, and medications not approved by the physician should be avoided by the breastfeeding mother.

KEY POINTS

1 Prepregnancy weight and pregnancy weight gain are significantly related to the birth weight and subsequent health of the baby.

2 Inadequate weight gain during pregnancy may be a result of various causes, including problems with depression, eating disorders, or food availability.

3 Pica during pregnancy can lead to serious complications including malnutrition, obesity, anemia, tooth decay, and intestinal obstruction.

4 A woman who will be breastfeeding needs to continue following an adequate diet, increasing calories by 500 kcal/day, and increasing fluids to 10 to 12 glasses/day.

SUGGESTED READINGS

Carruth BR, Skinner JD: Practitioners beware: regional differences in beliefs about nutrition during pregnancy, *J Am Diet Assoc* 91:435-440, 1991.

Fogel CI, Woods NF: *Women's health care: a comprehensive handbook,* Thousand Oaks, Calif, 1995, Sage Publications.

Horner RD et al: Pica practices of pregnant women, *J Am Diet Assoc* 91:34-38, 1991.

Institute of Medicine: *Nutrition during pregnancy: weight gain and nutrient supplements,* Washington, DC, 1991, National Academy Press.

Mahan LK, Arlin M: *Krause's food, nutrition and diet therapy,* Philadelphia, 1992, WB Saunders.

Newman V, Lee D: Developing a daily food guide for women, *J Nutr Ed* 23(2):76-82, 1991.

Story M: *Nutrition management of the pregnant adolescent,* Washington, DC, 1990, National Clearinghouse.

32

Prenatal Diagnosis and Teratology

THOMAS J. ALBERT, JR.

Major congenital anomalies are the leading cause of infant mortality in the United States and occur in 3% of all liveborn infants at term. Two thirds of all major congenital anomalies are the result of multifactorial (polygenic) or unknown causes, and 20% to 25% are caused by chromosomal (aneuploidy or less commonly polyploidy and structural gene defects) or monogenic (single gene or Mendelian) disorders. Fetal defor-

BOX 32-1

Common Indications for Genetic Counseling With the Potential Need for Prenatal Diagnosis

Advanced maternal age*
Elevated or low† maternal serum α-fetoprotein (MSAFP)
Ultrasonographically detected fetal abnormality
Family history of an inheritable disorder
- Multifactional traits (i.e., midline facial clefting, congenital heart disease, and NTDs).
- Monogenic disorders (i.e., cystic fibrosis, Duchenne/Becker muscular dystrophy, and hemophilia)
- Chromosomal disorders (i.e., aneuploidy; structural defects such as parental translocations, inversions, deletions, ring chromosomes, and isochromosomes; mosaicism; polyploidy)
- Unknown cause (i.e., some cases of mental retardation)
- Prior stillborn fetus or congenitally malformed fetus or neonate

High risk ethnic group
- Southeast Asian (α-thalassemia)
- Mediterranean extract (β-thalassemia)
- Black (sickle cell disease)
- Jewish (Tay-Sachs and Gaucher's diseases)

Exposure to teratogen
- Drug (i.e., isotretinoin)
- Environmental/occupational agent (i.e., lead)
- Infectious agent (i.e., toxoplasmosis)
- Physical agent (i.e., radiation and hyperthermia)

Habitual (recurrent) abortion
Maternal disease (i.e., diabetes mellitus, PKU, epilepsy, alcoholism, and myasthenia gravis)
Consanguinity

*Maternal age ≥35 years old at the expected date of confinement.
†Low MSAFP alone or in combination with abnormal values for HCG and uE3.

mation (as seen with chronic oligohydramnios) or disruption (i.e., amniotic band syndrome) are rare causes for congenital anomalies. Only a small percentage of birth defects are known to be caused by teratogenic exposure. Box 32-1 lists common indications for prenatal testing.

PRENATAL DIAGNOSIS

Maternal Serum Analyte Screening for Birth Defects

At 15 to 18 weeks gestation, physicians offer either MSAFP alone or the triple screening profile (or "triple analyte profile") consisting of MSAFP, unconjugated estriol (uE3), and HCG to all pregnant women. Box 32-2

BOX 32-2

Etiologies for Elevated Maternal Serum α-Fetoprotein

Incorrect dates	Oligohydramnios
Multifetal pregnancy	Omphalocele/gastroschisis
Spina bifida	Bladder exstrophy
Anencephaly	Sacrococcygeal teratoma
Encephalocele	Gastrointestinal obstruction
Fetal-maternal hemorrhage	Urologic obstruction
Fetal demise	Congenital nephrosis

lists several congenital abnormalities that may be associated with an elevated MSAFP.

The use of MSAFP testing as a means of screening for structural birth defects began in the 1970s. An elevated value may detect 80% to 90% of open neural tube defects (NTDs) and 50% of ventral abdominal wall defects (i.e., omphalocele and gastroschisis). Most centers use a "cut-off" value of 2.0 or 2.5 MoMs to signify an increased risk for structural congenital anomalies (the lower the cut-off value, the higher the sensitivity and the false positive rate). When an abnormal MSAFP value is obtained, an ultrasound is performed to ascertain the correct dates (unless an ultrasound was previously documented for gestational dating) and to rule out multifetal pregnancy or fetal demise. Abnormal MSAFP values that are associated with incorrect gestational dating may be recalculated by the laboratory using the correct gestational age. Several centers recommend repeating the MSAFP if it is mildly elevated and the pregnancy is not advanced, although other centers proceed with further evaluation after a single abnormally high value. The patient with an abnormal MSAFP then receives further genetic counseling and a comprehensive obstetric ultrasound with a detailed anatomic survey. Amniocentesis may abide in the diagnosis of a fetal abnormality (fetal karyotype and amniotic fluid α-fetoprotein [AF-AFP]) and is routinely offered to patients with an elevated MSAFP. When no abnormality can be identified as the cause for the abnormally elevated MSAFP, the patient then has an "unexplained elevated MSAFP," which has been associated with an increased risk of adverse perinatal outcome.

The use of MSAFP testing as a screening method for the detection of fetal aneuploidy, based on a "low" level (i.e., less than 0.5 MoM), was introduced in the 1980s. Low MSAFP values should not be repeated and require further evaluation. A numerical risk of aneuploidy (e.g., Down syndrome) may be calculated based on the MSAFP value and the maternal age, affording a 45% prenatal detection rate of this condition if the statistical risk equals that of a 35-year-old gravida at midpregnancy, that is, 1:270.

Use of the triple screening profile in clinical practice is more recent. Down syndrome is associated with low MSAFP and uE3 values and an elevated HCG level. Low values for all three analytes is associated with an increased risk of trisomy-18. The triple screening profile is more expensive than the MSAFP value alone; however, the combined profile increases the detection rate of Down syndrome to approximately 60%, with fewer false positive tests.

Although several ultrasonographic stigmata of Down syndrome have been described (i.e., nuchal fold thickness greater than 5 mm), over 50% of fetuses with this chromosomal abnormality may have no identifiable ultrasonographic abnormality. A minority of fetuses with trisomy-18 or trisomy-13 may also have no ultrasonographically identifiable structural lesion. For this reason, diagnosis rests on karyotype results obtained by amniocentesis.

Patients with advanced maternal age are currently universally offered diagnostic genetic amniocentesis for the detection of fetal aneuploidy. The appropriateness of the medical decision to alternatively offer the patient a screening test (e.g., triple screening profile) for the same purpose has yet to be fully determined.

Amniocentesis

Common indications for genetic amniocentesis are advanced maternal age and abnormal maternal serum analyte screening. Less common indications include an ultrasonographically detected fetal anomaly or a family or ethnic history of an inheritable disorder that is amenable to diagnosis by analysis of amniotic fluid. Traditionally, genetic amniocentesis has been offered at 15 to 18 weeks pregnancy. More recently, many centers are performing the procedure at 13 to 15 weeks gestation ("early" amniocentesis).

Three major collaborative trials of genetic amniocentesis have reported a procedure-related pregnancy loss rate of 1/200 for "traditional amniocentesis" and >99% cytogenetic diagnostic accuracy. The complication rate for "early" amniocentesis may be slightly higher. The performance of amniocentesis before 12 to 13 weeks gestation may be associated with a significantly higher risk of complications because of the relative small volume of amniotic fluid and incomplete fusion of the chorioamniotic membranes. Complication rates are directly proportional to an increasing number of needle insertions and operator inexperience. The most commonly reported complication is transient vaginal spotting or transvaginal leakage of amniotic fluid in approximately 1% to 2% of amniocenteses, although protracted fluid loss may result in pregnancy loss (or with certain fetal complications occasionally found in any condition associated with chronic oligohydramnios). The risk for chorioamnionitis is 1/1000 amniocenteses. After amniocentesis, patients who are Rh-negative should receive Rh hyperimmune globulin (300 μg) because of the potential of a procedure-associated fetal-maternal hemorrhage (FMH).

Chorionic Villus Sampling

Chorionic villus sampling (CVS) was first reported in 1983, and the indications for its usage are the same as for genetic amniocentesis except for analyses that require amniotic fluid for AF-AFP and AChE determination.

The advantage of CVS over amniocentesis is the availability of the procedure (and therefore the fetal karyotype) at an earlier gestational age (9 to 12 weeks). CVS is especially useful for DNA and metabolic testing for Mendelian disorders. In certain rare conditions, such as 21-hydroxylase deficiency, an earlier diagnosis may afford the opportunity for more timely and effective fetal therapy. The disadvantages of CVS as compared with amniocentesis include a slightly increased procedure-related pregnancy loss rate of 0.5% to 1% and an increased occurrence of mosaicism. Both confined placental mosaicism and true fetal mosaicism occur in 1% of CVS specimens. When mosaicism is found during CVS, amniocentesis or cordocentesis at a later gestational age may be of value. Pseudomosaicism, a laboratory artifact, occurs in 1% to 2% of CVS analyses.

CVS is commonly performed by either transabdominal or transcervical techniques using continuous ultrasonographic guidance at 9 to 12 weeks gestation. Rarely, transabdominal CVS for fetal karyotyping may be performed in the second or third trimesters of pregnancy (termed *placental biopsy*) for chromosome analysis if fetal growth restriction or a malformation associated with severe oligohydramnios is present. As with amniocentesis, patients who are Rh-negative should receive Rh hyperimmune globulin after CVS. Additionally, CVS is contraindicated (amniocentesis is preferred) in patients who are known to be isoimmunized.

Percutaneous Umbilical Blood Sampling

Percutaneous umbilical blood sampling (PUBS) was introduced in the 1980s and has been clinically useful in the management of fetal isoimmunization. The procedure may also be used for genetic testing, most commonly in the setting where a rapid karyotype is desirable, such as in a fetus diagnosed with a malformation or severe growth restriction after 20 weeks gestation. Cytogenetic analysis on fetal blood is usually available within 24 to 48 hours. Depending on the clinical indication, fetal blood may also be sent for metabolic and hematologic studies, acid-base values, viral cultures, and immunologic studies. A 1% fetal loss rate has been described with PUBS. The procedure requires technical expertise and should be performed only by an experienced operator.

Fetoscopic and Ultrasonographic Fetal Sampling

Rarely, fetal tissue sampling is indicated for certain conditions that cannot be diagnosed by conventional methods of invasive prenatal diagnostic testing. Fetoscopic methods have a high fetal loss rate of 1% to 3%. Fetoscopic and ultrasonographic fetal sampling should be performed only at centers experienced with such techniques. Fetal skin sampling has been performed for congenital ichthyosis and epidermolysis bullosa and fetal liver biopsy is performed for certain hepatic enzyme deficiencies.

TERATOLOGY

There are several major classifications of teratogens: drugs (and environmental or occupational chemicals), infectious agents, radiation, hyperthermia, mechanical deformation or disruption, and maternal metabolic disease. Teratogens may cause several potential embryofetal alterations such as structural malformation, decreased fertility, mutagenesis, carcinogenesis, growth alteration, fetal or neonatal death, and functional abnormalities (i.e., mental retardation, neurologic or behavioral abnormality, and developmental delay). When a conceptus is exposed to more than one agent at a time (e.g., abuse of multiple drugs), it may be difficult to establish teratogenicity of any individual agent because of the concurrent exposures.

Gestational age at the time of exposure to a teratogen is of critical importance, thus the term *critical periods.* The preorganogenesis period during the first 2 weeks after fertilization is known as the *all or none period* when teratogenic exposure causes either spontaneous abortion or embryonic resorption versus an unaffected conceptus. The time interval between days 15 to 60 postconception is the *embryonic period,* during which organogenesis occurs, and this is the time when exposure to a teratogen may cause a major morphologic defect. Beyond 9 weeks gestation, the conceptus enters the fetal period of growth and development, during which minor morphologic and functional deficits may be caused by a teratogen (i.e., mental retardation and growth restriction). Critical stages of human embryonic development have also been described for the various organ systems.

Of the thousands of drugs available, there are only approximately 30 known human teratogens (Box 32-3).

The general approach to drugs in pregnancy should be as follows: (1) unless medically indicated, avoid the use of drugs in the first trimester

BOX 32-3

Known Human Teratogens

DRUGS

ACE inhibitors
Alkylating agents (busulfan, cyclophosphamide)
Androgenic hormones (danazol, testosterone)
Carbamazepine, hydantoin, trimethadione, valproic acid
Antiepileptics
Coumarins
Diethylstilbestrol
Ethanol
Folic acid antagonists (aminopterin, methotrexate)
Isotretinoin, etretinate, vitamin A excess
Lithium
Lead
Methimazole
Organic mercury
Penicillamine
Polybrominated and polychlorinated biphenyls (PBB, PCB)
Tetracycline
Thalidomide

INFECTIOUS AGENTS

Cytomegalovirus, herpes simplex virus, varicella/zoster virus, rubella virus, toxoplasmosis, syphilis

PHYSICAL AGENT

Hyperthermia, ionizing radiation (>5 rad), radioactive iodine and treat nonpharmaceutically if possible (i.e., diet modifications for "morning sickness" as initial therapy); (2) any female of reproductive age is pregnant until proved otherwise; (3) never give "permission" for "recreational drugs"; (4) assess risks and benefits for all drugs and use the lowest effective dosage and duration of therapy; (5) if possible, avoid newer drugs and select those agents with which the greatest clinical experience exists; (6) if unsure regarding the indication, therapeutic use, or teratogenetic potential of any drug, a physician should research it and become familiar with the FDA classification system; and (7) of vast importance is documentation.

Ethanol

Ethanol ingestion during pregnancy is the most common preventable cause of mental retardation (MR) in the United States. From 1% to 2% of reproductive-age females are alcoholic, and overtly alcoholic mothers have a 30% to 40% risk of having a child with fetal alcohol syndrome (FAS) if more than two drinks are consumed per day. The incidence of FAS is 1300 to 2000 liveborns; sequelae include MR, microcephaly, growth restriction, midline facial hypoplasia, congenital heart and limb defects, and impaired speech, motor, and neurobehavioral function. More subtle neurobehavioral abnormalities are called *fetal alcohol effects.* The effect of "binge drinking" is unknown, and no safe level of ethanol consumption has been determined; therefore physicians should avoid giving patients "social permission" for alcohol ingestion.

Diethylstilbestrol

Diethylstilbestrol (DES) is a nonsteroidal synthetic estrogen approved by the FDA in 1942 to prevent abortions; an estimated 2 million women were exposed. In female offspring, benign cervicovaginal adenosis occurs in 32% to 90%, and 25% have cervicouterine structural abnormalities (such as a cervical "hood" or "comb," "T-shaped" uterus, or a uterine constriction band); these morphologic abnormalities account for an increased risk of preterm delivery, spontaneous abortion, and ectopic pregnancy. Clear cell adenocarcinoma of the vagina occurs rarely, a 1/1000 risk. Approximately 25% of male offspring may be affected with cryptorchidism, small testes, or epididymal cysts.

Coumadin

At 6 to 9 weeks gestation, the potent human teratogen Coumadin causes fetal warfarin syndrome (FWS) in 15% to 25% of exposed pregnancies. FWS is thought to be caused by microhemorrhages in the developing organs. Exposure may also result in spontaneous abortion or fetal or neonatal death. FWS consists of MR, ophthalmic abnormalities (i.e., optic nerve atrophy), hydrocephaly or microcephaly, midline facial hypoplasia, boney stippling (i.e., similar to chondroplasia punctata), growth restriction, and developmental delay. Some teratogenic effects, such as MR and ophthalmic abnormalities, may also be seen with exposure in the second and third trimesters of pregnancy. For this reason, heparin is the anticoagulant of choice in pregnancies complicated by thromboembolism. An exception to this may be in patients with highly thrombogenic artificial metallic heart valves in whom thrombosis may occur despite therapeutic administration of heparin.

Antineoplastic Drugs

The folic acid antagonists aminopterin and methotrexate cause a similar embryopathy consisting of hydrocephaly, craniosynostosis, limb and neural tube defects, and cleft palate. The risk of congenital malformation in the first trimester after methotrexate exposure is 25%. Aminopterin in the first trimester causes fetal resorption and is therefore contraindicated in pregnancy. The alkylating agents busulfan and cyclophosphamide are also known to be human teratogens and have been associated with imperforate anus, digital abnormalities, and abnormal arterial systems.

Research on antineoplastic drugs generally describes an approximate 15% risk of malformation with exposure in the first trimester. There is no increased risk of anomalies after second or third trimester exposure; however, a 40% risk of growth restriction may occur. Offspring may have an increased risk of sterility.

Thalidomide

Thalidomide, an anxiolytic/sedative, is quite possibly the most infamous of human teratogens, responsible for an epidemic of phocomelia in Europe in the 1960s. External ear defects, duodenal atresia, renal agenesis, and tetralogy of Fallot were also reported as teratogenic sequelae of this agent.

Isotretinoin

Isotretinoin, a vitamin A isomer, is used in the treatment of cystic acne. This drug is contraindicated during pregnancy because of the increased risk of spontaneous abortion and the 25% risk of congenital malformation in the first trimester. There is an additional 25% risk of MR. Megadosages of vitamin A cause a similar embryopathy. Called *retinoic acid embryopathy,* it includes microtia or anotia, ophthalmic abnormality (i.e., optic nerve atrophy and microphthalmia), hydrocephaly, congenital heart defect (i.e., transposition of the great vessels and ventriculoseptal defect), deafness, blindness, and thymic abnormality. Topical tretinoin (Retin-A) may be associated with lower systemic levels of the drug, and its use has not been associated with human malformation; however, there is insufficient human data and therefore its use is not recommended during pregnancy. A related drug, etretinate (Tegison), a highly lipophilic drug used for the treatment of psoriasis, has a long half-life and may cause embryopathy even with preconceptional usage; therefore a reliable form of contraception should be used for at least 6 months after dosing.

Antibiotics

Although there are few studies addressing the safety of specific antibiotics during pregnancy, many of these drugs (i.e., penicillin, cephalosporin, and clindamycin) have been deemed "safe" for use in pregnancy based on a wealth of clinical experience with the drug. The tetracyclines and the long-acting forms minocycline and doxycycline are contraindicated during pregnancy because they may cause staining of the decidual teeth and boney stippling with associated growth inhibition. With greater dosages of tetracyclines, maternal acute fatty liver and renal failure were reported. Streptomycin and kanamycin may cause cranial nerve VIII damage; however, gentamycin is commonly used to treat infections during pregnancy (with close attention to dosing with extended courses of treatment.) Fluoroquinolones cause an irreversible arthropathy in canines and therefore they are not a first-line antibiotic for use in pregnancy. Although sulfa drugs are not a human teratogen, their use should be avoided in patients with glucose-6-phosphate dehydrogenase deficiency, and because it displaces bound bilirubin its use is not recommended in the third trimester. Use of the combination drug trimethoprim (bacterial folic acid inhibitor) and sulfamethoxasole is not favored as a first-line drug for the treatment of UTIs during pregnancy because the former component is relatively contraindicated in the first trimester and the latter component is relatively contraindicated in the third trimester. The imidazoles (antifungals) and metronidazole (Flagyl) are associated with a positive Ames test for mutagenicity, causing some physicians to avoid their use in the first trimester even though they are not proved human teratogens.

Angiotensin Converting Enzyme Inhibitors

Angiotensin converting enzyme inhibitors, commonly used antihypertensive agents (i.e., captopril, enalapril, and lisinopril), may cause fetal (and neonatal) renal failure and consequent fetal anuria, severe oligohydramnios, and pulmonary hypoplasia. These agents are also embryocidal in animals. Their use is absolutely contraindicated in pregnancy.

Androgenic Hormones

In the first trimester, danazol and exogenous testosterone may cause virilization of a female fetus (i.e., labial fusion and phallic enlargement). Drugs containing androgenic compounds that have been chemically altered for their use as progestational agents (i.e., combination birth control pills and Depo-Provera) also have the small potential of causing virilization in a female fetus.

Lithium

Used for the treatment of bipolar affective disorder, lithium carries an 8% risk of congenital heart defect and a 2.7% risk specifically for Epstein's anomaly. Additionally, neonatal toxicity infrequently occurs in neonates after exposure in the third trimester and manifests as hypotonia, lethargy, poor feeding, hypothyroidism, goiter, bradycardia, cyanosis, and nephrogenic diabetes insipidus.

Antiepileptics

Epilepsy in pregnancy is associated with a twofold to threefold increase in the incidence of congenital malformations and MR. Ideally, the patient should receive preconceptional counseling regarding periconceptional usage of folate (NTD prophylaxis) and continuation or discontinuation of the antiepileptic agent before conception, depending on the status of the patient's seizure disorder. Because of the potential maternal and fetal risks with recurrent seizures, patients with an active seizure disorder would benefit from continuation of their antiepileptic regimen. Under a physician's care, an attempt should be made to convert patients on trimethadione or valproic acid to another antiepileptic agent. During pregnancy, the patient's drug levels should be followed approximately every month and patients should be counseled regarding the availability of prenatal diagnosis.

Use of valproic acid in the first trimester is associated with a 1% to 2% risk of NTD. The fetal valproate syndrome consists of craniofacial abnormalities (hypertelorism, shallow orbits, small nose and mouth, and low-set ears), congenital heart defect, brachycephaly, and hyperconvex nails with overlapping digits. Use of valproic acid in the first trimester of pregnancy is not recommended.

Trimethadione (and paramethadione) is contraindicated in pregnancy because its use has been associated with craniofacial abnormalities, speech difficulties, hearing loss, simian crease, cardiac abnormality, growth deficiency, MR, and microcephaly.

Hydantoin is associated with a 30% risk of a minor abnormality and less than a 10% risk of a major abnormality. The fetal hydantoin syndrome consists of craniofacial abnormality (cleft lip and palate), growth restriction, MR, congenital heart defect, limb defect, and hypoplastic nails/distal phalanges.

Carbamazepine was once considered to be the antiepileptic of choice in pregnancy; however, the teratogenic risk of this agent is similar to what occurs after hydantoin exposure. The fetal carbamazepine syndrome (which is similar to the fetal hydantoin syndrome) consists of craniofacial abnormality (upslanting palpebral fissures, short nose, and epicanthal folds), growth restriction, MR, developmental delay, 0.5% to 1% risk of NTD, and abnormal fingertips.

There are inconsistent data linking phenobarbital with major congenital abnormalities, though the use of this agent during pregnancy has been linked with minor abnormalities similar to those seen with fetal hydantoin syndrome.

Penicillamine

Penicillamine, a chelating agent, is used in the treatment of Wilson's disease (hepatolenticular degeneration), cystinuria, and severe rheumatoid arthritis. After 100 documented exposures during pregnancy, there have been six cases of connective tissue abnormalities reported (i.e., cutis laxa and venous fragility). After counseling patients regarding its risks and benefits, penicillamine may be appropriate in the management of pregnant patients with Wilson's disease.

Thyroid Drugs

When administered to a pregnant patient, radioactive iodine is associated with congenital hypothyroidism and goiter in the offspring because the fetal thyroid avidly begins to concentrate iodine by 7 to 10 weeks gestation; therefore its use is contraindicated in pregnancy. Saturated solution of potassium iodide (SSKI) may be used in the treatment of a patient with life-threatening thyroid storm, though its use may be associated with the occurrence of congenital goiter. Thyroid hormone replacement (Synthroid), commonly used for maternal hypothyroidism, has minimal transplacental passage and is safe for use in pregnancy. The related compounds, propylthiouracil (PTU) and methimazole (Tapazole), are commonly used in the treatment of maternal hyperthyroidism. PTU is preferred over methimazole because of the greater clinical experience with it and the initial linkage of methimazole with aplasia cutis. Congenital goiter and hypothyroidism have been reported as a rare side effect of these thioamide drugs; therefore the patient is managed by serial assessment of symptomatology and thyroid function tests using the lowest dosage of PTU to keep the patient in the upper euthyroid range.

Environmental Agents

Prenatal exposure to organic mercury, a fungicide that is associated with bioaccumulation and that was in use until the 1960s, is concentrated in the sensitive fetal brain and in breast milk. There is no obvious defect at birth, though devastating developmental sequelae ensue including MR, cerebral palsy, deafness, blindness, seizures, and growth restriction.

Polychlorinated and polybrominated biphenyls (PCBs, PBBs) also accumulate in fat and breast milk. They are industrial agents that are stable and bioaccumulate. Epidemics related to cooking oil use have been reported, linking exposure not only with an adult illness but with low birth weight and neuroectodermal dysplasia (consisting of skin and mucosal hyperpigmentation, natal teeth, gingival hyperplasia, acne, fragile teeth, deformed nails, exophthalmus, and delayed bone age).

KEY POINTS

1. Of all liveborn infants, 3% have a major congenital anomaly. The incidence increases with certain obstetric conditions. In the majority of cases, the etiology is multifactorial and is less commonly caused by a chromosomal or Mendelian disorder. Teratogenesis and fetal deformation are uncommon causes of birth defects.
2. Advanced maternal age and abnormal maternal serum α-fetoprotein screening (i.e., MSAFP) are the first and second most common indications for prenatal diagnostic testing, respectively. MSAFP and the triple screening profile are screening tests for birth defects.
3. Approximately 30 drugs are known human teratogens. The most potent teratogenic drugs include ethanol, DES, Coumadin, folic acid antagonists, thalidomide, isotretinoin, ACE inhibitors, androgenic hormones, trimethadione, valproic acid, and radioactive iodine.
4. The "critical period" of teratogenesis is the embryonic period during which organogenesis occurs, between 15 to 60 days after conception.
5. The prescribing physician should consider the risks and benefits of any drug used in pregnancy, with preference for drugs known to be safe in pregnancy.

SUGGESTED READINGS

American College of Obstetricians and Gynecologists: *Alpha-fetoprotein,* ACOG Technical Bulletin #154, Washington, DC, 1991, ACOG.

Assel BG et al: Single-operator comparison of early and mid-second trimester amniocentesis, *Obstet Gynecol* 79:940, 1992.

Burton BK, Schulz CJ, Burd LI: Limb anomalies associated with chorionic villus sampling, *Obstet Gynecol* 79:726-30, 1992.

Lippman A et al and Canadian Collaborative CVS-Amniocentesis Clinical Trial Group: Canadian multicenter randomized clinical trial of chorionic villus sampling and amniocentesis: final report, *Prenat Diag* 12:385, 1992.

33

Genetics

BETH ANN SCHMALZ

Significant genetic diseases or birth defects occur in 3% to 5% of all human live births. The incidence of diagnosed defects doubles by 8 years of age. (The box on p. 241 in Chapter 32 lists common indications for referral to a genetic center.)

Genetic counseling provides information to families regarding the occurrence and risk of recurrence of genetic disorders. Genetic evaluation and counseling also help the affected child reach its fullest potential and the family to adjust to the child's special needs. Genetic counseling is nondirective, educational, unconditional, and supportive.

A genetic evaluation allows the clinical geneticist to determine the *diagnosis* and *etiology* of a disorder in a family. The two may be definite, probable, suspected, sporadic, or unknown. Follow-up genetic visits allow monitoring of the patient's progress and sharing of new developments with the family.

TYPES

Genetic diseases are classified into four major categories: chromosomal, single gene, multifactorial, and somatic cell defects. Exceptions to classic Mendelian inheritance are included as nonclassical patterns.

Chromosome abnormalities (CAs) occur in 50% of spontaneous abortions and in 0.5% of live births. The most common CAs in abortuses are 45,X; triploidy; and trisomy 16. Trisomies 21, 18, and 13 are the most common CAs among live births. The risk for delivering a live birth with any CA increases from 1:526 to 1:63 between maternal ages 20 and 40 years, respectively. If a patient has a Down syndrome (DS) family member, her risk may also be increased. Trisomy 21 accounts for 95% of DS cases; 4% result from an unbalanced translocation and half are familial. The recurrence risk for trisomy 21 is 1% if the mother is under 40 years of age. When the mother is over 39, the recurrence risk is the maternal age-related risk. If the affected child has a translocation, chromosome analysis is recommended for the parents. The recurrence risk is about 10% when the mother is a translocation carrier, but less than 5% when the father is a carrier.

Box 33-1 lists several single-gene disorders.

The most common pattern of inheritance is autosomal dominant (AD). An individual with an AD gane has a 50-50 chance of transmitting it to a child. The mutant gene occurs equally in both sexes. Because the gene is dominant, the condition manifests itself when only one copy is present. Reduced penetrance and variable expressivity of an AD gene may affect the phenotype, even within the same family. A woman with mild neurofibromatosis, for example, may produce a child with a plexiform neurofibroma causing serious deformities.

BOX 33-1

Selected Single-Gene Disorders Listed by Pattern of Inheritance

Autosomal dominant	Autosomal recessive	X-Linked
Achondroplasia	21-Hydroxylase deficiency	Becker muscular dystrophy
Adult polycystic kidney disease	Cystic fibrosis	Duchenne muscular dystrophy
Apert's syndrome	Diastrophic dysplasia	Fragile X syndrome
Ehlers-Danlos syndrome types I, II, and III	Gaucher's disease	Hemophilia A (factor VIII deficiency)
Familial hypercholesterolemia	Hurler's syndrome	Hemophilia B (factor IX deficiency)
Huntington's disease	Limb-Girdle muscular dystrophy	Hunter's syndrome
Marfan syndrome	Meckel-Gruber syndrome	Menkes' syndrome
Myotonic dystrophy	Phenylketonuria (PKU)	OTC deficiency (ornithine transcarbamylase)
Neurofibromatosis type 1 and 2	Sickle cell disease	
Osteogenesis imperfecta types I, II and IV	Tay-Sachs disease	
Saethre-Chotzen syndrome	Werdnig-Hoffman disease (SMAI)	
Tuberous sclerosis	Wilson's disease	
Waardenburg's syndrome		

In autosomal recessive (AR) disorders, an affected individual has two copies of the mutant gene. If both parents carry the same AR gene, the chance is 1:4 that they will produce an affected child.

The mutant gene for an X-linked (XL) disorder is located on the X chromosome. XL recessive disorders are passed on by carrier females to, theoretically, half of their sons. A daughter of an affected male is an obligate carrier. Male-to-male transmission does not occur.

Fragile X syndrome is the most common cause of inherited mental retardation. The XL inheritance pattern is atypical. A female fragile X carrier may be unaffected or she may have symptoms, including mental retardation. Her daughters and sons are at risk of inheriting the gene. A transmitting male carries the fragile X gene but does not express symptoms and is able to pass on the gene.

Nonclassic Patterns

Some genetic disorders have heterogeneous inheritance patterns. Retinitis pigmentosa is a common cause of visual impairment. Charcot-Marie-Tooth disease is a relatively common polyneuropathy syndrome. Ehlers-Danlos syndrome causes increased tissue elasticity and fragility because of an underlying defect of collagen structure. Each of these conditions occurs in AD, AR, and XL forms.

Mitochondria possess unique, maternally inherited DNA. The following disorders are encoded in the mitochondrial genome: Kearns-Sayre syndrome, Leber's hereditary optic atrophy, mitochondrial encephalomyopathy with lactic acidosis and stroke-like episodes, and myoclonus epilepsy with ragged red fibers.

In mosaicism, two genetically different cell lines, derived from a single zygote, are present. A phenotypically normal, germline-mosaic parent may produce more than one child with an AD disorder. The mutation occurs in some of the parent's germ cells; it may be passed on to any of the offspring.

The expression of a disease phenotype depends on whether the gene is inherited from the mother or the father. If the gene for myotonic dystrophy is maternally inherited, the child is at risk for a severe, early-onset form of the disease. The onset of symptoms of Huntington's disease is relatively early when the gene is paternally inherited.

In uniparental disomy, one parent contributes both members of a pair of chromosomes to a child. Uniparental disomy offers an explanation for cases in which a cystic fibrosis (CF) child is born to one CF carrier and one CF noncarrier.

Multifactorial conditions result from the interaction of maternally and paternally inherited genetic factors with environmental factors. Examples include anencephaly, spina bifida, cleft lip, cleft palate, club foot, and many congenital heart defects.

Somatic cell disorders, such as cancer, develop only in specific somatic cells. Mutations in the genes that control cellular growth lead to malignancy.

DIAGNOSIS

The Family Pedigree

Gathering accurate and thorough family history information is a fundamental component of the genetic evaluation. The pedigree is a diagram of the family history. Collection of the following data is suggested:

1. Any infertility or miscarriages (gestational age of)
2. Stillbirths or neonatal deaths (autopsy results)
3. Health status of family members: birth defects, mental retardation or learning disabilities, or chronic health problems
4. Familial traits (for example, if patient has short stature, ask about heights of family members)
5. For deceased family members: age at and cause of death
6. For family members with anomalies: age of onset, severity, and any pertinent history

Ethnic or religious background may affect the risk for a genetic disease (Table 33-1). Preconceptional genetic counseling alleviates much of the anxiety and time constraints imposed during pregnancy.

Physical Examination

Other medical specialists play a substantial role in the care of individuals with genetic disorders. An ophthalmologist and a cardiologist follow a patient with Marfan syndrome because of the risks of severe myopia, lens dislocation, valvular incompetence, and problems of the aorta. An individual undergoing presymptomatic testing for Huntington's disease must be provided with genetic counseling, as well as psychologic and neurologic evaluations.

Laboratory Assessment

Karyotype

A peripheral blood karyotype is recommended for an individual with multiple congenital anomalies, mental retardation of unknown etiology, or abnormal sexual development. Blood karyotypes should be offered to couples who have experienced three or more unexplained spontaneous abortions. In approximately 6% of these couples, one partner carries a chromosomal rearrangement that increases the risk for chromosomally unbalanced gametes.

A karyotype may be prepared from cultured cells derived from several tissue sources, particularly when a blood sample is unobtainable. Chromosome abnormalities occur in 6% to 11% of stillborn babies and babies who die in the neonatal period. A karyotype should be obtained to help identify the cause and recurrence risk for the family. It is useful to examine tissue cultured from the products of conception or spontaneous abortions. A skin biopsy of an individual with suspected mosaicism should be studied.

A fluorescence in situ hybridization (FISH) analysis utilizes DNA probes that are hybridized to metaphase chromosomes spread on a slide; the hybridization signals are then visualized as bright spots under the microscope. FISH probes are used for rapid preliminary karyotyping and to determine the origin of unusual chromosomal variants in blood or tissue

TABLE 33-1
At-Risk Ethnic Groups

Population	Genetic disease	Population	Genetic disease
African Americans, Greeks, Asiatic Indians	Sickle cell disease	European and United States Caucasians	Cystic fibrosis
Ashkenazi Jews*, French Canadians	Tay-Sachs disease	French Canadians and Lebanese	Familial hypercholesterolemia
Ashkenazi Jews	Gaucher's disease	Scottish	Phenylketonuria (PKU)
Mediterraneans, Africans, Indians, Southern Chinese, Indonesians	Thalassemia	Irish, Welsh, and Northern Chinese	Neural tube defects (NTDs)
Danish	Alpha-1-antitrypsin deficiency	White South Africans	Porphyria

*Ashkenazi Jews are of Eastern European ancestry.

samples. FISH is useful in the identification of microdeletion syndromes (Angelman's, cri du chat, DiGeorge, Miller-Dieker, Prader-Willi, Smith-Magenis, velocardiofacial [Shprintzen's], Williams, and Wolf-Hirschhorn) and cancer cell rearrangements.

Carrier screening tests

Many carrier screens become obsolete as DNA analysis becomes available for more genetic disorders. Still informative are hemoglobin electrophoresis for sickle cell disease, hemoglobin SC disease, and thalassemias; hexosaminidase A activity for Tay-Sachs disease; CBC for thalassemias; and Pi typing for alpha$_1$-antitrypsin deficiency. In addition, measurement of factor VIII levels for hemophilia A, factor IX levels for hemophilia B, and serum creatine kinase levels for Duchenne muscular dystrophy is currently performed.

DNA analysis

DNA analysis is currently available to establish carrier status and/or to rule out certain genetic diseases. If the location of the mutation is known, a direct gene test may be available. DNA from potentially affected or carrier individuals is examined to identify or rule out a specific mutation. For some diseases, the results of DNA analysis alter an individual's risk but do not rule out the risk. One example is cystic fibrosis, for which over 300 mutations have been identified.

If the exact location of a gene has not been identified, a DNA linkage analysis may be available. The DNA of various family members is examined for specific markers. A family is referred to as *informative* when the affected and unaffected individuals can be distinguished using markers. Some families, though, are unfortunately found to be *uninformative.* The current testing protocol for a particular disease may be obtained via a genetic center.

TREATMENT

Surgery provides treatment in some cases for multifactorial conditions such as open spina bifida and cleft lip and palate. Treatment for single-gene disorders may be successful when the basic biochemical defect is known. A patient with PKU can escape the risk for severe mental retardation if dietary phenylalanine is avoided. Galactosemia can be treated by dietary limitation of galactose to avoid the risk for mental retardation and liver failure. Another treatment strategy is the replacement of an essential factor that is deficient because of a genetic disease. Thyroid hormone replacement prevents the mental retardation associated with congenital hypothyroidism. An effective treatment for individuals with hemophilia A involves the infusion of plasma fractions enriched with factor VIII. Transplantation represents still another treatment strategy. Examples are bone marrow transplantation for β-thalassemia and liver transplantation for alpha$_1$-antitrypsin deficiency.

Unfortunately, the basic defect is currently unknown for the majority of single-gene diseases. The number of known biochemical defects will increase dramatically with anticipated technologic advances. One newer treatment strategy is gene transfer therapy.

KEY POINTS

1 Cytogenetic records are essential in ruling out a familial versus a nonfamilial chromosome abnormality. A FISH analysis offers rapid results in some cases, but confirmation by conventional chromosome analysis may be necessary.

2 Single-gene disorders are catalogued into autosomal dominant, autosomal recessive, and X-linked inheritance patterns. Some diseases, however, exhibit different forms that follow different patterns of inheritance.

3 Mitochondrial inheritance, mosaicism, imprinting, and uniparental disomy are nonclassic patterns of inheritance.

4 Certain ethnic groups have an increased incidence of specific genetic diseases.

5 DNA analysis and carrier screening are available for some genetic diseases.

SUGGESTED READINGS

Emery AEH, Rimoin DL, eds: *Principles and practice of medical genetics,* vol 1 & 2, ed 2, Edinburgh, 1990, Churchill Livingstone.

Gelehrter TD, Collins FS: *Principles of medical genetics,* Baltimore, 1990, Williams & Wilkins.

Jones KL: *Smith's recognizable patterns of human malformations,* ed 4, Philadelphia, 1988, WB Saunders.

Milunsky A, ed: *Genetic disorders and the fetus: diagnosis, prevention, and treatment,* ed 3, Baltimore, 1992, Johns Hopkins University Press.

34

Ultrasound

Normal

JEFFREY G. BOYLE AND PAMELA M. FOY

Obstetric ultrasound has become an important part of prenatal care for diagnosis, therapy, and fetal surveillance. Performed early in pregnancy, an ultrasound examination can accurately establish or confirm a patient's EDC. In addition, physicians can rely on ultrasound to follow fetal growth serially, to assess fetal well-being, and to detect anomalies. Ultrasonography has also made diagnostic and therapeutic procedures such as amniocentesis, chorionic villus sampling, percutaneous umbilical blood sampling (PUBS), and fetal therapy safer and easier to perform.

Ultrasonography employs high-frequency sound waves in the range of 2 to 10 megahertz (MHz). Higher frequency sound waves improve image resolution but have reduced penetration. The most commonly used transducers are curvilinear and 3.5 to 5 MHz. Various crystals in the transducer produce ultrasound energy and also receive the reflected signals. A real-time ultrasound image is produced by mapping out reflections from internal organs, vessels, bones, and soft tissue. Doppler and color flow technologies have added to the diagnostic capabilities of real-time ultrasound.

The indications for obstetric ultrasonography have been debated. In addition to establishing an accurate EDC, other advantages of an ultrasound examination include the detection of fetal anomalies, multiple gestations, growth abnormalities, abnormalities in amniotic fluid volume, and placental location. Yet some research suggests that ultrasound should be performed only for specific indications because of the costs involved, potential risks, differences in level of training among physicians and sonographers, and lack of evidence to indicate an improvement in perinatal outcome (Box 34-1). The three types of obstetric ultrasound are basic, limited, and comprehensive. A basic examination is adequate for most pregnancies to establish or confirm due dates and to provide a general anatomic fetal survey. A limited examination is used to obtain specific information either in an emergency situation or to assess fetal surveillance. A comprehensive examination is used to diagnose fetal anomalies

BOX 34-1

Indications for an Obstetric Ultrasound Examination

Unknown or uncertain clinical dates
Confirmation of dates for scheduled repeat cesarean or induction of labor
Fetal growth assessment for acute and chronic maternal medical diseases
Late initial visit
Uterine size or dates discrepancy
Vaginal bleeding
Uncertain fetal presentation
Suspected multiple gestation
Pelvic or adnexal mass suspected on clinical exam
Suspected abnormalities in amniotic fluid volume
Biophysical evaluation
Fetal weight and presentation in cases of preterm labor or premature rupture of membranes
Fetal growth assessment for multiple gestation
Abnormal prenatal diagnostic screening test
History of maternal congenital anomaly
Advanced maternal age
External version and breech extraction

and should be performed by a sonographer or physician with advanced training.

The safety of obstetric ultrasound has been an important issue regarding the frequency of serial and prolonged examinations. Studies performed with long-term follow-up have found no biologic, developmental, neurologic, or psychologic effects on fetuses exposed in utero to diagnostic ultrasound.

THE FIRST TRIMESTER

The introduction of vaginal probe technology 10 years ago permits visualization of the embryo or fetus and surrounding structures with unsurpassed detail. This technique is widely accepted by women and is more desirable than the transabdominal approach because the maternal bladder need not be full for the examination. Evaluation of the adnexa and uterus is easiest at this point in gestation, and much information can be obtained about uterine anomalies that can be difficult to visualize with sonography during the second and third trimesters. Ovarian masses may also be readily evaluated, since frequently they still present in the true pelvis.

Although diagnostic ultrasound is not performed on all pregnant women, much clinical information can be obtained from a first-trimester scan. Specifically, transvaginal sonography (TVS) can confirm or establish dates, determine the location of a pregnancy (intrauterine or extrauterine), detect embryonic or fetal life, and establish a cause for bleeding (20% to 50% of women may experience bleeding in the first few weeks of pregnancy). TVS performed at 10 to 12 weeks gestation detects certain anomalies such as cystic hygroma, anencephaly, and generalized edema, which previously could only be visualized during the second trimester. With closer proximity to the uterus, TVS affords an exquisite view of the gestational sac, yolk sac, and embryo or fetus, which is not consistently appreciated with the transabdominal approach to scanning.

Gestational Sac

The gestational sac is the first definitive sign of early pregnancy and represents the chorionic cavity. With the TVS approach, the gestational sac can be visualized at 4.5 menstrual weeks and is consistently seen by 5 menstrual weeks when it should measure 5 mm in diameter. Once visualized, growth is constant, with a rate of 1 to 2 mm/day during early pregnancy. Normal features of the gestational sac include location near the fundus eccentrically positioned relative to the endometrial stripe, round or oval with a smooth contour, and initially surrounded by an echogenic ring that represents the trophoblasts and the decidual reaction.

Yolk Sac

The secondary yolk sac is the earliest embryonic landmark recognized within the gestational sac at the beginning of the fifth menstrual week. As the amniotic cavity increases in size to surround the embryo, the yolk sac is situated between the amnion and the chorion. Sonographically, the yolk sac will be visualized as a rounded hypoechoic structure with an echogenic ring, measuring between 3 and 4 mm in size. In general, a yolk sac can be demonstrated within the gestational sac by TVS when the sac is approximately 10 mm in size.

Fetal Cardiac Activity

By 6 weeks gestational age, the fetal heart rate is identifiable with TVS. Although cardiac rate varies with gestational age, the mean cardiac rate increases from 128 bpm at 6.4 weeks to a peak of 174 bpm at 9 weeks. The cardiac rate subsequently declines to 161 bpm at 11 weeks and 147 bpm at 14 weeks. Slow heart rates (<90 bpm) carry a poor prognosis. The likelihood of death is high when the heart rate is between 80 to 90 bpm and almost certain when the rate is below 80 bpm. Clinically, this information is helpful for patient counseling and follow-up. If a sonogram demonstrates a heart rate <90 bpm, the woman can be informed of the prognosis and a follow-up scan may be performed in 1 to 2 weeks. Although the repeat ultrasound examination will not affect the outcome of the pregnancy, the patient may benefit by a more timely diagnosis of intrauterine death.

Crown-Rump Length

The crown-rump length (CRL) is generally considered the most accurate sonographic measurement for determining gestational age during the first trimester. This measurement can have a range of error of 3 days. Previously, with the transabdominal approach, measurement errors were more commonly seen. CRL measurement could be underestimated if the embryo or fetus is not measured in full extension, or overestimated if extremities or yolk sac are included. Improved visualization with TVS reduces these measurement errors.

SECOND AND THIRD TRIMESTERS

A detailed evaluation of fetal anatomy can be adequately performed at 18 to 20 weeks gestation when parameters for fetal growth can be accurately assessed and fetal organs are of sufficient size to visualize both major and a variety of minor defects. In addition, appropriate diagnostic and therapeutic measures can be taken including termination, additional testing, or fetal therapy as necessary. Some abnormalities may not be visualized until after 24 weeks. This must be considered in determining the timing of the initial study, the indications for the exam, and the need for repeat testing. After a comprehensive ultrasound examination has been performed, repeat studies to verify the initial findings are not justified except for specific clinical indications.

Most normative data used for comparing growth parameters were obtained from clinically dated pregnancies in different populations. Variations in measurements can be accounted for by ultrasound technique, maternal race, altitude, and equipment. Physicians should become familiar with reference tables and their appropriate application to various patient populations. The ultrasound study should be used to assist in clinical management, not to direct it. In addition, a due date should be changed only if the ultrasound estimated date is outside the range of error for the gestational age in which the dating scan is being performed. To ensure accuracy, multiple measurements of each parameter should be obtained and compared.

A systematic method for performing an ultrasound examination is recommended so that important growth parameters and organ systems are not omitted. The following guidelines for fetal anatomy evaluation are recommended:

1. Fetal cardiac activity. Record the fetal heart rate and rhythm.
2. Fetal presentation.
3. Placental location. Record the proximity of the placenta to the cervix.
4. Amniotic fluid volume. This can be reported subjectively or quantitatively with an amniotic fluid index.
5. Confirm number of fetuses. Describe placentation including chorionicity in multiple gestations.
6. Evaluation of uterus and adnexa. Look for adnexal masses and müllerian defects.
7. Estimate of gestational age. Use a combination of BPD, HC, FL, and AC* to determine gestational age. Compare measurements and estimated fetal weight from previous exams to determine trends in fetal growth and accuracy of gestational age. Additional measurements including humerus length (HL), outer orbital diameter (OOD), and transcerebellar diameter (TCD) can be helpful.
8. Evaluation of fetal anatomy. This should include the following:

Head

1. Head shape. Look for oval shape in contrast to "lemon"-shaped skull, dolichocephalic, or brachycephalic.
2. Biparietal diameter (BPD) (Fig. 34-1, *A*). This measurement is the largest transverse diameter of the fetal cranium, taken at the level of the thalami, cavum septum pelucidum, and frontal and posterior horns of the lateral ventricles. Measure from the outer skull of one side to the inner skull of the other. Most reference tables are based on outer skull to inner skull measurements by convention. Look for symmetry of parietal bones and oval head shape. In cases of dolichocephaly or brachycephaly, the BPD measurement may be inaccurate. The cephalic index (BPD/OFD) should be .75 to .85 for BPD to be valid. If it is less than .75, the HC measurement should be used.
3. Occipitofrontal diameter (OFD). Taken at the same level as the BPD from leading edge to leading edge of the skull.
4. Head circumference (HC). Circumference measurement including soft tissue obtained at the same level as the BPD.
5. Posterior cerebral ventricle diameters. These measurements are obtained from a transverse axial plane by locating the choroid plexus. The width of the anterior and posterior horns of the lateral ventricles is measured perpendicular to the ventricle axis, not the head axis.

**BPD*, Biparietal diameter; *HC*, head circumference, *FL*, femur length; *AC*, abdominal circumference.

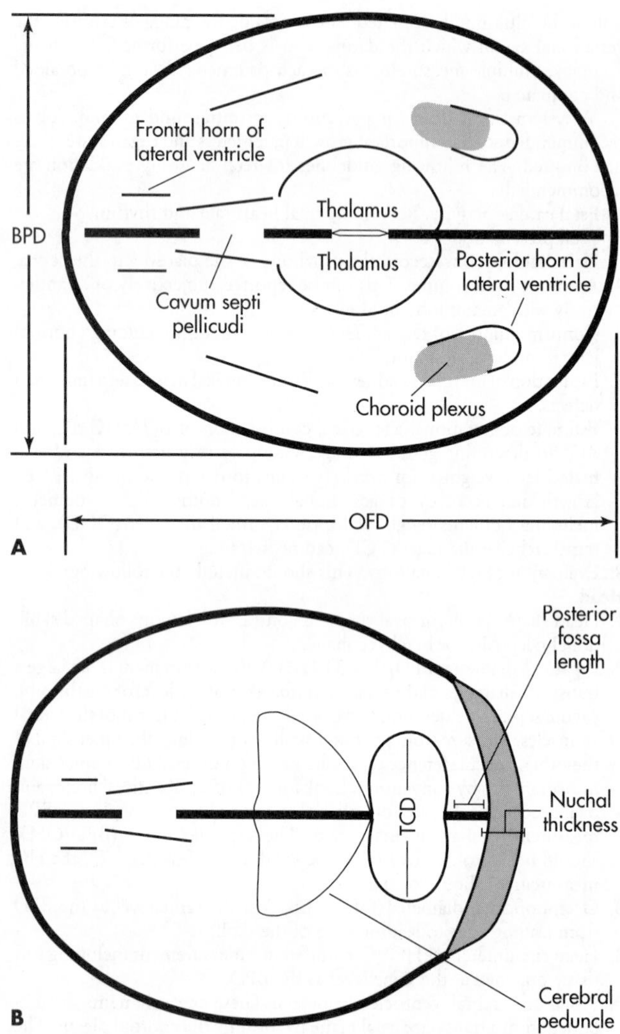

FIG. 34-1 A, BPD and occipitofrontal diameter *(OFD)* are measured from the leading edge to the leading edge of the cranial vault, excluding the soft tissue of the scalp. The head circumference measurement is at the same level as the BPD, but includes the soft tissue of the scalp. **B,** The cerebellum and cisterna magna. The transcerebellar diameter (TCD) can be used to estimate gestational age.

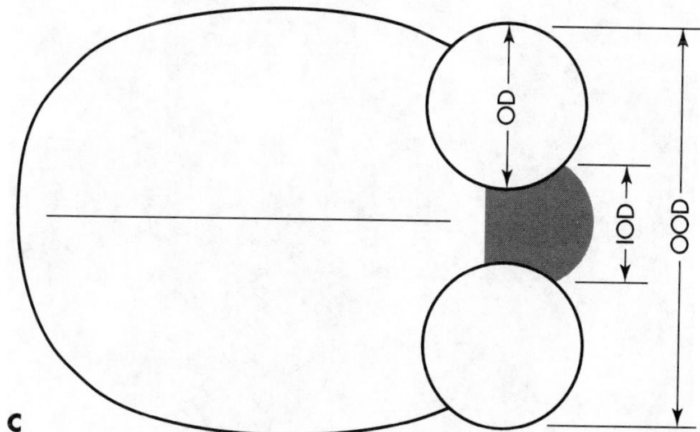

FIG. 34-1, cont'd C, Orbital diameters can be used to calculate gestational age. *OOD,* Outer orbital diameter; *IOD,* interorbital diameter, *OD,* ocular diameter.

6. Transcerebellar diameter (TCD) (Fig. 34-1, *B*). To obtain this measurement, the transducer should be rotated slightly caudad from the BPD plane at the level of the thalami. The TCD should be measured at the level of the cavum septum pellucidum, cerebral peduncles, and cerebellar hemispheres. The measurement is taken from outer hemisphere to outer hemisphere.
7. Posterior fossa. Measurement is made posterior to cerebellum to inner cranial vault. Referred to as *cisterna magna.*
8. Face. Evaluate upper and lower lips, palate, and profile.
9. Outer orbital diameter (OOD) (Fig. 34-1,*C*).

Extremities

1. Humerus length (HL). Measure end to end.
2. Hands. Locate hands and visualize digits if possible.
3. Femur length (FL) (Fig. 34-2, *A*). Longest metaphysis length, measured end to end.
4. Feet. Identify both feet and measure heel to longest toe. Compare foot length to femur length in evaluation of skeletal dysplasia.

Thorax

1. Cardiac evaluation includes four chamber view (Fig. 34-2, *B*), aortic outflow, pulmonary outflow, ventricular and atrial symmetry, ventricular and atrial septa, and visualization of AV valves.
2. Lungs. Look for symmetry, echogenicity, and extrathoracic compression.

Abdomen

1. Abdominal circumference (AC) (Figure 34-2, *C*). Measurement of the AC is obtained in the plane perpendicular to the fetal spine or abdominal aorta at the level of the liver, stomach, and umbilical vein.

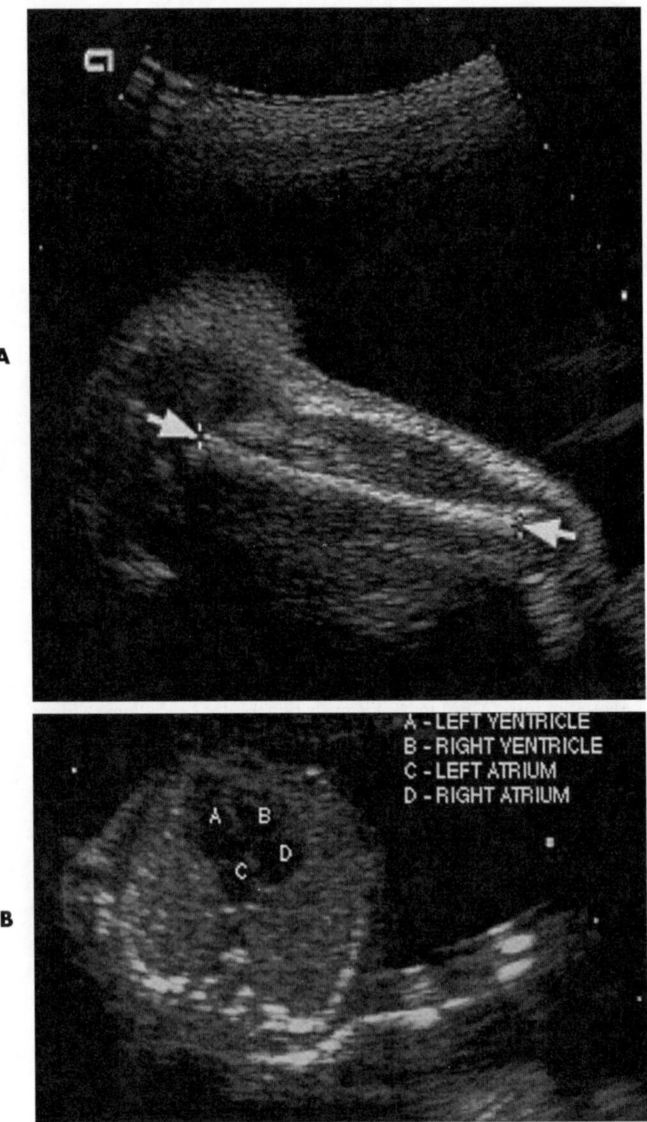

FIG. 34-2 A, Measurement of the femur including only the ossified diaphysis. **B,** Four-chamber heart. Sonogram through the thorax demonstrates the normal cardiac axis and position as well as the four cardiac chambers.

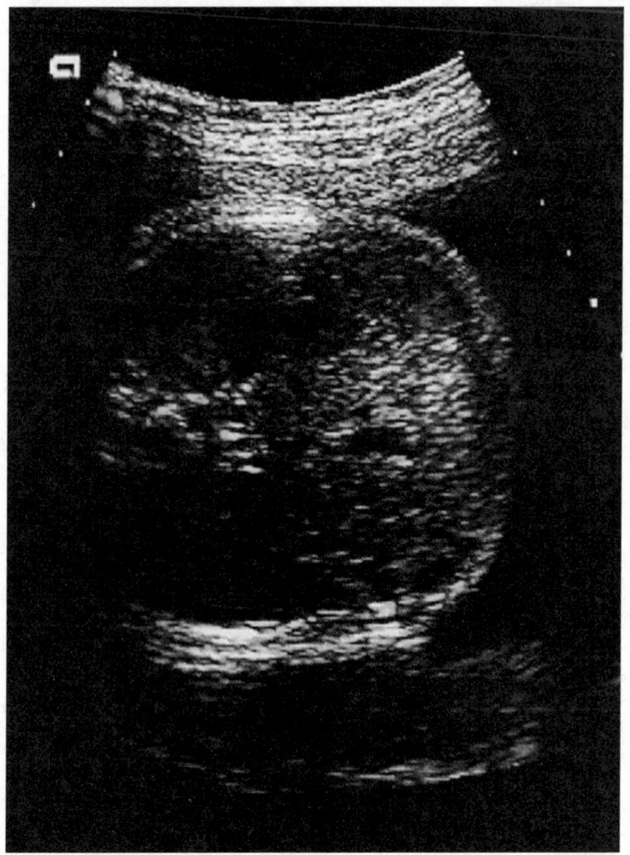

C

FIG. 34-2, cont'd **C,** Transverse scan of the fetal abdomen illustrates the standard plane of measurement for the abdominal circumference; the fetal stomach, liver, and ascending left portal vein are seen on the plane section.

2. Size and location of stomach.
3. Umbilical cord insertion. Should be identified in the midabdomen.
4. Size and echogenicity of large and small bowel.
5. Presence, size, and echogenicity of the kidneys.

Pelvis

1. Bladder. Record presence and size.
2. Genitals.

Umbilical cord

1. Vessels. Identify three-vessel cord (two arteries and one vein).

Placenta

1. Location. Determine anterior, posterior, fundal, or previa. Avoid references to "placenta previa" in first and second trimesters.
2. Thickness and cord insertion.

THE BIOPHYSICAL PROFILE

During the third trimester of pregnancy, real-time sonography can provide information about parameters that reflect fetal well-being. Fetal assessment by the biophysical profile (BPP) should be performed on women with recognized fetal or maternal high-risk factors. Hypoxemia or CNS asphyxia may produce alterations in the frequency and patterns of fetal biophysical activities. The incorporation of several variables to predict fetal biophysical states may be evaluated by dynamic real-time sonography. The variables are assessed and then coded numerically as normal or abnormal according to fixed criteria (Table 34-1). The fetus should be evaluated with sonography at least 30 minutes, as fetal sleep states change over a 20- to 40-minute period.

Clinical Interpretation

The clinical management of a patient having had a BPP is based on the test score and the obstetric factors affecting the pregnancy. (Table 34-2). The BPP provides an estimate of the risk of fetal death. Testing may be weekly or twice weekly in high-risk groups such as postdates patients and diabetic and alloimmunized women. Severe cases may require daily testing of the BPP. If the risk is low, as with a normal test score, intervention should be for obstetric and maternal factors only. If the risk is high with an abnormal score (6 or less) or oligohydramnios, labor should be induced.

DOPPLER ULTRASOUND

Once considered investigational in obstetrics, Doppler is now an important component of the ultrasound examination when assessing fetal well-being. The Doppler principle is used to measure the velocity of blood flow in vessels. The peak velocity, as well as the shape of the spectral waveform, can be analyzed to yield information about blood flow and resistance in a given vessel.

There are two types of spectral Doppler probes, continuous-wave (CW) and pulsed-wave with real-time imaging (duplex). More commonly used in obstetrics are pulsed Doppler systems. With pulsed Doppler, a short burst of sound energy is used rather than a continuous wave; however, the basic principles of Doppler still apply. This duplex system is capable of providing simultaneous Doppler and real-time imaging from a single probe. The depth of Doppler detection is determined by a gate that is superimposed with a cursor over the real-time image and positioned by the operator. Now, many fetal vessels may be examined under direct ultrasound visualization with Doppler that were not visible with a CW probe.

TABLE 34-1
Fetal Biophysical Profile Score

Variable	Normal (Score = 2)	Abnormal (Score = 0)
Fetal breathing movements (FBM)	The presence of at least 30 sec of sustained FBM in 30 min of observation	Less than 30 sec of FBM in 30 min
Gross body movements	Three or more gross body movements in 30 min of observation; simultaneous limb and trunk movements are counted as a single movement	Two or less gross body movements in 30 min of observation
Fetal tone	At least one episode of motion of a limb from a position of flexion to extension and a rapid return to flexion	Fetus in a position of semi- or full-limb extension with no return to flexion with movement; absence of fetal movement is counted as absent tone
Fetal heart rate (FHR)	The presence of two or more fetal heart-rate accelerations of at least 15 beats/min that last at least 15 sec and are associated with fetal movement in 30 min	No acceleration or less than two accelerations of the fetal heart rate in 30 min of observation
Amniotic fluid volume (AFV)	A pocket of amniotic fluid that measures at least 2 cm in two perpendicular planes	Largest pocket of amniotic fluid measures <2 cm in two perpendicular planes
Maximal score	10	
Minimal score		0

Modified from Manning F et al: *Am J Obstet Gynecol* 140:289, 1981.

Although flow volume in large vessels may be calculated, this is difficult in obstetrics because the uterine vessels and umbilical arteries are coiled (Fig. 34-3). Angle-independent indices using ratios of peak systolic to end diastolic frequencies can be used as indicators of resistance to flow (Fig. 34-4). Usually, reduction in end diastolic flow indicates increased resistance downstream.

By far, most clinical evaluations have been carried out on the umbilical artery. This Doppler examination provides information on the placental

TABLE 34-2
Biophysical Profile Scoring: Management Protocol

BPS score	Interpretation	Recommended management
10	Normal nonasphyxiated	No fetal indication for intervention; repeat test weekly except in diabetic patient and postdate pregnancy (twice weekly)
8/10 normal fluid 8/8	Normal nonasphyxiated	No fetal indication for intervention; repeat testing as per protocol
8/10 decreased fluid	Chronic fetal asphyxia suspected	Deliver
6	Possible fetal asphyxia	Deliver if AFV is abnormal or if normal fluid at >36 wk with favorable cervix; if gestation is <36 wk or L/S <2/1 or cervix unfavorable, repeat test in 24 hr; if repeat test score is ≤6, deliver; if repeat test score is >6, observe and repeat per protocol
4	Probable fetal asphyxia	Repeat testing same day; if BPS is ≤6, deliver
0-2	Almost certain fetal asphyxia	Deliver

From Manning FA et al: *Am J Obstet Gynecol* 157: 881, 1987.
BPS, Biophysical profile scoring; *AFV,* amniotic fluid volume; *L/S,* lecithin/sphingomyelin ratio.

circulation and placental resistance. Normal umbilical artery values, obtained from the angle-independent ratios, vary with gestational age with increasing end diastolic flow in the third trimester (measurements charts are available). The two most common pregnancy complications, which may have abnormal umbilical artery flow velocity waveforms, include intrauterine growth restriction (IUGR) and maternal hypertension. Diabetes mellitus, systemic lupus erythematosus, twin gestation, and fetuses with anomalies may also exhibit an abnormal umbilical artery flow velocity waveform with Doppler. Typically, the abnormal umbilical artery wave-

A

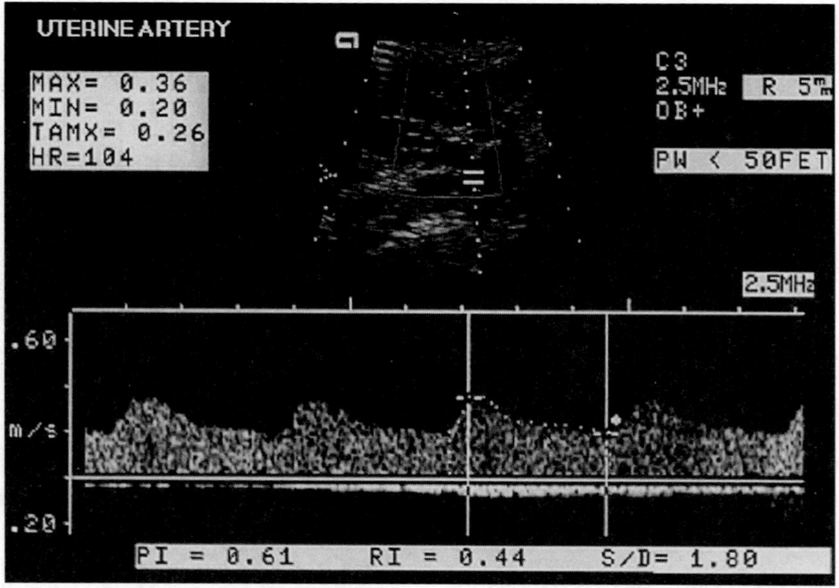

FIG. 34-3 A, Normal pulsed-Doppler waveform of a maternal left uterine artery.

Continued

B

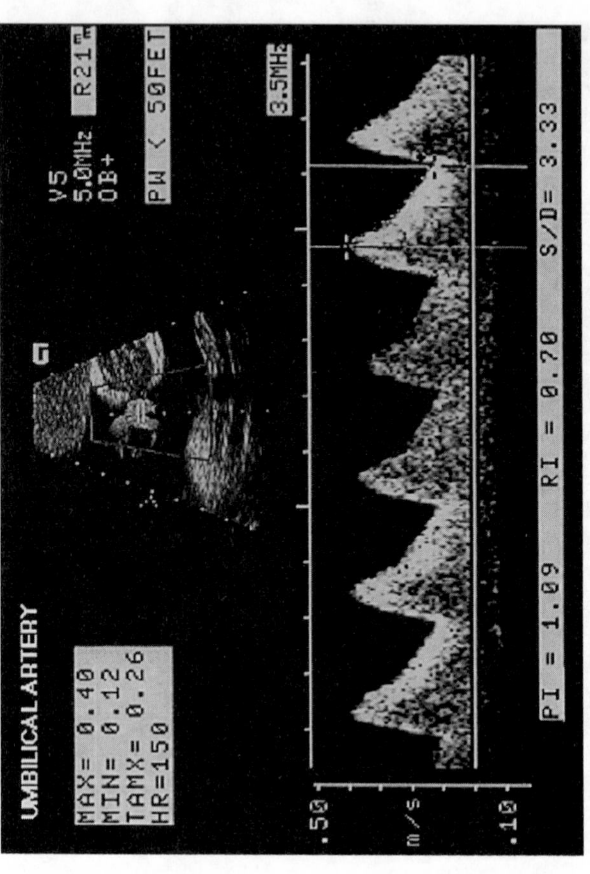

FIG. 34-3, cont'd B, Pulsed Doppler waveform of an umbilical artery reveals a normal systolic to diastolic ratio of approximately 3.33 at 34 weeks gestation.

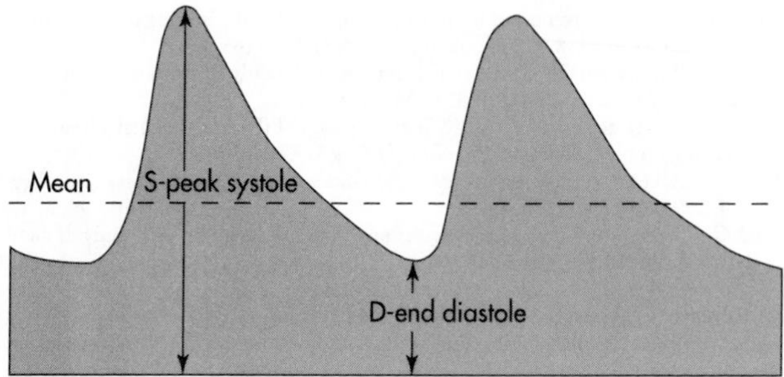

FIG. 34-4 Angle-independent indices. Increases in these ratios above normal ranges suggest increased downstream resistance: S/D ratio, systole/diastole; resistance index (RI), systole-diastole/systole; pulsatility index (PI), systole-diastole/mean.

form will exhibit decreased diastolic flow or in some extreme cases absent end diastolic flow.

Maternal volume studies at present have an uncertain clinical role. However, in cases of severe IUGR and maternal hypertension uterine flow velocity waveforms will demonstrate a high systolic to diastolic ratio, with a notch frequently seen in early diastole after 27 weeks gestation.

KEY POINTS

1. With a transvaginal ultrasound, the gestational sac can be visualized at 4.5 menstrual weeks.
2. By 6 weeks gestation, the fetal heart rate is identifiable with transvaginal sonography.
3. The optimum time for a comprehensive ultrasound examination is 18 to 20 weeks gestation.
4. The range of error for assessing fetal age changes with advancing gestation.
5. The physician or sonographer performing diagnostic ultrasound examinations should have appropriate training in the detection of fetal abnormalities.

SUGGESTED READINGS

ACOG: *Ultrasonography in pregnancy,* ACOG Technical Bulletin, Publication No. 187, Washington DC, 1993, ACOG.

AIUM: Guidelines for performance of the antepartum obstetrical ultrasound examination guidelines, *J Ultrasound Med* 10:576, 1991.

Bonilla-Musoles FM et al: Early detection of embryonic malformations by transvaginal and color Doppler sonography, *J Ultrasound Med* 13:347-355, 1994.

Chitty LS et al: Effectiveness of routine ultrasonography in detecting fetal structural abnormalities in a low risk population, *Br Med J* 303:1165, 1992.
Doubilet PM, Benson CB: Embryonic heart rate in the early first trimester: what rate is normal? *J Ultrasound Med* 14:431-434, 1995.
Ewigman BG et al and the RADIUS study group: Effect of prenatal ultrasound screening on perinatal outcome, *N Engl J Med* 329:821, 1993.
Fleischer AC et al: *The principles and practice of ultrasonography in obstetrics and gynecology,* ed 4, 1991, Appleton & Lange.
Luck C: Value of routine ultrasound scanning at 19 weeks: a four year study of 8849 deliveries, *Br Med J* 304:1474, 1992.
Maslak SH, Fruend JG: *Color Doppler instrumentation: vascular imaging by color Doppler and magnetic resonance,* 1991, Springer-Verlag.
Newnham JP et al: Effects of frequent ultrasound during pregnancy: a randomized controlled trial, *Lancet* 342:887, 1993.
Nicolaides K et al: Ultrasonographically detectable markers of fetal chromosome defects, *Ultrasound Obstet Gynecol* 3:56, 1993.
Nyberg DA et al, eds: *Transvaginal ultrasound,* St. Louis, 1992, Mosby.
Pretorius DH, Mahony BS: The role of obstetrical ultrasonography. In Nyberg DA, Mahony BS, Pretorius DH: *Diagnostic ultrasound of fetal anomalies: text and atlas,* St. Louis, 1990, Mosby.
Shirley IM, Bottomley F, Robinson VP: Routine radiographer screening for fetal abnormalities by ultrasound in an unselected low risk population, *Br J Radiol* 65:564, 1992.

Abnormal

Pamela M. Foy and Steven G. Gabbe

Diagnostic ultrasound in the past 10 years has virtually given the obstetrician a view inside the fetus as well as its surrounding environment. With a thorough knowledge of normal anatomy, physiology, and pathology, imagers can now detect a multitude of major anomalies as well as many minor anomalies. Previously, these anomalies were recognized only at the time of delivery. The antenatal sonographic detection of anomalies permits the opportunity to counsel patients, change the management of the pregnancy or delivery, and optimize the care of the newborn.

AMNIOTIC FLUID

Amniotic fluid is a major component of the intrauterine environment. This fluid normally increases in volume until the middle of the third trimester and then declines. Maintaining a normal amount of amniotic fluid is a dynamic process that reflects a balance between production (fetal urination) and consumption (fetal swallowing and GI absorption).

Polyhydramnios or excessive fluid may be associated with congenital anomalies, maternal causes such as diabetes mellitus, or it may be idiopathic. NTDs, obstruction of the fetal GI tract, multiple gestations, and fetal hydrops are also associated with increased fluid. Oligohydramnios, a reduction in amniotic fluid volume, may be associated with premature rupture of the membranes, intrauterine growth restriction, and/or postmaturity. Genitourinary anomalies involving decreased urine production include bilateral renal agenesis, infantile polycystic kidney disease, distal urinary tract obstruction, and bilateral multicystic dysplastic kidneys.

Sonographic attempts to measure amniotic fluid volume use either subjective or semiquanitative techniques. The subjective assessment, using the operator's own visual criteria, is quick and efficient for the experienced. Visually, oligohydramnios will present as fetal crowding with a lack of fluid. With polyhydramnios, the fetal abdomen will be completely surrounded with amniotic fluid (normally, the abdomen will be in contact with the anterior and posterior wall of the uterus). The semiquanitative assessment measures one or more pockets of amniotic fluid. With the single deepest pocket assessment, a vertical measurement is made of the biggest pocket. A measurement of less than 1 to 2 cm is representative of oligohydramnios, whereas a measurement of greater than 8 cm reflects polyhydramnios. Phelan's four quadrant method, the amniotic fluid index (AFI), divides the uterus into four quadrants by sagittal and transverse lines at the level of the umbilicus. A vertical measurement of the largest pocket in each quadrant is made. The total of each of these measurements is used to obtain the AFI in cm. An AFI of less than 5 cm is considered to represent oligohydramnios and an AFI of greater than 18 to 20 cm indicates polyhydramnios. Clinically, the subjective assessment is initially applied to verify that the amniotic fluid volume is normal, and the AFI is used when the subjective assessment indicates an abnormal fluid volume. The AFI can be followed with serial examinations. After 35 weeks gestation, an AFI may be warranted to accurately assess amniotic fluid volume.

CENTRAL NERVOUS SYSTEM

CNS anomalies are frequently encountered and in most instances are easily detected with sonography. Some of the more common yet most devastating of congenital anomalies are cerebral malformations. The vast majority of major cerebral anomalies may be detected with prenatal sonography. Diagnostic ultrasound is quite useful in evaluating intracranial anatomy during the second and third trimesters of pregnancy. The ventricular system, a major cerebral landmark, is used to define the normal position and normal echo pattern of other intracranial structures.

Hydrocephalus or ventriculomegaly is easily detectable with sonography. Various nomograms exist for portions of the ventricular system. Measurement of the atria of the lateral ventricle is less than 10 mm from 16 weeks gestation to term (Fig. 34-5, *A*). Enlargement of the lateral ventricles and third ventricle with a normal posterior fossa is usually aqueductal stenosis or communicating hydrocephalus (Fig. 34-5, *B*). Ventriculomegaly is associated with other cerebral anomalies, most frequently NTDs. Thirty percent of all fetuses identified with ventriculomegaly have spina bifida. The Dandy-Walker malformation is characterized by a posterior fossa cyst that communicates with the fourth ventricle through a defect of the midline cerebellar vermis. Enlargement of the lateral ventricles with this condition is variable.

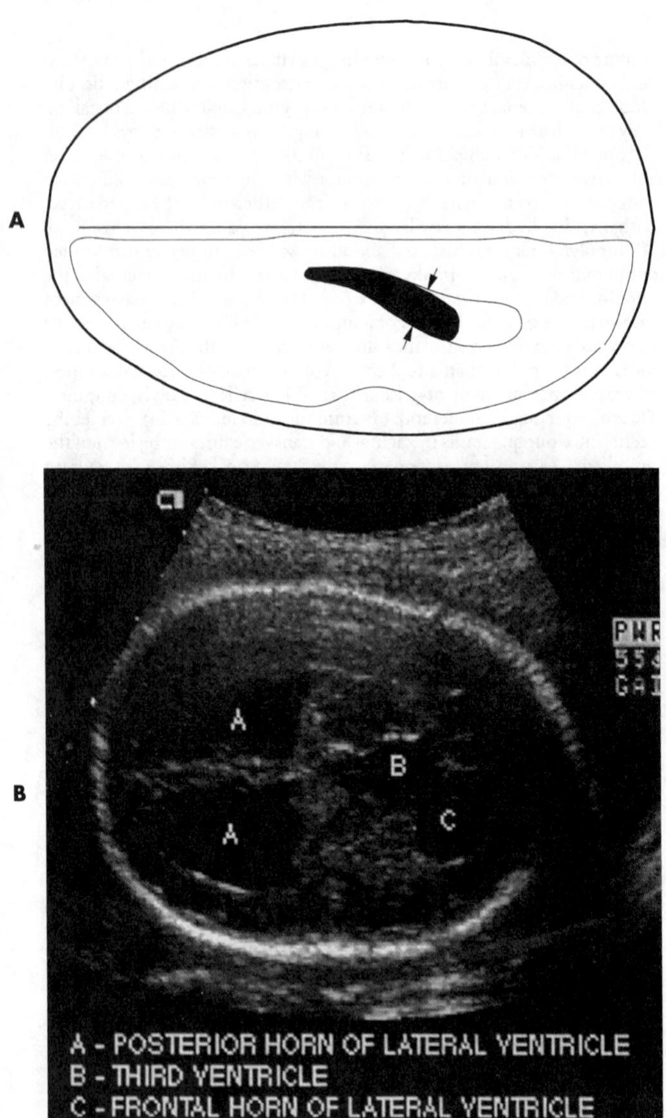

FIG. 34-5 A, Measurement of the transverse diameter of the posterior horn of the lateral ventricle. Normal measurement <10 mm. **B,** Dilated lateral ventricles and a third ventricle. This fetus also has a dilated fourth ventricle. This is an example of communicating hydrocephalus.

Anencephaly is the most common NTD, with an occurrence rate of 1/1000 live births. Risk factors may include family history and twins. An elevated MSAFP will be found with this malformation. Sonographically, the diagnosis can be made in the early second trimester and is highly reliable. By 12 weeks gestation, the cranial vault should be developed and sonographically is extremely echogenic. Anencephaly is characterized by absence of the cerebral hemispheres and cranium. When evaluating the fetal face, absence of the cranial vault cephalad to the orbits will be demonstrated (Fig. 34-6). Polyhydramnios is seen in approximately half of the cases, appearing to be related to menstrual age. Frequently, amniotic fluid volume is normal during the second trimester but increased during the third trimester. This malformation is uniformly fatal.

Spina bifida is a defect that can occur anywhere along the spine but most commonly involves the lumbosacral region. It is characterized by a defect of the soft tissues and vertebral arches. Detection rates for spina bifida vary. However, accuracy at referral centers where comprehensive ultrasound examinations are performed is close to 99%.

Sonographically, indirect cranial signs are evaluated before evaluation of the spine because spinal defects can be obscured when the spine

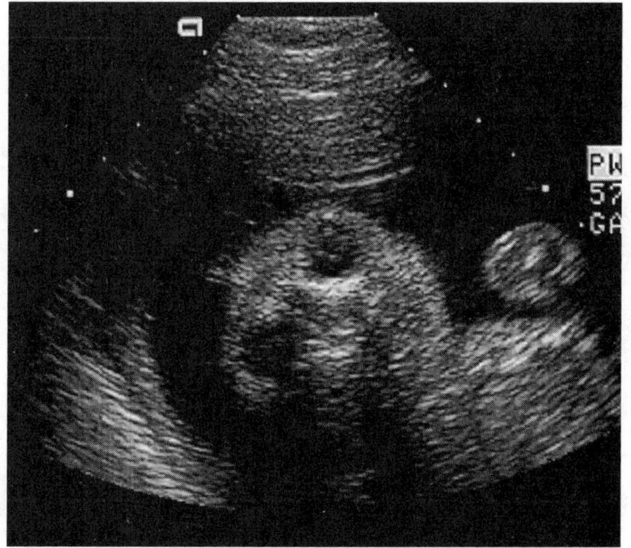

FIG. 34-6 Typical sonographic appearance of a coronal view of the fetal face of an anencephalic fetus. Notice the absence of the cranial vault superior to the orbits.

is adjacent to the uterine wall, the placenta, or when a patient is obese. The cranial findings associated with spina bifida include reduced BPD, ventriculomegaly, lemon sign, banana sign, and nonvisualization of the cisterna magna. Ventricular dilation is present in 75% of fetuses with spina bifida before 24 weeks gestation. The lemon sign, a concave deformity of the cranium at approximately the level of the coronal suture, is demonstrated in the majority of fetuses examined before 24 weeks gestation (Fig. 34-7, *A*). This cranial sign is less reliable after 24 weeks. The banana sign describes the shape of the cerebellar hemispheres as they wrap around the midbrain. They resemble a banana lying on its side. The cisterna magna should be visualized in virtually all fetuses during the second and early third trimester. Failure to visualize this cisterna suggests downward displacement of the cerebellum. The lemon sign in conjunction with ventricular dilation and/or a banana sign should be viewed as highly suspicious for spina bifida. When evaluating the spine, transverse views of the spine will define the defect of the vertebral arches, whereas sagittal views are most useful in assessing the extent of the lesion (Fig. 34-7, *B*).

The term *encephalocele* describes a cranial defect that involves herniation of the brain and meninges. Encephaloceles are frequently found midline at the level of the occipital bone but they may also arise from the frontal or parietal bones. Ventricular dilation is frequently found, and true encephaloceles with massive externalization of brain tissue may be associated with microcephaly. Many anomalies have been reported with this condition, including ventriculomegaly (65% of the time with occipital encephaloceles, 15% of the time with frontal encephaloceles), spina bifida (7% to 15% of fetuses), and, facial clefts (with frontal encephaloceles only). Encephaloceles are also associated with multiple anomaly syndromes including Meckel-Gruber syndrome. This autosomal recessive disorder is characterized by renal cystic dysplasia (100%) and therefore oligohydramnios, occipital encephalocele (80%), and polydactyly.

FETAL HEART

Congenital heart disease (CHD) is the most common congenital anomaly found among newborns, with an incidence estimated to be 8/1000 live births. The sonographic accuracy for detecting cardiac malformations during a screening obstetric ultrasound for routine clinical indications has been poor when compared with detection rates for other major anomalies. Factors affecting detection accuracy include experience of the operator, type of equipment used, and the gestational age of the fetus. Other technical factors include maternal body habitus, fetal position, and the amount of amniotic fluid present.

Correctly interpreted, a four-chamber view of the heart can rule out approximately 60% of cardiac defects. Once fetal position is determined, a transverse section of the thorax at the level of the four chambers should be obtained. The apex of the heart should point toward the left anterior chest wall, with the descending aorta visualized in cross section on the left, adjacent to the spine. The right ventricle, the most anterior chamber, is adjacent to the anterior chest wall. The two ventricles and the two atria are

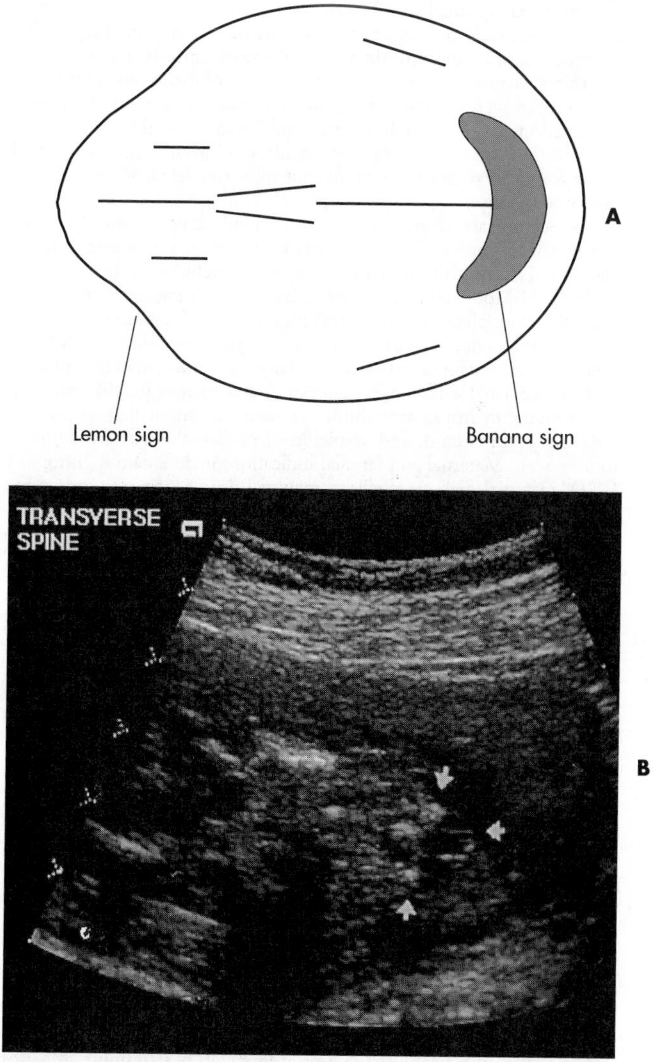

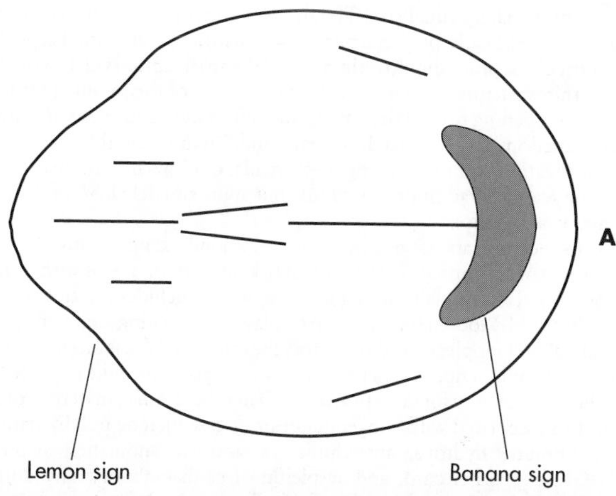

B

FIG. 34-7 A, The lemon sign (frontal indentation) and the banana sign (curvature of the cerebellum). **B,** A transverse view of the distal spine revealing a dysraphic defect. The distal posterior ossification centers are divergent (U sign). The meningomyelocele sac is also demonstrated.

of approximately equal size. The two well-moving atrioventricular valves are oriented nearly perpendicular to the ventricular and atrial septa. The ventricular septum should be intact, and the atrial septum will be visualized as a thin structure separating the atria. The flap of the foramen ovale will be seen opening toward the left atrium. Subjective assessment of ventricular function and normal heart rate and rhythm should be obtained. Visualization of the left and right ventricular outflows may be incorporated in the scan; this addition would rule out approximately 80% of the major cardiac anomalies.

In recent years, targeted cardiac ultrasound examinations have been considered appropriate for patients at risk for carrying a fetus with a cardiac anomaly. This specialized examination, which includes multiple views of the heart, M-Mode, a time-motion display for evaluating fetal arrhythmias, and pulsed Doppler recordings across the cardiac valves, is often performed by or in conjunction with a pediatric cardiologist. The indications for fetal echocardiography for detection of CHD may be familial, maternal, or fetal. Factors associated with congenital heart disease include polyhydramnios, nonimmune hydrops, arrhythmia, extracardiac anomalies, symmetric IUGR, two-vessel cord, and suspicion of cardiac abnormality during a routine scan. Maternal and familial indications include family history of CHD, maternal diabetes mellitus, maternal drug exposure during pregnancy (e.g., lithium or phenytoin), maternal infections, collagen vascular disease, and, maternal PKU.

Hypoplastic Left Heart

A mild form of hypoplastic left heart (HLH) syndrome may result from aortic and mitral stenosis. The most severe form reveals complete absence of the left heart, with atresia of the aortic and mitral valves and hypoplasia of the left ventricle and ascending aorta. This congenital anomaly should be easily detected on a four-chamber view of the fetal heart. Prognosis is always extremely poor, and management approaches vary.

Cardiac Arrhythmias

Using real-time sonography, pulsed Doppler techniques, and M-Mode, fetal cardiac imaging can be used to diagnose fetal cardiac arrhythmias. Irregular patterns of fetal heart rhythms will frequently be detected in the physician's office with a hand-held Doppler device. Brief periods of tachycardia, bradycardia, and ectopic beats are commonly seen. These intermittent rhythm disturbances are usually not of significant hemodynamic consequence and may account for 80% of all fetal arrhythmias detected by ultrasound. Weekly Doppler examinations will confirm that the rhythm disturbances remain intermittent. Sustained fetal arrhythmia is hemodynamically more troublesome. Sustained fetal tachycardia results in a fetal heart rate of at least 240 beats/minute. Most of these fetuses will have a structurally normal heart. Sustained fetal bradycardia is the most ominous of the fetal arrhythmias. The most common fetal bradycardia is complete heart block with heart rates of 60 beats per minute or less. One half to two thirds of fetuses with congenital heart block will have associated major structural CHD. The majority of these fetuses die.

ABDOMEN

The stomach, a left-sided organ, can be visualized sonographically as early as 12 weeks but should be seen consistently on all fetuses by 16 weeks gestation. Variations in stomach size are routine among fetuses and even within the same fetus during an examination. Nonvisualization of a stomach with normal amniotic fluid volume is probably transient and caused by the dynamic filling and emptying nature of the stomach. Nonvisualization of a fetal stomach, in its usual location and with polyhydramnios, can have many different etiologies, including esophageal atresia, diaphragmatic hernia, facial cleft, and, CNS disorder.

The small bowel is less commonly identified by ultrasound than the stomach. It can be seen centrally located in the abdomen and often will exhibit transient peristalsis. The large bowel appears sonographically as a hypoechoic tubular structure around the perimeter of the abdomen, and should be identified in all fetuses by 28 weeks gestation.

Duodenal atresia is the most common type of congenital small bowel obstruction (Fig. 34-8). The sonographic diagnosis is suggested by demonstration of polyhydramnios and a fluid-filled double bubble in the abdomen. The double bubble is a distended stomach within the left upper quadrant connecting with an enlarged duodenum located to the right of midline. Duodenal atresia is associated with other anomalies including CHD, esophageal atresia, imperforate anus, and renal and vertebral anomalies. In addition, approximately 25% to 30% of the fetuses will have trisomy 21.

The two main types of abdominal wall defects easily detected by sonography include omphalocele and gastroschisis. Both are associated with external herniation of the abdominal contents, but omphalocele is a midline defect, whereas gastroschisis is paraumbilical and usually to the right of midline.

Gastroschisis is usually an isolated condition that is rarely associated with other anomalies. The fetus has a normal abdominal cord insertion site with an abdominal wall defect to the right of the umbilicus. A variable amount of bowel can protrude through the defect and float in the surrounding amniotic fluid. Because the abdominal organs are in direct contact with the amniotic fluid, the MS-AFP level will be elevated. The sonographic diagnosis of this condition is highly reliable. Although small bowel is always eviscerated through the abdominal wall defect, it is often accompanied by large bowel. Linear measurements of a cross section of a small bowel can be obtained and should be less than 12 mm. Serial ultrasound examination should be performed to evaluate fetal growth and to detect possible bowel complications such as obstruction, atresia, and necrosis.

A

TRANSVERSE
PWR = 0dB
54dB 1/2/6
GAIN= -1dB
A - STOMACH
B - DUODENUM

B

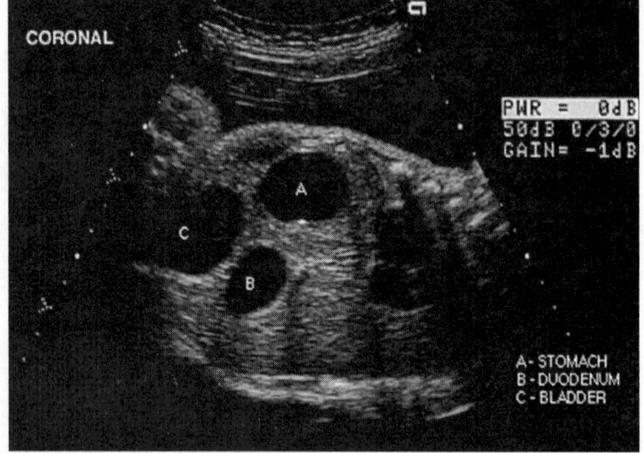

FIG. 34-8 Duodenal atresia. **A,** Transverse scan of the fetal abdomen revealing the fluid-filled stomach communicating with the duodenum. **B,** Coronal view of the same fetus demonstrates the fluid-filled stomach, duodenum, and bladder.

Omphalocele is a midline defect that results in herniation of the intraabdominal structures into the base of the umbilical cord. These abdominal structures are limited by a membrane and will not be seen freely floating as with gastroschisis. This membrane presents a limiting barrier to leaking of AFP into the amniotic fluid, so that MS-AFP levels associated

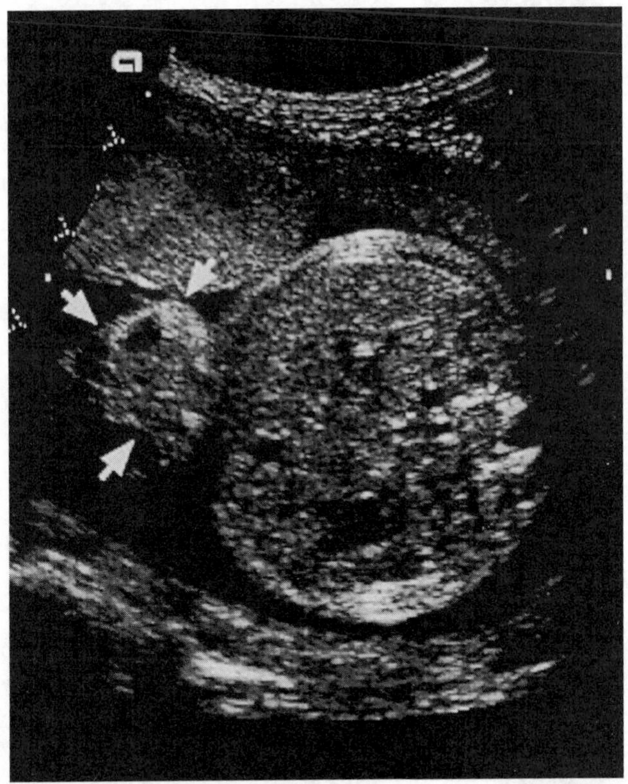

FIG. 34-9 Transverse sonogram at 27 weeks gestation reveals a supraumbilical omphalocele. Mild polyhydramnios is present.

with omphalocele are generally lower than those observed with gastroschisis. In omphaloceles eviscerated organs can include liver, stomach, and small and large bowel (Fig. 34-9). The sonographic appearance can demonstrate variability depending on the size of the ventral abdominal wall defect, type of eviscerated organs, presence of ascites, and associated anomalies. Polyhydramnios may be seen in approximately one third of the cases. Omphaloceles are associated with anomalies of other organ systems (50% to 70%) and chromosome abnormalities (30% to 40%). When the prenatal ultrasound examination reveals an omphalocele, prenatal testing should be offered to the patient to facilitate accurate DNA analysis.

KEY POINTS

1 The antenatal sonographic detection of anomalies permits the opportunity to counsel patients, change the management of the pregnancy or delivery, and optimize the care of the newborn.

2 The sonographic accuracy for detecting cardiac malformations during a screening obstetric ultrasound for routine clinical indications has been poor compared with detection rates for other abnormalities.

3 The two main types of abdominal wall defects easily detected by sonography include omphalocele and gastroschisis.

SUGGESTED READINGS

Babcook CJ et al: Gastroschisis: can sonography of the fetal bowel accurately predict postnatal outcome? *J Ultrasound Med* 13:701-706, 1994.

Fleischer AC et al: *The principles and practice of ultrasonography in obstetrics and gynecology,* ed 4, 1991, Appleton & Lange.

Kirk JS et al: Prenatal screening for cardiac anomalies: the value of routine addition of the aortic root to the four-chamber view, *Obstet Gynecol* (84)3, Sept 1994.

Nyberg DA, Mahony BS, Pretorius DH: *Diagnostic ultrasound of fetal anomalies,* Chicago, 1990, Year Book Medical Publishers.

Paidas MJ, Crombleholme TM, Robertson FM: Prenatal diagnosis and management of the fetus with an abdominal wall defect, *Semin Perinatol* (18)3, June 1994.

Wheller JJ: Diagnosis of arrhythmias and congenital heart disease. In *Heart disease in infants, children and adolescents including the fetus and young adult,* ed 5, Baltimore, 1995, Williams & Wilkins.

35

Antenatal Testing

Cynthia Shellhaas

The goal of antenatal fetal assessment is to accurately assess fetal well-being and thereby decrease perinatal morbidity and mortality by determining the need for delivery versus continued testing without unnecessary intervention. Any patient at increased risk for adverse outcome should undergo testing. The most common indications are those related to uteroplacental insufficiency such as postdate pregnancy, IUGR, oligohydramnios, growth disorders, and maternal conditions such as diabetes, hypertension, and cyanotic heart disease.

FETAL MOVEMENT COUNTING

Fetal movement is reported by most women by the 20th week of gestation, with the maximum level of activity being at 28 to 32 weeks gestation. Maternal perception of fetal activity, or more specifically, alterations in an established pattern of activity have been used to screen for a compromised fetus. Fetal activity is diurnal and most prominent in the early evening. Ultrasound observation of the fetus and maternal perception of fetal movement correlate about 80% to 90% of the time but an objective record of fetal movement is still needed.

There are several different methods of counting fetal movement. Each involves either counting and recording movements during a fixed time or counting a specific number of movements and then recording the time span. Over a 12-hour period, only 2.5% of women will notice less than 10 movements. This is the underlying principle in using fetal movement counting as a screening tool in both high- and low-risk obstetric populations.

NONSTRESS TESTING

Nonstress testing is currently the mainstay of antenatal fetal assessment. The nonstress test is performed in a standardized manner with the patient in the semi-Fowler position. External abdominal transducers monitor fetal heart rate and uterine activity. The patient is given an event marker so that she can register any perceived movements. The most commonly accepted criterion for reactivity requires two accelerations of 15 beats/minute in any 20-minute period. Each acceleration should last at least 15 seconds. The test may be affected by factors such as prematurity, medications, and fetal sleep state. Approximately 65% of fetuses demonstrate fetal heart rate reactivity by 28 weeks gestation, about 95% by 34 weeks gestation. Although fetal sleep states occur, most normal third trimester fetuses will demonstrate reactivity after 70 minutes. A high false positive rate of 75% to 90% is a major disadvantage to the test.

The third trimester fetus responds to many different external stimuli such as sound or light vibration with gross body movements. Transabdominal application of vibroacoustic stimulation (VAS) using an electronic artificial larynx may be used to evoke a fetal response both antenatally and during delivery. These responses are as valid as those seen spontaneously. Primary uses of VAS are to decrease the incidence of nonreactive tests, to shorten testing time, to induce fetal movement on ultrasound to promote better visualization, and to decrease scalp sampling during delivery. If the test remains nonreactive, the fetus must be further evaluated either by a BPP or contraction stress test.

BIOPHYSICAL PROFILE

The BPP includes the nonstress test with the addition of fetal behavioral states as viewed on ultrasound (see Chapter 34).

There is an inverse and linear relationship between a recent BPP score and subsequent fetal distress, NICU admission, IUGR, 5-minute Apgar score less than 7, and cord pH less than 7.2. There is also an inverse and exponential relationship between a recent BPP score and perinatal mortality.

One modification of the biophysical profile involves use of the nonstress test and ultrasound assessment of amniotic fluid volume using the AFI. The complete BPP may be performed if either the nonstress test or amniotic fluid volume are abnormal; this modification is designed to make testing easier than doing a full BPP and more effective than a nonstress test alone. There is a relationship between oligohydramnios, nonreactivity of the nonstress test, and fetal heart rate decelerations.

CONTRACTION STRESS TEST

The contraction stress test has long been considered the gold standard of antenatal testing. Like the nonstress test, it involves monitoring the fetal heart rate but under the condition of regular contractions. Its underlying premise is that a compromised fetus will decompensate under the stress of contractions and respond to the temporary decrease in placental perfusion with a decrease in fetal heart rate (a late deceleration).

TABLE 35-1
Interpretation of the Contraction Stress Test

Interpretation	Description	Incidence (%)
Negative	No late decelerations appearing anywhere on the tracing with adequate uterine contractions (3 in 10 min)	80
Positive	Late decelerations that are consistent and persistent are present with the majority (greater than 50%) of contractions without excessive uterine activity; if persistent late decelerations are seen before the frequency of contractions is adequate, test is interpreted as positive	3-5
Suspicious	Inconsistent late decelerations	5
Hyperstimulation	Uterine contractions closer than every 2 min or lasting more than 90 sec or five uterine contractions in 10 min; if no late decelerations are seen, test interpreted as negative	5
Unsatisfactory	Quality of the tracing is inadequate for interpretation, or adequate uterine activity cannot be achieved	5

From Gabbe SG et al: *Obstetrics: normal and problem pregnancies,* ed 2, New York, 1986, Churchill Livingstone.

This decrease begins at the peak of the contraction and continues after the contraction concludes.

The test may be performed either of two ways: with the intravenous administration of exogenous oxytocin (OCT) or with the endogenous release of oxytocin in response to breast nipple stimulation. In both cases the patient is placed in the semi-Fowler or left lateral recumbent position and is hooked up to an external fetal heart rate monitor and tocodynamometer to obtain a baseline fetal heart rate tracing. An oxytocin challenge is begun using either intravenous oxytocin infusion or unilateral nipple rolling until three contractions of at least 40 seconds occur in a 10-minute interval. Care must be taken to avoid uterine hyperstimulation. Interpretation criteria of the contraction stress test are shown in Table 35-1. The contraction stress test has a high sensitivity but also a high false positive rate of at least 50%. It is a cumbersome test to perform because it is best done on the labor and delivery unit and may take several hours.

DOPPLER VELOCIMETRY

Doppler velocimetry is a specialized form of ultrasound used to study the circulatory system and especially resistance to blood flow. Since it appears that decreased uteroplacental perfusion is a major contributor to fetal morbidity and mortality, Doppler velocimetry is potentially useful as a tool in fetal evaluation. When an ultrasound beam intersects blood flow in a vessel it is scattered in all directions, including back to the transducer. This scattering is probably caused by changes in red cell concentration. The velocity of the red cell is determined by measuring the change in frequency in a sound wave reflected off that red cell. Waveforms are obtained in which the vertical dimension represents the Doppler-shifted sound frequencies and the horizontal dimension represents time. In vessels that are coiled (e.g., umbilical and uterine) the angle between the Doppler beam and vessel can't be accurately measured so angle-independent indices such as the ratios of peak systolic to end diastolic frequencies are used as indicators of resistance to flow. Results normally show decreasing resistance with increasing gestational age. End diastolic flow is consistently present by 15 weeks gestation. The absence of end diastolic flow and the reversal of end diastolic flow are both reflective of increased placental vascular resistance and are associated with increased perinatal morbidity and mortality. Reversal of end diastolic flow is considered the more ominous of the two findings. It is not clear as to whether reversal of flow in and of itself is an indication for delivery. Neither of these findings are usually found without some other nonreassuring fetal test results. The role of Doppler in fetal assessment remains controversial. The presence of abnormal Doppler does signal the need for more intensive fetal monitoring on an in-patient basis with either daily or twice daily nonstress tests or BPPs (Fig. 35-1).

CORDOCENTESIS

Percutaneous umbilical blood sampling (PUBS, also called *cordocentesis*) may be done under direct ultrasound guidance as early as 18 to 20 weeks

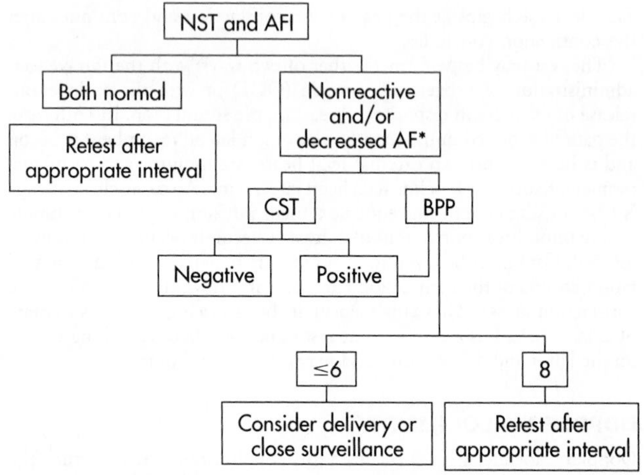

FIG. 35-1 Antepartum fetal surveillance in which the nonstress test (NST) and amniotic fluid index (AFI) are used as the primary methods for fetal evaluation. A nonreactive NST and/or decreased amniotic fluid (AF) are further evaluated using either the contraction stress test (CST) or the biophysical profile (BPP). *If the fetus is mature and amniotic fluid volume is reduced, delivery should be considered before further testing is undertaken. (From Gabbe S: *Obstetrics: normal and problem pregnancies,* ed 3, 1996, Churchill Livingstone; modified from Finberg HJ et al: *J Ultra Med* 9:583, 1990.)

and throughout gestation. This technique provides a unique opportunity to directly assess the fetal blood gas and acid-base status of either the umbilical artery or vein as a measure of fetal well-being. However, cordocentesis is highly invasive with a procedure-related fetal loss rate of 1%. Indications are few, especially given the wide array of other less invasive modalities available for fetal assessment. One of its few applications may be in conjunction with other tests such as rapid fetal karyotyping, especially in the very preterm fetus.

KEY POINTS

1 Ultrasound observation of the fetus and maternal perception of movement correlate 80% to 90% of the time.

2 Nonstress testing monitors fetal heart rate and uterine activity. The BPP involves nonstress testing and fetal behavioral states obtained through ultrasound.

3 The contraction stress test monitors fetal heart rate with contractions present.

4 Doppler velocimetry and cordocentesis are less common procedures used to monitor fetal condition.

SUGGESTED READINGS

American College of Obstetricians and Gynecologists: *Antepartum fetal surveillance,* Technical Bulletin #188, January 1994, ACOG.

Divon MY: Umbilical artery Doppler velocimetry: clinical utility in high-risk pregnancies, *Am J Obstet Gynecol* 174:10, 1996.

Manning FA et al: Fetal assessment based on fetal biophysical profile scoring: an analysis of perinatal morbidity and mortality, *Am J Obstet Gynecol* 162:703, 1990.

Smith CV: Vibroacoustic stimulation for risk assessment, *Clin Perinatol* 21:797, 1994.

Wing DA et al: How frequently should the amniotic fluid index be performed during the course of antepartum testing? *Am J Obstet Gynecol* 174:33, 1996.

36

Medical Diseases in Pregnancy

Carcinoma of the Cervix

JOHN G. BOUTSELIS

When carcinoma of the cervix is diagnosed during pregnancy, the following factors must be addressed: (1) termination of pregnancy, (2) without termination, how long can treatment be deferred until fetal maturity is attained without compromising maternal cure rate, (3) can tumor metastasize to the products of conception, (4) will pregnancy accelerate the cancerous growth, and (5) will cancer of the cervix affect pregnancy or optimal therapy?

Cancer complicating pregnancy occurs in 1/1200 pregnancies, and the most common malignancies in pregnancy in order of frequency are breast, leukemias/lymphomas, cervical carcinoma, melanomas, and bone malignancy. Cervical cancer may be the most common malignancy in women during the reproductive years. The overall survival rates in pregnant and nonpregnant patients with cervical cancer are similar.

PATHOLOGY

Carcinoma In-Situ of the Cervix

- Incidence: 1/800 pregnancies.
- Symptoms: 95% asymptomatic.
- Gross appearance of cervix is normal in 95% of patients.

- Detection: A proper Pap smear includes the cervical brush and cervical scrape. False negative rates are 5% to 20%. Evaluation of the abnormal Pap smear includes colposcopy and biopsy (Fig. 36-1).
- Diagnosis: Colposcopy and cervical biopsy. An endocervical curettage is contraindicated. A cervical cone is seldom necessary, and the only absolute indication for conization is suspected microinvasive carcinoma. Complications of cervical conization in pregnancy are 26% to 28% and pregnancy loss 9%.
- Treatment: No definitive therapy until the postpartum period and then treat as in the nonpregnant patient with an excision (e.g., LEEP) procedure rather than a destructive procedure (e.g., laser vaporization, cryosurgery). Cesarean delivery is recommended for obstetric indications.
- Recurrence rate for residual disease when treated during pregnancy by conization is 20% to 60% depending on in which trimester conization was performed. When treated during the postpartum period, the recurrence rate should be 3% to 4%, providing surgical margins are free of tumor.

Microinvasive Carcinoma

The histologic criteria as to what constitutes microinvasion is of the utmost importance, particularly as described by the Society of Gynecologic Oncologists (SGO) and FIGO.

- SGO criteria: Depth of stromal invasion not to exceed 3 mm below the basement membrane, no LVSI, and no coalescing of tumor tongues that invade the underlying stroma.
- FIGO criteria: Stage IA-1, minimal stromal invasion. Stage IA-2, depth of invasion does not exceed 5 mm, and horizontal spread does not exceed 7 mm. (NOTE: Not included by FIGO is no LVSI).
- Incidence: Unknown but best estimates are less than 5% of invasive cancers are microinvasive.
- Symptoms: 90% asymptomatic.
- Gross appearance of cervix: Normal in 85% of the patients.
- Diagnosis: Made by conization of cervix.
- Treatment: Varies from conization to hysterectomy and modified radical hysterectomy. The current recommendation for treatment would be to permit the pregnancy to reach term, anticipate a vaginal delivery, and provide definitive postpartum therapy. Treatment should be the same as that used with the nonpregnant patient:
  1. Patient desires future reproduction: Cone and follow when depth invasion is 3 mm or less. Modified radical hysterectomy and node dissection are indicated when depth of invasion is 4 to 5 mm.
  2. No future reproduction desired: Simple hysterectomy with depth of invasion 3 mm or less. A modified radical hysterectomy and node dissection with invasion depth of 4 to 5 mm.

There is a 5-year survival rate of 95% to 99%, depending on depth of invasion.

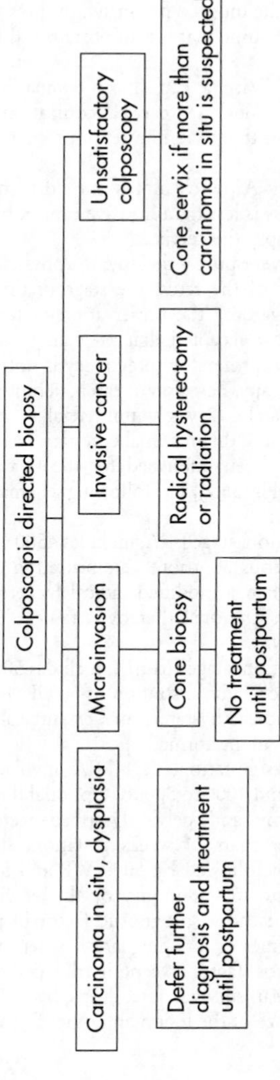

FIG. 36-1 Management of the abnormal pap smear. (Modified from DiSaia P, Creasman W: *Clinical gynecologic oncology*, ed 4, St. Louis, 1993, Mosby.)

Invasive Carcinoma of Cervix

- Incidence: With an incidence of 1/1000 to 2200 pregnancies, invasive carcinoma of the cervix is the most common malignancy encountered during pregnancy.
- Symptoms: By far the most common symptom is vaginal bleeding, and one must not assume that it is of obstetric etiology.
- Diagnosis
  No visible lesion: With a Pap smear compatible with invasive cancer and no visible lesion, a cervical conization is indicated and should be done after the first trimester of pregnancy or at 16 weeks gestation.
  Gross visible lesion: A punch biopsy should be performed; if the pathologic diagnosis is less than invasive cancer, perform a cervical conization or rebiopsy the cervix.
- Treatment: To deliver optimal therapy, the physician must consider the gestational age of the fetus, the stage of the lesion, and the patient's wishes regarding the preservation or termination of the pregnancy. It is now accepted that pregnancy will not accelerate the cancerous growth, therefore pregnancy is not a factor in determining optimal therapy. Based on research, definitive therapy can be deferred approximately 12 weeks until fetal maturity is obtained without compromising the maternal cure rate.

Many schemas have been published for the treatment of cervical carcinoma in pregnancy (Fig. 36-2). The following schema is recommended by DiSaia and Creasman:

Up to 24 weeks gestation, stage I-IIA, includes 4500 whole pelvis (WP) radiation; after spontaneous abortion, administration of 6000 B. If no spontaneous abortion, then a modified radical hysterectomy (no node dissection) is performed. Optional therapy is radical hysterectomy and pelvic lymphadenectomy.

Up to 24 weeks gestation, stage IIB-IIIB, includes 5000 WP radiation; after spontaneous abortion, administration of 5000B. If no spontaneous abortion, a modified radical hysterectomy *or* surgical evacuation and administration of 5000B are performed.

Longer than 24 weeks gestation, stage I-IIA, involves C-section near term, 5000 to 6000 WP and 4000 to 5000B. Optional therapy is C-section and radical hysterectomy and pelvic lymphadenectomy in a near-term pregnancy. Longer than 24 weeks gestation, stage IIB-IIIB, involves C-section at term followed by 5000 WP and 5000 B.

For delay of therapy in carcinoma of the cervix in pregnancy, the method of delivery is not a prognostic factor in patient curability rate. Similarly, the trimester of pregnancy when the diagnosis is made is not a prognostic factor except in the first six months post partum, where the 5-year survival rate drops by 15%. This may be attributed to the larger size of the lesion and other factors. More research is needed.

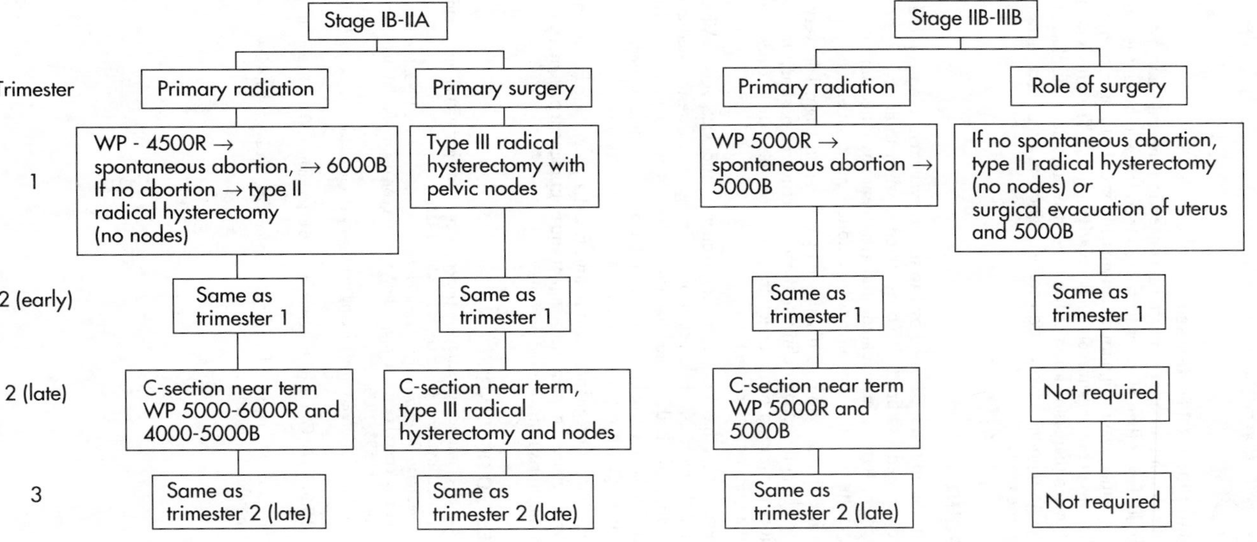

FIG. 36-2 Treatment for cervical carcinoma in pregnancy. *WP*, Whole pelvic radiation (cGy); *B*, brachytherapy (2T + C) mg HR. (Modified from DiSaia P, Creasman W: *Clinical gynecologic oncology*, ed 4, St. Louis, 1993, Mosby.)

Fetal and Placental Metastasis

Metastatic lesions to the product of conception are rare and poorly understood. Fewer than 50 cases have been reported, and by far the most common primary was malignant melanoma, followed by breast cancer, and combinations of breast cancer and leukemia/lymphoma. The fetus is rarely involved when there is invasion only on the maternal side of the placenta. There are no reported cases of gynecologic cancer in pregnancy metastasizing to the fetus.

KEY POINTS

1. Carcinoma in situ is detected by Pap smear, evaluated colposcopically, and diagnosed by directed biopsy or cone when indicated. Vaginal delivery at term is anticipated, and treatment instituted during the postpartum period is the same as for a nonpregnant patient.
2. Microinvasive carcinoma is diagnosed by conization, vaginal delivery is anticipated at term, and definitive therapy is rendered post partum and includes conization or hysterectomy based on the patient's desire to maintain reproductive function.
3. Invasive cancer has no effect on pregnancy and vice versa. When diagnosed before 24 weeks gestation, the pregnancy is terminated and treatment instituted. When diagnosed after 24 weeks gestation, the pregnancy is delivered near term and definitive therapy instituted. Primary surgery is recommended for stage IB-IIA lesions.
4. The method of pregnancy termination is not a prognostic factor, and survival rates are similar in the pregnant and nonpregnant patient, except when diagnosis is made post partum.

SUGGESTED READINGS

Cooper R et al: A multicenter study on preterm weight and gestational age specific neonatal mortality, *Am J Obstet Gynecol* 168:78-84, 1993.

DiSaia P, Creasman W: *Clinical gynecologic oncology*, ed 4, St. Louis, 1993, Mosby.

Duggan B et al: Cervical cancer in pregnancy: reporting on planned delay in therapy, *Obstet Gynecol* 82:598, 1993.

Hacker N, Veldon J: Conservative therapy in early gynecologic cancer, *Cancer* 71:91, 1993.

Hopkins M, Morley G: Cancer of the cervix, stage IB in pregnancy, *Obstet Gynecol* 80:9, 1992.

Morrow C, Curtin J, Townsend D: *Synopsis of gynecologic oncology*, ed 4, New York, 1993, Churchill Livingstone.

Cardiac and Pulmonary Diseases

Michael C. Gordon

Pregnancy causes profound physiologic changes to the cardiovascular and respiratory systems that can influence the diagnosis, management, and prognosis of cardiac and pulmonary diseases. These changes result in increasing stress to both systems, which can lead to serious problems in women with preexisting cardiac or pulmonary disease.

By eight weeks gestation cardiac output has begun to increase, and by 24 to 28 weeks gestation it peaks at 30% to 50% above nonpregnant values where it then remains relatively unchanged until delivery (4.3 to 6.2 L/min). During labor, further demands are placed on the heart because cardiac output can rise an additional 50% above baseline pregnancy values. With each uterine contraction there is a 300- to 500-ml autotransfusion of blood into the central circulation, and immediately after delivery even greater increases in the cardiac output can occur. This increase may peak at 80% above the prelabor values.

Cardiac output is the product of stroke volume and the heart rate, and blood pressure is the product of cardiac output and systemic vascular resistance. Increased cardiac output in pregnancy is due to the increase in both the stroke volume and the maternal heart rate. During pregnancy there is a 17% increase in stroke volume and an increase in the maternal heart rate of 12 to 20 beats per minute (Table 36-1). In spite of this increase in cardiac ouput, maternal blood pressure is decreased until late in pregnancy as a result of a greater decrease in the systemic vascular resistance (SVR). The SVR decreases 21% as a result of a generalized arteriolar dilation caused by hormonal changes of pregnancy and the development of a large venous capacitance system within the placenta.

TABLE 36-1
Central Hemodynamic Changes During Pregnancy

	Nonpregnant	Pregnant	% Change
Cardiac output (L/min)	4.3	6.2	+43%
Heart rate (bpm)	71	83	+17%
Systemic vascular resistance (dyne/cm/sec^5)	1530	1220	–21%
Pulmonary vascular resistance (dyne/cm/sec^5)	119	78	–34%
Mean arterial pressure (mm Hg)	86	90	n.s.
Colloid osmotic pressure (mm Hg)	21	18	–14%

Note: Measurements made during the third trimester with the women in the lateral decubitus position.

Modified from Clark SI et al: Central hemodynamic assessment of normal term pregnancy, *Am J Obstet Gynecol,* 161:1439, 1989.

Maternal blood pressure decreases by the seventh gestational week, with a maximal decrease in the diastolic blood pressure of 10 mm Hg at 28 weeks followed by increases toward nonpregnant levels by term. Both maternal cardiac output and blood pressure are very dependent on maternal position by 24 weeks of gestation. The gravid uterus causes significant obstruction of the vena caval blood flow in 90% of women when they are in the supine position, which results in a decrease in the central venous return to the heart. This can result in decreased cardiac output, decreased uterine and placental blood flow, a sudden drop in blood pressure, bradycardia, and syncope in up to 10% of women.

In normal pregnancy, maternal plasma volume begins to increase by 10 weeks gestation and continues until there is a 50% expansion at 30 to 34 weeks. This results in a 1.5 L increase in blood volume. The expansion in the blood volume is compensated for by an increase in venous capacitance.

Pregnancy also affects the respiratory system. The enlarging uterus causes a 4 cm elevation in the diaphragm, which leads to a decrease in the functional residual capacity within the lungs of 10% to 25% by the fifth month of pregnancy. However, as a result of the increased flaring of the lower ribs, widening of the rib cage, and enhanced diaphragmatic function, the inspiratory capacity of the lungs increases. Therefore the vital capacity and the total lung volumes are not changed despite the decrease in the residual capacity. Because of increased progesterone levels, pregnancy causes a state of chronic hyperventilation as reflected by an increased tidal volume and minute ventilation. The respiratory rate does not change. Maximal breathing capacity, forced vital capacity, peak flow rates, forced expiratory volume in 1 second (FEV_1), and lung compliance are not affected by pregnancy.

A marked increase in minute ventilation (20% to 50%) from 7.5 to 10.5 L/min occurs during the first trimester and then it remains fairly constant for the remainder of gestation. This results in a 70% increase in alveolar ventilation, which is reflected by a change in the normal blood gases during pregnancy. The hyperventilation results in a chronic respiratory alkalosis with an arterial pH of 7.4 to 7.45, a decreased Pco_2 to 28 to 30 mm Hg, and a decreased Hco_3 to 18 to 21 mEq/L. Early in pregnancy the arterial Po_2 increases (106 to 108) as the Pco_2 decreases, but by the third trimester there is a slight decrease in the Po_2 (101 to 104) as a result of the enlarging uterus.

As the minute ventilation increases, there is a simultaneous but lesser increase in the oxygen consumption during pregnancy. The increase in O_2 consumption is only 50% that of the increase in minute ventilation and is caused by the oxygen requirements of the fetus, placenta, increased maternal tissue, and the increase in cardiac and respiratory work. With exercise or during labor an even greater increase in both minute ventilation and O_2 consumption occurs. During a contraction, the O_2 consumption can triple. As a result of the increased oxygen consumption and the decreased functional residual capacity, the oxygen reserve is lower and the pregnant women is more susceptible to the effects of apnea or transient hypoxia. With apnea, such as during intubation, a more rapid onset of hypoxia, hypercapnia, and respiratory acidosis develops.

The physiologic changes of pregnancy lead to a number of changes in maternal physical signs and symptoms that can mimic cardiac or respiratory disease and make it more difficult to determine if true disease is present. Dyspnea is common during normal pregnancy, and about 50% of women complain of dyspnea before 20 weeks of gestation and 75% experience it by the third trimester. Certain distinguishing features differentiate the dyspnea of pregnancy from the much less common dyspnea of pulmonary or cardiac disease. First, the dyspnea of pregnancy occurs early in pregnancy and does not worsen significantly as the pregnancy progresses, whereas the symptoms of heart disease usually become more severe in the latter half of pregnancy. Second, physiologic dyspnea is usually only mild, does not stop women from performing their normal daily activities, and does not occur at rest. Other normal symptoms in pregnancy that can mimic disease include fatigue, reduced exercise tolerance, occasional orthopnea, syncope, and chest discomfort. Symptoms that should not be attributed to a normal pregnancy and need a more thorough investigation include hemoptysis, syncope or chest pain with exertion, progressive orthopnea or paroxysmal nocturnal dyspnea, and dyspnea associated with a cough or that limits daily activities. Normal physical findings during pregnancy that could be mistaken as evidence for pulmonary or cardiac disease include peripheral edema, mild tachycardia, jugular venous distention after 20 weeks of gestation, lateral displacement of the left ventricular apex, brisk left and right ventricular function, early or midsystolic or continuous systolic murmurs, increase in the amplitude of peripheral pulses, transient pulmonary basilar rales, persistent splitting of the heart sounds, and the presence of the third heart sound (S3). Certain physical signs when found in pregnancy require a thorough evaluation because of their association with pulmonary or cardiac disease. These include cyanosis, clubbing, prominent jugular venous distention, systolic murmur greater than grade 3/6, diastolic murmur, cardiomegaly, sustained arrhythmia, diffuse wheezes, rhonchi or rales, and a left parasternal lift.

PULMONARY DISEASES

Asthma

Asthma is one of the most common illnesses that affect pregnant women, with an incidence in pregnancy of between 1% and 7%. Although typically a mild disease, asthma causes 4000 deaths annually within the United States, and the incidence of status asthmaticus approaches 0.15% to 0.2% during pregnancy. Status asthmaticus is defined as severe asthma of any type not responding to treatment after 30 to 60 minutes of intensive therapy. During pregnancy, the risk of uncontrolled asthma is more dangerous than the medications used to treat it.

The effects of pregnancy on asthma are variable. No evidence exists that pregnancy has a predictable effect on asthma or that it has any long-term adverse effects. Women with more severe asthma before pregnancy are more likely to worsen during pregnancy.

If well controlled, asthma poses minimal risk to the pregnancy or the fetus. If uncontrolled, it can cause maternal and fetal injury. Studies have consistently shown an increased risk of preterm birth, low birth weight, fetal growth restriction, fetal demise, and neonatal hypoxemia. The significance of the fetal risk directly correlates with the severity of the maternal asthma, with the fetal risk being highest in the group of women on chronic oral corticosteroids. Maternal risk includes the need for systemic steroids, mechanical ventilation, and death from status asthmaticus. Labor and delivery will exacerbate asthma for approximately 10% of women.

Asthma can be subdivided into types based on symptoms and need for treatment. Mild asthma is defined as an individual having symptoms less than twice weekly or nocturnal symptoms less than twice monthly and in between episodes is symptom free. Moderate asthma is defined as requiring the use of a β-adrenergic agonist more than three times weekly or individuals with pulmonary function tests at 60% to 80% of predicted. Individuals with severe disease have continuous symptoms, limited activity levels, frequent nocturnal symptoms, severe exacerbations, and impaired lung function (<60% predicted).

Diagnosis

Diagnosis of asthma is based on establishing a history of recurrent episodic airway bronchospasm with recovery, along with the characteristic symptoms that may be nocturnal, seasonal, or occur after exposure to various environmental stimuli. Characteristic symptoms include cough, wheezing, dyspnea, and chest tightness. Wheezing can be confirmed with chest auscultation. The use of pulmonary function tests, which demonstrate reversible airway obstructive disease, are helpful in distinguishing between asthma and other causes of pulmonary complaints during pregnancy.

Since the patient's and the physician's perception of asthma severity are often insensitive and inaccurate, objective measures of lung function are essential for assessing and monitoring the patient's condition. These can be made by using a spirometer to measure vital capacity, forced vital capacity, and FEV_1; peak flow meters to measure the peak expiratory flow rate (PEFR); or an arterial blood gas. The single best predictor of pulmonary function is FEV_1, but the PEFR correlates well with the FEV_1. The advantage of the PEFR is that it is inexpensive, easily obtainable, and can be monitored at home by the patient to assess the response to therapy and to detect early signs of worsening asthma. The PEFR needs to be obtained when the patient is healthy to obtain a baseline for later comparison. Predicted values are in the range of 380 to 550 L/min. In patients with moderate to severe asthma, the PEFR should be recorded at least daily, and they should bring the records to their clinic visits so that determinations on therapy can be made. The PEFR can also be used by the patient to determine how severe her asthma is during an exacerbation. If the PEFR is 70% to 90% of baseline, then the patient should initiate an increase in the frequency of the inhaled β-2 agonist. If compromise persists, additional therapy should be added. If the PEFR is 50% to 70% of baseline, the patient should contact her physican or go to the clinic or emergency room. If the PEFR is less than 50% of baseline, the individual should go immediately to the emergency room.

In patients with severe asthma, serial ultrasound to assess fetal growth should be performed from 24 weeks until delivery, and antepartum testing should be used during the third trimester to evaluate the fetus. Since the pregnant patient and her fetus are less tolerant of hypoxemia, continuous fetal monitoring may be indicated during periods of asthma exacerbations if the fetus is past 24 to 26 weeks of gestation.

Treatment

Asthma should be treated as aggressively during pregnancy as in the nonpregnant state. The goal of treatment is to maintain normal lung function, control symptoms, maintain normal activity levels, prevent exacerbations, and avoid adverse effects of medications. Pharmacologic treatment is aimed at decreasing inflammation and at preventing acute exacerbations. The number of medications used and the frequency of use are established on a step-care approach based on the severity of the patient's asthma. Based on symptoms, the number and frequency of medications are either increased or decreased. The two basic categories of drugs used in treating asthma are bronchodilators and antiinflammatory medications. Fortunately, the majority of drugs used in treating asthma are safe during pregnancy, and pregnancy will have little effect in influencing the choice of medications to be used. Inhalants are preferred, and using older drugs with a long history of use during pregnancy is also preferred. The delivery of inhaled medications to the respiratory tract can be optimized by appropriate inhaler technique and by the use of spacer devices.

All patients with asthma must have an inhaled β-2 agonist available for treatment of acute symptoms. In patients with mild asthma, this may be the only medication needed. In managing individuals with moderate to severe disease, the current emphasis is to use antiinflammatory drugs as a maintenance medication to decrease airway inflammation in addition to the use of inhaled β-2 agonist. This will frequently limit the patient's symptoms and the need for frequent use of inhaled β-2 agonist. The different antiinflammatory drugs include cromolyn sodium, inhaled steroids, or oral steroids. In individuals who are not controlled by any combination of bronchodilators, cromolyn sodium, or inhaled steroids, the use of oral corticosteroids is indicated. Initially, the patient is usually started on 30 to 60 mg daily of prednisone for 3 to 7 days with a rapid taper over 1 to 2 weeks. If the individual needs long-term oral prednisone, attempts should be made to reduce it to the lowest possible dose, and alternate-day therapy may be tried. Recently the use of oral β-2 agonist, atropine, and theophylline have been deemphasized except in the individual with severe asthma.

Management of acute exacerbation of asthma includes the use of supplemental oxygen, bronchodilators, and intravenous corticosteroids to maintain a Po_2 of at least 60 to 65 mm Hg with an O_2 saturation of greater than 90%. Inhaled metaproterenol (0.3 cc in 3 cc saline) or albuterol (0.5 cc in 3 cc saline) from a hand-held nebulizer, or subcutaneous epinephrine (0.3 cc of a 1/1000 solution) or terbutaline (0.25 mg) given every 20 minutes for up to 3 times is the initial treatment for severe asthma exacerbations. If there is a poor or only a partial response to the bronchodilators, then intravenous steroids should be added early in the course of treatment. Either prednisone (75 to 150 mg) or methylprednisolone (60 to 120 mg) can be given every 6 to 8 hours for 1 to 3 days followed by a short course of oral prednisone. Intravenous theophylline (aminophylline) can be used in individuals with poor responses to the previously mentioned medications but is no longer the mainstay of therapy for acute asthma. Patients should be evaluated for antibiotic therapy if there is an infectious etiology to the acute asthma exacerbation.

In labor, women with asthma should continue their scheduled asthma medications and may need supplemental oxygen. Labor is not a trigger for asthma, and the need for intravenous steroids or aminophylline is uncommon. The use of 15-methyl prostaglandin F_2-α (hemabate) is contraindicated in women with asthma, but the use of prostaglandin E_2 suppositories has not been reported to cause bronchospasm.

Pneumonia

Pneumonia is one of the most common nonobstetric infections that causes serious maternal morbidity and mortality during pregnancy. The incidence during pregnancy is 1 to 2/1000 deliveries. Certain types of pneumonia have greater virulence and mortality during pregnancy, in particular viral pneumonia. Studies show an increased risk of preterm delivery and fetal loss.

Pneumonia is defined as inflammation affecting the lung parenchyma distal to the larger airways and involving the respiratory bronchioles and alveolar units. Pneumonia can be subdivided into typical and atypical types. Typical pneumonia is characterized by the abrupt onset of fever, chills, purulent sputum, and a lobar infiltrate on a chest x-ray and is usually caused by *Streptococcus pneumoniae* or *Haemophilus influenzae. S. pneumoniae* is the most common bacterial pathogen to cause pneumonia in pregnancy. Atypical pneumonia has a lower fever, less toxicity, a dry cough with a mucoid sputum, and a patchy or interstitial infiltrate. The pathogens that cause atypical pneumonia are more likely to be *Mycoplasma pneumoniae, Chlamydia pneumoniae, Legionella pneumophila,* and viruses.

A serious cause of pneumonia in pregnancy is aspiration, which typically occurs during the intrapartum period and is associated with endotracheal intubation. If a women in the postpartum period develops respiratory failure, there should be a high index of suspicion for aspiration as well as for a pulmonary embolism. Viruses also cause pneumonia in pregnancy, and evidence exists that maternal prognosis with varicella or influenza pneumonia is significantly worse. Varicella pneumonia occurs 2 to 5 days after the onset of the rash, and mortality is 11% to 35%.

Diagnosis

The clinical features of pneumonia are not affected by pregnancy. Typically, there is a preceding URI and the individual has a fever, cough, and more rarely dyspnea. The diagnosis of pneumonia is based on the history and physical examination and is corroborated by radiologic findings. On physical examination there may be evidence of pulmonary consolidation with dullness to percussion, tubular or decreased breath sounds, inspiratory crackles, and increased tactile fremitus; however, the lung examination can be more normal if there is an interstitial or atypical pneumonia. All pregnant women with suspected pneumonia need a chest x-ray with shielding of the fetus.

A sputum specimen for a gram stain and culture helps determine the etiology of the infection and the correct antibiotic treatment. In addition, a blood culture for both aerobic and anaerobic organisms and an arterial blood gas should be obtained. Clinically, it can be difficult to distinguish viral from bacterial pneumonia. Classically, the viral infection will present as an atypical pneumonia without consolidation, without an elevated white blood count, and bacteria will not be seen on a gram stain of the sputum. Women with suspected *M. pneumoniae* can be tested for complement-fixing antibodies to mycoplasma and the presence of cold agglutinins.

Treatment

Treatment of the pregnant woman with pneumonia is only slightly altered by the pregnancy. Certain antibiotics cannot be used during pregnancy; these include tetracycline, the quinolones, and potentially sulfonamides during the third trimester. All pregnant patients with pneumonia need to be hospitalized for intravenous antibiotics and need to be evaluated for supplemental oxygen requirements. If it is after 20 to 22 weeks gestation, the patient should be monitored for preterm labor, and fetal heart rate monitoring should be considered.

The choice of intravenous antibiotics depends on the severity of the infection and the factors affecting the likely etiology of the infection. If the patient is severely ill or at risk for a nosocomial infection, she should be empirically treated for *S. pneumoniae, H. influenzae, L. pneumophila,* and gram-negative organisms with broad spectrum antibiotics such as a second/third generation cephalosporin or amoxicillin-clavulanate and potentially an aminoglycoside. If the patient is at risk for developing an aspiration pneumonia, then coverage of anaerobic bacteria needs to be added. In the individual with a community-acquired pneumonia, the initial choice of antibiotics can include erythromycin, amoxicillin, penicillin, or a first-generation cephalosporin, based on the presentation of the illness and the likelihood of *H. influenzae, S. pneumoniae,* or *M. pneumoniae.* The results of the gram stain may allow for a more empirical choice of antibiotics.

In patients with suspected viral pneumonia, antibiotic treatment may be needed if a superimposed bacterial infection develops or if the patient's condition worsens. In women with varicella pneumonia, the use of intravenous acyclovir has been reported. The use of antiviral agents such as amantadine and ribaviran should be considered in the severely ill individual with influenza pneumonia.

Sarcoidosis

Sarcoidosis is a chronic, multisystem, granulomatous disease of unknown etiology. It is characterized by an accumulation of T lymphocytes and phagocytes within caseous granulomas in a perivascular pattern. All parts of the body can be affected, but the lungs are the most commonly affected site. Other areas affected more frequently include the lymph nodes, skin, eyes, and the liver. This disease can affect individuals differently and is often acute and subacute and self-limiting, but can also be chronic with periods of remission or exacerbations. The overall lifetime prognosis is good in the majority of individuals. In 50% of patients, the disease spontaneously resolves; however, about 10% of individuals die because of the sarcoidosis. Most patients develop symptoms between the ages of 20 and 40, and in the United States the majority of patients are African-Americans.

The incidence of sarcoidosis in pregnancy is 2 to 6/10,000 women, and pregnancy does not appear to adversely affect the clinical course of the disease. In most pregnant women with sarcoidosis there is no change or a slight improvement in the individual's symptoms. In the majority of women with sarcoidosis no increase in the incidence of fetal or obstetric complications occurs unless there is severe preexisting disease.

Diagnosis

Most commonly, a patient experiences respiratory symptoms of dyspnea with or without exertion, a nonproductive cough, and nonspecific chest pain that develops insidiously over months or abruptly over 1 to 2 weeks. In 10% to 20% of cases, an asymptomatic patient is diagnosed after having a chest x-ray for an unrelated reason. Lymphadenopathy is very common and usually involves the hilar nodes. Ninety percent of individuals with sarcoidosis have abnormal chest x-rays with the classical presentation of bilateral hilar adenopathy with parenchymal infiltrates. The diagnosis cannot be based solely on the findings of the x-ray, and instead is based on a combination of clinical, radiographic, and histologic findings. Biopsy is helpful in making a definitive diagnosis of sarcoidosis. No blood tests are diagnostic of the disease. The angiotensin-converting enzyme is elevated in two thirds of patients, but levels do not appear to reliably reflect disease activity. The differential diagnoses of individuals with possible sarcoidosis include neoplastic diseases (lymphoma) and other granulomatous diseases such as tuberculosis or fungal infections.

Treatment

Treatment of individuals with sarcoidosis is unchanged by pregnancy. The mainstay of therapy is corticosteroids, to which the disease is usually very responsive. Treatment is indicated for symptomatic patients or if there is significant vital organ involvement. The workup for pregnant women with sarcoidosis should include pulmonary function tests, an arterial blood gas, and possible echocardiogram for women with severe disease. Ideally, patients should be evaluated before pregnancy. During pregnancy, serial monitoring of pulmonary function is indicated as well as the use of fetal monitoring to include ultrasound and antepartum testing.

Tuberculosis

The incidence of tuberculosis (TB) increased in the United States from 1985 to 1990 by 16%, with 25,701 new cases in 1990. TB is caused by *Mycobacterium tuberculosis,* and there is an increasing trend in the incidence of TB at younger ages. Before 1985 TB was rare in pregnant women in the United States, but these new trends imply that TB in pregnancy may become an increasing problem. TB infection occurs in two stages: the preclinical and the clinical stage. The preclinical stage is defined as the time when the individual has a positive tuberculin skin test (purified protein derivative [PPD]) but has no symptoms and no evidence of active disease on chest x-ray. The bacilli multiply within the lungs for several weeks and can spread to other organs. After 1 to 3 months, the host develops cell-mediated immunity and the areas of infection heal, but viable bacilli persist within these lesions for many years if not treated. The clinical stage (the term *tuberculosis* usually refers to the clinical disease) occurs when manifestations of pulmonary or extrapulmonary TB become evident. The time period between these two stages may be several weeks or many years. This typically occurs if the individual becomes immune suppressed. Without specific treatment, 5% to 10% of individuals with a positive PPD will develop tuberculosis. In general, environmental factors influence the likelihood of acquiring TB infection, whereas host-related factors determine the chance of TB infection progressing to disease.

Tuberculosis is not more common or more serious during pregnancy, and pregnancy does not increase the risk of progression from preclinical infection to disease. However, women with active TB can pass the infection to the fetus and cause congenital TB in 3 out of 100 infected pregnancies. Neonatal mortality is 22% despite treatment of the newborn. Pregnant women have the same cure rates as nonpregnant individuals when treated with chemotherapy (antituberculosis medications) and the rate of progression from the preclinical infection in properly treated subjects is less than 1%. There is no evidence that properly treated patients with clinical TB infection have a worse outcome in pregnancy when compared with uninfected women. TB is not a teratogen.

Diagnosis

Patients with subclinical TB are usually asymptomatic, but occasionally the patient may experience a fever, cough, and pleuritic pain. Pregnant women with active TB are more often symptom-free than are nonpregnant individuals. Common symptoms of active TB include cough with minimal sputum production, low-grade fever, hemoptysis, and weight loss. Five percent to 10% of individuals have extrapulmonary TB. The chest x-ray is usually abnormal with a variety of infiltrative patterns, or there may be cavitations or mediastinal lymphadenopathy. The diagnosis of active TB infection is established when TB bacilli are identified in sputum or other body fluids by culture or the finding of acid-fast bacilli on smear.

In the past, some authorities recommended tuberculin skin testing for all pregnant women; however, this appears unnecessary. Instead, women in high-risk groups should be tested using the Mantoux method of TB skin test using 0.1 ml of 5 tuberculin unit strength PPD. Pregnancy does not affect the interpretation of the PPD, and the test is read as the amount of induration at 48 to 72 hours.

Interpretation of the test is based on risk factors. In individuals with low risk, greater or equal to 15 mm is considered positive. In individuals with the highest risk factors, a reaction is positive if it is greater or equal to 5 mm. This includes individuals with exposure to TB-infected persons, an abnormal chest x-ray, clinical evidence of TB, or HIV infection. For the other high risk groups (residents of correctional institutions, nursing homes, or homeless persons; poor or medically indigent persons in urban areas; IV drug users or alcoholics; foreign-born persons from areas with a high TB prevalence; health care workers; persons with medical risk factors known to increase the risk of disease if infection has occurred; and persons on immunosuppressive therapies), a reaction ≥10 mm is positive. If the PPD is positive, a chest x-ray is needed to rule out active disease and patients should be thoroughly questioned about symptoms of TB infection.

Treatment

In nonpregnant women less than 35 years old with a positive PPD but no evidence of active disease, isoniazid (INH), 300 mg daily, is recommended for 6 to 12 months. In pregnancy, the decision to treat is more controversial. Most authorities recommend deferring treatment until 3 to 6 months post partum. Exceptions to this are the women with known recent PPD conversion (<2 years) or with recent exposure to active infection in which, if left untreated, there is a 2% to 4% incidence of developing active disease in the first year. Also, women with HIV infection or who are immunocompromised should be treated.

INH crosses the placenta and is considered safe during pregnancy (category C drug). However, some physicians recommend withholding its use until after 12 weeks gestation in asymptomatic women to decrease fetal exposure risks. INH can cause serious and occasionally life-threatening hepatitis, and the risk appears to be increased during pregnancy and in the first 3 months post partum. Therefore when using INH in pregnancy, baseline and monthly liver function tests should be measured. Pyridoxine 50 mg daily (vitamin B_6) is recommended for pregnant women on INH.

Recommendations for treatment of pregnant women with active infection are unchanged. The risk of TB is far greater than the risk of drug toxicity to the mother or the fetus. Active TB is always treated with at least two tuberculostatic drugs. The current recommendation by the CDC during pregnancy is to use INH and rifampin for 9 months with the addition of ethambutol if there is a chance of isoniazid resistance. In nonpregnant patients, the CDC recommends the use of INH and rifampin for 6 months with the addition of pyrazinamide for the first 2 months. The use of this 6-month treatment in pregnancy is controversial because of the unknown fetal risk of pyrazinamide, but several international TB organizations recommend this regimen. The use of the other antituberculosis drug is considered safe during pregnancy and with lactation. The only widely used antituberculosis drug with known fetal teratogenicity is streptomycin.

CARDIAC DISEASES

Although both maternal and cardiovascular mortality have declined significantly in the past two decades, the apparent prevalence of cardiac disease in the pregnant patient has remained relatively constant at 0.5% to 1% in the United States. The major change is in the type of cardiac disease now being seen, with an increased proportion of heart disease as a result of congenital causes. The majority of women with cardiac disease can now expect a safe pregnancy with low maternal and fetal mortality rates. However, cardiac disease is still a leading cause of indirect maternal death during pregnancy.

The problems encountered by pregnant women with cardiac disease are secondary to four principal physiologic cardiovascular changes of pregnancy: (1) The increase in the intravascular volume and the cardiac output may be poorly tolerated in women whose cardiac output is limited by intrinsic myocardial disease, valvular lesions, or ischemic cardiac disease. This increase can lead to congestive heart disease or ischemia. (2) The decrease in the systemic vascular resistance may lead to a worsening of a right to left shunt and worsen cyanotic heart disease. This decrease may also increase the likelihood of systemic hypotension, which can be poorly tolerated in women with aortic stenosis or pulmonary hypertension. (3) The hypercoagulability of pregnancy increases the risk of thromboembolism in women with cardiac lesions that cause an increased risk of arterial thrombosis (artificial valves, atrial fibrillation, and pulmonary hypertension). (4) Marked and rapid changes occur in the intravascular fluid volumes during labor and delivery, and such shifts may be poorly tolerated by women whose cardiac output is highly dependent on maintaining a certain precise preload to avoid either congestive heart failure (CHF) or systemic hypotension.

Currently two classification schemes are used to better clarify the risks of pregnancy in women with specific cardiac lesions. The New York Heart Association (NYHA) classification is based on the woman's functional status before or early in pregnancy: class I is asymptomatic, class II indicates symptoms with greater than normal activity, class III indicates symptoms with normal activity, and class IV indicates symptoms at bed rest. Generally women in functional classes I and II have a favorable prognosis in pregnancy, with maternal mortality less than 1%. Women in classes III and IV have a maternal mortality of 6.8%. However, the functional status may deteriorate during pregnancy regardless of the class, and up to 40% of patients developing CHF and pulmonary edema during pregnancy began the pregnancy in class I or II.

The second and newer classification scheme is based on the specific maternal risk of each individual cardiac lesion found in past studies (Box 36-1). The goal of this classification system is to utilize a more complex descriptive system encompassing the etiologic, anatomic, and physiologic diagnosis to establish a more useful way of counseling the patient regarding the advisability of becoming or continuing a pregnancy. Women in group 1 are considered to have a negligible risk of maternal mortality (<1%), but a risk that is higher than the background maternal mortality rate of 9/100,000 in the United States. Individuals in group 2 have a substantial increased risk of maternal mortality (5% to 15%) if the pregnancy is carried to term, but the risk is generally not so excessive that pregnancy is contraindicated in all cases after a thorough evaluation has been conducted. Group 2 is subdivided into those women with the risk of mortality secondary only to the intrinsic cardiac lesion (group 2A) and those women with the additional risk of the complications from the need of anticoagulant therapy (group 2B). Women in group 3 are subject to a risk of maternal mortality exceeding that seen with almost any other condition in obstetrics (25% to 50%), and pregnancy should be strongly discouraged. Women with lesions in group 3 should be encouraged to undergo sterilization if not

BOX 36-1
Maternal Mortality Risk Associated With Pregnancy

GROUP 1—MORTALITY <1%

Atrial septal defect
Ventricular septal defect
Patent ductus arteriosus
Pulmonic/tricuspid disease
Tetralogy of Fallot, corrected
Bioprosthetic valve
Mitral stenosis, NYHA class I and II

GROUP 2—MORTALITY 5% TO 15%

2A

Mitral stenosis, NYHA III and IV
Aortic stenosis
Coarctation of aorta, uncomplicated (without valvular involvement)
Uncorrected tetralogy of Fallot
Previous myocardial infarction
Marfan syndrome with normal aorta (may be Group 1)

2B

Mitral stenosis with atrial fibrillation
Artificial valve

Group 3–Mortality 25% to 50%

Pulmonary hypertension
Marfan syndrome with aortic involvement (aortic root ≥40 mm)
Coarctation of aorta, with valvular involvement

pregnant; if in the first trimester, abortion should be strongly considered. The risk of termination of pregnancy in the second trimester is probably also safer than proceeding to term in this group of women, but the data are scant.

These two classifications are complementary and should be used together to better predict the risk for a specific patient. Within a group of individuals with a similar cardiac lesion, the NYHA classification can be used to place the patient at either a higher or lower risk for complications within the range specified for the type of lesion. Finally, because the prevalence of each specific cardiac lesion is relatively uncommon in pregnancy and because the risk of maternal mortality is frequently based on data from studies conducted before 1975, the exact risk for each lesion is only an estimate. Therefore it would seem there is a good chance that the exact risk for a specific disease may be overestimated.

Depending on the etiology of the heart disease, the specific cardiac lesion, and the severity of the disease, the fetal risk in women with heart disease varies. Women with congenital heart disease have a 5% to 10% risk of fetal cardiac lesions with a range of 2.5% to 18%, depending on the type of lesion. Fetuses of women with left ventricular outflow abnormalities appear to be at the highest risk. Overall, perinatal morbidity and mortality in women with cardiac disease do not appear to be much higher than the general obstetric population. However, the risk of perinatal complications is greatly increased in women with cyanotic heart lesions, decreased cardiac output, or if cardiac surgery is performed during the pregnancy. The greatest risk appears to be in women with cyanotic heart disease, where fetal mortality exceeds 50%, and a successful pregnancy is rare if the maternal hematocrit exceeds 65%.

Diagnosis

Rarely does cardiac disease arrive de novo in pregnancy. Echocardiography is one of the most useful clinical tools in diagnosing heart disease in pregnancy and in monitoring the progress of the heart during pregnancy. Other tests that can be used to diagnose or monitor heart disease include electrocardiography (ECG), stress test, and the use of invasive hemodynamic monitoring (Swan-Ganz catheter). Occasionally the use of cardiac catheterization with fluoroscopy or radionuclide studies will be needed during pregnancy. A fetal echocardiogram should be done at 16 to 20 weeks gestation. In all women with significant heart disease (in particular women with decreased cardiac output, hypoxia, or polycythemia), antepartum testing during the third trimester and serial fetal ultrasounds should be performed to assess for appropriate fetal growth.

Treatment

Ideally the patient with cardiac disease would be seen for preconception counseling and maternal and fetal risks could be explained. In women with certain types of cardiac diseases, surgery may be indicated before pregnancy, such as in patients with severe aortic or mitral stenosis. If the individual is not seen before pregnancy, which unfortunately is the more common presentation, then an evaluation of the risks needs to be accomplished during the first trimester when a therapeutic abortion could be more safely performed if needed.

General antepartum guidelines in these women include activity restriction, treatment of other medical conditions that could lead to further cardiac stress (infection, anemia, hyperthyroidism, and hypertension), and use of prophylaxis for subacute bacterial endocarditis (SBE) when indicated. These women should be closely assessed for the development of worsening of their cardiac function. In women with decreased cardiac output or with deterioration in their NYHA functional status, prolonged hospital bed rest may be needed.

General guidelines for labor management include liberal use of supplemental O_2, use of the right or left lateral recumbent position, avoidance of fluid overload, use of epidural anesthesia, SBE prophylaxis, and consideration for shortening the second stage of labor with forceps or vacuum. Epidural anesthesia should be used in any patient with a significant cardiac lesion to reduce the increase in the cardiac output that occurs with labor. In patients with cardiac lesions at risk for sudden cardiac death caused by hypotension, such as aortic stenosis or pulmonary hypertension, the use of epidural anesthesia is more controversial. In these patients the use of epidural narcotics can be used to minimize the risk of maternal hypotension. Patients with cardiac lesions in group 2 or 3 will usually benefit from the use of a Swan-Ganz catheter during labor. In the majority of cardiac diseases, the route of delivery should be influenced mainly by obstetric factors as there is no evidence cesarean delivery reduces morbidity and may instead increase it. The exception to this rule is when invasive monitoring is not available when needed and then a cesarean delivery may be necessary.

Specific Cardiac Defects

The incidence of myocardial infarction (MI) in pregnancy has been reported to be 1/10,000, and fewer than 100 cases have been reported. The mortality rate in the largest series of 68 women was 37%, with an increased risk of death if the infarction occurred in the third trimester or at the time of delivery (45%). The highest risk was seen if the MI occurred within 2 weeks of delivery (50%). No maternal deaths occurred if delivery was greater than two weeks after the initial or recurrent infarction. The fetal loss rate was high at 34%. The amount of residual cardiac function after the infarction appears to be a major prognostic factor of pregnancy outcome. If the MI occurs at less than 14 to 16 weeks gestation, pregnancy termination should be considered because of the potential for reinfarction and the ability to perform the procedure with minimal difficulty. If the pregnancy is continued, efforts need to be made to decrease myocardial O_2 demand by using medical therapy and by limiting maternal exertion with adequate bed rest. The use of β-blockers, calcium channel blockers, digoxin, nitrates, or antiarrhythmic agents is not altered by the pregnancy. The delivery and the immediate puerperium represent the period of greatest risk. These patients may need Swan-Ganz catheterization, and as with the majority of cardiac diseases the route of delivery should be influenced mainly by obstetric factors because there is no evidence cesarean delivery reduces morbidity.

Mitral stenosis is the most common rheumatic valvular lesion that complicates pregnancy. The primary hemodynamic problem caused by mitral stenosis involves the obstruction of ventricular diastolic filling caused by the narrowed mitral valve orifice. This can lead to a decrease in cardiac output and a rise in the pulmonary capillary wedge pressure (PCWP) and can result in pulmonary edema and cardiac failure. Cardiac output in individuals with mitral stenosis largely depends on maintaining an adequate diastolic filling time and an adequate left ventricular preload. The diastolic filling time is greatly affected by the maternal heart rate, and in patients with mitral stenosis tachycardia may contribute significantly to hemodynamic instability. A major risk to these women is the development of atrial fibrillation, which frequently will result in CHF. In the presence of mitral stenosis, the PCWP is not an accurate reflection of the left ventricular preload, and these individuals often require a high-normal or elevated PCWP to maintain an adequate left ventricular preload and cardiac output. The greatest risk to these patients during pregnancy is the development of CHF, which can result in maternal death. The increase in cardiac output during pregnancy can exceed the heart's capacity to pump blood across the narrowed mitral valve and result in CHF. Approximately 25% of women with mitral stenosis develop symptoms for the first time during pregnancy. The third trimester, labor and delivery, and the immediate puerperium are the periods during pregnancy with the greatest increase in maternal cardiac output, and this is when the risk of developing CHF is highest. Overall, 12% to 20% of women develop CHF, with an associated maternal mortality rate of 14% to 17%. The risk of maternal mortality with NYHA class I or II is ≤1%, but increases to 4% to 5% with class III or IV and 15% with preexistent atrial fibrillation. Women with rheumatic heart disease are at increased risk for redeveloping rheumatic fever and therefore should receive prophylaxis with either monthly intramuscular benzathine penicillin or daily oral penicillin. The time of greatest risk is in the immediate postpartum period. In patients in NYHA class III or IV or with moderate to severe stenosis, the use of a Swan-Ganz catheter is recommended. It should be placed either before an induction or early in labor. To prevent maternal tachycardia in women with significant mitral stenosis, oral β-blocker therapy should be given if the maternal pulse exceeds 90 beats/minute at the start of labor. Rarely, intravenous β-blockers will be needed to control acute tachycardia. Because of the increase in cardiac output during labor, these patients are often functioning at maximum cardiac output and may not be able to handle the rapid increase in the preload that occurs immediately after delivery. This postpartum autotransfusion is felt to be the result of the release of vena caval obstruction and the return of blood back into the central circulation from the uterus as a result of the uterine contractions after delivery. This can result in an increase in the PCWP of 10 to 16 mmHG and result in acute pulmonary edema unless the patient's PCWP is maintained at 14 to 16 mmHg before delivery.

Aortic stenosis can be either rheumatic or congenital (bicuspid aortic valve), and both are rarely encountered during pregnancy. Fortunately, when aortic stenosis does complicate pregnancy, the lesions are usually not severe. Severe disease is uncommon during the childbearing years because of its slow, progressive nature, with the average age of clinical presentation being 48. Clinical signs of critical aortic stenosis are angina, syncope, and dyspnea. Because of the hypervolemia of pregnancy, which increases the preload to the left ventricle and thus improves cardiac output, most women with aortic stenosis tolerate pregnancy well. If the mitral valve is normal and physical activity is limited, pulmonary edema is rare. The exception to this occurs with critical aortic stenosis when the lesion is so severe it prevents an increase in the cardiac output. Women with aortic stenosis are at greatest risk from a decrease in the cardiac output, which can lead to sudden death. Any factor that causes a decrease in venous return or hypotension will cause an increase in the valvular gradient and result in a diminished cardiac output. Therefore these women are at the greatest risk during delivery because of increased risk of hypotension from blood loss, epidurals, or occlusions of the vena cava by the uterus in the supine position. The perinatal mortality rate of continued pregnancies is 4%. Women with shunt gradients exceeding 100 mm Hg are at greatest risk, and women with shunts less than 50 mm Hg usually tolerate pregnancy well. Labor management encompasses the goal of avoiding maternal tachycardia and maintaining hemodynamic parameters within a narrow therapeutic window. Small decreases in the preload may result in decreased cardiac output and sudden death, whereas increases in the vascular volume can produce an increase in the PCWP and result in pulmonary edema. The use of Swan-Ganz catheter is warranted in these patients. Because the risk of hypovolemia is a far greater threat to the patient than is pulmonary edema, the PCWP should be maintained in the range of 18 mm Hg to maintain a margin of safety against unexpected peripartum blood loss.

Atrial septal defects are the most common congenital lesions seen during pregnancy. Atrial septal defects are usually asymptomatic and rarely cause problems during pregnancy unless associated with arrhythmias or the rare occurrence of pulmonary hypertension. The size of the ventricular septal defect is the most important predictor of pregnancy outcome. Small defects rarely cause problems, whereas larger defects more frequently cause CHF, arrhythmias, or pulmonary hypertension. For the patient with uncomplicated septal defects, labor and delivery is well tolerated and minimal intervention is required.

Women with pulmonary hypertension or Eisenmenger syndrome are always in danger of sudden death; however, pregnancy is a time of particular hazard, especially during labor and delivery and the early postpartum period when maternal mortality is 50%. Eisenmenger syndrome occurs when a congenital left-to-right shunt causes progressive pulmonary hypertension that leads to shunt reversal (right-to-left) with resultant hypoxemia and cyanosis. Unlike the majority of other cardiac defects, which have shown improved maternal survival in recent years, these cardiac lesions continue to have a dismal prognosis. Causes of maternal death include thromboembolic disorders, acute heart failure from hypovolemia, and idiopathic deaths at 4 to 6 week post partum. These deaths are thought to be the result of worsening of the pulmonary hypertension secondary to the loss of pregnancy-associated hormones and appear to be unpreventable. The overall fetal loss rate in these women is between 50% to 75%, with an increased risk of fetal growth restriction, prematurity, and neonatal cardiac defects. These women should be strongly advised against pregnancy and need to be advised that pregnancy termination is probably safer than continuing the pregnancy during the first half of gestation. If these women plan to attempt a successful pregnancy, hospitalization for the duration of pregnancy is recommended. In addition, supplemental oxygen may need to be used to maintain a maternal Po_2 at 60 to 70 mmHg. A Swan-Ganz catheter should be used during labor and delivery if technically possible. The primary concern needs to be the avoidance of hypotension to maintain pulmonary blood flow even at the risk of developing some degree of pulmonary edema. Because of the risk of sudden postpartum cardiac decompensation, these patients need to be carefully followed in the initial weeks after delivery.

Marfan syndrome is a variably expressed autosomal dominant disorder characterized by a generalized weakness of connective tissue resulting in skeletal, ocular, and cardiovascular abnormalities. The connective tissue weakness in the aorta can result in aortic aneurysms, rupture, or dissection. In women with an aortic root diameter of more than 40 mm, the maternal mortality rate is up to 50% and pregnancy should be avoided. If the aortic root is less than 40 mm Hg and there is not moderate to severe aortic regurgitation, then the mortality rate is less than 5% (0/21 in one study). In this group of women, pregnancy does not seem to affect the long-term prognosis. In women choosing to risk pregnancy, the aortic root should be measured every 8 to 12 weeks by echocardiogram. If there is a rapidly expanding aortic root, then consideration for pregnancy termination is required. The use of β-blockers during the third trimester and at delivery has been recommended previously; however, there is no evidence they prevent complications in women with aortic roots <40 mm. Genetic counseling is necessary; the risk of the neonate developing Marfan syndrome is 50% and prenatal diagnosis is not available.

KEY POINTS

1 The physiologic changes of pregnancy lead to a number of changes in maternal physical signs and symptoms that can mimic cardiac or respiratory disease and make it more difficult to determine if true disease is present.

2 Asthma is one of the most common illnesses that affects pregnant women. The risk of uncontrolled asthma is more dangerous than the medications used in treating it.

3 Pneumonia is one of the most common nonobstetric infections to cause serious maternal morbidity and mortality.

4 Cardiac disease is still a leading cause of indirect maternal death during pregnancy.

5 Two classification schemes are used to better clarify the risks of pregnancy in women with specific cardiac lesions. The first is the New York Heart Association (NYHA) classification and is based on the women's functional status before or early in pregnancy. The second is based on the specific maternal risk of each individual cardiac lesion found in past studies.

SUGGESTED READINGS

ACOG: *Cardiac disease in pregnancy,* Technical bulletin number 168, June 1992, ACOG.

American Thoracic Society: Treatment of tuberculosis and tuberculosis infection in adults and children, *Am J Respir Crit Care Med* 149:1359, 1994.

Bhagwat AR, Engel PJ: Heart disease and pregnancy, *Cardiol Clin* 13(2):163, 1995.

Clark SL: Asthma in pregnancy, *Obstet Gynecol* 82:1036, 1993.

Clark SL: Cardiac disease in pregnancy, *Obstet Gynecol Clin North Am* 18(2):237, 1991.

Lao TT et al: Congenital aortic stenosis and pregnancy: a reappraisal, *Am J Obstet Gynecol* 169:540, 1993.

Patton DE et al: Cyanotic maternal heart disease in pregnancy, *Obstet Gynecol Surv* 45(9):594, 1990.

Perlow JH et al: Severity of asthma and perinatal outcome, *Am J Obstet Gynecol* 167:963, 1992.

Richey SD et al: Pneumonia complicating pregnancy, *Obstet Gynecol* 84:525, 1994.

Zeldis SM: Dyspnea during pregnancy: distinguishing cardiac from pulmonary causes, *Clin Chest Med* 13(4):567, 1992.

Diabetes

MARK B. LANDON

Fetal and neonatal mortality rates have been reduced from approximately 65% before the discovery of insulin to 2% to 5% at present. Excluding major congenital malformations, the perinatal mortality rate for the insulin-dependent woman receiving optimal care is nearly equivalent to that observed in normal pregnancies.

Gestational diabetes mellitus (GDM), a state of carbohydrate intolerance restricted to pregnant women whose disorder is discovered during pregnancy, is a controversial diagnosis. GDM represents nearly 90% of the cases of diabetes complicating pregnancy and affects 1% to 3% of the pregnant population. The association of various neonatal morbidities common to preexisting insulin-dependent diabetes with GDM has made screening and treatment common in the United States.

PATHOPHYSIOLOGY

In normal pregnancy, early rises in maternal estrogen and progesterone levels lead to B cell hyperplasia and increased insulin secretion. Relative maternal fasting hypoglycemia accompanies an increased peripheral utilization of glucose. Increased HPL levels stimulate lipolysis in adipose tissue. HPL is responsible in part for the diabetogenic state of pregnancy. In normal pregnant women, glucose homeostasis is maintained by increased insulin secretion to counteract the decreased sensitivity to insulin at the cellular level. Glucose crosses the placenta by carrier-mediated facilitated diffusion. Insulin and other protein hormones do not cross the placenta. Fetal blood glucose levels usually remain 20 to 30 mg/dl lower than maternal levels. Elevation of maternal glucose levels (raised glycosylated hemoglobin concentration) during the first trimester has been associated with an increased risk for congenital anomalies in the offspring of women with preexisting diabetes. The overall rate of anomalies is approximately three times higher than in nondiabetic population. Although excess glucose is an apparent teratogen, other factors may contribute to the high malformation rate. Persistently elevated levels of maternal glucose lead to fetal hyperglycemia and result in fetal B cell hyperplasia and hyperinsulinemia. Excessive growth or macrosomia may result (Pedersen hypothesis). Fetal hyperglycemia and hyperinsulinemia may contribute to an increased risk of stillbirth and neonatal morbidities such as RDS, hypoglycemia, hyperbilirubinemia, hypocalcemia, polycythemia, and cardiomegaly.

Table 36-2 presents a classification of diabetes in pregnancy. Renal disease (class F) is observed in 5% to 10% of patients. This includes those with reduced creatinine clearance and/or proteinuria of at least 400 mg in 24 hours measured during the first 20 weeks gestation. These pregnancies are at increased risk for preterm delivery, fetal growth restriction, and preeclampsia. Pregnancy probably does not affect the progression of diabetic nephropathy. Pregnancy conveys a greater than twofold independent risk for the progression of retinopathy. Progression to prolif-

TABLE 36-2
White Classification of Diabetes in Pregnancy

Class	Age of onset (years)		Duration (years)	Vascular disease	Insulin
A_1	Any		Any	None	0
A_2	Any		Any	None	+
B	Over 20		<10	None	+
C	10-19	or	10-19	None	+
D	<10		>20	Benign retinopathy	+
F	Any		Any	Nephropathy	+
R	Any		Any	Proliferative retinopathy	+
H	Any		Any	Heart disease	+

erative retinopathy is rare in women with background retinal changes or those with normal exams. Proliferative eye disease should be treated before conception.

DETECTION

The majority of cases of diabetes during pregnancy are gestational diabetes. These women represent a group with significant risk for overt diabetes in later life (greater than 50% at 15-year follow-up). Controversy exists as to whether all pregnant women should be screened for gestational diabetes. Reliance on risk factors (e.g., age, previous stillbirth, previous large infant) will detect only 50% of cases. Screening is performed at 24 to 28 weeks of gestation with a 50 g oral glucose load, followed by a plasma glucose determination 1 hour later. An abnormal screening value (135 to 140 mg/dl) necessitates a diagnostic 3-hour oral glucose tolerance test.

TREATMENT (Fig. 36-3)

Treatment involves self-monitoring of glucose with frequent glucose assessments (fasting, preprandial, and postprandial). Fasting levels are maintained at <100 mg/dl and postprandial (2 hours) at less than 120 mg/dl. Multiple insulin injection regimens will be employed by the majority of patients to achieve these goals. An insulin pump is maintained for women well controlled with this therapy. Diet therapy is critical to successful glucoregulation. A program of three meals and several snacks is employed. Dietary composition is 50% to 60% carbohydrate, 20% protein, and 25% to 30% fat. Caloric intake is based on prepregnancy weight, with caloric restriction (less than 1600 kcal/day); and weight loss is not advised. Ophthalmologic and renal status are evaluated each trimester at a minimum. Fetal surveillance consists of MSAFP at 16 to 18 weeks gestation, sonogram at 18 to 20 weeks to rule out anomalies, fetal echocardiography

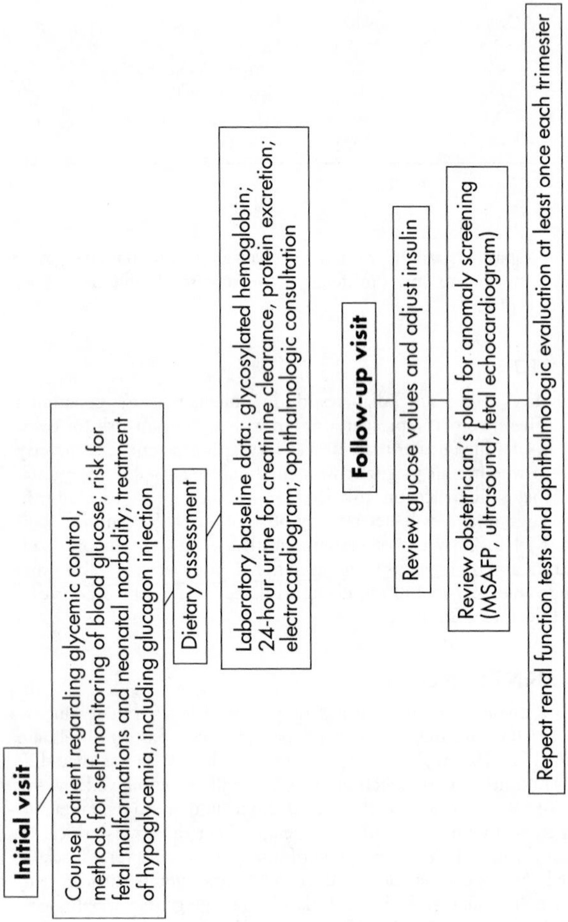

Initial visit

Counsel patient regarding glycemic control, methods for self-monitoring of blood glucose; risk for fetal malformations and neonatal morbidity; treatment of hypoglycemia, including glucagon injection

Dietary assessment

Laboratory baseline data: glycosylated hemoglobin; 24-hour urine for creatinine clearance, protein excretion; electrocardiogram; ophthalmologic consultation

Follow-up visit

Review glucose values and adjust insulin

Review obstetrician's plan for anomaly screening (MSAFP, ultrasound, fetal echocardiogram)

Repeat renal function tests and ophthalmologic evaluation at least once each trimester

FIG. 36-3 Management of the pregestational diabetic pregnancy.

at 20 to 22 weeks, and serial sonography to assess fetal growth. Antenatal detection of macrosomia is limited by the error of ultrasound measurements of fetal weight. Fetal heart rate testing (nonstress test [NST]) or biophysical profiles (BPP) are performed during the third trimester, and daily fetal movement counting is done by women with insulin-dependent diabetes.

TIMING AND MODE OF DELIVERY

Elective delivery is often planned at 38 weeks after ensuring fetal lung maturity by amniocentesis. In well-controlled patients without vasculopathy and with secure dating, delivery may be delayed until 39 to 40 weeks. Amniocentesis is not generally performed in such cases. Preterm delivery is indicated for suspected fetal jeopardy, worsening maternal vascular disease, and preeclampsia. Cesarean delivery rates are declining for women with insulin-dependent diabetes mellitus. An arrest pattern in labor should alert the obstetrician to the possibility of cephalopelvic disproportion (CPD) and/or fetal macrosomia. Shoulder dystocia is more common in diabetic pregnancies. Euglycemia should be maintained throughout labor. Continuous insulin infusion and frequent glucose testing are mandatory.

MANAGEMENT OF GESTATIONAL DIABETES

For gestational diabetes, dietary therapy of 2000 to 2500 kcal/day without concentrated sweets is recommended. As a guideline, insulin therapy is reserved for repeated fasting hyperglycemia (>105 mg/dl) and/or postprandial hyperglycemia (>120 mg/dl at 2 hours postprandial). Women with GDM are at low risk for an intrauterine fetal demise. Patients with a history of stillbirth, preeclampsia, or those requiring insulin should undergo the same fetal testing as insulin-dependent women. Finally, ultrasound assessment of fetal size before delivery is recommended (Fig. 36-4).

COUNSELING

A reduced rate of congenital malformations is observed in women seeking prepregnancy consultation and care for their disease. Glycosylated hemoglobin levels obtained during the first trimester may be used to counsel diabetic women regarding the risk for an anomalous infant. Although the diabetic population has not been studied specifically, folic acid dietary supplementation with a dose of at least 0.4 mg daily should be prescribed to reduce the frequency of NTDs. Low-dose oral contraception appears to be safe in insulin-dependent women without vascular disease and in former GDM women. Lipid profiles should be obtained in each case. Little information is available concerning long-acting progestins in women with diabetes or previous GDM.

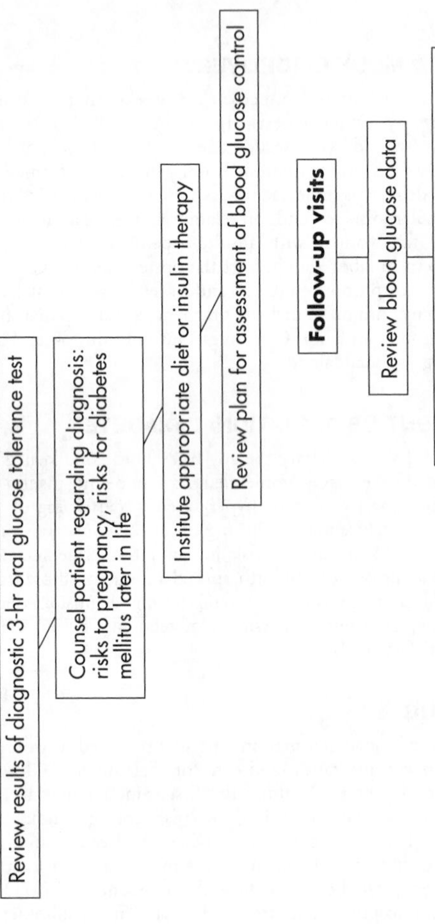

FIG. 36-4 Management of the gestational diabetic pregnancy.

KEY POINTS

1 During pregnancy in the insulin-dependent diabetic woman, periods of maternal hyperglycemia lead to fetal hyperglycemia and thus fetal pancreatic stimulation. The resulting fetal hyperinsulinemia is associated with excessive fetal growth and other morbidities.

2 Congenital malformations are two to four times more common in the offspring of insulin-dependent diabetic women.

3 Women with diabetic nephropathy are at increased risk for preeclampsia, fetal growth restriction, and early delivery. Management involves control of maternal hypertension and intensive fetal surveillance.

4 Screening for gestational diabetes, a disorder of carbohydrate intolerance discovered during pregnancy, should be undertaken at 24 to 28 weeks gestation.

5 Delivery of the insulin-dependent diabetic patient should be delayed until fetal maturation has taken place, provided that the patient is well controlled and that antepartum fetal surveillance remains reassuring.

SUGGESTED READINGS

ACOG: *Diabetes and pregnancy,* Technical bulletin number 200, December, 1994, ACOG.

Chew EY et al: Metabolic control and progression of retinopathy: the diabetes in early pregnancy study, *Diabetes Care* 18:631, 1995.

Gordon M et al: Perinatal outcome and long-term follow-up associated with modern management of diabetic nephropathy (class F), *Obstet Gynecol,* 87:401-409, 1996.

Greene MF: Prevention and diagnosis of congenital anomalies in diabetic pregnancies, *Clin Perinatol* 20:533, 1993.

Greene MF, Benacerraf B: Prenatal diagnosis in diabetic gravidas: utility of ultrasound and MSAFP screening, *Obstet Gynecol* 77:420-425, 1991.

Jovanovic-Peterson L, Peterson CM: Nutritional management of the obese gestational diabetic pregnant woman, *J Am Coll Nutr* 11:246-250, 1992.

Landon MB et al: Fetal surveillance in pregnancies complicated by insulin-dependent diabetes mellitus, *Am J Obstet Gynecol* 167:617-621, 1992.

Perinatal mortality and congenital malformations in infants born to women with insulin dependent diabetes, *MMWR* 29:363, 1990.

Summary and recommendations of the Third International Workshop Conference, *Diabetes* (Suppl 2), 1991.

Endocrine Abnormalities

MARK B. LANDON

PATHOPHYSIOLOGY

The thyroid gland is functioning maximally during normal pregnancy. Basal metabolic rate is elevated in pregnant women. Enlargement of the thyroid gland during gestation is believed to be a compensatory mechanism to maintain gland activity despite a decrease in plasma inorganic iodine.

Laboratory assessment of thyroid function is altered by pregnancy. Under estrogen stimulation, hepatic synthesis of thyroid-binding globulin (TBG) rises to levels twice normal by 12 weeks gestation. Measurements of total serum thyroxine (T_4) include bound as well as the minute fraction of biologically active free T_4. Minor elevations of free T_4 and T_3 can be demonstrated in early pregnancy and then decline with advancing gestation. However, serum levels of free T_4, free T_3, and TSH remain in the normal nonpregnant range during gestation. When assays for free T_3 and T_4 are not available, an estimate of free hormone activity is generally obtained by employing the T_3 resin uptake test.

Hyperthyroidism

Hyperthyroidism complicates 0.2% of pregnancies. Although pregnancy does not worsen the disease, uncontrolled disease does increase neonatal morbidity as a result of preterm birth and low birthweight. Approximately 1% of offspring of women with Graves' disease demonstrate hyperthyroidism through placental passage of thyroid-stimulating immune globulin.

Graves' disease is the most common cause of hyperthyroidism, resulting in diffuse glandular enlargement. *Toxic nodular goiter, thyrotoxicosis factitia,* and *gestational trophoblastic disease* are less common etiologies.

Normal symptoms of pregnancy may be confused with hyperthyroidism (e.g., heat intolerance, nervousness, and mild tachycardia). Resting tachycardia (>100 bpm) or weight loss should suggest possible hyperthyroidism. Ophthalmologic signs such as exophthalmos and lid lag are helpful diagnostic clues. Patients with hyperemesis may also have underlying biochemical hyperthyroidism. It is unusual for such women to have clinical signs of hyperthyroidism. The biochemical abnormalities generally return to normal by 18 weeks gestation. Laboratory diagnosis consists of elevated free thyroxine levels. As T_4 increases with normal pregnancy, FT_4I must be calculated if free thyroxine levels are not available.

Treatment involves medical therapy consisting of propylthiouracil (PTU) or methimazole. PTU is preferred because methimazole has been associated with aplasia cutis of the scalp of newborns. Surgery is indicated only in cases refractory to medical therapy. Thyroid function should be assessed every 2 weeks and PTU dosage adjusted accordingly. In one third of cases, PTU may be discontinued during the second half of pregnancy. PTU crosses the placenta and may cause fetal hypothyroidism. Prompt therapy in the newborn period probably prevents neurologic sequelae.

Thyroid storm is an uncommon endocrinologic emergency. It is seen in undiagnosed and partially treated patients. It may result in cardiovascular collapse. Hyperpyrexia (>102° F), tachycardia, and agitation are symptoms. Treatment consists of propranolol administration, vigorous fluid replacement, antipyretics, and antithyriod medication (sodium iodide or oral SSKI solution followed by PTU therapy).

Hypothyroidism

Hypothyroidism is rare in pregnancy because most hypothyroid women are infertile. The effect on pregnancy is controversial. The rate of stillbirth, miscarriage, preeclampsia, and fetal growth restriction may be increased.

The diagnosis is made in the presence of low FT_4I and an elevated TSH level. Treatment of hypothyroidism begins with 0.05 to 0.1 mg/day of L-thyroxine (Synthroid) with the dose increased to a maximum of 0.2 mg/day. Therapy is guided by following TSH levels, which may take weeks to return to baseline. The outcome of treated pregnancies is generally good.

Postpartum Thyroid Dysfunction

The usual pattern of postpartum thyroid dysfunction is hyperthyroidism followed by transient hypothyroidism with subsequent recovery. Postpartum thyroid dysfunction is characterized by destructive lymphocytic thyroiditis. Thyrotoxicosis develops as a result of gland destruction, making PTU ineffective and peripheral beta-blockade the treatment if symptoms are severe. Approximately two thirds of women who develop transient hyperthyroidism return to a euthyroid state, whereas one third develop hypothyroidism.

Hyperparathyroidism

It is rare to encounter hyperparathyroidism in pregnancy, though detection may increase with automated serum Ca determinations. It is associated with increased perinatal morbidity and mortality. Stillbirth is increased, as are neonatal deaths (2%) from tetany (15% of cases). Neonatal tetany results from fetal hypercalcemia and subsequent fetal parathyroid suppression.

Symptoms include fatigue, muscle weakness, constipation, abdominal pain, bone pain, fractures, and nephrolithiasis signifying progressive disease. Laboratory diagnosis consists of elevated serum Ca^{++} and reduced serum phosphate levels. Marked phosphaturia may be present. PTH levels that are increased in normal pregnancy are elevated out of proportion to serum calcium levels.

Medical therapy employing oral phosphate may be attempted in mild cases, particularly if delivery can be accomplished. Surgical therapy is indicated if marked hypercalcemia and progressive symptoms are present.

Hypoparathyroidism

Hypoparathyroidism is also an uncommon disorder resulting from inadvertent parathyroidectomy or as an autoimmune process. The principal concern in pregnancy is inadequate transfer of calcium to the fetus with subsequent secondary hyperparathyroidism in the fetus (bone demineralization). The diagnosis is established by the presence of hypocalcemia, hyperphosphatemia, prior neck surgery, irritability, and tetany. Trousseau's sign (carpopedal spasm) is also indicative. Treatment is medical with supplemental calcium 1 to 4 g/day and 100,000 to 150,000 IU vitamin D or calcitriol 2 to 3 mg/day.

Prolactin-Producing Adenomas

With use of ovulation induction and prolactin suppression by bromocriptine, pregnancy is becoming more common in women with prolactinomas. Most women with microadenomas (<1 cm) have uneventful pregnancies, but 5% will experience symptoms of headache and visual disturbance.

Visual field and ophthalmologic examinations are reserved for symptomatic patients. Bromocriptine therapy is indicated if these symptoms appear. Transsphenoidal surgery is rarely necessary. Breastfeeding is not contraindicated in these women.

In women with macroadenomas (>1 cm) definitive therapy (surgery or radiation) is preferred before attempting pregnancy because more than one third of patients will experience symptoms during pregnancy. Visual field and ophthalmologic examination should be performed at least each trimester. Symptoms are treated primarily with bromocriptine. If fetal maturity is established in a symptomatic patient, delivery should be accomplished.

Diabetes Insipidus

Diabetes insipidus (DI) is a rare disorder of inadequate antidiuretic (vasopressin) production by the protein pituitary gland and rarely complicates pregnancy. Massive polyuria and dilute urine (sp. grav <1.005) are characteristic findings. Polyuria and urinary hyposmolarity continue despite water restriction. DI may worsen during pregnancy because of the increased glomerular filtration rate. Treatment consists of intranasal L-deamino-8-d-arginine (DDAVP) administration.

Pituitary Insufficiency

Sheehan's syndrome is postpartum ischemic necrosis of the anterior pituitary, which is typically observed after severe postpartum hemorrhage and hypotensive shock. Delayed diagnosis is extremely common. Failure to lactate is often an early finding. Progression of disease leads to loss of axillary and pubic hair, oligomenorrhea or amenorrhea, and senile vaginal atrophy. Hypothyroidism is present with advanced disease. Treatment consists of replacing the multiple deficient hormones, and patients may conceive with replacement hormonal therapy (87% live-birth rate).

Cushing's Syndrome

Characterized by excess glucocorticoid production, Cushing's syndrome is usually secondary to excess ACTH production by a pituitary adenoma. Other etiologies include adrenal tumor, neoplastic ectopic ACTH production, nodular adrenal hyperplasia, and exogenous corticosteroid therapy. Clinical features may initially be difficult to distinguish from normal pregnancy (e.g., weakness, weight gain, edema, striae, hypertension, and impaired glucose tolerance). Early-onset hypertension, early bruising, and proximal myopathy suggest Cushing's syndrome. Pregnancy in women with Cushing's syndrome is marked by a high rate of preterm delivery and stillbirths in cases not terminated. Women with adenomas almost invariably develop hypertension during pregnancy.

The diagnosis of Cushing's syndrome is established by laboratory assays. Elevated serum cortisol with failure to suppress with dexamethasone indicates Cushing's syndrome. Pregnant individuals may fail to suppress with a 1 mg (low dose) suppression test. Identification of the course of hormone production is necessary before treatment can be undertaken. Pituitary disease is treated surgically. Abdominal CT to rule out adrenal tumor is indicated if there is failure to suppress cortisol with a high dexamethasone test (8 mg). Fetal loss rates exceed 30% when definitive treatment is delayed.

Adrenal Insufficiency

Adrenal insufficiency may be primary (Addison's disease) or secondary to pituitary disease or exogenous adrenal suppression. Fatigue, weakness, anorexia, hypotension, hypoglycemia, and skin hyperpigmentation are common presenting complaints. Diagnosis is confirmed by decreased plasma cortisol levels and failure to stimulate cortisol production with Cortrosyn (synthetic ACTH) administration. Glucocorticoid replacement with prednisone and mineralocorticoid replacement with Florinef constitute treatment. Dosages may need to be adjusted during pregnancy, labor, and delivery.

Pheochromocytoma

This catecholamine-producing tumor arises from adrenal medulla or sympathetic nervous tissue and may be malignant in 10% of cases. Pheochromocytoma may present as hypertensive crisis with cerebral hemorrhage or severe congestive failures. The diagnosis is not established until postmortem in 30% of cases.

Symptoms mimic severe preeclampsia. Paroxysmal hypertension onset before 20 weeks and lack of significant proteinuria may be helpful in the differential diagnosis. Definitive diagnosis is made by laboratory measurement of catecholamines and metabolites (vanillylmandelic acid) in 24-hour urine collection. Phentolamine (L-adrenergic blocker) test should not be used in pregnancy because it may provoke severe hypotension.

Treatment includes localization of the tumor by CT scan, prompt surgical excision, and stabilization of the patient on α-blockers. Beta-blockade is reserved for treatment of arrhythmias. Cesarean delivery is preferred in untreated cases. Adrenal exploration may be performed.

KEY POINTS

1. Uncontrolled maternal hyperthyroidism is associated with an increased incidence of neonatal morbidity resulting from preterm birth and low birthweight.
2. The rates of stillbirth, miscarriage, preeclampsia, and growth restriction appears to be increased in hypothyroid women.
3. The usual pattern of postpartum thyroid dysfunction is hyperthyroidism followed by transient hypothyroidism with subsequent recovery.
4. Uncontrolled hyperparathyroidism is associated with an increased risk of stillbirth.
5. The vast majority of women with a prolactin-secreting pituitary microadenoma have uneventful pregnancies. Women with pituitary macroadenomas are more likely to experience symptomatic tumor enlargement during pregnancy.

6 Cesarean delivery is preferred for pheochromocytoma because it minimizes the potential catecholamine surges associated with labor and vaginal delivery.

SUGGESTED READINGS

Buescher MA, McClamrock HD, Adashi EY: Cushing's syndrome in pregnancy, *Obstet Gynecol* 79:130, 1992.

Davis LE et al: Thyrotoxicosis complicating pregnancy, *Am J Obstet Gynecol* 160:63, 1989.

Mandel SJ, Brent GA, Larsen PR: Review of antithyroid drug use during pregnancy and report of a case of aplasia cutis, *Thyroid* 4:129, 1994.

Sweeney WF, Katz VL: Recurrent pheochromocytoma during pregnancy, *Obstet Gynecol* 835:829, 1994.

Hematologic Complications

PHILIP SAMUELS

Hematologic complications are among the most common problems encountered in pregnancy. Although anemia is the most frequently encountered pregnancy-related hematologic abnormality, platelet disorders and aberrations in the coagulation cascade are also seen occasionally during pregnancy. Fig. 36-5 depicts one of many ways to evaluate the pregnant patient with anemia.

IRON DEFICIENCY ANEMIA

Arbitrarily using a hematocrit of 32% as a cutoff for anemia, approximately 50% of pregnant women are anemic. Roughly 75% of anemias that occur during gestation are classified as being caused by iron deficiency.

During a singleton pregnancy, the maternal plasma volume gradually expands by approximately 50%. During the same time, the total red blood cell (RBC) mass only increases by 30%. Because there is a relative deficiency of RBCs, this is often classified as an *iron deficiency anemia.* This anemia, however, is physiologic and not pathologic. It becomes pathologic if the patient has decreased iron stores from situations such as frequent conception, inadequate diet, or excessive blood loss. Such patients cannot mount a reticulocytosis as their hematocrit falls, and therefore the dilutional effect is exaggerated, leading to a more profound anemia. In the patient with normal iron stores, hemoglobin concentrations return to normal by 6 weeks post partum.

To clinically distinguish the normal physiologic changes of pregnancy from pathologic iron deficiency anemia, one must be familiar with the iron requirements of pregnancy and the proper use of laboratory parameters. The increased RBC mass requires 450 mg, the fetus and placenta require 360 mg, vaginal delivery requires 190 mg, and lactation necessitates 1 mg/day of elemental iron. A major storage form of iron is ferritin, which comprises approximately 25% of the 2 g of iron stores found in healthy

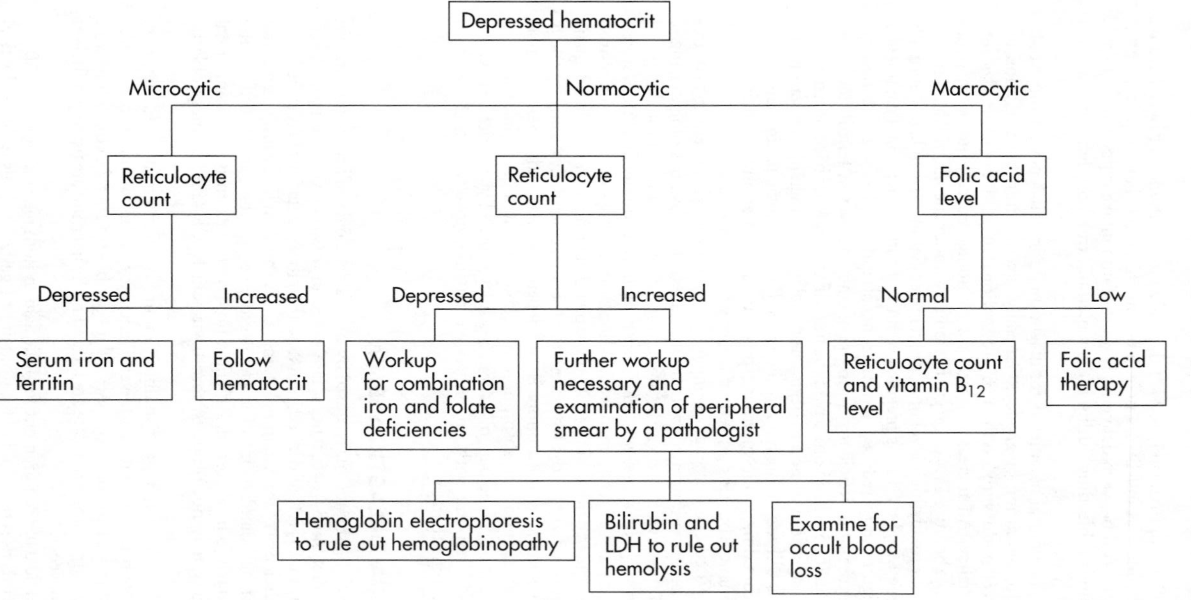

FIG. 36-5 Complex evaluation of anemia during pregnancy.

women. Approximately 65% of the body's iron is found in RBCs. Because of the increase in RBCs, a pregnant woman's iron balance is precarious. If the interval between deliveries is short, if iron intake is poor, or if there is significant bleeding during the puerperium, true iron deficiency anemia readily develops.

The normal parameters for diagnosing iron deficiency anemia can be confusing during pregnancy. Generally, a serum iron concentration less than 60 mg/dl with less than 16% saturation is suggestive of pathologic iron deficiency. An increase in total iron binding capacity, however, is not reliable because 15% of pregnant women without anemia will demonstrate an abnormally high level of this parameter. Serum ferritin levels normally decrease slightly during pregnancy, but stay within the normal parameters. A significantly reduced ferritin concentration is the best parameter to diagnose iron deficiency during pregnancy. However, ferritin levels can fluctuate 25% from one day to the next. If a woman has been iron depleted for a significant time and begins iron replacement therapy, her serum iron levels will rise before her ferritin levels. If hematologic parameters remain confounding, bone marrow aspiration can be performed safely during pregnancy, but this procedure is rarely necessary or indicated.

Whether all pregnant women need iron prophylaxis remains controversial. In a primigravida with mild anemia caused by physiologic changes, iron therapy other than the amount in prenatal vitamins probably is not necessary. In those who are at risk of having diminished iron stores, prophylaxis is recommended. Although many physicians prescribe iron three times daily, a single 325-mg tablet daily usually results in adequate prophylaxis. For those who need iron therapy, twice daily dosing is usually sufficient. Iron absorption is pH-dependent. Antacids therefore may decrease duodenal absorption of iron, and vitamin C may increase absorption. If the patient's anemia is soley caused by iron deficiency, she should respond with an impressive reticulocytosis within 2 weeks of beginning therapy.

MEGALOBLASTIC ANEMIA

Megaloblastic anemia is caused by either a deficiency of folate or of vitamin B_{12}. Vitamin B_{12} deficiency is rare, especially in women of childbearing age. Vitamin B_{12} is found in red meats and therefore vegetarians may suffer from a deficiency of this vitamin. Vitamin B_{12} is absorbed in the distal ileum and must be bound to intrinsic factor produced by the parietal cells of the stomach to be absorbed. Patients who have had extensive gastrointestinal surgery may not properly absorb vitmain B_{12}, leading to megaloblastic anemia.

Folic acid is a water-soluble vitamin found in green vegetables, dark yellow fruits, peanuts, and liver. Deficiency of this vitamin is responsible for the vast majority of cases of megaloblastic anemia coinciding with pregnancy. Stores of folate are located in the liver and are usually sufficient for 6 weeks.

The daily requirement for folic acid in nonpregnant women is 50 μg, and this rises threefold to fourfold during gestation. This is caused by fetal demands and the decrease in gastrointestinal absorption of folate during pregnancy. Most diets contain adequate folic acid, and nonprescription prenatal vitamins contain 0.8 mg of folic acid whereas prescription vitamins contain 1 mg. Therefore most pregnant women receive adequate folic acid. It is recommended that women at risk of giving birth to a child with NTD take 4 mg of folic acid daily. Women with significant hemoglobinopathies, patients receiving phenytoin and other liver-metabolized anticonvulsants, women carrying multiple gestations, and those with frequent conceptions are at risk of folic acid deficiency. If the patient is truly folic acid–deficient, she should respond with a reticulocytosis about 3 days after beginning therapy. Testing for serum folate is now rapid and readily available. This immunoassay is often linked with an assay for vitamin B_{12} so that both results are obtained even if only a folate level is ordered.

Iron deficiency is frequently concomitant with folic acid deficiency. These patients usually have normocytic normochromic anemia. If a patient with folate deficiency does not respond to therapy within a week, iron therapy should also be instituted after the appropriate tests for iron deficiency have been obtained.

HEMOGLOBINOPATHIES

Hemoglobin is a tetrameric protein comprised of two pairs of polypeptide chains with a heme group attached to each chain. Hemoglobin A_1 comprises 95% of hemoglobin in the adult with a hemoglobinopathy. The remaining 5% consists of hemoglobin A_2 and/or hemoglobin F. In the fetus, fetal hemoglobin (hemoglobin F) declines during the third trimester, reaching its permanent nadir several months after birth. Hemoglobinopathies occur when there is a change in the structure of a peptide chain or an inability to synthesize a specific polypeptide chain in the usual amount. The genetics of these hemoglobinopathies is often straightforward. The prevalence of the most common hemoglobinopathies in adult blacks is shown in Table 36-3.

TABLE 36-3
Frequency of Common Hemoglobinopathies in Adult Blacks in the United States

Type	Frequency
Hemoglobin AS	1 in 12
Hemoglobin SS	1 in 708
Hemoglobin AC	1 in 41
Hemoglobin CC	1 in 4790
Hemoglobin SC	1 in 757
Hemoglobin S/β-thalassemia	1 in 1672

Hemoglobin S

Hemoglobin S is a variant of hemoglobin A_1 with substitution of valine for glutamic acid in the sixth position of the β-chain. This single amino acid substitution causes the RBC to assume a sickle shape at low oxygen tensions, resulting in sludging in small vessels and microinfarction of the affected organs. Sickled RBCs have a lifespan of 5 to 10 days compared with 120 days for a normal RBC. Sickling is triggered by hypoxia, acidosis, and/or dehydration.

Patients with hemoglobin AS generally have 35% to 45% hemoglobin S and are usually asymptomatic. Because sickle cell disease (hemoglobin SS) is an autosomal recessive disorder, the child of two individuals who have hemoglobin AS has a 50% chance of having hemoglobin AS and a 25% chance of having symptomatic sickle cell disease (hemoglobin SS). Women at risk for having hemoglobin S should be screened at their first prenatal visit. If the screen is positive, these individuals and their partners should undergo hemoglobin fractionation (hemoglobin electrophoresis) to determine if it is appropriate to offer prenatal diagnosis. Prenatal diagnosis of sickle cell disease can be performed by DNA analysis with PCR and southern blotting.

Painful vasoocclusive episodes involving multiple organ systems as well as the bones and joints are the clinical hallmark of sickle cell anemia. No organ system is immune to these painful crises. Osteomyelitis is not rare in these patients, and salmonella osteomyelitis is found almost exclusively in conjunction with sickle cell disease. There is an increased incidence of pyelonephritis in patients with sickle cell disease, especially during pregnancy. In severe cases, sickling can occur in the renal medulla, resulting in papillary necrosis. Because these patients have decreased RBC survival and chronic hemolysis, they often demonstrate mild jaundice, and bilirubin gallstone can be found in 30% of women with sickle cell disease. The chronic anemia can also result in left ventricular hypertrophy and eventually high-output CHF. Analgesia, oxygen, and hydration are the clinical foundation for treating painful crises regardless of the organ system involved, and this is also true during pregnancy.

Sickle cell disease (hemoglobin SS) is associated with poor pregnancy outcomes. The rate of spontaneous abortion may be as high as 25%. The perinatal mortality rate is approximately 15%. Much of the perinatal mortality is related to preterm birth, which may occur secondary to idiopathic preterm labor, maternal indications, or fetal indications (such as growth restriction and nonreassuring fetal well-being). About one third of infants born to mothers with sickle cell disease weigh less than 2500 g at birth, some a result of prematurity and others IUGR. IUGR may be caused by sickling in the smaller uterine vessels, resulting in a chronic decrease in fetal oxygenation and thus delayed fetal growth.

There is an increased risk of third trimester stillbirth in patients with hemoglobin SS, with rates approaching 8%. These fetal losses do not occur only at times of sickle cell crisis, but may occur with no maternal symptoms whatsoever. Because of this finding, stringent antepartum fetal testing, including serial sonography to assess fetal growth, is encouraged.

A care plan for each trimester is shown in Fig. 36-6. Patients should be

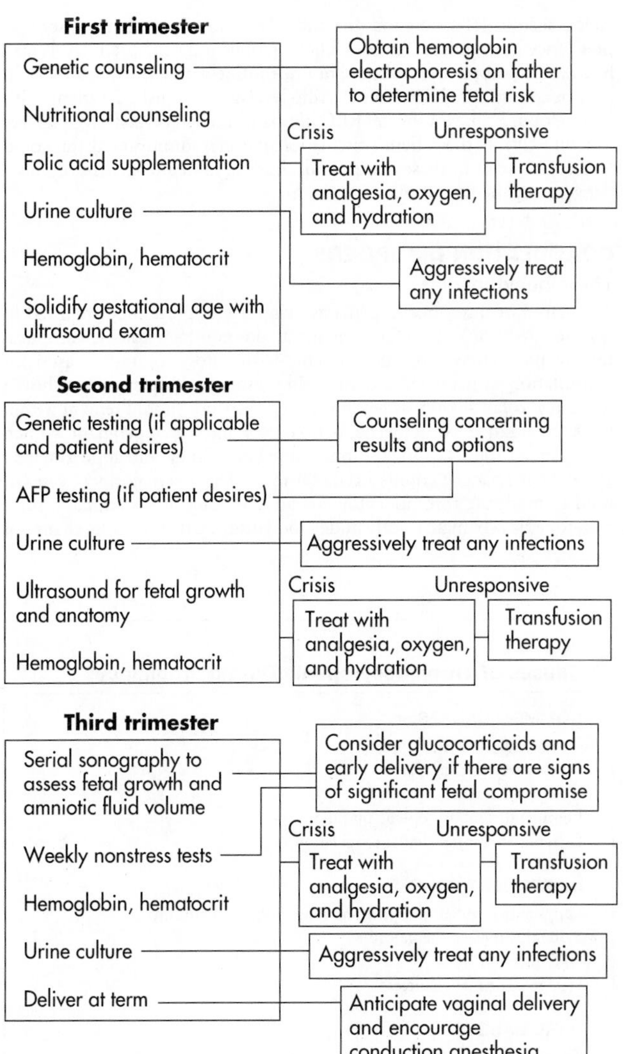

FIG. 36-6 Systemic approach to prenatal care in a patient with sickle cell disease.

encouraged to follow a good diet and take folate supplements as soon as pregnancy is diagnosed. Although hemoglobin and hematocrit levels may be low, iron supplements should not be routinely prescribed. Iron should only be administered if iron and ferritin levels are diminished. Patients with hemoglobin SS have a shorter RBC lifespan, and hemolyzed RBCs release iron directly into the patient's circulation. If iron is administered, this could lead to an excess of these compounds, leading to hemosiderosis or, more dangerously, hemochromatosis.

COAGULATION DISORDERS

Thrombocytopenia

The causes of thrombocytopenia associated with pregnancy are listed in Box 36-2. Although anemia is the most common hematologic complication of pregnancy, thrombocytopenia is the most common reason for consultation with a hematologist during gestation. Platelet counts show a tendency to fall slightly as gestation progresses but should remain within the normal range. Nonetheless, between 4% and 7% of pregnant women have platelet counts $<150,000/mm^3$ during pregnancy, and approximately 1% will have platelet counts $<100,000/mm^3$. The vast majority of cases of mild to moderate thrombocytopenia are the result of gestational thrombocytopenia, a benign, poorly understood disorder that has little chance of

BOX 36-2

Causes of Thrombocytopenia During Pregnancy

COMMON CAUSES

Gestational thrombocytopenia
Severe preeclampsia
HELLP syndrome
Immune thrombocytopenic purpura
Disseminated intravascular coagulation

INFREQUENT CAUSES

Lupus anticoagulant/antiphospholipid antibody syndrome
Systemic lupus erythematosus
HIV infection
Hematologic malignancies

RARE CAUSES

Thrombotic thrombocytopenic purpura
Hemolytic uremic syndrome
Type IIb von Willebrand's disease
Folic acid deficiency
May-Hegglin anomaly (congenital thrombocytopenia)

causing maternal or neonatal problems. Obstetricians, however, are obliged to rule out other forms of thrombocytopenia that are associated with severe maternal and/or perinatal morbidity. In general, lower platelet counts are more likely to represent a more serious condition.

Gestational Thrombocytopenia

Patients with gestational thrombocytopenia usually have mild (platelet count 100,000/mm^3 to 149,000/mm^3) or moderate (platelet count 50,000/mm^3 to 99,000/mm^3) thrombocytopenia. These patients usually require no therapy, and the fetus appears to be at little, if any, risk of being born with profound thrombocytopenia (platelet count <50,000/mm^3). The decrease in platelet count in patients with gestational thrombocytopenia is not merely the result of dilution of platelets with increasing blood volume. It appears to be caused by an acceleration of the normal increase in platelet destruction that occurs during pregnancy.

Immune Thrombocytopenic Purpura

Immune thrombocytopenic purpura (ITP) affects 2 to 3/1000 pregnancies and can lead to profound neonatal thrombocytopenia in 20% of cases. In this disorder, platelets are coated with platelet-bound antibodies, and these platelets are removed from the circulation by binding to Fc receptors in the reticuloendothelial system.

Treatment of a gravida with ITP depends on clinical signs as well as the platelet count. Spontaneous bleeding usually does not occur until the platelet count falls below 20,000/mm^3, and increased surgical bleeding usually does not occur until the platelet count falls below 50,000/mm^3. Glucocorticoids are the mainstay for raising the platelet count in a patient with ITP. Any steroid that has glucocorticoid effects may work, but intravenous methylprednisolone and oral prednisone are ideal because they have very little mineralocorticoid effect and thus little risk of disturbing electrolyte balance. The ususal dose of methylprednisolone is 1.0 to 1.5 mg/kg total body weight/day administered intravenously in divided doses. If the physician chooses to start with oral medication, prednisone can be administered in a dose of 60 to 100 mg/day. It can be given as a single dose, but there is less gastrointestinal upset if it is given in divided doses. The initial dose of medication should be maintained until the platelet count approaches 100,000/mm^3. Then the dose can be rapidly tapered while trying to maintain the patient's platelet count at about 100,000/mm^3. There is little risk that methylprednisolone or prednisone will cause neonatal adrenal suppression because only about 10% of this medication crosses the placenta. The maternal response rate for glucocorticoids is 70%. Side effects from glucocorticoids include fluid retention, hirsutism, acne, striae, poor wound healing, and monilial vaginitis. Rare, serious side effects include aseptic necrosis of the hip, osteoporosis, and cataract formation. Because very little of these medications reaches the fetus unaltered, prednisone and methylprednisolone do not have teratogenic effects.

Because 30% of severely thrombocytopenic patients will not respond to glucocorticoids, obstetricians must be familiar with the use of intravenous immune globulin (IVIG). This agent probably works by binding to the Fc receptors on the reticuloendothelial cells, thus preventing platelet binding and destruction. Liquid and lyophilized forms of this medication are available. The usual dose is 0.4 gm/kg/day for 3 to 5 days, but larger doses are occasionally necessary. The response usually begins in 2 to 3 days and often peaks in 5 days. Because the length of response varies, the timing of dosing is extremely important. If the obstetrician is attempting to raise the platelet count for delivery, therapy should be instituted 5 to 8 days before the planned delivery.

If the physician is unable to keep the patient's platelet count above $20{,}000/mm^3$ with other forms of therapy, splenectomy can be safely performed during pregnancy. It is best carried out in midtrimester when there is the least chance of inciting preterm labor. Platelet transfusions should be reserved for patients having clinically significant bleeding while waiting for other forms of therapy to take effect. They should also be administered before a vaginal delivery if the mother's platelet count is less than $20{,}000/mm^3$ or before a cesarean delivery if the maternal platelet count is less than $50{,}000/mm^3$. Because ITP is a disorder resulting in platelet destruction, the life span of the transfused platelets is very short. The transfusion should be administered as close to the time of delivery as possible so the patient will receive maximum benefit from the transfusion. Each transfused unit of platelets will initially raise the maternal platelet count $10{,}000/mm^3$. Platelets are usually available from the blood bank in packs of 4 to 6 units. Fig. 36-7 outlines the treatment of the pregnant woman with severe thrombocytopenia.

Neonatal Alloimmune Thrombocytopenia

Neonatal alloimmune thrombocytopenia is a rare disorder in which the mother lacks a common specific platelet antigen and develops antibodies against that antigen. The disease is somewhat analogous to Rh isoimmunization, except that it involves platelets. If the fetus inherits the antigen from the father, maternal IgG directed against that antigen attacks the fetal platelets, resulting in severe intrauterine thrombocytopenia. The antibodies involved are usually directed against PLA-1 or BAK. There is a high risk of intracranial hemorrhage in these fetuses. Treatment often involves maternal administration of IVIG and cesarean delivery. Occasionally, cord platelet counts are determined in utero and the fetus is transfused with maternal platelets because they do not have the target antigen. Maternal platelets are often infused into the neonate soon after birth.

Disseminated Intravascular Coagulation

Disseminated intravascualr coagulation (DIC) is a term used to describe a widespread hematologic process of accelerated fibrin formation and lysis. DIC occurs when regulatory systems that control the fine balance between the coagulation cascade and the fibrinolytic system are upset.

The most common cause of DIC is probably underestimation of blood loss with inadequate replacement by crystalloid or colloid. In these cases, vasospasm occurs, with resultant endothelial damage and initiation of DIC. Also, hypotension results in decreased perfusion that leads to local

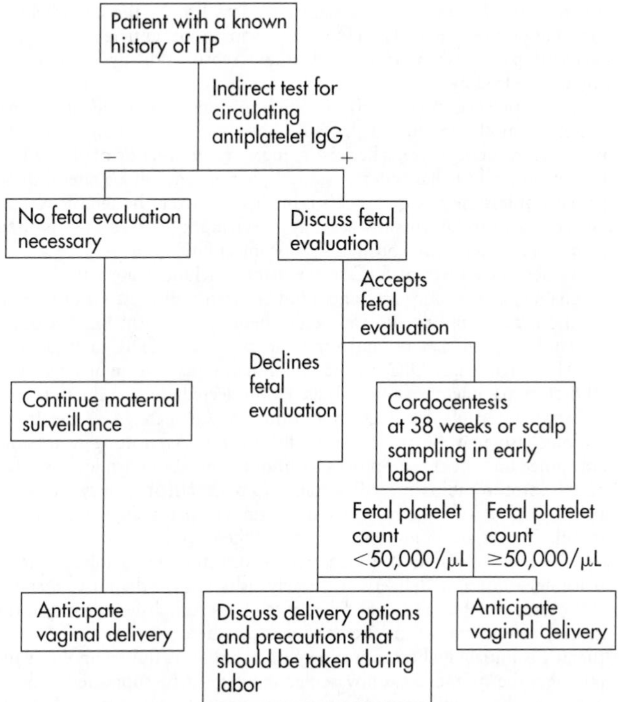

FIG. 36-7 Management of low platelet count during pregnancy.

hypoxia and acidosis at the tissue level, thus starting the DIC cascade. By keeping the patient volume replete, DIC can often be avoided, even when there is severe anemia.

Although every medical student is taught that a retained dead fetus can cause DIC, this is unusual. This process must continue for at least 3 weeks before any DIC can occur. The exception, of course, is fetal death caused by placental abruption. In this situation, the abruption initiates DIC–not the deceased fetus. When the retroplacental blood clot forms and expands, it consumes coagulation factors and may result in a consumptive coagulopathy. This takes place if delivery does not occur in a timely fashion or if coagulation factors are not administered when needed. The coagulation profile in these cases usually begins as an isolated fall in fibrinogen with an increase in fibrin degradation products.

Both gram-negative and gram-positive bacteria can lead to sepsis resulting in DIC. In these rare cases, endotoxin or cytokines may lead to loss of normal hemostatic mechanisms controlled by the endothelium throughout the body. Therefore DIC should be anticipated in any pregnant patient who has overwhelming sepsis and any evidence of abnormal bleeding.

Severe preeclampsia and HELLP syndrome can result in DIC if delivery is not promptly conducted. Usually, however, these patients show an isolated thrombocytopenia because of increased destruction of platelets by the reticuloendothelial system. Clinically significant DIC is rare in these patients unless the disease process is unchecked. Even though there is no evidence of overt DIC in most severely preeclamptic patients, there is often laboratory evidence demonstrating subclinical DIC.

Other rare causes of DIC in pregnancy include acute fatty liver of pregnancy, aseptic abortion, and adult respiratory distress syndrome. In addition, autoimmune diseases, acute hemolytic transfusion reactions, hematologic malignancies, and tumors are rare causes of DIC in pregnancy.

The diagnosis of DIC can be preliminarily made from any sensitive laboratory parameter of fibrinolysis. Fibrin degradation products are the most widely available gauge of fibrinolysis. An increase in the fibrin D-dimer also may be predictive of fibrinolysis. As clotting factors are consumed and the disease process continues, the fibrinogen level will fall and the prothrombin time will become prolonged. In pregnancy, however, there is such a wide normal range for fibrinogen that a single value is not useful. The physician must serially follow these levels.

The basic treatment of DIC involves correcting the inciting event. In placental abruption, delivery in a timely fashion is the definitive therapy. If the fetus is stable, a vaginal delivery can be accomplished as long as the mother's fluid status and hematologic parameters are monitored and therapy is initiated when appropriate. If an amniotic fluid embolus is the etiology, the mother's cardiovascular status must be supported and the coagulopathy rapidly treated because cardiovascular collapse and DIC are the most frequent causes of maternal mortality. In the case of the retained dead fetus, delivery should be accomplished after DIC is diagnosed, but this does take several weeks to develop. In the case of DIC related to severe preeclampsia/HELLP, the definitive treatment is delivery. Vaginal delivery is preferable, but if the fetus is unstable, or if the mother is deteriorating, cesarean delivery should be strongly considered.

Treating the patient with DIC secondary to sepsis requires rapid care. Wide-spectrum antibiotics should be given, and the choice of antibiotics depends on the site of the suspected underlying infection. If the infection is caused by an abscess (including intrauterine infection), the site should be drained even if this means a very premature delivery. If the infection is caused by an indwelling intravascular or urethral catheter, these must be removed.

Plasma replacement therapy should be considered when the prothrombin time is approximately 1.5 times the control value. This test is a rough indicator of the extent to which the extrinsic clotting system has been activated. The goal is to keep the prothrombin time within 2 to 3 seconds of the control value. When administering plasma, the physician must carefully evaluate the patient's volume status and renal function to prevent fluid overload. If the fibrinogen is <100 mg/dl, cryoprecipitate should be administered because each unit of cryoprecipitate raises the fibrinogen level about 10 mg/dl. In patients with DIC and a fibrinogen level of <100 mg/dl, the usual transfusion regimen is 10 units of cryoprecipitate for every two to three units of plasma. This infuses maximal fibrinogen in a small volume. If the patient develops clinically significant anemia, RBCs should be replaced as indicated. Platelets should be transfused if the platelet count is <20,000/μL or if clincially significant bleeding occurs with a platelet count between 20,000/L and 50,000/L. The usual rate of transfusion is 1 to 3 units/10 kg/day.

KEY POINTS

1 Iron deficiency anemia is the most common hematologic complication of pregnancy.

2 Iron supplements taken once daily are adequate for prophylaxis and twice daily is usually sufficient for treatment.

3 Approximately 8% of adult blacks in the United States have sickle cell trait (hemoglobin AS).

4 The keystones of treating sickle crisis in pregnancy are analgesia, hydration, and oxygen.

5 Approximately 4% to 7% of pregnant women will have platelet counts <150,000/mm^3 at term.

6 The most common cause of DIC in pregnancy is probably underestimation of surgical blood loss with inadequate crystalloid and colloid replacement.

SUGGESTED READINGS

Burrows RF, Kelton JG: Thrombocytopenia at delivery: a prospective survey of 6715 deliveries, *Am J Obstet Gynecol* 162:731, 1990.

Burrows RF, Kelton JG: Low fetal risks in pregnancies associated with idiopathic thrombocytopenic purpura, *Am J Obstet Gynecol* 163:1147, 1990.

Burrows RF, Kelton JG: Fetal thrombocytopenia and its relation to maternal thrombocytopenia, *N Engl J Med* 329:1463, 1993.

Hoffman R et al, eds: *Hematology basic principles and practice,* New York, 1991, Churchill Livingstone, pp 1394-1405.

Kaplan C et al: Fetal platelet counts in thrombocytopenic pregnancy, *Lancet* 336:979, 1990.

Martin JN et al: The natural history of HELLP syndrome: patterns of disease progression and regression, *Am J Obstet Gynecol* 164:1500, 1991.

McCrae KR, Samuels P, Schreiber AD: Pregnancy-associated thrombocytopenia: pathogenesis and management, *Blood* 80:1697, 1992.

Samuels P et al: Estimation of the risk of thrombocytopenia in offspring of pregnant women with presumed immune thrombocytopenic purpura, *N Engl J Med* 323:229, 1990.

Tchernia G et al: Antiplatelet antibodies in mothers of severely thrombocytopenic neonates, *Br J Haematol* 84:457, 1993.

Autoimmune Disease

ROSEMARY E. REISS

Autoimmune disorders include a broad spectrum of illnesses caused by derangement of humoral or cell-mediated immune responses. These disorders frequently coincide with pregnancy. The spontaneous exacerbations and remissions that characterize autoimmune disorders make it difficult to determine how their course is affected by pregnancy.

Clinical abnormalities in autoimmune disorders are produced through many mechanisms. Antibodies may block or stimulate specific membrane-bound receptors. In other cases, antibodies have cytotoxic effects. Autoantibodies may be tissue specific or they may target many end organs to cause multisystem disease. Nonspecific tissue damage may also occur when circulating complexes of antibodies and antigen (immune complexes) deposit in tissues such as the skin or kidney to cause inflammation and fibrosis. Antilymphocyte antibodies may cause abnormalities in cell-mediated immunity.

SYSTEMIC LUPUS ERYTHEMATOSUS

Systemic lupus erythematosus (SLE) is a multisystem disorder in which B and helper T lymphocyte hyperactivity lead to sustained production of autoantibodies and immune complexes. Approximately 90% of cases occur in women, and onset is usually in the reproductive years. The prevalence is 15 to 50/100,000 and varies among populations, with black women affected about three times as often as white women.

Pregnancy is not believed to affect the course of SLE, and 20% to 40% of patients experience flares during pregnancy, comparable to flare frequency during other 9-month intervals. Women who are in remission at the onset of pregnancy usually do well. However, patients with active renal disease at conception, especially those with an elevated creatinine level, have high complication rates in pregnancy, with some reports of permanent renal failure developing during pregnancy. Conception should therefore be postponed until 6 months to 1 year after remission of lupus nephritis has been achieved. There is still some controversy as to whether SLE symptoms flare post partum. Prophylactic corticosteroids are probably unnecessary in the patient in remission, though any woman with SLE should be closely monitored during the first few weeks post partum.

Diagnosis

Almost all SLE patients have antinuclear antibodies (ANA), but since patients with other autoimmune disorders often have ANAs, a positive titer is not pathognomonic. Anti-DNA antibodies are more specific for active SLE, but these wane when the disease is in remission. One or more serious systemic manifestations are eventually present in about half of SLE patients. These may include glomerular nephritis (characterized by protein, red cells, and casts in the urine), pleural or pericardial inflammation with effusions, and CNS manifestations such as stroke, seizures, memory loss, or mood changes (Box 36-3). The distribution of symptoms does not appear to be affected by pregnancy.

To standardize diagnosis of SLE, the American Rheumatologic Association has established as criteria for definitive diagnosis the presence of 4 of 11 manifestations of disease:

1. Malar rash
2. Discoid lupus
3. Photosensitivity
4. Oral or nasal ulcers
5. Arthritis (nondeforming)
6. Pleuritis/pericarditis
7. Renal diseases
   Cellular casts
   Proteinuria
8. Neurologic disorder (seizures/psychosis)
9. Cytopenia or hemolytic anemia

BOX 36-3
Clinical Manifestations of SLE and Percentage of Patients Affected

MANIFESTATION
Arthrtis and arthralgias (92%)
Fever (84%)
Skin eruptions (72%)
Lymphadenopathy (59%)
Renal disease (53%)
Anorexia, nausea, vomiting (53%)
Myalgia (48%)
Pleuritis (45%)
CNS abnormality (26%)

LAB ABNORMALITY
ANA (95%-99%)
Anti-dsDNA (70%)
Hypocomplementemia (75%)
Globulin (60%-77%)
RF (20%)
False positive STS (15%)
Anemia (72%)
Leukopenia (61%)
Thrombocytopenia (15%)
Positive direct Coombs (14%)
Antiphospholipid antibodies (10%)

10. Immunologic disorders
    LE cells
    False positive STS
    Anti-DNA
    Anti-Sm
11. ANA

These need not be present simultaneously. Before clinically symptomatic SLE is present, associated autoantibodies, including the lupus anticoagulant or anti-SSA and SSB, may be present and may cause pregnancy complications.

Effects on Pregnancy

Fertility is not reduced in SLE except in patients with chronic renal failure. Rates of first- and second-trimester spontaneous abortion and intrauterine fetal death are all increased. Although active systemic disease increases the risk of late fetal loss, women with the so-called *lupus anticoagulant* are at high risk of fetal wastage throughout pregnancy, even if they have no other findings suggestive of SLE.

Fetal growth restriction and fetal demise are increased in SLE patients. Though medications used to treat lupus may directly inhibit fetal growth, placental insufficiency is probably more often the cause, since several manifestations of SLE may impair placentation. Hypertension predisposes to vasoconstriction in placental bed vessels. Cytotoxic antilymphocyte antibodies may cross react with trophoblast. Immune complexes can cause placental vasculitis. Lupus anticoagulants are associated with endothelial injury and placental infarction.

The same mechanisms that can create placental insufficiency also predispose to preeclampsia. The incidence of preeclampsia in SLE is estimated at 20% to 25%. SLE flares can mimic preeclampsia, making it especially difficult to diagnose SLE if it appears de novo during the third trimester of pregnancy. It is important to differentiate a lupus flare, which can be managed medically, from preeclampsia, which may warrant delivery (Table 36-4). If proteinuria and hypertension increase rapidly in the third trimester, especially in the absence of a urinary sediment indicating nephritis, preeclampsia is likely.

Transplacental passage of maternal IgG autoantibodies sometimes causes symptoms in the neonate. Antibodies to Ro (SSA) antigen or the associated La (SSB) antigen are present in mothers of affected infants. Symptoms are usually transient and resolve completely in a few months as the newborn clears maternal antibodies. Malar erythema and discoid or annular skin lesions may be present, usually located on the face or scalp. Transient hemolytic anemia, leukopenia, or thrombocytopenia can also occur, but do not usually require treatment.

Irreversible congenital complete heart block (CCHB) of autoimmune origin complicates about 1% of pregnancies in women with SLE and about 5% of pregnancies in women with Sjögren's syndrome. Autoimmune CCHB can also occur in infants whose mothers have no previously detected autoimmune disease. In any setting, the mother invariably has antibodies to Ro (SSA) and/or La (SSB) antigens. Risk of

TABLE 36-4
Differentiation of Lupus Nephritis From Preeclampsia

Finding	SLE nephritis	Preeclampsia
Hypertension	+	+
Proteinuria	+	+
Urinalysis	+ cellular casts, RBC	Usually inactive sediment; may have muddy brown casts if ATN present
Thrombocytopenia	±/–	+/–
dsDNA	Present	Absent
C_3, C_4	Usually low	Usually normal
Antithrombin III	Normal	Often low
Responds to corticosteroids and immune suppressants	Yes (may take 2-3 weeks for corticosteroids)	No

recurrence in subsequent pregnancies after the delivery of an affected infant is about 33%.

Autoimmune CCHB is believed to be caused by binding of antibody to the cardiac conducting system, with resulting fibrosis and calcification in the area of the AV node. Diagnosis is made by finding fetal heart rate fixed at 50 to 90 bpm, with M-mode ultrasound confirming the dissociation of atrial and ventricular contractions. Bradycardia begins before 24 weeks gestation. A transient pericarditis manifested by pericardial effusion may initially be present. Some have proposed that since inflammatory changes precede the onset of bradycardia, fetal treatment with corticosteroids might prevent the development of permanent heart block, but efficacy of this approach has not yet been convincingly demonstrated.

In utero, the bradycardia is usually well tolerated and is not a contraindication to vaginal delivery. However, if the fetus develops hydrops, a sign of fetal heart failure, cesarean delivery is warranted. Even infants who tolerated bradycardia in utero may require permanent cardiac pacing after delivery.

Treatment

Corticosteroids effectively suppress most SLE manifestations. Long-term steroid therapy has significant side effects, but because of potential fetal effects of prostaglandin inhibitors and antimalarials, corticosteroids are often used as first-line agents during pregnancy.

Both physicians and patients should be cautious in tapering medications to spare fetal effects. Side effects of medications are usually less threatening to the pregnancy than a flare of systemic lupus symptoms. Corticosteroid doses may need to be increased, at least transiently, if other medications are stopped. In the case of a flare of systemic lupus, treatment should be as aggressive in the pregnant woman as in a nonpregnant one,

BOX 36-4
Management of Systemic SLE Flare

GOALS

Suppress acute flare of nephritis, hemolysis, organic brain syndrome, thrombocytopenia, or pleuritis
Prevention of irreversible end-organ damage

MATERNAL MANAGEMENT

Admit patient
Laboratory evaluation:
CBC, platelet count, electrolytes, BUN, creatinine, LFTs, ANA, complement levels, double-stranded DNA, 12- or 24-hour urine for protein and creatinine.
Use C_3, C_4, dsDNA to assess response; proteinuria responds more slowly and may first worsen
Prednisone 60-200 mg/day until clinical and laboratory evidence of remission

OR

If life-threatening complications, consider "pulse" therapy: 1 g methylprednisolone IV daily for 3 to 7 days, then 40-60 mg prednisone orally
If patient is unresponsive to pulse therapy, add azathioprine 1-2 mg/kg/day or cyclophosphamide 2-3 mg/kg/day.
Once control is achieved, taper steroids by 10% every 7 days to maintenance level, continuing to monitor for reactivation of flare
Screen frequently for glucose intolerance

FETAL MANAGEMENT

If in 3rd trimester, perform NST and estimate amniotic fluid volume twice weekly; deliver if test results are nonreassuring

with only minor adjustments in drug choice necessary. Management of SLE in pregnancy is summarized in Box 36-4.

LUPUS ANTICOAGULANT (LAC)/ANTIPHOSPHOLIPID ANTIBODY (APA) SYNDROME

LAC/APA is an ill-defined term that describes patients with predilection to thrombosis, recurrent pregnancy loss, autoantibodies to phospholipids, and sometimes thrombocytopenia. LAC syndrome was first described in patients with SLE. However, for 50% of affected women, no other symptoms or serologies suggestive of lupus may be present. These autoantibodies cause arterial and venous thrombosis in vivo, but prolong the aPTT in vitro (thus the term *lupus anticoagulant*). Diagnosis and management of the syndrome have been hampered by technical difficulties in the assays for antiphospholipid antibodies (APA), the lack of strict definitions for the syndrome, and the absence of controlled trials of therapies.

Nonetheless, this syndrome plainly causes significant morbidity in pregnancy. Untreated patients may have spontaneous abortion rates as high as 65%, and stillbirth rates are almost 30%. Even with treatment, less than 60% of pregnancies end in normally grown live borns (spontaneous abortion 13%, stillbirth 17%, IUGR 13%). Risk of preeclampsia is high. Pregnancy complications are presumed to be caused by vascular thrombosis and secondary infarction in the placenta or decidua caused by interaction of antiphospholipid antibodies with phospholipids in vascular endothelium and/or platelets that promote thrombosis.

Diagnosis

The syndrome is considered in patients with unexplained habitual abortion, any unexplained pregnancy loss after 14 weeks, and preeclampsia in the second or early third trimester or severe preeclampsia.

Unexplained intrauterine growth restriction and oligohydramnios, recurrent placental abruption, SLE, false positive serologic test for syphilis, and history of arterial or venous thrombosis are other indicators.

Ideally, diagnostic tests are peformed in a lab with a special interest in the syndrome because false positives are common and can lead to overtreatment, which itself has significant morbidity. Lupus anticoagulant assay (aPTT, kaolin clotting time, dilute Russell viper venom time, tissue thromboplastin neutralization, platelet neutralization procedure) is a battery of tests designed to assess the anticoagulant behavior of antiphospholipid antibodies in vitro, and to distinguish their presence from other causes of prolongation of the PTT such as factor deficiencies. APA are enzyme-linked immunoassays (ELISAs) used to detect IgG, IgM, or IgA against cardiolipin or other phospholipids. Some patients test positive for both LAC and APA assays, some only for one. The presence of LAC functional activity is rare and highly suggestive of clinically significant disease. Positive ELISAs for APA are more common and harder to interpret. To be significant, APA must be present in moderate to high titers. IgG antibodies are more clearly associated with poor pregnancy outcomes than IgM.

Treatment

Because of the lack of randomized prospective trials, optimal therapy remains controversial. Therapeutic approaches include prednisone, low-dose aspirin (65 to 80 mg/day), and intravenous immunoglobulins and immunosuppressants. Side effects can be significant.

One approach is to treat those patients without overt SLE or history of thrombosis who have APA but not LAC with low-dose aspirin alone. Patients with a history of thrombosis or with positive LAC assays are usually treated with low-dose aspirin and heparin at low therapeutic levels. If such a patient has an elevated baseline aPPT, activated Factor X levels are assayed to determine therapeutic heparin levels. Patients who have SLE and no history of thrombosis can be treated with low-dose aspirin and prednisone if corticosteroids are needed for control of their lupus symptoms or with prophylactic doses of heparin and low-dose aspirin if not. An effort should be made to avoid using heparin with prednisone because of the additive effects on osteopenia.

All patients with LAC/APA syndrome require careful monitoring of fetal well-being, with early delivery if testing suggests deterioration. NSTs and ultrasound to evaluate growth and amniotic fluid volume should be performed during the third trimester. Doppler velocimetry to assess placental resistance may also help identify those patients who remain at high risk for stillbirth or IUGR despite treatment.

RHEUMATOID ARTHRITIS

Rheumatoid arthritis (RA) is characterized by progressively deforming symmetrical polyarthritis. Extraarticular manifestations may also be present, including subcutaneous rheumatoid nodules, vasculitis, fever, and, more rarely, pulmonary involvement, neutropenia, or splenomegaly. Estimates of the prevalence of RA range from 0.2% for persistent disease to 2.5% if all suspected cases are included. Women are 2.5 to 3 times more likely to develop RA than men; however, systemic manifestations are less common in women. Adult RA is uncommon in obstetric patients because the peak time of onset is after age 40. However, juvenile rheumatoid arthritis (JRA) or the joint deformities it produces can persist until adulthood and may complicate pregnancy.

Diagnosis

The diagnosis of RA is based primarily on clinical findings, the most common of which are morning joint stiffness, arthritis of three or more joint areas simultaneously, arthritis of hand joints, symmetric arthritis, rheumatoid nodules, serum rheumatoid factor, and radiographic changes (erosion or decalcification). The presence of four of seven criteria is considered diagnostic of RA, though patients in early stages of the disease may not initially meet criteria.

Pregnancy

Symptoms of RA usually improve during pregnancy. Half of all patients feel better by the first trimester and another 25% improve by the second trimester. Response is usually similar in successive pregnancies. However, weight gain and postural changes accompanying pregnancy may aggravate symptoms.

RA does not appear to increase fetal wastage or other pregnancy complications. However, if arthritic changes have reduced the woman's range of spine or hip movement, this may pose problems at delivery. If regional anesthetics are used, extreme caution must be observed when positioning the patient for delivery to avoid trauma to the joints. If the patient is unable to flex or abduct her thighs, cesarean delivery may be necessary. To avoid complications or delay in the event of emergency cesarean delivery, patients with spine involvement should be evaluated antepartum by an anesthesiologist for airway access and to plan the safest mode of anesthesia. Although regional anesthesia is preferable, if this cannot be achieved while the patient is awake, intubation or local anesthesia for cesarean delivery may be necessary in extreme cases.

Treatment

Goals of treatment of RA are to relieve pain and reduce the inflammation that leads to permanent joint deformity and decreased function. All of the useful medications (whether analgesic, antiinflammatory, or immune suppressive) have potential fetal side effects. In the nonpregnant woman, aspirin is the mainstay of therapy. Though this drug is not teratogenic, potential for fetal effects, including premature constriction of the ductus arteriosus and salicylate toxicity, discourage its use in the third trimester. Similar to treatment of SLE during pregnancy, the use of prednisone may need to be liberalized to allow tapering of NSAIDs. Fortunately, since RA usually remits during pregnancy, most medications can be used sparingly. Patients with severe symptoms should be comanaged with a rheumatologist.

SCLERODERMA (SYSTEMIC SCLEROSIS)

Diagnosis

The hallmark of scleroderma is excessive fibrosis of the skin or viscera caused by increased synthesis of collagen by fibroblasts in the affected organs. Though clinical expression of disease varies widely depending on the organ system affected, the skin is almost always involved. Initially there is puffiness, especially of the hands, with loss of skin creases and nonpitting edema. Development of thickened, taut, "hidebound" skin follows. Flexion contractures and subcutaneous calcifications may develop. Vascular abnormalities are also common, with Raynaud's phenomenon present in 95% of patients. Pulmonary involvement, manifesting as interstitial fibrosis, pleuritis, and pulmonary hypertension, is a frequent cause of death. Scleroderma can involve the heart, producing myocardial fibrosis that can cause arrhythmias, heart block, and CHF. Gastrointestinal involvement, especially esophageal motility problems, is common.

Subgroups of scleroderma have been classified by prognosis. Localized scleroderma with only patchy skin involvement has excellent prognosis and should be considered a separate disorder. Generalized scleroderma, also called *systemic sclerosis,* may be divided into two groups. The first, limited cutaneous scleroderma, includes the CREST syndrome (**c**alcinosis, **R**aynaud's phenomenon, **e**sophageal hypomotility, **s**clerodactyly, **t**elangiectasis) and has less visceral involvement and slow progression. Diffuse scleroderma is characterized by truncal skin involvement, widespread visceral disease, and rapid progression.

Treatment

Treatment of scleroderma is directed at symptom relief. No regimen has been found that slows the progressive fibrosis. Patients with diffuse scleroderma who show rapid progression of skin disease are at higher risk for development of scleroderma renal crisis, characterized by malignant hypertension, encephalopathy, retinopathy, microangiopathic hemolytic anemia, and azotemia–a frequently fatal syndrome.

Management

Despite female predominance, scleroderma is infrequent in pregnancy because its onset usually follows the reproductive years. The course of the disease is usually not altered by pregnancy. However, pregnancy may acclerate progression of scleroderma renal failure. Scleroderma renal crisis has been present in most reported maternal deaths and was sometimes mistaken for preeclampsia. ACE inhibitors, which are the treatment of choice for scleroderma hypertension, are contraindicated in pregnancy because they have been documented to cause fetal wastage, growth restriction, renal failure, and fetal demise in humans as well as animals.

The impact of scleroderma on pregnancy depends on disease severity. Evidence of high rates of fetal wastage and prematurity is not consistent. Physiologic changes in pregnancy may exacerbate scleroderma symptoms such as esophageal reflux or CHF.

SJÖGREN'S SYNDROME

Sjögren's syndrome, a complex of keratoconjunctivitis sicca (dry eyes), xerostomia (dry mouth), and episodic salivary gland enlargement, can be found alone or in association with many autoimmune or connective tissue disorders, notably RA, SLE, and scleroderma. Sjögren's is noteworthy in pregnancy because it is characterized by the presence of SSA (antiRo) and SSB (antiLa) antibodies, which can cross the placenta to cause neonatal lupus syndromes.

PREGNANCY CONSIDERATIONS FOR DRUG THERAPY IN AUTOIMMUNE DISEASE

Corticosteroids usually effectively suppress symptoms of SLE and other autoimmune disorders. Because prednisone is inactivated in the placenta, fetal effects of this drug are minimal.

Antimalarials are contraindicated in pregnancy except in areas where malaria is endemic. These agents bind to DNA and inhibit nucleic acid repair. In animal studies they are concentrated in fetal eye structures, and retinal toxicity is observed in adults. Small studies of women treated with chloroquine or hydroxychloroquine in the first trimester found no teratogenic effect and no hearing or vision problems in offspring. Wide experience with weekly use of these drugs for malaria prophylaxis suggests that at least low doses are safe.

In nonpregnant patients, azathioprine, cyclosporine A, and cyclophosphamide are often used in autoimmune disease in concert with corticosteroids to treat life- or organ-threatening nephritis, cerebritis, or thrombocytopenia, or to modify the course of RA. Response is more rapid than with corticosteroids alone, and immunosuppressants can preserve renal function in patients with lupus nephritis. Since these cytotoxic agents are always used in combination with corticosteroids, it is difficult to evaluate their independent effects in pregnancy. No increase in fetal malformation rate has been documented with azathioprine, but it may be associated with slowed fetal growth. Little information is available about cyclophosphamide in pregnancy; azathioprine is preferred because it has less toxicity. Cyclosporine A is not an animal teratogen, but human effects are insufficiently reported.

Sulfasalazine can also be used to modify the course of RA. It can be safely used during pregnancy, though near term it may increase neonatal jaundice.

KEY POINTS

1 SLE and related disorders occur in women in reproductive years and may increase fetal wastage, growth restriction, and preeclampsia.

2 Symptoms of SLE should be aggressively treated during pregnancy.

3 Rheumatoid arthritis is usually well tolerated during pregnancy.

SUGGESTED READINGS

Branch DW et al: Outcome of treated pregnancies in women with antiphospholipid antibody syndrome: an update of the Utah experience, *Obstet Gynecol* 80:614-20, 1992.

Carreira PE, Gutierrez-Larraya F, Gomez-Reino JJ: Successful intrauterine therapy with dexamethasone of fetal myocarditis or heart block in a woman with systemic lupus erythematosus, *J Rheumatol* 20:1204-7, 1993.

Gimovsky ML, Montoro M: Systemic lupus erythematosus and other connective tissue diseases in pregnancy. *Clin Obstet Gynecol* 34:35-50, 1991.

Out HG et al: A prospective controlled multicenter study on the obstetric risk of pregnant women with antiphospholipid antibodies, *Am J Obstet Gynecol* 167:26-32, 1992.

Hepatic and Gastrointestinal Disease

Christopher L. Mabee and John J. Fromkes

Pregnancy requires physiologic adaptation to fully support the requirements of fetal homeostasis. Approximately 75% of pregnancies have associated clinical or subclinical hepatic or gastrointestinal pathology. Fig. 36-8 outlines the steps in evaluating hepatic and gastrointestinal disease in pregnancy.

HEPATIC DISEASE

Intrahepatic Cholestasis of Pregnancy

Intrahepatic cholestasis of pregnancy (ICP) is characterized by intense pruritus and cholestasis that usually appears in the third trimester of pregnancy, persists until parturition, and remits shortly thereafter. The disease is usually benign for the mother, causing no long-term sequelae. However, ICP may induce fetal distress and prematurity and has been associated with stillbirths. Intrahepatic cholestasis of pregnancy character-

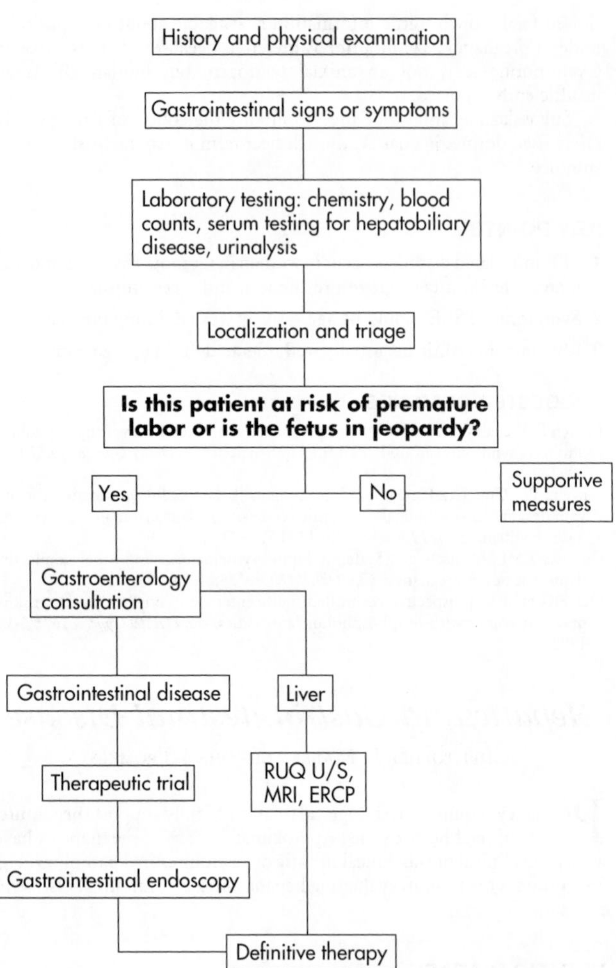

FIG. 36-8 Evaluating hepatic and gastrointestinal disease in pregnancy.

istically recurs in future pregnancies even though the patient's biochemical cholestasis completely remits after delivery. In the United States, the disease is present in 1 to 2 patients/10,000 deliveries.

ICP should be suspected in patients complaining of generalized pruritus with nocturnal exacerbations with or without jaundice. It appears in most women after the 30th week of pregnancy and, though rare, can occur earlier. Jaundice occurs in only about 20% of patients. Most women describe a darkening of their urine that coincides with direct hyperbilirubinemia. The diagnostic criteria most widely used include pruritus, mild to moderate increases in serum aminotransferases from 2 to 10 times normal, elevations in total and direct bilirubin to 100 times normal, and disappearance of biochemical cholestasis after delivery. Physical examination usually is unremarkable for signs of acute or chronic liver disease. However, if the gravid uterus permits, the liver edge can often be palpated as soft and slightly tender.

The differential diagnosis includes acute viral hepatitis, acute fatty liver of pregnancy, primary biliary cirrhosis, and biliary tract obstruction. These entities usually can be diagnosed based on associated risk factors, exposures, acuity of illness, or persistence of cholestasis after parturition.

Therapeutic measures should be taken to relieve the patient's symptoms and to obtain a normal, spontaneous delivery at term. Low-fat diets and rest seem to coincide with partial remission of pruritus and jaundice and are recommended. Pharmacologic approaches include cholestyramine, antihistamines and benzodiazepines, low-dose phenobarbital, and ursodeoxycholic acid. The first two approaches appear ineffective. Phenobarbital is contraindicated in the last weeks of pregnancy. Treatment with ursodeoxycholic acid appears promising, but more data are needed.

Preeclampsia

Preeclampsia, a vascular endothelial disease of unknown etiology, occurs in 5% to 8% of all pregnancies. It affects multiple areas of the body, including the brain, heart, lungs, liver, kidneys, and hematologic and reproductive systems. It may produce varying combinations of organ dysfunction and is characterized by its clinical variability and appearance during the last trimester of pregnancy. This disease is a risk for maternal and fetal morbidity and mortality.

Criteria for diagnosis include pregnancy-induced hypertension, proteinuria, and edema. Preeclampsia is usually classified as mild or severe depending on the magnitude of hypertension and proteinuria. Preeclampsia is considered mild if blood pressure is <160/110 mm Hg and proteinuria is <5 g/24 hours. However, if the patient experiences oliguria, neurologic changes, pulmonary edema, abdominal pain, altered liver function tests, or thrombocytopenia, they are considered to have severe disease.

The differential diagnosis includes chronic hypertension, chronic hypertension with superimposed preeclampsia, and gestational hypertension. These entities do not have significant proteinuria, although they may be associated with edema and should be differentiated from pregnancy-induced hypertension and preeclampsia.

The standard treatment is bed rest and delivery. Intravenous magnesium sulfate is given to prevent seizures in the patient, which is a known complication of preeclampsia. Patients with significant epigastric or right upper quadrant pain should be considered for an abdominal CT scan to rule out subcapsular or intraparenchymal hematoma of the liver. Antihypertensive therapy should be instituted with two main objectives, to reduce the maternal morbidity and mortality secondary to cerebrovascular accidents, and to reduce perinatal IUGR and abruptio placentae. Although several agents have been shown to be safe for use during pregnancy, methyldopa, hydralazine, and labetalol appear to be preferred by most obstetricians.

HELLP Syndrome

HELLP syndrome, or microangiopathic intravascular *h*emolysis, *e*levated *l*iver enzymes, and *l*ow *p*latelets, is found in about 5% of patients with preeclampsia. The etiology of the disease is unknown.

The predominant diagnostic criteria include a lactate dehydrogenase (LDH) level >600 IU/L, an aspartate aminotransferase (AST) level >72 IU/L, and a platelet count <100,000/mm^3. Elevations of the LDH and AST are secondary to microangiopathic changes in the vasculature with its attendant hemolysis. This process results in the development of schistocytes, evident on the peripheral blood smear, which can be helpful in making the diagnosis. The presentation of HELLP is variable and may be quite subtle. The patient may be in the second trimester and hypertension may be absent; however, most patients have evidence of preeclampsia, with elevations in blood pressure, proteinuria, and edema.

The differential diagnosis of HELLP syndrome includes gastroenteritis, cholelithiasis, idiopathic thrombocytopenic purpura (ITP), thrombotic thrombocytopenic purpura (TTP), and acute viral hepatitis. It is particularly difficult to differentiate TTP from HELLP syndrome because of their diagnostic similarities. TTP is a disorder characterized by fever, mental status changes, acute renal dysfunction, microangiopathic hemolysis, and thrombocytopenia. Patients with HELLP syndrome usually have improvements in their LDH level and platelet counts during the first week after parturition, which distinguishes these patients from those with TTP.

Therapeutic options are limited and controversial for mothers before delivery. If the patient is remote from term, hospitalization with close observation and delivery after fetal lung maturation is complete is usually advocated. Treatment with parenteral corticosteroids between the 24th and 37th weeks of gestation is helpful in reducing maternal morbidity and postponing premature delivery. Plasmapheresis has been utilized in HELLP syndrome with success but is indicated in less than 10% of patients, is expensive, and should not be utilized indiscriminately. Treatment after parturition, where most morbidity and mortality associated with HELLP syndrome occurs, is less constricted. Administration of parenteral dexamethasone over the first 36 hours post partum seems promising.

Liver Hematoma

Localized hepatic hemorrhage and blood clot formation are potential risks associated with preeclampsia and HELLP syndrome. The disorder is rarely encountered today because of improvements in therapy for toxemia of pregnancy. Hepatic subcapsular hematomas occur infrequently in these patients; however, they may become very large and complicated, resulting in sympathetic pleural effusions, rupture, and further bleeding. Liver hematoma should be suspected in any patient with pregnancy-induced hypertension, significant abdominal discomfort, and liver function abnormalities.

Management of patients with liver hematomas with or without rupture varies. Patients with large hematomas with marked pleural effusions or infected hematomas should undergo operative evaluation of the clot. Other patients can be managed conservatively with serial CT scans or ultrasound examination.

Acute Fatty Liver of Pregnancy

Acute fatty liver of pregnancy, a life-threatening complication of pregnancy, is of unknown etiology and is characterized by hepatic dysfunction, jaundice, coagulopathy, and encephalopathy. The disease usually occurs in the last trimester, although it may begin post partum. Prognosis is very poor, particularly in patients with significant encephalopathy or coma, where the mortality rate is approximately 80%.

Diagnosis is based on a histologic examination of the liver that shows microvesicular and macrovesicular fat deposition. Clinical presentation is often nonspecific, and it is often difficult to differentiate patients with HELLP and preeclampsia from those with acute fatty liver of pregnancy. Therapy consists of expeditious delivery with supportive maternal and fetal care.

Acute Viral Hepatitis

In the United States, the most common cause of jaundice during pregnancy is viral hepatitis. Viral agents most likely to infect patients during childbearing years are hepatitis A, B, C, D, and E. Cytomegalovirus, Epstein-Barr virus, and herpes simplex also routinely cause significant hepatic injury during pregnancy. The clinical manifestations and course of disease are the same as in nonpregnant patients. Therapeutic measures for women with acute viral hepatitis are supportive, requiring only rest and good nutritional support in the majority. The most important viral entity in terms of significant risk for vertical transmission and long-term morbidity and mortality in the fetus is hepatitis B. The CDC recommends that all pregnant women be screened for this virus. Most pregnant women with hepatitis B are chronic asymptomatic carriers. The incidence of hepatitis B during pregnancy is about 1%. If the patient harbors the organism and has serologic evidence of the surface antigen, both active and passive immunization should be administered to the neonate within the first 24 hours of life. The passive immunization is in the form of specific hepatitis B immunoglobulin (HBIG). The active vaccine should then be readministered to the infant at 1 month and 6 months to complete the vaccination series. This regimen prevents transmission to the fetus in at least 90% of cases. Hepatitis B can be transmitted by breastfeeding, which is discouraged in developed countries because of the supply of adequate substitutes. Preventive measures for hepatitis D are the same as for hepatitis B.

The transmission of hepatitis A only represents a threat to the fetus if the mother becomes acutely infected during the last 2 weeks before parturition; therefore if there is potential vertical transmission, a single dose of pooled immunoglobulin should be administered within 24 hours of delivery.

Hepatitis C immunoprophylaxis is recommended but only on an empiric basis. The current standard of care is to administer within 24 hours of delivery one dose of pooled immunoglobulin. There is no active form of immunization.

Chronic Viral Hepatitis

Pregnancy in patients with chronic liver disease often correlates with the severity of the disease. Usually pregnancy does not worsen the liver disease, and the chronic hepatic dysfunction does not markedly increase the risks associated with carrying a fetus, with certain exceptions. In patients with cirrhosis, there are likely to be complications such as varicella bleeding, spontaneous bacterial peritonitis, ascites, encephalopathy, hepatorenal syndrome, and prematurity with the potential for increased fetal mortality. There also appears to be an increase in maternal mortality in cirrhotics. Thus pregnancy in patients with cirrhotic liver disease should routinely be avoided.

Patients with known chronic liver disease should be evaluated by a gastroenterologist or hepatologist along with an obstetrician before conception if possible so that the risk of pregnancy can be discussed and a logical plan for future pregnancy attained.

Hepatic Tumors

Many patients experience abdominal pain during the course of a pregnancy. On ultrasonographic evaluation of these patients, hepatic mass lesions are frequently noted. It is often possible to wait through the pregnancy to determine the nature of a mass, particularly if it is relatively asymptomatic, is not associated with liver function abnormalities, and is not expanding. However, if the mass is expanding or there is evidence of bleeding or abnormal laboratory studies, then a more intensive investigation is necessary.

Primary hepatic cysts are the most common lesions recognized and present sonographically as homogenous water densities. Solitary hemangiomas, usually localized to the right lobe of the liver, are also common. These lesions rarely require operative therapy; however, surgical extirpation has been advocated by some if the lesion is associated with considerable pain and expansion. Of interest, hepatic hemangiomas have been associated with high-output cardiac failure, particularly during pregnancy.

These lesions are usually seen ultrasonographically, although they are occasionally missed or not fully qualified with this diagnostic modality. Hepatic lesions are most definitively assessed with MRI, which is the diagnostic modality of choice during pregnancy.

Amebic liver abscesses have been diagnosed during pregnancy and can rupture. These lesions are usually amenable to conservative therapy with antibiotics. Pyogenic abscesses are also possible but are decidely rare. In patients from Mediterranean countries, a painful cystic liver mass should prompt a search for echinococcal disease. Operative intervention may be necessary in these patients, particularly if the lesion is expansive. Orthotopic liver transplantation has been advocated by some for patients with advanced cystic disease not amenable to more conservative measures, although tumor recurrence is possible.

Focal nodular hyperplasia and liver cell adenoma are both increased in patients during pregnancy. Although these lesions are both associated with birth control pills and pregnancy, they are morphologically distinct and represent different forms of risk for the patient and fetus. Liver cell adenoma is a true neoplasm associated with spontaneous rupture and intraperitoneal hemorrhage in approximately 25% of cases. Focal nodular hyperplasia is a hypervascular lesion associated with increased estrogen states; however, it is not known to represent a significant risk for bleeding during pregnancy. Liver function remains normal, and the diagnosis is made by MRI. Management of these lesions may require arteriography (if MRI is nondiagnostic) and surgical exploration. Surgical treatment is recommended in many patients, however there is a mortality of about 5% associated with major hepatic resections. Newer surgical techniques designed to enucleate the tumor may replace the more time-consuming dangerous lobectomies.

Primary hepatocellular carcinoma is very rare in patients during pregnancy unless cirrhosis is present. Serum AFP levels provide a useful marker for this malignancy, even in pregnant patients. Levels are typically greater than 500 ng/ml, distinguishing this entity from normal gestation, multiple gestations, or pregnancies involving fetal NTDs. Therapeutic options are limited. Chemotherapy and radiation have not proved to be of significant benefit in patients with hepatocellular carcinoma, and resection should be considered. The morphologically distinct fibrolamellar variant of hepatocellular carcinoma is found almost exclusively in young women. Although therapy is the same, these patients have a more favorable prognosis.

GASTROINTESTINAL DISEASE

Nausea and Vomiting

Approximately 75% of patients experience nausea and vomiting during the first trimester of pregnancy. The symptoms usually ocur in the morning, are mild, and disappear during the second trimester. Most of these patients can be managed conservatively, although a small percentage require hospitalization. There is a direct association between the onset of nausea and elevations in chorionic gonadotropin levels. Frequently, patients with the most severe symptoms have multiple gestations or molar pregnancies, conditions known to have higher levels of this hormone than normal single gestations. Interestingly, there also has been an association between hyperthyroidism and nausea and vomiting during pregnancy, with approximately 70% of patients with hyperemesis gravidarum having hyperthyroxinemia.

Hyperemesis Gravidarum

Hyperemesis gravidarum is a term defined as intractable nausea and vomiting that occurs in about 1% of all pregnancies. The disorder is more commonly found in whites during their first pregnancy and is seen less frequently in blacks and Eskimos. The disorder tends to recur with subsequent pregnancies. It is more commonly found in patients characterized as immature and from oppressive cultures.

The diagnosis is based on historical information and physical findings consistent with significant dehydration. Mild elevations of aspartate aminotransferase and bilirubin may be seen. The condition is usually self-limited but occasionally requires hospitalization for total parenteral nutrition if there is persistent weight loss or ketosis. Eneteral feeding is an effective modality for nutritional support and should be attempted before parenteral routes. Patients should be told to avoid foods that are particularly emetogenic; a dietary diary can be helpful in this regard. Antiemetics should be avoided if possible. Esophagogastroduodenoscopy is indicated to evaluate patients not responding to typical conservative therapy or those who complain of dysphagia or odynophagia. The prognosis overall is very good.

Irritable Bowel Syndrome

Irritable bowel syndrome is a common disorder resulting in episodic cyclical patterns of diarrhea or constipation with lower abdominal pain. Diagnosis is based on normal routine laboratory studies, including a thyroid panel and ESR, and a normal flexible sigmoidscopy in a patient with typical complaints. Most patients usually are in their 20s to 40s, but occasionally are asymptomatic until later in life. The disorder is usually managed conservatively in pregnant patients and represents no risk to the patient or fetus.

Gastroesophageal Reflux Disease

Pregnancy represents a significant risk for gastroesophageal reflux for several reasons. The lower esophageal sphincter tone decreases as the pregnancy lengthens because of continued increases in serum progresterone levels. The intragastric pressure increases secondary to the abdominal pressure from the gravid uterus and the intraesophageal pressure decreases, all of which facilitate the reflux of gastric contents into the esophagus, resulting in inflammation and pyrosis or heartburn. Symptoms typically associated with gastroesophageal reflux disease include substernal burning after meals and water brash, which is the development of a salty liquid in the mouth because of increased salivation. Water brash is thought to be a response to the esophagosalivary reflex, which occurs secondary to reflux of gastric contents into the esophagus. These symptoms are exacerbated by large meals (especially at bedtime), fats, tomato-based products, alcohol, greasy foods, chocolate, coffee products (caffeinated or decaffeinated), and artificial sweeteners or carminatives. The diagnosis is based on symptoms and response to therapy; however, if symptoms of dysphagia or odynophagia are present, upper GI endoscopy should be done to rule out potential complications. Therapeutic options are conservative and frequently include refraining from bedtime snacks, elevating the head of the bed, and using antacids, alginic acid, and histamine-2 receptor antagonists.

Peptic Ulcer Disease

Peptic ulcer disease is uncommon during pregnancy but should be suspected in a patient with significant epigastric pain relieved by eating. Esophagogastroduodenscopy should be reserved for the patient not responding to conventional therapy with antacids or in those with a suspected complication such as obstruction or bleeding. Barium radiographs are contraindicated in all cases. *Helicobacter pylori* is associated with approximately 95% of patients with a duodenal ulcer. Subsequently, patients resistant to diagnostic endoscopy during or after pregnancy should undergo a full diagnostic workup of their symptoms should they recur after parturition.

Mendelson's Syndrome (Acid-Aspiration Syndrome)

Pregnant patients are at increased risk for developing aspiration syndromes during parturition because of delayed gastric emptying and increased intraabdominal and intragastric pressure. Significant pulmonary parenchymal damage can take place if 25 ml of fluids is aspirated with a pH of <2.5. This damage is most likely in the right lower or middle lobe and is usually a segmetal or subsegmental injury rather then a lobar process. Primary preventive therapy directed against aspiration is the most important and appropriate intervention. Antacids can increase the intragastic pH but also increase the volume of potential refluxant, thus their use before labor is discouraged. Antisecretory therapy with histamine-2 receptor blocking agents can increase the pH of the gastric contents without increasing the refluxant and thus are the drugs of choice.

Gastrointestinal Bypass and Pregnancy

Patients with jejunoileal bypass represent a special though unusual problem to the obstetrican. With these patients, fat absorption is decreased from 30% to 80%, with significant effects on water and electrolyte balance. Liver disease is common in patients with jejunoileal bypass secondary to steatosis and the potential for cirrhosis. Management is typically conservative, consisting of dietary supplementation of fat and fat-soluble vitamins. Particular attention is paid to avoiding dehydration. Total parenteral nutrition is rarely necessary.

Inflammatory Bowel Disease

Inflammatory bowel disease or ulcerative colitis and Crohn's disease are idiopathic disorders resulting in abdominal pain, diarrhea, weight loss, fever, and other uncommon extraintestinal manifestations. Crohn's disease is decidely more toxic to pregnant patients, putting them at risk for poor nutrition; anal, perineal, and rectovaginal fistula formation; prematurity; and fetal loss. Infectious etiologies should be considered in patients who initially complain of abdominal pain with blood diarrhea. *Campyblobacter, Salmonella, Shigella, Escherichia, Yersinia,* and *Entamoeba* should all be considered, and stool cultures for these organisms should be done. The definitive diagnosis is usually made by colonoscopy with biopsies. Treatment of inflammatory bowel disease is the same for pregnant and nonpregnant patients and includes mesalamine, sulfasalazine, metronidazole, and corticosteroids. Treatment with oral 5-aminosalicylic acid is safe and effective for patients with active inflammatory bowel disease during pregnancy without any risk to the fetus. Metronidazole is not recommended for use during the first trimester of pregnancy because of the possible cytotoxic effects associated with its use in mice. There is no evidence in humans that metronidazole causes carcinogenesis with short-term therapy. The management of surgical complications during pregnancy is the same as in nonpregnant patients, although there is a substantial risk for premature birth.

For patients with quiescent disease at the onset of pregnancy, about 33% of patients with ulcerative colitis will have an exacerbation during the course of their pregnancy, and the others will remain the same or go into further remission. Approximately 15% to 40% of patients with Crohn's disease will relapse during the course of pregnancy.

Appendicitis

Most patients with acute appendicitis complain of abdominal pain, nausea, vomiting, and anorexia. The diagnosis is often difficult because of considerable overlap with symptoms of pregnancy. The normal position of the appendix changes throughout pregnancy. As the gravid uterus increases in size, the appendiceal position moves superiorly. Furthermore, the broad ligament blocks its position for palpation. Subsequently, palpation of the lateral abdominal wall will often be more revealing, If appendicitis is suspected, surgery should not be postponed; however, most clinicians would recommend a vertical incision unless the diagnosis is certain, in which case a transverse incision is advised. If the patient is near term, a cesarean delivery need not be performed unless indicated by the fetal condition because the recent appendiceal surgical scar represents no risk for spontaneous vaginal delivery.

Gallbladder Disease

Cholelithiasis is increased during pregnancy secondary to increases in estrogen production. This does not correlate, however, with the development of cholecystitis. Cholecystectomy should be avoided during pregnancy if at all possible. This procedure should be performed during two circumstances: when bile duct obstruction produces severe pancreatitis or if ascending cholangitis develops. If cholecystectomy is performed during the second or third trimesters, there is less than 5% mortality of the fetus. Endoscopic retrograde cholangiopancreatography (ERCP) with therapeutic sphincterectomy can be performed during pregnancy, although most clinical endoscopists have limited experience.

Pancreatitis

Pancreatitis during pregnancy is usually secondary to underlying hepatobiliary disease and not alcohol use. Symptoms include epigastric pain with elevations of serum amylase and/or lipase, although the absolute level of amylase is usually lower in pregnant patients secondary to increased glomerular filtration rates. Pancreatic pseudocysts and abscesses represent a considerable risk for prematurity, but should be managed similarly to those in nonpregnant patients.

KEY POINTS

1 Knowledge of developing therapeutic options is paramount in high-risk obstetrics with respect to hepatic and gastrointestinal disease during pregnancy.

2 When diagnostic or therapeutic uncertainty exists, obtain a gastroenterology consultation.

3 Gastrointestinal endoscopy is a safe and efficacious diagnostic and therapeutic modality during pregnancy.

SUGGESTED READINGS

Boyce RA: Enteral nutrition in hyperemesis gravidarum: a new development, *J Am Diet Assoc* 92(6):733-736, 1992.

Dubner H, Fromm H: Ursodeoxycholic acid treatment of intrahepatic cholestasis of pregnancy: observations on efficacy and safety, *Gastroenterology* 104(2):660-661, 1993.

Eckhauser FE et al: Enucleation combined with hepatic vascular exclusion is a safe and effective alternative to hepatic resection for liver cell adenoma, *Am Surg* 60(7):466-471, 1994.

Habal FM, Hui G, Greenberg GR: Orla 5-aminosalicyclic acid for inflammatory bowel disease in pregnancy: safety and clinical course, *Gastroenterology* 105(4):1057-60, 1993.

Magann EF et al: Antepartum corticosteroids: disease stabilization in patients with the syndrome of hemolysis, elevated liver enzymes, and low platelets, *Am J Obstet Gynecol* 171(4):1148-1158, 1994.

Mishra L, Seett LB: Viral hepatitis, A through E, complicating pregnancy, *Gastroenterol Clin North Am* 21(4):873-935, 1992.

Olans LB, Woof JL: Gastroesophageal reflux in pregnancy, *Gastrointest Endosc Clin N Am* 4(4):699-712, 1994.

Palma J et al: Effects of ursodeoxycholic acid in patients with intrahepatic cholestasis of pregnancy [preliminary report], *Rev Med Chil* 119:169-171, 1991.

Usta IM et al: Acute fatty liver of pregnancy: an experience in the diagnosis and management of fourteen cases, *Am J Obstet Gynecol* 171(5):1342-1347, 1994.

Chronic Hypertension

FREDERICK P. ZUSPAN

The hypertensive diseases of pregnancy constitute the most common medical problems seen in pregnancy (8% to 11%). The most common hypertensive problem is preeclampsia/eclampsia, seen in approximately 6% to 7% of patients. Chronic hypertension is seen in 4% to 5% of all pregnancies.

Chronic hypertension in pregnancy is diagnosed if there is a sustained elevation of arterial blood pressure >140/90 mm Hg *before* the 20th week of gestation. Often the diagnosis of chronic hypertension is made restrospectively and can be suspected if the diastolic blood pressure during pregnancy before the 20th week of gestation is >80 mm Hg.

TABLE 36-5
Chronic Hypertensive Disease (Severity)

	Blood pressure level	End-organ damage	Response to therapy	Number of therapies to control
Mild	>140/90 <150/100	0	+	0-1
Moderate	>150/100 <170/110	±	+	1
Severe	>170/110	+	±	>2

Classification of chronic hypertension in pregnancy can be mild, moderate, or severe and depends on the absolute level of blood pressure with or without evidence of end organ damage on existing chronic hypertension. One of the most severe problems the patient and the fetus will encounter is antecedent chronic hypertension with superimposed preeclampsia/eclampsia (Table 36-5).

PATHOPHYSIOLOGY AND BLOOD PRESSURE REGULATION

The brachial artery blood pressure is highest when the patient is in the sitting position and lowest when the patient is on her side. Uterine size, compression of the inferior vena cava and aorta, and change in vascular resistance are factors that alter blood pressure readings as the uterus enlarges. Blood pressure should be taken in the sitting position after several minutes of rest.

Utilizing a sphygmomanometer, the blood pressure recording may differ between different observers by as great as ±10 mm Hg. The best reading is obtained by the patient in the home environment utilizing an automated device.

If the mean arterial blood pressure [Systolic – $\frac{2}{3}$(D) or Diastolic + (S – $\frac{D}{3}$)] is persistently >110, the prognosis for the fetus worsens. Fetal loss is directly proportional to the elevation of the mean arterial blood pressure, but systolic blood pressure is also important.

The circadian rhythm of all humans for blood pressure recordings indicates that during sleep the blood pressure is lowest and it is next lowest on awakening. It is highest in the afternoon and then gradually decreases as activity decreases. Pregnant women on antihypertensive therapy may have a reversal in these findings, with higher readings at night.

DIAGNOSIS

If a patient does not have overt hypertension (i.e., a blood pressure of >140/90 before the 20th week of gestation), identifying chronic hypertension as an underlying factor is difficult, especially if she is nulliparous. If one or more of the following signs are present, the physician should suspect chronic hypertension or an underlying tendency for the disease:

(1) diastolic blood pressure in a nonpregnant state or before the 20th week of gestation that consistently exceeds 80 mm/Hg, (2) history of hypertension during pregnancy or after a stress event, (3) history of secondary causes of hypertension (e.g., chronic renal disease), (4) a positive family history of hypertension, (5) and history of hypertension when not pregnant. For the differential diagnosis, preeclampsia should be assumed until proved otherwise and appropriate management instituted. Chronic hypertension in the absence of a negative history is difficult to diagnose in a nulliparous patient.

THERAPY AND MANAGEMENT

Ideally, preconceptional counseling is obtained for a woman with chronic hypertension (Fig. 36-9). Experience with previous pregnancies should be ascertained, and baseline data including prepregnancy laboratory work are needed. Instruction in monitoring of blood pressure before conception is recommended. If the patient is on a specific type of medication and contemplating pregnancy, her medication should be changed to one acceptable during pregnancy. Chronic diuretic therapy should gradually be diminished and eventually eliminated before conception.

Evaluation of the pregnant patient with hypertension includes a search for the etiology and the severity of the disease. Those with mild disease need only baseline studies such as documentation that hypertension exists with the use of home blood pressure monitoring; laboratory tests, including CBC, detailed urinalysis, and serum creatinine level; a careful examination, including evaluation of heart size and murmurs; and a funduscopic examination. If the hypertension is moderate to severe, additional studies should include ECG, chest x-ray for heart contour, electrolytes, creatinine clearance, and ultrasound examination to rule out unilateral small kidney. If hypertension is episodic, urinary catecholamine testing can rule out a pheochromocytoma.

An appropriate diet that curtails heavy salt use is also recommended. The patient is encouraged to use fresh or frozen food and avoid liquids or foods in cans or bottles, which will result in a daily intake of 4 g of sodium chloride, sufficient restriction for the pregnant, chronic hypertensive patient. At least 70 g of protein should be consumed daily.

In addition, the patient should be seen at least every 2 weeks during the prenatal period. Self-monitoring of blood pressure should be performed before and after the patient's 45 minutes of bed rest at noontime. If this is not possible, additional bed rest of at least 1 hour before preparation of the evening meal is encouraged. Lying on the side is the only acceptable method to increase renal blood flow to the kidney. If the self-monitored blood pressure recording is consistently >90 mm Hg in the first half of pregnancy, pharmacotherapy should be considered. Although this may not alter fetal salvage or prevent preeclampsia, it should control major alterations in maternal blood pressure and be protective for the mother. Other measures include confirming EDC with ultrasound and accurate symphysis to fundal height measurements. Ultrasound is usually performed three times: in the first trimester for pregnancy dating, at 28 weeks,

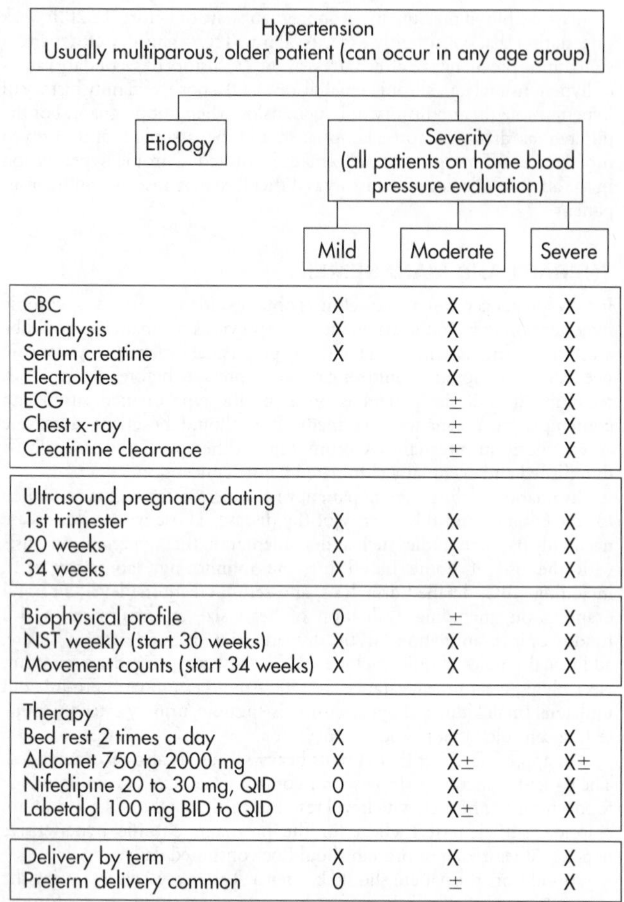

	Mild	Moderate	Severe
CBC	X	X	X
Urinalysis	X	X	X
Serum creatine	X	X	X
Electrolytes		X	X
ECG		±	X
Chest x-ray		±	X
Creatinine clearance		±	X
Ultrasound pregnancy dating			
1st trimester	X	X	X
20 weeks	X	X	X
34 weeks	X	X	X
Biophysical profile	0	±	X
NST weekly (start 30 weeks)	X	X	X
Movement counts (start 34 weeks)	X	X	X
Therapy			
Bed rest 2 times a day	X	X	X
Aldomet 750 to 2000 mg	X	X±	X±
Nifedipine 20 to 30 mg, QID	0	X	X
Labetalol 100 mg BID to QID	0	X±	X
Delivery by term	X	X	X
Preterm delivery common	0	±	X

FIG. 36-9 Diagnosis of chronic hypertension in pregnancy.

and again at 32 to 34 weeks to rule out IUGR. Decreased amniotic fluid should be one sign to assess for IUGR. Careful dating of gestational age is important to prevent the patient from progressing beyond term. The development of preeclampsia, seen as an increase in blood pressure and the development of proteinuria, is often discovered by the patient who is self-monitoring. Prevention of preeclampsia is the focus.

The major therapy for women who have chronic hypertensive disease of pregnancy is bed rest. This should be encouraged for 45 minutes at midday and for 1 hour before preparation of the evening meal. This is the only modality that will increase uterine blood flow.

Uterine blood flow also is increased by the left lateral recumbent position. The mechanism for this increased flow most likely is to decrease the excretion of stress hormone (i.e., epinephrine, noreinephrine), to increase renal plasma flow, and to increase glomerular filtration rate to the kidneys, which presents more sodium to the kidney and promotes the physiologic diuresis of sodium, which in turn decreases cardiovascular reactivity and maintains a stable or decreased blood pressure. All of this ultimately ends up promoting fetal growth and health.

The roles of calcium and low-dose aspirin to prevent preeclampsia are not definitive. Limited research findings show some prevention, but dosage, timing, and overall use of these agents are not clear.

All agree that the "normal" pregnant patient should not be treated with low-dose aspirin. The real question to be answered is, which patients, if any, deserve low-dose aspirin. The only randomized prospective study of high-risk patients with chronic hypertension shows no benefit from low-dose aspirin.

The incidence of eclampsia varies in different parts of the world, being consistently high in India, Jamaica, Thailand, and Columbia and less in Ethiopia, the United States, and Guatemala. Investigators have looked at the relationship between the intake of calcium/person/day and the incidence of eclampsia in different countries and have identified that inverse relationships exist between an increased calcium intake and the incidence of eclampsia. Studies used 1 g/day and 2 g/day of calcium supplementation. There was a significant difference if patients used the 2g/day supplementation in decreasing the incidence of preeclampsia and the numbers of positive angiotensin sensitivity tests that indicated alterations in cardiovascular reactivity. The only randomized prospective study done in the multi-centered maternal-fetal medicine network shows no benefit from the use of calcium to treat chronic hypertension.

When diastolic blood pressure exceeds 90 mm Hg, therapy is specifically for the mother and will not improve fetal salvage or prevent preeclampsia. The drug of choice is methyldopa (Aldomet) in divided doses of 750 to 2000 mg/day. Labetalol, a beta blocker with an alpha component, has been useful as have calcium channel blockers. No commonly used drug has proved to be the drug of choice (Table 36-6). ACE inhibitors should not be used because of fetal effects. Parenteral hydralazine is the drug of choice for acute hypertensive episodes, but IV Labetalol and oral nifedipine are also useful. Overuse causes fetal distress.

All drugs cross the placenta and enter the fetal circulation. Newborns usually make good adjustments to these drugs unless prematurity is a factor. These drugs have not been known to cause birth defects. Parlodel should *not* be used for lactation suppression if the patient has hypertension because of a possible association with strokes and CVA.

TABLE 36-6
Commonly Used Drugs

Drug	Type	Usual oral dose
Aldomet	Central effect (drug of choice)	750-2000 mg qd
Atenolol	Beta blocker (reports of IUGR)	25-50 mg bid to tid
Hydralazine	Direct action on vessels (tachyphylaxis, excellent IV)	20-30 mg bid to qid
Labetalol	Beta blocker with alpha component (most-used drug in Europe)	100 mg bid to tid
Nifedipine	Calcium channel blocker (good results in oral therapy)	20-120 mg qd
Propranolol	Beta blocker (off patent) (not popular in pregnancy)	20-40 mg bid to qid

ANTEPARTUM FETAL EVALUATION

Antepartum fetal evaluation includes fetal growth assessment. Biochemical testing has been of no value, and only biophysical testing is currently used, usually after 30 weeks of gestation. Nonstress tests should be done at each visit from 30 weeks on. An oxytocin contraction test (OCT) may be needed if the nonstress test is unsatisfactory. The vibroacoustic stimulation test will facilitate the nonstress test. In addition, fetal movement activity counting is utilized after the 32nd week of gestation (see Chapter 35). IUGR is usually not seen until after the 30th to 32nd week of gestation. Chronic hypertension also is associated with a fourfold to eightfold increase in abruptio placenta. If the patient complains of abdominal discomfort, this diagnosis must be considered.

If preterm delivery and lack of pulmonary maturity are present, glucocorticoids utilizing betamethasone or dexamethasone may be given to decrease RDS. A waiting period of 48 hours is desirable after medication administration to enhance pulmonary maturity.

LABOR AND DELIVERY CONSIDERATIONS

Continuous electronic fetal monitoring during labor is advised. Early rupture of membranes is performed for scalp clip application and judicious use of scalp pH or scalp stimulation as needed. Regional anesthesthesia with epidural is satisfactory and ideal, but guard against hypotension if the patient has had antihypertensive medication during pregnancy. A pediatrician should be available for evaluation of the newborn. All antihypertensive agents should be assumed to cross the placenta. The newborn usually does quite well if not premature.

POSTPARTUM CONSIDERATIONS

Reevaluation of the need, amount, and type of antihypertensive medication is necessary. The patient should be encouraged to continue self-monitoring of her blood pressure. Women who have chronic hypertension should *not* be placed on oral contraceptives once they leave the hospital or at their 6-week examination. Some form of barrier contraception is preferable. Many of these women have completed their childbearing and can be offered a permanent form of contraception.

KEY POINTS

1 Hypertensive diseases of pregnancy are the most common medical problems in pregnancy. Classification of severity is important–the higher the blood pressure, the worse the prognosis.

2 Preconceptional counseling is important, with adjustment of drugs in preparation for pregnancy necessary.

3 The recommended position for taking blood pressure is the sitting position. Home blood pressure monitoring is an important part of management and decreases the need for antihypertensive therapy and hospitalization.

4 The cornerstone of therapy is bed rest to decrease catecholamines and increase uterine blood flow. Consider antihypertensive drugs if DBP >90. Avoid ACE inhibitors. Drugs *do not* prevent preeclampsia.

5 Monitor the patient to allow diagnosis of superimposed preeclampsia at early stage. This is the worst condition for the fetus. The patient on home blood pressure monitoring often helps make the diagnosis.

6 Antepartum fetal evaluation includes good prenatal care (every 2 weeks), periodic ultasound to assess fetal growth and fluid, fetal activity count, and delivery no later than term. During labor, utilize continuous electronic fetal monitoring as soon as artificial rupture of membranes is done. Administer regional anesthesia with epidural and have pediatrician present.

SUGGESTED READINGS

Belizan JM et al: Calcium supplementation to prevent hypertensive disorders of pregnancy, *New Engl J Med* 325:1399-1404, 1991.

Caritus SN et al: SPO abstract #7 [NICHD MFMU Network]: Low-dose aspirin does not prevent pre-eclampsia in high-risk women, *Am J Obstet Gynecol* 176:53, 1997.

The Eclampsia Collaborative Group: Evidence from the Collaborative Eclampsia Trial: which anti-convulsant for women with eclampsia? *Lancet* 345:1455, 1995.

National high blood pressure education program working group report on high blood pressure in pregnancy, *Am J Obstet Gynecol* 163:1689-1712, 1990.

Levine RJ et al: SPO Abstract #1: Calcium for pre-eclampsia prevention: a double-blind, placebo-controlled trial in healthy nulliparas, *Am J Obstet Gynecol* 176:52, 1997.

Sibai BM, Sarinoglu C, Mercer BM: Eclampsia VII: Pregnancy outcome after eclampsia and long-term prognosis, *Am J Obstet Gynecol* 166:1757-63, 1992.

Sibai BM et al: A randomized prospective comparison of nifedipine and bed rest alone in the management of preeclampsia remote from term, *Am J Obstet Gynecol* 167:879-884, 1992.

Sibai BM et al: Prevention of preeclampsia with low dose aspirin in nulliparous pregnant women, *New Engl J Med* 329:1213, 1993.

Zuspan FP, Rayburn WF: Blood pressure self monitoring during pregnancy, *Am J Obstet Gynecol* 164:2-6, 1991.
Zuspan FP, Samuels P: Preventing preeclampsia, editorial, *N Engl J Med* 329:(17)1265, 1993.

Renal Complications

John M. Davison

RENAL ALTERATIONS IN NORMAL PREGNANCY

Glomerular filtration rate (GFR) and renal plasma flow increase 50% to 70% above prepregnancy values. GFR, as 24-hour creatinine clearance, increases immediately in early pregnancy, and serum levels of creatinine and urea, which average 73 µmol/L (9.82 mg/dl) and 4.3 mmol/L (25 mg/dl), respectively, in nonpregnant women, decrease to mean values of 51 µmol/L (0.58 mg/dl) and 3.3 mmol/L (20 mg/dl) in pregnancy. Creatinine values of 75 µmol/L (0.85 mg/dl) and urea levels of 4.5 mol/L (27 mg/dl), which are acceptable in nonpregnant women, are suspect in pregnancy. Caution is necessary when serially assessing renal function on the basis of serum creatinine levels alone (especially in the presence of renal disease) because even when up to 50% of renal function has been lost, serum creatinine can still be less than 130 mmol/L (145 mg/dl).

The kidneys enlarge because both vascular volume and intestinal space increase, with a 70% increase overall in renal volume by the third trimester. The calyces, renal pelves, and ureters dilate markedly, changes that are invariably more prominent on the right side and evident in 90% of women by the third trimester. There are important clinical complications. It should not be mistaken for obstructive uropathy. Stasis or urine within the ureters may contribute to the tendency in pregnant women with asymptomatic bacteriuria to develop frank pyelonephritis. There may be errors in tests based on timed urine collections. Finally, postpartum x-ray assessment of the renal tract should be delayed until at least 4 months postpartum to allow changes to resolve.

URINARY TRACT INFECTIONS

Urinary tract infections (UTIs) are common in both pregnant and nonpregnant women. Susceptibility relates to basic immunologic differences, structural/functional abnormalities, and socioeconomic factors and may be further increased in pregnancy because of ureteropelvic dilation and increased urinary nutrient content (glucose and amino acids). Since diagnosis is difficult because normal pregnancy-related symptoms include urinary frequency, dysuria, nocturia, and urgency, it must be based on laboratory evidence. A standard definition of infection is a colony count >100,000 bacteria/ml of urine, although counts as low as 20,000 may represent active infection in pregnancy. Urinary white cell count tends to increase in pregnancy such that moderate pyuria may be normal. *E. coli* is the predominant infecting organism (75% to 90% of cases); *Klebseilla, Proteus* and *Enterobacter* account for most of the remainder.

Asymptomatic Bacteriuria

In pregnancy, 5% of women will have a covert urinary infection, 30% of whom will develop a symptomatic infection if untreated. Urinary infection confers an increased risk of pregnancy complications, including premature labor, fetal growth restriction, and preeclampsia. Most obstetricians advocate routine screening at antenatal booking, with additional screening (monthly) in women with a history of urinary infections and/or renal disorders, a policy that would predict 70% of those destined to have symptomatic infections. Treatment should be governed by organism sensitivity and continued for at least 7 to 10 days for initial infections and 21 days for recurrences. Regardless of the antimicrobial used or duration of treatment, 30% of women will relapse. Some authorities advocate prophylactic therapy after reinfection.

There is no evidence that asymptomatic infections cause permanent renal damage in adults with normal urinary tracts. Radiologic abnormalities of the urinary tract are present in 20% of pregnant women with asymptomatic bacteriuria, although the association in some is incidental.

Cystitis

Acute cystitis occurs in 2% of pregnancies, often in women who initially had negative screening in early pregnancy. It probably has a different pathogenesis than asymptomatic bacteriuria or acute pyelonephritis. Infection may be introduced by bladder catheterization, a procedure commonly employed on labor wards and after cesarean delivery. Treatment reduces the risk of ascending infections.

Acute Pyelonephritis

Ureteric dilation may increase susceptibility to pyelonephritis in pregnancy; despite routine screening, it still complicates 1% of pregnancies (3% in unscreened populations). High fever (often fluctuating), vomiting, rigors, and severe loin pain are common findings, but may be absent in the early stages. Diagnosis should be supported by urine microscopy and culture. Severe infections can have serious sequelae, including septic shock, adult RDS, and perinephric abscess formation.

The differential diagnosis is similar to that in nonpregnant subjects but, in addition, loin pain may be caused by acute hydroureter/hydronephrosis or it may be referred from the lumbosacral vertebrae or sacroiliac joints (because of increased lumbar lordosis and softening of pelvic ligaments). Abdominal pain may also be caused by abruptio placentae, degenerating fibroids, chorioamnionitis, or acute appendicitis, the latter presenting atypically in late pregnancy when the uterus is maximally enlarged.

Treatment should be aggressive and undertaken in the hospital. Fluid and electrolyte balance should be monitored and intravenous fluids given to correct hypovolemia. Fetal tachycardia is common, making fetal heart monitoring difficult to interpret. There is a risk of premature labor, although prevention by treatment with beta sympathomimetics may exacerbate endotoxin-induced cardiovascular effects and increase the risk of respiratory complications. A penicillin or cephalosporin should be administered intravenously pending confirmation of organism sensitivity and oral therapy continued for 2 weeks. Failure to respond to treatment may indicate an underlying pelviureteric or ureteric obstruction or the presence of calculi and warrants further investigation.

If gram-negative sepsis is suspected, blood cultures should be taken and an aminoglycoside (gentamycin or tobramycin) added to the regimen, although the new penicillins (e.g., piperacillin) appear to be equally effective, with reduced risk to the fetus. Blood levels of an aminoglycoside should be monitored, since its clearance is altered in pregnancy.

HYDROURETER/HYDRONEPHROSIS

Ureteropelvic dilation is common in pregnancy and may cause loin pain. Urine microscopy demonstrates few or no red cells, repeat urine cultures are negative, and diagnosis is confirmed by ultrasound. Positioning the patient in the knee-chest position may relieve discomfort and promote spontaneous drainage. Rarely is ureteric catheterization (stenting) or nephrostomy necessary to preserve renal function, unless there is a solitary kidney.

UROLITHIASIS (RENAL TRACT CALCULI)

Although factors associated with renal stone formation are known to increase in pregnancy (e.g., urinary stasis, ascending infections, and excretion of stone-forming salts (such as calcium, urate, and cystine), the incidence of renal calculi is low (1/2000 pregnancies). Furthermore, pregnancy does not appear to increase symptomatic calculi in known "stone formers." Enhanced excretion of inhibitors of calcium stone formation such as magnesium, citrate, and nephrocalcin, as well as increased alkalinity of the urine, may afford some protection.

The presentation of renal calculi is similar to that in nonpregnant women. Most ureteric colic occurs in the second or third trimester when ureteric dilation is greatest and perhaps previously as stones pass into the ureter, only to become stuck at the pelvic brim. The mainstay of diagnosis of calculi is ultrasound. Interpretation of findings and visualization of the ureter can be difficult but may by enhanced with color flow Doppler scanning. Radiologic examination is undesirable because of potential effects on the fetus, although limited exposure may be warranted. Renal function should be assessed and infection excluded, but any in-depth analysis of urine and plasma biochemistry to determine the cause of stone formation should be delayed until 4 months after delivery when nonpregnant "norms" can be applied. Conservative management is usually successful or delivery can be effected before undertaking surgical or minimally invasive intervention. Any definitive surgery should be delayed until at least 4 months post partum. The safety of lithotripsy has not been validated in pregnancy. Drugs used to treat "stone formers" (thiazides, xanthine oxidase inhibitors, D-penicillamine) are best avoided.

PREGNANCY IN WOMEN WITH CHRONIC RENAL DISEASE

Fertility and the ability to sustain an uncomplicated pregnancy generally relate to the degree of functional impairment and the presence or absence of hypertension rather than to the renal lesion. Patients are arbitrarily considered in three categories: those with (1) *preserved or only mildly impaired renal function* (serum creatinine ≤1.4 md/dl [≤125 μmol/L]) and no hypertension, (2) *moderate renal insufficiency* (serum creatinine 1.5 to 3 mg/dl or 133 to 275 μmol/L [some use 2.5 mg/dl or 221 μmol/L as the cut-off]), and (3) *severe renal insufficiency* (serum creatinine ≥3 mg/dl or 275 μmol/L) (Table 36-7).

Women in the first category usually have successful obstetric outcomes, and pregnancy does not appear to adversely affect the underlying disease; perinatal mortality in this group is now less than 3%, and evidence of irreversible renal function loss in the mother is even lower. This generalization, however, may not hold true for certain kidney diseases (Table 36-8).

Renal Function

If renal function deteriorates significantly at any stage of pregnancy, reversible causes, such as UTI, subtle dehydration, or electrolyte imbalance (occasionally precipitated by inadvertent diuretic therapy) should be sought. Near term, as in normal pregnancy, a decrease in function of 15% to 20%, which affects blood creatinine minimally, is permissible. Failure to detect a reversible cause of a significant decrement is grounds to end the pregnancy by elective delivery. When proteinuria occurs and persists but

TABLE 36-7

Severity of Renal Disease and Prospects for Pregnancy

	Category		
Prospects	Mild (%)	Moderate (%)	Severe (%)
Pregnancy complications	26	47	86
Successful obstetric outcome	96 (85)	90 (59)	25 (71)
Long-term sequelae	<3 (9)	25 (71)	53 (92)

Estimates are based on 2310 women/3425 pregnancies (1973 to 1995) and do not include collagen diseases. Numbers in parenthesis refer to prospects when complication(s) develop before 28 weeks gestation. (Davison JM and Baylis C, unpublished data).

A very recent analysis of 67 women/82 pregnancies (Jones and Hayslett, 1996) with moderate and severe disease from six tertiary centers is important. Although maternal complications occurred in 70% of cases, and pregnancy-related renal function loss in almost 50% (10% progressed rapidly to end stage failure), the infant survival rate was over 90%, presumably reflecting the specialist obstetric and neonatal care in those centers.

TABLE 36-8
Specific Kidney Diseases and Pregnancy

Renal disease	Effects and outcomes
Chronic glomerulonephritis	Usually no adverse effect in the absence of hypertension. One view is that glomerulonephritis is adversely affected by the coagulation changes of pregnancy. UTIs may occur more frequently.
IgA nephropathy	Risks of uncontrolled and/or sudden escalating hypertension and worsening of renal function.
Pyelonephritis	Bacteriuria in pregnancy can lead to exacerbation. Multiple organ system derangements may ensue, including adult RDS.
Reflux nephropathy	Risks of sudden escalating hypertension and worsening of renal function.
Urolithiasis	Infections can be more frequent, but ureteral dilation and stasis do not seem to affect natural history. Limited data exists on lithotripsy, thus it is best avoided.
Polycystic disease	Functional impairment and hypertension are usually minimal in childbearing years.
Diabetic nephropathy	Usually no adverse effect on the renal lesion, but there is increased frequency of infection, edema, and/or preeclampsia.
Systemic lupus erythematosus (SLE)	Controversial; prognosis most favorable if disease in remission >6 months before conception. Steroid dosage should be increased post partum.
Periarteritis nodosa	Fetal prognosis is dismal and maternal death often occurs.
Scleroderma (SS)	If onset occurs during pregnancy, there can be rapid overall deterioration. Reactivation of quiescent scleroderma may occur post partum.
Previous urinary tract surgery	Might be associated with other malformations of the urogenital tract. UTIs are common during pregnancy. Renal function may undergo reversible decrease. No significant obstructive problem but cesarean delivery often needed for abnormal presentation and/or to avoid disruption of the continence mechanism if artificial sphincter present.
After nephrectomy, solitary kidney, and pelvic kidney	Might be associated with other malformations of urogenital tract. Pregnancy well tolerated. Dystocia rarely occurs with pelvic kidney.
Wegener's granulomatosis	Limited information. Proteinuria (with or without hypertension) is common from early in pregnancy. Immunosuppressives are safe but cytotoxic drugs are best avoided.
Renal artery stenosis	May present as chronic hypertension or as recurrent isolated preeclampsia. If diagnosed, transluminal angioplasty can be undertaken in pregnancy if appropriate.

blood pressure is normal and renal function is preserved, pregnancy can be allowed to continue.

Blood Pressure

Most of the specific risks of hypertension in pregnancy appear to be related to superimposed preeclampsia. There is confusion about the true incidence of superimposed preeclampsia in women with preexisting renal disease. This is because the diagnosis cannot be made with certainty on clinical grounds alone; hypertension and proteinuria may be manifestations of the underlying renal disease. Treatment of mild hypertension (diastolic blood pressure >95 mm Hg in the second trimester or <100 mg Hg in the third) is not necessary during normal pregnancy, but many would treat women with underlying renal disease more aggressively, believing that this preserves kidney function.

Fetal Surveillance and Timing of Delivery

Serial assessment of fetal well-being is essential because renal disease can be associated with IUGR and, when complications do arise, the judicious moment for intervention can be assessed by changes in fetal status. Current technology should minimize the incidence of intrauterine fetal death as well as neonatal morbidity and mortality. Planned preterm delivery may be necessary if there are signs of impending intrauterine fetal death, if renal function deteriorates substantially, if uncontrollable hypertension supervenes, or if eclampsia occurs.

ACUTE OBSTETRIC RENAL FAILURE

Complications of pregnancy used to be a common cause of acute renal failure (ARF) but are now rare, except in third world countries. Improved obstetric management, particularly of preeclampsia and acute hemorrhage, as well as liberalization of abortion laws that prevent the need for illegal procedures that may lead to sepsis, have dramatically reduced the incidence of ARF. Most cases are now related to preeclampsia and its complications, although any cause of ARF may arise in pregnancy.

Acute tubular necrosis is usually the underlying lesion, but a higher proportion of cases are caused by renal cortical necrosis than in nonpregnant subjects. Nevertheless, when ARF is associated with pregnancy-specific conditions such as preeclampsia and HELLP syndrome, spontaneous recovery can be surprisingly rapid after delivery.

Invariably the pregnancy has advanced far enough for the fetus to be viable, and coordination with the neonatal team allows timing of delivery. In the obstetric setting, however, the current pregnancy may represent the best chance of perinatal success so, with the exclusion of preeclampsia, many would advocate early and frequent dialysis to prolong the pregnancy.

Preeclampsia

In preeclampsia, a common condition characterized by generalized vasoconstriction and often associated with minor renal dysfunction, ARF is rare unless there are other complications such as HELLP syndrome or abruptio placentae.

Uterine Sepsis and Pyelonephritis

Serious postpartum and postabortion sepsis is now rare. Improved supportive therapy and evacuation of retained products of conception usually prevent serious sequelae. Clostridial infection can rapidly supervene, resulting in ARF, hemolysis, coagulopathy, and hypocalcemia, although death is usually caused by overwhelming sepsis rather than renal failure. Surgical removal of the uterus is often recommended, but some prefer conservative management, stating that complications make surgery too risky.

Acute primary pyelonephritis is rarely associated with renal dysfunction or ARF in nonpregnant women. In pregnancy, however, decrements in creatinine clearance are common and the risk of ARF appears to be greater, perhaps because of increased sensitivity of renal vasculature to bacterial endotoxins.

Acute Fatty Liver of Pregnancy

Acute fatty liver of pregnancy (AFLP) occurs in late pregnancy or early puerperium and is associated with severe hepatic dysfunction and coagulopathy. Renal dysfunction may be mild, although ARF is not uncommon. Despite its rarity, awareness of AFLP is essential because its initial presentation may be subtle (nausea, vomiting, mild jaundice) or complicated by other conditions such as preeclampsia, in which case there may be rapid progress to severe maternal and fetal compromise. Mortality rates for both mother and baby have been quoted at greater than 70%, although earlier recognition leads to earlier intervention and reduces mortality rates to less than 20%. Other causes of hepatic dysfunction must be excluded and delivery effected immediately, followed by maximal supportive care.

Idiopathic Postpartum Renal Failure

Idiopathic postpartum renal failure is rare but is a recognized cause of ARF in the first few weeks after delivery. Its etiology is obscure, but there are histologic similarities with hemolytic uremic syndrome and malignant nephrosclerosis. The outcome of this condition is poor, few women make a complete recovery.

PREGNANCY IN WOMEN ON LONG-TERM DIALYSIS

Despite reduced libido and relative infertility, women on hemodialysis and peritoneal dialysis can conceive and must therefore use contraception if they wish to avoid pregnancy. Although conception is not common (an incidence of 1/200 patients has been quoted), its true frequency is unknown because most pregnancies in dialyzed patients probably end in early spontaenous abortion and there is a high therapeutic abortion rate in this group of patients.

Some women do achieve delivery of a viable infant, but most physicians do not advise attempts at pregnancy or its continuation if present when the patient has severe renal insufficiency. These patients are prone to volume overloads, severe exacerbations of their hypertension, and/or superimposed preeclampsia and polyhydramnios. They also have high fetal wastage at all stages in pregnancy. Pregnancy poses excessive risks for the mother, and even when therapeutic terminations are excluded the live birth outcome at very best is 40% to 50%.

Women on dialysis frequently present for care in advanced pregnancy because pregnancy was not suspected. Irregular menstruation is common in dialysis patients, and missed periods usually are ignored. Urine pregnancy tests are unreliable (even if there is any urine available). Ultrasound is needed to confirm and date the pregnancy.

The dialysis strategy for a pregnant patient involves a 50% increase in hours and frequency. Plasma urea levels are maintained at <20 mmol/L (120 mg/dl). Intrauterine fetal death is more likely if levels are much in excess of 20 mmol/L. Success has occasionally been achieved despite levels of 25 mmol/L (150 mg/dl) for many weeks. Hypotension during dialysis, which could be damaging to the fetus, is prevented. In late pregnancy the uterus and the supine posture may aggravate this by decreasing venous return. Rigid control of blood pressure is ensured, and rapid fluctuations in intravascular volume are prevented by limiting interdialysis weight gain to about 1 kg until late pregnancy. Signs of preterm labor are assessed; dialysis and uterine contractions are associated. In addition, calcium levels are evaluated to prevent hypercalcemia. Drug therapy is reduced to maintenance levels: prednisone 15 mg/day or less and azathioprine 2 mg/kg body weight/day or less. Safe doses of cyclosporin-A have not yet been established.

In most women, renal function is augmented during pregnancy, but permanent impairment occurs in 15% of pregnancies. In some there may be transient deterioration in late pregnancy (with or without proteinuria). If complications (usually hypertension, renal deterioration and/or rejection) occur before 28 weeks gestation, successful obstetric outcome is reduced by 20%. There is a 30% chance of developing hypertension, preeclampsia, or both. Preterm delivery occurs in 46% to 60% of cases, and IUGR occurs in at least 20% of pregnancies. Despite its pelvic location, a transplanted kidney rarely produces dystocia and is not injured during vaginal delivery. Cesarean delivery should be reserved for obstetric reasons only. Neonatal complications include RDS, leucopenia, thrombocytopenia, adrenocortical insufficiency, and infection. More information is needed about the intrauterine effects and neonatal aftermath of immunosuppression, which at maintenance levels is apparently harmless. From the limited data available, it seems that pregnancy does not necessarily compromise long-term renal outlook.

KEY POINTS

1 Urinary tract infection are the most frequent renal complications during an otherwise normal pregnancy.

2 With chronic renal disease, pregnancy is not contraindicated and a successful and healthy obstetric outcome is attained with no adverse effect on the course of the renal disease if prepregnancy kidney dysfunction is minimal and hypertension does not occur.

3 Treatment of renal failure aims to prevent uremic symptomatology, acid-base and electrolyte disturbances, and volume problems.

4 With dialysis, pregnancy is probably contraindicated because of major risks of the mother and an uncertain and low chance of success.

5 In renal transplantation, the overall complication rate is 46% and chances of success exceed 90%.

SUGGESTED READINGS

Baylis C, Davison JM: The urinary system. In Hytten FE, Chamberlain GVP, eds: *Clinical physiology in obstetrics,* London, 1991, Blackwell Publications, pp. 245-302.

Davison JM, Lindheimer MD: Renal disorders. In Creasy RK, Resnik R, eds; *Maternal fetal medicine: principles and practice,* Philadelphia, 1994, WB Saunders, pp 844-864.

Hou SH: Pregnancy in women on haemodialysis and peritoneal dialysis, *Balliere's Clin Obstet Gyanecol* 8:481-500, 1994.

Jones DC, Hayslett JP: Outcome of pregnancy in women with moderate or severe renal insufficiency, *N Engl J Med* 335:226-232, 1996.

Lindheimer MD, Katz AI: Gestation in women with kidney disease: prognosis and management, *Balliere's Clin Obstet Gynaecol* 8:387-404, 1994.

Petruiset N, Grunfeld JP: Acute renal failure in pregnancy, *Balliere's Clin Obstet Gynecol* 8:333-351, 1994.

Twickler DM et al: Ultrasonic evaluation of central and end-organ hemodynamics in antepartum pyelonephritis, *Am J Obstet Gynecol* 170:814-818, 1994.

37

Perinatal Infections and Immunizations

Kevin A. Ault

CONGENITAL INFECTIONS

Congenital infections of the fetus and newborn are caused by a diverse group of viruses, bacteria, and protozoa. Previously, "TORCH" titers were often ordered in response to certain clinical situations such as intrauterine fetal demise. However, this approach does not take into account new diagnostic methods such as polymerase chain reaction (PCR) and "new" diseases such as varicella, HIV, and parvovirus B19. An estimated 15% of abnormal ultrasounds are the result of congenital infection, with suggestive findings of intracranial calcifications, microcephaly, hydrops fetalis, ascites, IUGR, intrahepatic and intraabdominal calcifications, and hepatosplenomegaly. Additionally, the availability of cordocentesis allows direct diagnostic testing of the fetal bloodstream.

Cytomegalovirus

Cytomegalovirus (CMV) is one of the family of herpes viruses that are characterized by asymptomatic infection with periods of latency and reactivation with intermittent viral shedding. CMV is spread by a variety of mechanisms and is present in many bodily secretions. This infection is nearly always asymptomatic in the immunocompetent host. Antibody response will not clear this virus, and the presence of IgG antibodies in an enzyme-linked immunoabsorbent assay (ELISA) indicates prior infection. IgM antibodies are not a reliable indicator of acute infection because IgM may be present weeks after the initial infection and may reappear at times of reactivation. Any individual may be infected with several strains of CMV.

Because this virus is widespread, serologic evidence of prior infection can be found in 50% to 85% of reproductive-age women. Higher rates of infection are found in women with lower socioeconomic status. Because of this large reservoir of virus, asymptomatic seroconversion is common during pregnancy. Approximately 1% to 2% of women will seroconvert during pregnancy. Risk factors for seroconversion include the presence of a young child in the home, Caucasian race, young maternal age, and middle to upper socioeconomic status. Being a health care worker with occupational exposure to CMV does not appear to increase the risk of either seroconversion during pregnancy or congenital infection.

CMV is the most common perinatal infection, but a vast majority (>90%) of infections of the newborn are asymptomatic. The fetus can be infected in utero by transplacental passage of the virus. Also, the neonate may be infected by CMV present in vaginal secretions. Maternal seroconversion (a primary infection with CMV) during pregnancy will result in a 30% to 40% rate of transmission to the newborn. Women previously infected with CMV will transmit the virus to approximately 1% of their neonates. Infected neonates can display a wide variety of symptoms including petechiae, deafness, hepatosplenomegaly, jaundice, chorioretinitis, and microcephaly. CMV is relatively easy to grow in the diagnostic microbiology laboratory, and urine culture of neonates is the best test for infection. If the diagnosis of intrauterine infection is suspected, amniocentesis with culture of the amniotic fluid should be performed. Cordocentesis has been suggested for detection of fetal IgM; however, this test may be falsely negative because of the immaturity of the fetal immune system.

Routine maternal screening for CMV infection is futile because of the high prevalence of antibodies and the very small likelihood of clinical disease in newborns. Prior exposure to CMV (seropositive for IgG antibodies) greatly lowers the risk of congenital infection but does not offer complete protection. No vaccine is available. Although the antiviral drug ganciclovir has been useful in treating CMV in immunocompromised patients, it is not helpful in congenital infection. In the unlikely event that maternal seroconversion is documented, termination of pregnancy is not indicated because significant neonatal disease is unlikely.

Rubella

Since the introduction of the rubella vaccine almost three decades ago, the total number of cases of both rubella and congenital rubella have dropped dramatically. The rubella virus crosses the placenta, and rates of congenital rubella depend on the stage of gestation. Fetal defects can occur in 90% of infants born to mothers who had rubella at less than 11 weeks gestation. This transmission rate drops quickly as gestational age advances, and cases of congenital rubella related to late second- and third-trimester infection are rare.

The classic triad of findings in a neonate with congenital rubella includes deafness, patent ductus arteriosus, and cataracts. Long-term sequelae relate to CNS damage. Accidental vaccination during pregnancy does not cause congenital rubella.

Several strategies exist to prevent congenital rubella. First, children should be vaccinated against rubella as part of routine pediatric health care. Additionally, all pregnant women should be screened for rubella immunity. Seronegative women should be counseled to avoid children with rubellalike viral illnesses. Postpartum vaccine should be administered to all seronegative women. This vaccine is safe in women who are breastfeeding.

Herpes Simplex Virus

Herpes simplex virus (HSV) is another member of the herpes virus family. The clinical disease caused by this virus is recurrent genital ulcers. Most genital infections are caused by HSV type 2. Generally, the initial outbreak is characterized by multiple painful ulcers of the vulva, vagina, and/or cervix that are 3 or 4 mm in size. Systemic symptoms include fever, headache, myalgia, and urinary retention. This primary outbreak is usually followed by recurrences at unpredictable intervals, and these outbreaks are generally less severe. This is an example of the latency and reactivation of this family of viruses. Also similar to other members of this family, IgG antibodies are not protective, and a positive serologic test indicates prior exposure. Serologic evidence of prior infection can be found in 35% of middle-class, reproductive-age women. Therefore asymptomatic infection with intermittent shedding of this virus is very common.

Neonatal infection can be devastating, especially when there is CNS involvement. A majority of infected infants will exhibit the typical vesicular rash. Fatality rates in cases of disseminated disease are 15% to 50%, with many of the survivors having long-term neurologic damage. Neonatal herpes is acquired when the infant passes through an infected birth canal. In rare cases, HSV can cross the placenta and cause intrauterine infection.

In the past, cesarean-delivery was routinely performed to prevent neonatal exposure to infected vaginal secretions. This strategy was found lacking because most women have asymptomatic infection and shed HSV unpredictably. Antepartum cultures of asymptomatic women do not predict which women will be shedding the virus at the time of delivery. Because of the large reservoir of women exposed to HSV and the asymptomatic shedding of the virus, women giving birth to an infected newborn will not usually give a clinical history of genital herpes. The current recommendation is to perform a cesarean delivery only if active herpetic lesions are present. Women with a clinical history of genital herpes should undergo speculum examination with visualization of the cervix and vagina and an external exam of the vulva to locate herpetic lesions. If no lesions are found, a vaginal delivery should be anticipated.

Syphilis

In the late 1980s and early 1990s, syphilis rates in women soared to their highest level since the widespread availability of penicillin. Congenital infection with syphilis has been recognized since the 16th century. Primary syphilis is a difficult diagnosis to make in women because the syphilis chancre is painless and can be located in the upper vagina or on the cervix. The palmar/plantar rash of secondary syphilis is pathognomonic. Many other symptoms of secondary syphilis include nonspecific signs and symptoms of systemic illness such as fevers, malaise, adenopathy, mucous patches, alopecia, and various other skin lesions. Darkfield microscopy will show motile spirochetes if lesions such as the chancre are sampled. Nonspecific (or nontreponemal) serologic tests such as the VDRL or RPR are also useful for diagnosis. Latent syphilis can be defined as positive serologic tests with signs and symptoms of syphilis. In the early stages of syphilis, 80% to 90% of transmission to the fetus takes place via transplacental infection.

Many of the ultrasound findings suggestive of congenital infections can occur in intrauterine infections with syphilis, especially nonimmune hydrops. Spirochetes may be found in the amniotic fluid. Two classic presentations of syphilis during pregnancy are late intrauterine fetal demise and delivery of a small-for-gestational-age neonate. Approximately half of newborns with congenital syphilis are asymptomatic. Findings consistent with congenital syphilis of the neonate include rhinitis or "snuffles," various rashes, and hematologic abnormalities. Long bone radiographs are useful diagnostic tests in the workup of suspected congenital syphilis and will show periostitis and metaphysitis.

Penicillin is the treatment of choice for syphilis during pregnancy. Pregnant women should be treated with the dose of penicillin appropriate for the stage of the disease. For primary, secondary, and early latent syphilis, the treatment is 2.4 million units of benzathine penicillin given as an intramuscular injection. This dose of penicillin will prevent the congenital sequelae of syphilis as well. Doxycycline and erythromycin are not reliable therapies for syphilis during pregnancy. For pregnant women with a penicillin allergy and who require therapy for syphilis, penicillin desensitization should be done.

Varicella Zoster

Every physician can recognize the widespread vesicular rash of chickenpox, a common childhood disease caused by the varicella zoster virus, also from the herpes virus family. This virus is latent in the nerve ganglia and can recur in later life as herpes zoster or "shingles." It can cause congenital infection, with resultant limb hypoplasia, cutaneous scarring, microcephaly, and other CNS damage.

Because of the highly infectious nature of varicella, most reproductive-age women will give a reliable history of prior childhood illness. Even in the absence of a clinical history, 80% to 90% of women will have serologic evidence of prior infection by ELISA. Varicella in adulthood can be a serious illness. Of special concern in pregnant women is varicella pneumonia. This complication occurs when the typical skin lesions are at their peak. Symptoms are typical of pneumonia and include cough, tachypnea, dyspnea, and chest pain. Mortality in the absence of antiviral therapy is 40%.

Two potential interventions for management of varicella exposure during pregnancy exist. Once testing and/or history have not ruled out previous varicella infection, varicella zoster immune globulin (VZIG) can be given at one vial (125 mg)/10 kg to a maximum of five vials. The ability of VZIG to prevent congenital infection is unproved, but it is believed to decrease the likelihood of serious maternal illness. The VZIG must be given within 96 hours to prevent a potential infection. For women with varicella pneumonia, intravenous acyclovir should be given at a dose of 5 to 10 mg/kg divided into three doses.

Parvovirus B19

Parvovirus B19 is the causative agent of the childhood illness erythema infectiosum or "fifth" disease. This disease is notable for the "slapped cheek" rash it causes in the infected child. Because of the epidemic nature of this disease, 50% to 70% of reproductive-age women will have serologic evidence of prior childhood infection. Acute infection in adults is often asymptomatic.

This virus can cross the placenta, and its pathology is based on its ability to infect erythrocyte precursor cells in the fetus. Infection of these stem cells can lead to fetal anemia and nonimmune hydrops. No other abnormality has been consistently reported with this virus. Intrauterine infection in the second trimester can cause elevation of maternal serum AFP.

Diagnosis of acute maternal infection can be made by demonstrating IgM antibodies. PCR to identify parvovirus DNA can be performed on maternal sera, fetal blood, and amniotic fluid. In women exposed to this virus, sera should be tested by ELISA for virus-specific IgG and IgM antibodies. If IgG antibodies are positive and IgM antibodies are negative, this is consistent with a prior childhood illness and no further workup is indicated. If IgM antibodies are found, fetal surveillance with serial ultrasound examinations is warranted. If hydrops fetalis is found, intrauterine blood transfusion to correct fetal anemia can be considered.

Hepatitis B

In 1988 the CDC recommended screening all pregnant women for hepatitis B surface antigen, a serologic marker potentially indicating chronic carriage and infectivity. At approximately the same time, routine neonatal vaccination was recommended. These measures were undertaken because perinatal transmission of hepatitis leads to chronic liver disease in up to 90% of affected infants.

Newborns acquire hepatitis B through exposure to infected maternal body fluids and blood via maternal-fetal hemorrhage. This leakage of blood is common in the late third trimester and in labor. There are no congenital syndrome or ultrasound-associated findings with this disease. Presence of the "E" antigen (HBeAg) indicates a high degree of infectivity. In mothers with HBeAg, neonatal transmission of hepatitis B is 85% to 90%.

The key to this disease is prevention. All pregnant women should be screened at their first prenatal visit with a serologic test for hepatitis B surface antigen. A positive finding must be communicated to the newborn nursery. The exposed newborn should be given 0.5 ml of hepatitis immune globulin within 12 hours of birth. Additionally, the usual neonatal doses of vaccine should be given.

Toxoplasmosis

Toxoplasma gondii is a protozoan and the causative agent of congenital toxoplasmosis. Most clinicians associate toxoplasmosis with cats, the definitive host for this microorganism. However, *T. gondii* can infect a wide variety of animals, including human beings. Additionally, the oocyst stage is stable for long periods (years) in variable environmental conditions. Therefore toxoplasmosis can be acquired from poorly cooked meat and ordinary garden soil.

Fetal infection occurs after acute maternal infection and parasitemia. The estimated rate for acute toxoplasmosis during pregnancy is 0.2% to 1% in the United States. Maternal infection before pregnancy protects against congenital toxoplasmosis except when there is significant maternal immunosuppression. Acute toxoplasmosis is asymptomatic in adults in 90% of cases. The likelihood of transplacental infection of the fetus depends on gestational age, with the highest rates late in gestation. Estimated rates of infection for first trimester are 10%, second trimester 30%, and third trimester 60%. However, the earlier in gestation fetal infection occurs, the higher likelihood of fetal damage. Ultrasound findings suggestive of congenital toxoplasmosis are similar to findings for other congenital infections. Overall, approximately 85% of congenitally infected neonates are asymptomatic at birth. Sequelae of congenital infection are related to CNS damage and include seizures, psychomotor and mental retardation, and blindness caused by chorioretinitis.

The difficulty in diagnosing maternal toxoplasmosis is the result of unreliable serologic testing, especially false positive IgM tests. More specific laboratory tests are now available, and testing for IgA and IgE is promising. When intrauterine infection is suspected, cordocentesis may be done for serologic testing and tissue culture for isolation of the protozoan. Amniotic fluid for PCR is also a useful test. When maternal seroconversion is documented, antiparasitic therapy decreases the likelihood of fetal damage. Fetal infection occurs several weeks after maternal infection, so therapy is appropriate. Seroconversion is more likely to result in fetal infection after 26 weeks gestation. Consequently, pyrimethamine with sulfadiazine is the indicated initial therapy at this later gestation age.

Because no established system for laboratory diagnosis of congenital toxoplasmosis exists, all pregnant women should be educated about primary prevention methods. These include avoiding contact with cat litter. If cat litter is handled, disinfection is performed by covering litter with near-boiling water for 5 minutes. Patients should also wear gloves while gardening, cook meat to an internal temperature of 150° F, and wash fruits and vegetables before eating them.

Human Immunodeficiency Virus (HIV)

Reproductive-age women are increasingly becoming a part of the HIV/AIDS epidemic. HIV preferentially attacks CD4 positive lymphocytes, causing a gradual depletion of these essential immune cells and leading to opportunistic infections and unusual neoplasms. The clinical syndrome of AIDS is defined by a low CD4 count along with these infections and neoplasms. Since AIDS is usually preceded by years of asymptomatic HIV infection, there are several women with an undiagnosed subclinical HIV infection for every woman with clinically identified AIDS. Most cases of HIV/AIDS in women are acquired by heterosexual activity. The HIV both crosses the placenta and is present in vaginal secretions. Neonatal HIV and AIDS are similar illnesses to the adult diseases, characterized by immunosuppression and opportunistic infections.

Research indicates that zidovudine can be used to prevent perinatal infection. Prevention of neonatal transmission of HIV includes identifying seropositive women by voluntary universal screening. For seropositive women, zidovudine is administered during the second and third trimesters at a dosage of 100 mg five times daily. Intrapartum zidovudine (intravenous) is administered (2 mg/kg loading dose with 1 mg/kg/hour). For the first 6 weeks of life, zidovudine is given at 2 mg/kg orally every 6 hours beginning 8 to 12 hours after birth. Research shows a neonatal transmission rate of 8.3% versus approximately 25.5% in untreated women. Because of the transplacental passage of maternal IgG, neonatal testing for HIV will always be positive by the usual ELISA test. Other potential tests include culture for the HIV virus, PCR, and detection of HIV antigens such as p24. All these tests have been relatively insensitive for detecting neonatal HIV, and an improved test is needed for this clinical situation.

Group B β-Hemolytic Streptococcus

Group B β-hemolytic streptococcus (GBS), a gram-positive cocci, is part of the vaginal flora in 15% to 40% of women. It causes no symptoms, and it is therefore difficult to identify women who are at risk for carriage. Carriage is often transient, and the source for GBS is the rectal flora. The standard method for detection of GBS is a maternal rectovaginal culture in Todd-Hewitt broth, a selective culture media.

GBS is the leading cause of early onset neonatal sepsis, with an attack rate of 1 to 4/1000 live births. Other neonatal diseases caused by this bacteria are pneumonia and meningitis. These infections are acquired as the infant passes through the birth canal. Skin colonization takes place in a majority of infants that pass through a colonized vagina, but only a few develop invasive disease. Factors that put an infant at risk for more serious infection include prematurity, prolonged rupture of membranes (more than 18 hours), maternal fever or amnionitis, and a sibling with GBS disease.

Prevention of GBS is one of the most controversial areas in obstetrics. Antepartum treatment of colonization will not reduce transmission because of reseeding of the vagina from the rectal flora. Intrapartum administration of intravenous ampillicin reduces perinatal transmission of GBS, but it has been difficult to identify women who need this intervention. Antepartum cultures done at 24 to 28 weeks are poorly predictive of maternal colonization at delivery with both false negative and false positive results, probably because vaginal colonization is often transient. Additionally, rectovaginal cultures in selective broth take 48 hours. Rapid tests are relatively insensitive when compared to culture.

ADULT IMMUNIZATIONS

Missed opportunities for adult immunizations are one of the biggest public health challenges facing the primary care physician. An estimated 50,000 to 70,000 adults die each year in the United States from vaccine-preventable diseases. Utilization of these vaccines in at-risk patients is quite low, ranging from 10% to 40%. Guidelines for adult immunization are presented in Table 37-1.

As a general guideline, live virus vaccines should be avoided during pregnancy. Killed or antigen-only vaccines may be given as indicated. For example, completion of the hepatitis B series should not be delayed because of pregnancy. It is prudent to give influenza vaccine to pregnant women with underlying chronic disease. Some experts have recommended that pregnant women be immunized if they are in the third trimester during the flu seasons because of the increased risk of post-viral pneumonia in late pregnancy.

KEY POINTS

1 CMV is the most common perinatal infection; however, most cases are asymptomatic.

2 Penicillin is the treatment of choice for syphilis during pregnancy. For women who are allergic to penicillin, desensitization should be performed.

3 GBS is the most common cause of neonatal sepsis. Suggested strategies for prevention include giving antibiotics to women with positive rectovaginal cultures or to women with risk factors.

4 Perinatal transmission of HIV is prevented by antepartum, intrapartum, and neonatal administration of zidovudine.

5 Adult immunization is one of the most underused tools available to a primary care physician.

TABLE 37-1
Guidelines for Adult Immunizations

Vaccine	Indications	Dosage	Comments
Pneumococcal	Age greater than 65 yr; other adults at increased risk because of underlying diseases (e.g., diabetes, HIV)	0.5 ml intramuscular or subcutaneous	
Influenza	Age greater than 65 yrs, especially those with underlying diseases, health care workers	0.5 ml intramuscular	Must be given annually before flu season with current vaccine
Hepatitis A	Health care workers, food handlers, and other occupational risks, endemic populations		
Hepatitis B	Health care workers, sexual exposure, including prior STDs or multiple partners; household contacts; institutional settings	1 ml given intramuscular in three doses (second dose at 1 month and third at 6 months)	
Measles-mumps-rubella (MMR)	Women without documented immunity or vaccination, college students (measles)	0.5 ml subcutaneous	In most adult cases, MMR is preferred to monovalent vaccine
Tetanus-diphtheria	Every 10 years routinely	0.5 ml intramuscular	Certain classes of wounds may require administration of tetanus immune globulin

SUGGESTED READINGS

American College of Physicians: *Guide for adult immunizations,* ed 3, Philadelphia, 1994, The College.

Berry M, Dajani A: Resurgence of congenital syphilis, *Infect Dis Clin North Am* 6:19-29, 1992.

Connor E et al: Reduction of maternal-infant transmission of human immunodeficiency virus type with zidovudine treatment, *N Eng J Med* 331:1173-1180, 1994.

Enders G et al: Consequences of varicella and herpes zoster in pregnancy: prospective study of 1739 cases, *Lancet* 343:1547-1550, 1994.

Gratacos E et al: The incidence of human parvovirus B19 infection during pregnancy and its impact on perinatal outcome, *J Infect Dis* 171:1360-1363, 1995.

Pastorek JG: The ABCs of hepatitis in pregnancy, *Clin Obstet Gynecol* 36:843-854, 1993.

Raynor BD: Cytomegalovirus infection in pregnancy, *Semin Perinat* 17:394-402, 1993.

Wong SY, Remington JS: Toxoplasmosis in pregnancy, *Clin Infect Dis* 18:853-862, 1994.

38

Common Dermatologic Disorders

Michael C. Gordon and Mark B. Landon

SKIN CHANGES DURING NORMAL PREGNANCY

Physiologic changes in the skin during gestation may result in hyperpigmentation, hirsutism, hair loss, and several vascular abnormalities. Some of these conditions are believed to result from alterations in the hormonal milieu of pregnancy, yet for most skin changes in pregnancy there is little information concerning their precise etiology. The obstetrician must be able to distinguish common skin changes of pregnancy from primary cutaneous diseases that may predate or develop during pregnancy.

Hyperpigmentation

Hyperpigmentation can be found in approximately 90% of pregnancies. Darkening of the areolae, umbilicus, vulva, and perianal skin may occur as early as the first trimester. The linea alba often becomes the hyperpigmented linea nigra. Hyperpigmentation on the face, known as *melasma* or *chloasma,* will often prompt complaints from pregnant women. Chloasma is usually manifested by well-defined, hyperpigmented, centrofacial patches and appears in various shades of brown. Chloasma normally regresses or disappears in the majority of women. During pregnancy some nevi may increase in size and new nevi may develop. This may necessitate performing a biopsy if there is clinical suspicion for melanoma.

Hair Changes

Mild degrees of hirsutism are common during pregnancy. The face is frequently affected, although hair growth may be pronounced on the extremities as well. Mild hirsutism rarely requires therapy. Excessive hirsutism with virilization should warrant investigation for an androgen-secreting tumor.

Telogen effluvium, or hair loss after a shift of anagen (growing phase) follicles to telogen (resting phase), is often seen during the postpartum period. Patients may report hair loss for three to four months after delivery, and should be reassured that normal hair growth will occur 6 to 15 months post partum.

Striae Distensae

Striae distensae begin to appear in the late second trimester in up to 90% of pregnant women. Striae are thin, atrophic, pink or purple linear bands that are found on the abdomen, breasts, and thighs. Although many creams and ointments have been employed to treat striae distensae, these therapies are not thought to have any benefit. Striae persist permanently, although the purplish color fades with time.

Vascular Changes

Vascular changes are evident within the skin of most pregnant women. High levels of estrogen are believed to be responsible for proliferation of blood vessels and congestion. Erythema of the midpalm, hypothenar, and thenar eminences may occur as early as the first trimester as a result of sixfold increase in blood flow to the hands during pregnancy. Increased capillary fragility also is common during later pregnancy. Scattered petechiae are not uncommon over the lower extremities and are the result of a combination of increased capillary hydrostatic pressure and increased capillary fragility. Proliferation of blood vessels results in the formation of spider angiomata and capillary hemangiomas.

DERMATOLOGIC CONDITIONS ASSOCIATED WITH PREGNANCY

Pruritus

Pruritus is a common symptom in pregnancy, occurring in 3% to 14% of all women. Pruritus is also the common symptom of the majority of pregnancy-specific dermatologic diseases as well as nonpregnancy-specific diseases. One of the most common causes of pruritus in pregnancy is cholestasis of pregnancy, which occurs in 0.5% of pregnancies and is caused by intrahepatic cholestasis, which results in increased levels of serum bile salts. The itching is a result of the increased deposition of bile salts found in the skin and occurs in the third trimester of pregnancy. Classically the diagnosis of cholestasis is refuted if cutaneous lesions are present, and cholestasis is therefore not classified as a dermatologic disease of pregnancy. However, since skin lesions (excoriations) are frequently caused by scratching, it must be considered in the differential of skin lesions causing pruritus.

The differential diagnosis of dermatologic disorders specific to pregnancy that present with pruritus as a common symptom includes herpes gestationis, pruritic urticarial papules and plaques of pregnancy (PUPPP), prurigo gestationis, and pruritic folliculitis of pregnancy (Table 38-1 and Fig. 38-1). The difficulty in diagnosing these disorders can be attributed to a confusing nomenclature and the lack of specific diagnostic criteria for each of the disorders, with the exception of herpes gestationis. Multiple different terms have been used to classify similar skin lesions.

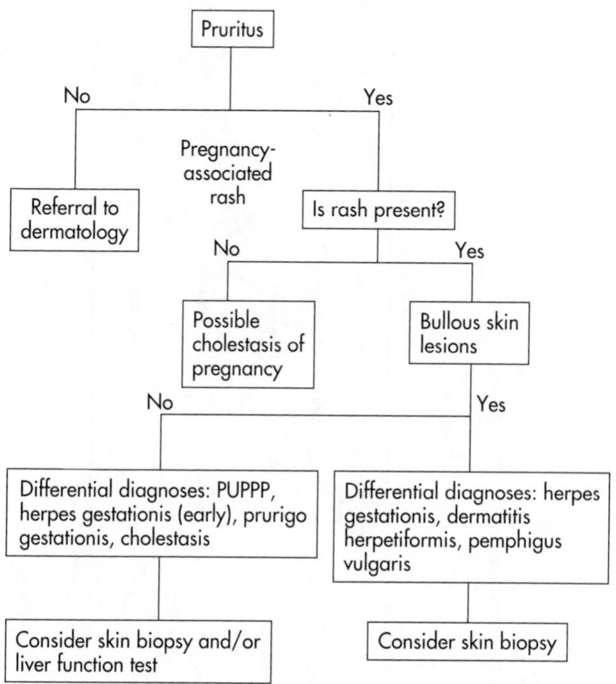

FIG. 38-1 Diagnosis and management of pruritus.

TABLE 38-1
Pruritic Dermatoses of Pregnancy

Disease	Onset	Degree of pruritus	Types of lesions	Distribution	Increased incidence of fetal morbidity or mortality
Herpes gestationis	First month to postpartum	Moderate to severe	Erythematous papules, vesicles, bullae	Abdomen, extremities, generalized	Unresolved
Prurigo gestationis	Fourth to ninth month	Moderate	Excoriated papules	Extensor surfaces of extremities	No
Impetigo herpetiformis	First to ninth month	Minimal	Pustules	Genitalia, medial thighs, umbilicus, breasts, axillas	Yes
Pruritic urticarial papules and plaques of pregnancy (PUPPP)	3rd trimester	Severe	Erythematous urticarial papules and plaques	Abdomen, thighs, buttocks, occasionally arms and legs	No
Cholestasis of pregnancy	3rd trimester	Moderate to severe	None or excoriations	Generalized	Unresolved

HERPES GESTATIONIS

Herpes (pemphigoid) gestationis is a pruritic, autoimmune, bullous disease of the skin that occurs only during pregnancy events and the puerperium. Bullous dermatologic diseases are rare and are considered the classical presentation of autoimmune diseases of the skin. The name *herpes* comes from the Greek word *herpein,* meaning "to creep," and became widely used long before virology and immunology changed the concept of the name *herpes* and has nothing to do with the herpes simplex virus. The disease is rare, with a reported incidence of 1/1700 to 50,000 pregnancies. Herpes gestationis does not increase the risk of maternal mortality.

Pathophysiology

Herpes gestationis is IgG mediated and the so-called *herpes gestationis factor (HG factor)* is a circulating IgG autoantibody with complement-fixing capability found in the serum of the majority of women with herpes gestationis. The HG factor can cross the placenta, has been shown to bind with the basement membrane of amnion and chorion laeve, and can be deposited in fetal skin. A genetic predisposition is suggested by an increased frequency of certain HLA antigens, which has been found in association with other autoimmune disorders. A hormonal influence seems to be operable because this disorder may recur with menses and oral contraceptive use. Histology reveals extensive necrosis of the basal cell layer and edema of the papillary dermis. A chronic inflammatory response with infiltrates of eosinophils admixed with lymphocytes is present around the bullae in a perivascular distribution.

Diagnosis

The initial symptom is pruritus, characteristically extreme, followed by erythema and edema of the subcutaneous tissue. Within days or weeks papules and plaques form, and these have been described as having an urticarial quality. The lesions are often present on the trunk, back, buttocks, forearms, palms, and soles and initially develop around the umbilicus in 50% of patients. The face, scalp, and mucosa are infrequently involved (<10% of women). Vesicles and tense, serum-filled bullae develop at the margins of the edematous, erythematous plaques or can appear de novo in otherwise clinically uninvolved skin within 2 to 4 weeks of the initial onset of the disease. This represents the final stage of the disease and does not always develop. The lesions tend to heal without scarring if secondary infection is prevented. The onset is usually during the second or third trimester with a mean onset of 21 weeks of gestation, although patients may present with recurring crops of blisters at any time during gestation. Herpes gestationis occurs for the first time during the early postpartum period (<4 days) in about 20% of cases. An inconsistent clinical finding is the tendency for spontaneous improvement during the last 6 to 8 weeks of pregnancy. However, the puerperium is often marked by exacerbation of this condition in the majority of women within 24 to 48 hours of delivery. The duration post partum is variable. Herpes gestationis may be recurrent and is usually more severe and has an earlier onset in subsequent pregnancies.

Differential Diagnosis

Clinically the disease presents with lesions that initially may closely resemble PUPPP and later, when bullae or vesicles develop, may closely resemble dermatitis herpetiformis, pemphigus vulgaris, and bullous pemphigoid. The diagnosis of herpes gestationis may be made with reasonable assurance if there is a typical clinical presentation and recurrence with pregnancy, as well as peripheral eosinophilia. Absolute confirmation is made by biopsy and immunopathologic studies that reveal complement C3 in a bandlike distribution along the basement membrane between the epidermis and dermis. This complement deposition is now accepted as the sine qua non of herpes gestationis and is demonstrable in essentially 100% of cases.

Treatment

The treatment for herpes gestationis is aimed at controlling pruritus, suppressing the formation of new vesicles and bullae, and preventing secondary infection of skin lesions. Topical steroids and antihistamines may be used initially if the symptoms are mild. Most patients will, however, require systemic corticosteroids. Prednisone is often begun in doses of 40 to 60 mg/day. The dose of steroid may be tapered as clinical improvement is noted, frequently to doses of 10 to 20 mg/day. Azathioprine, dapsone, and rarely plasmapheresis have been employed in cases that fail to respond to corticosteroids.

Fetal Risks

Studies have consistently shown an increased risk of preterm birth and fetal growth restriction with herpes gestationis, but the majority of studies did not find an increased incidence of stillbirths or miscarriages. This increased risk is believed to be secondary to possible abnormal immune reactions within the placenta related to the HG factor, and antepartum testing is currently recommended. Transient newborn herpes gestationis has also been reported along with the presence of circulating HG factor in 10% of newborns. Neonatal herpes gestationis is usually mild and may be marked only by erythematous papules or frank bullae. Presumably, passive transfer of antibody is the stimulus for this process, which generally resolves within a short period of time.

PUPPP SYNDROME

In 1979 the nomenclature *pruritic urticarial papules and plaques of pregnancy (PUPPP)* was first used to describe seven women with a severe pruritic eruption that first occurred during the third trimester of pregnancy. It was initially believed this eruption could be differentiated by clinical presentation and histologic findings from any other previously described dermatologic condition associated with pregnancy. In the United Kingdom the term *polymorphic eruptions of pregnancy (PEP)* was developed in an attempt to better describe the polymorphic features of this skin disease, and some dermatologists have suggested that this nomenclature be used instead of PUPPP. The incidence of PUPPP is 1/200 to 250 pregnancies, and PUPPP is the most common dermatosis of pregnancy. No increased maternal or fetal mortality or morbidity has been found in pregnancies complicated by PUPPP, but the maternal pruritus can be intense and there may be only partial relief with treatment.

Pathophysiology

The etiology and pathogenesis of PUPPP are unknown. No hormonal or autoimmune abnormalities have been found in women with PUPPP. Since the majority of women affected by PUPPP are primigravidae with prominent striae or those who have uterine overdistention with twins or hydramnios, it has been hypothesized that abnormal skin distention resulting in skin damage may play a role in the etiology of PUPPP. Histologic findings of this disorder consist of a normal epidermis accompanied by a superficial perivascular infiltrate of lymphocytes and histiocytes associated with edema of the papillary dermis. Immunofluorescence studies are negative for both immunoglobulins and complement.

Diagnosis

PUPPP lesions typically begin on the abdomen and initially consist of 1 to 2 mm erythematous papules surrounded by a narrow, pale halo that coalesce into urticarial plaques. The lesions typically begin in the abdominal striae. Small vesicles can also develop on the plaques. The lesions usually spread to the thighs and possibly the buttocks and arms within 2 to 3 days. The face is not affected. Most patients complain of intense pruritus that improves rapidly after delivery, with resolution in 1 to 2 weeks. The average onset of the skin lesions is 36 weeks gestation, and PUPPP rarely develops post partum. There are limited data on recurrence rates with subsequent pregnancies, but classically it is thought to not recur.

Differential Diagnosis

The histologic findings of PUPPP are nonspecific and may be associated with any urticarial allergic response as well as several viral exanthems. Therefore it is essential to obtain a complete drug history and to consider skin biopsy with immunofluorescent studies to exclude early or atypical herpes gestationis before making the diagnosis of PUPPP and starting treatment. There is no clear means of differentiating PUPPP from prurigo gestationis, and by using the nomenclature *PEP* this diagnostic problem can be eliminated.

Treatment

Therapy employing topical steroids is generally successful in the vast majority of women, but some women will require systemic steroids. Antipruritic drugs such as hydroxyzine or diphenhydramine may be helpful. The response to treatment may be difficult to evaluate because abatement of cutaneous lesions and pruritus typically accompanies delivery. Antepartum testing has been recommended in pregnancies with

PUPPP. The main goal of therapy is symptomatic relief of the intense pruritus. In some women the pruritis will be significant enough to warrant induction of labor once fetal lung maturity is assured.

PRURIGO GESTATIONIS (PAPULAR DERMATITIS)

Prurigo gestationis consists of pruritic, excoriated papules usually limited to the extensor surfaces of the extremities. The disease is said to occur in 1 out of 200 pregnancies, but since the diagnostic criteria are so poorly described and because of the potential overlap with PUPPP, the exact incidence is unknown. Papular dermatitis probably represents a more severe and widespread form of this condition, but in the past was considered a separate skin disorder because of the original reports of increased fetal risks and abnormal biochemical findings of elevations of urinary chorionic gonadotropin and decreased plasma levels of hydrocortisone in patients. The majority of current authors do not recognize this as a separate category. Maternal and fetal condition are not affected, and recurrence during subsequent gestations is uncommon.

Pathophysiology

No laboratory or biologic abnormalities have been consistently found in these women; the etiology and pathogenesis of these papular lesions are unknown, although there is some evidence of an atopic diathesis. Histologic findings show a nonspecific dermal perivascular lymphohistiocytic infiltrate.

Diagnosis

Prurigo gestationis lesions are small 1 to 2 mm papules that are distributed symmetrically on extensor surfaces of the extremities. Vesicle or bullae and plaque formation do not occur. Lesions generally appear during the second half of gestation. Two types of prurigo of pregnancy have been described. The early form that presents between 25 and 29 weeks of gestation is marked by intensely pruritic papules of the proximal extremities and trunk. The late form typically appears close to term, with papules often located in abdominal striae. The disease usually resolves after delivery.

Differential Diagnosis

The diagnosis of prurigo gestationis is made by the clinical appearance of a primary papular eruption in women without laboratory evidence of cholestasis of pregnancy. Because of the lack of major clinical, biologic, histologic, or hormonal features that can be used to distinguish this dermatitis, this condition cannot be reliably differentiated from PUPPP.

Treatment

The pruritus responds to calamine lotion and oral antipruritics. Corticosteroids are rarely necessary for the treatment of prurigo gestationis. No antepartum fetal testing appears necessary.

IMPETIGO HERPETIFORMIS

Pathophysiology

Although not a typical cause of pruritus, impetigo herpetiformis is a rare, pustular skin disease that has only been reported in less than 100 pregnancies. There is disagreement among various authors as to whether impetigo herpetiformis is a distinct entity caused by pregnancy or simply a form of pustular psoriasis triggered by pregnancy. In the typical woman with impetigo herpetiformis, there is no prior history of skin disease, there is no family history of psoriasis, and after the pregnancy the lesions do not recur except with subsequent pregnancies. The histopathologic features are indistinguishable from pustular psoriasis.

Diagnosis

The disorder usually occurs in the second half of gestation and begins with the appearance of groups of painful, sterile pustules on an erythematous base typically in the groin and inner thighs. These lesions coalesce and spread to the trunk and extremities and may become secondarily impetiginized. Bullae formation is uncommon. Unlike many of the dermatoses of pregnancy, the mucous membranes are frequently affected. Impetigo herpetiformis may be accompanied by systemic symptoms including fever, chills, arthralgias, vomiting, diarrhea, and lymphadenopathy. Prostration with septicemia may follow. Cardiac and renal failure have occurred in severe cases. The disease usually remits after delivery, but may recur in future pregnancies at an earlier gestational age. Impetigo herptiformis must be differentiated from impetigo, herpes gestationis, and pemphigus.

Treatment

Successful treatment of impetigo herpetiformis includes the administration of systemic corticosteroids and antibiotics for secondary infection, although only a moderate response to the corticosteroid treatment has been reported. Maternal fatalities and increased fetal wastage have been observed in the few reported cases. Therefore fetal surveillance with antepartum testing and elective delivery after fetal maturity has been documented are recommended.

KEY POINTS

1. Several physiologic changes of the skin that may concern the pregnant woman include hyperpigmentation, mild hirsutism, striae distensae, and vascular changes.
2. Pruritus is a relatively frequent symptom in pregnancy, is infrequently caused by a serious dermatologic disease, and usually resolves immediately post partum.
3. The most common causes of pruritic rashes in pregnancy are pruritic urticarial papules and plaques of pregnancy (PUPPP), prurigo gestationis (papular dermatitis), and cholestasis of pregnancy.

4 Rare dermatologic lesions associated with pregnancy are herpes gestationis and impetigo herpetiformis.

5 The only dermatologic diseases of pregnancy that have been shown to cause fetal morbidity are herpes gestationis and impetigo herpetiformis.

SUGGESTED READINGS

Borradori L, Saurat J: Specific dermatoses of pregnancy, toward a comprehensive view? *Arch Dermatol* 130:778, 1994.

Dacus JV: Pruritus in pregnancy, *Clin Obstet Gynecol* 33(4):738, 1990.

Murray JC: Pregnancy and the skin, *Dermatol Clin* 8(2):327, 1990.

Roger D et al: Specific pruritus diseases of pregnancy, a prospective study of 3192 pregnant women, *Arch Dermatol* 130:724, 1990.

Shornick JK, Black MM: Fetal risks in herpes gestationis, *J Am Acad Dermatol* 26:63, 1992.

Yancy KB: Herpes gestationis, *Dermatol Clinic* 8(4):727, 1990.

39

Premature Birth

JAY D. IAMS

Premature birth is the single largest cause of perinatal mortality and morbidity in nonanomalous infants in developed nations; complications of prematurity account for more than 70% of fetal and neonatal deaths annually in babies without anomalies and contribute disproportionately to developmental delay, visual and hearing impairment, chronic lung disease, and cerebral palsy. Babies born before 37 weeks gestation (259 days from the first day of the mother's last menstrual period, or 245 days after conception) are *premature,* regardless of birth weight. An infant who weighs less than 2500 g at birth is said to be *low birth weight* (LBW), regardless of gestational age. Very-low-birth-weight (VLBW) infants weigh less than 1500 g at birth. Rates of LBW and VLBW newborns in blacks are consistently about twice as high as corresponding rates in nonblacks, even when corrected for maternal age and income. The neonatal mortality rate is higher for male than for female VLBW infants. Rates of survival to hospital discharge are shown in Fig. 39-1 for infants weighing less than 1500 grams. Types of morbidity in premature infants who survive include respiratory distress syndrome (RDS), intraventricular hemorrhage (IVH), bronchopulmonary dysplasia (BPD), patent ductus arteriosus (PDA), necrotizing enterocolitis (NEC), sepsis, apnea, and retinopathy of prematurity (ROP). Long-term neurologic morbidity is a

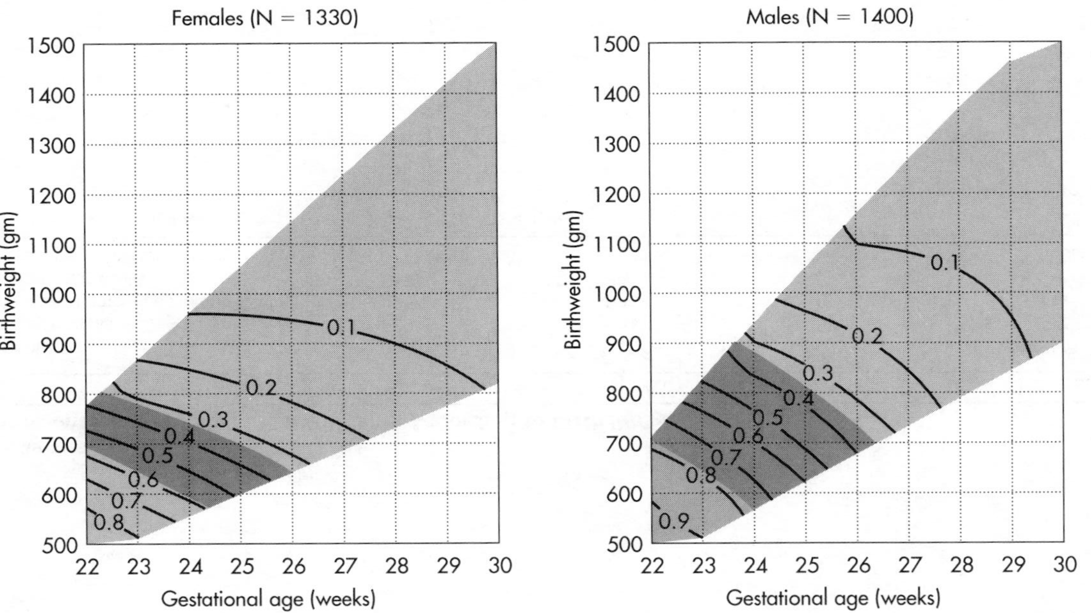

FIG. 39-1 Estimated mortality by birth weight, gestational age, and gender. (From Fanaroff AA et al: *Am J Obstet Gynecol* 173:1423, 1995.)

TABLE 39-1
Major Neonatal Morbidity in VLBW Infants According to Birth Weight

	501-750 g	751-1000 g	1001-1250 g	1251-1500 g
Number of infants	869	982	1153	1275
Respiratory distress	89%	83%	58%	39%
Intraventricular hemorrhage (grade III/IV)	25%	16%	8%	3%
Necrotizing enterocolitis	6%	6%	5%	4%
Hospital stay (average) for survivors	123 days	89 days	64 days	44 days

Data modified from Fanaroff AA et al: *Am J Obstet Gynecol* 173:1423–31, 1995.

significant concern for VLBW infants who survive. Table 39-1 displays the incidence of major morbidity for VLBW infants from 1991 to 1992 by birth weight as stated by the National Institute of Child Health and Human Development.

EPIDEMIOLOGY AND PATHOGENESIS

Prematurity is often called a *multifactorial problem.* Diagnoses that may lead to a preterm delivery include preterm labor, preterm ruptured membranes, preeclampsia, abruptio placentae, multiple gestation, placenta previa, fetal growth restriction, excessive or inadequate amniotic fluid volume, fetal anomalies, amnionitis, incompetent cervix, and maternal medical problems such as diabetes, asthma, drug abuse, and pyelonephritis may all lead to preterm delivery. Maternal characteristics associated with preterm delivery include maternal race (blacks at higher risk than nonblacks), poor nutrition and low prepregnancy weight, a history of previous preterm birth, absent or inadequate prenatal care, strenuous work, high personal stress, anemia (hemoglobin <10 g/dl), cigarette smoking, bacteriuria, genital colonization or infection (e.g., bacterial vaginosis, *N. gonorrhoeae, Chlamydia trachomatis,* mycoplasma, and ureaplasma), cervical injury or abnormality (e.g., in utero exposure to diethylstilbestrol or a history of cervical conization or second trimester induced abortion), uterine anomaly or fibroids, excessive uterine contractility, and premature cervical dilation of >1 cm or effacement ≥80%.

Spontaneous Versus Indicated Preterm Delivery

The clinical disorders listed have been usefully organized into two broad categories called **spontaneous** and **indicated** preterm births, based on the clinical presentation that led to premature delivery. Approximately 75% of preterm births occur "spontaneously" after preterm labor (PTL), preterm prematurely ruptured membranes (preterm PROM), or related diagnoses. The **spontaneous preterm delivery** category also includes deliveries after amnionitis, with or without preterm PROM, and as described in the next chapter, patients with reduced competence of the cervix. **Indicated preterm births** follow medical or obstetric disorders that place the fetus at risk (e.g., acute or chronic maternal hypertension, diabetes, placenta previa or abruption, and IUGR). Indicated preterm births account for 20% to 30% of births before 37 weeks. The distinction between indicated and spontaneous preterm births is useful because it has led to an understanding of spontaneous preterm birth as a syndrome that includes PTL, preterm PROM, amnionitis, and low or abnormal cervical competence. Spontaneous preterm births are more common among women who are indigent, poorly nourished, black, and/or who have a history of genital infection, in particular bacterial vaginosis. In parous women, the risk of spontaneous preterm birth is increased if there is a history of prior preterm delivery. The recurrence risk rises as the number of prior preterm births increases, and rises still further as the gestational age at delivery of the prior preterm birth decreases. The risk factors associated with spontaneous preterm birth have relatively high prevalence in the population and consequently a low predictive value for spontaneous preterm births. More than half occur in women who have no obvious risk factors.

How do these diverse risk factors influence the rate of premature delivery? The traditional view, that each risk factor or disease produces preterm birth in a unique and independent fashion, is being replaced by a model of interactive risk factors that act in concert to create an "injury" or inflammation at the maternal-fetal interface. In this model, the fetal membranes and decidua, in response to an inflammatory insult (usually infectious or ischemic, but occasionally traumatic or even "allergic" in origin) produce cytokines that elicit production of bioactive lipids (e.g., prostaglandin E_2, prostaglandin $F_{2\alpha}$, thromboxane-A_2) that stimulate myometrial contractions and may initiate release of proteases that can injure the membranes and underlying decidua, finally resulting via prostaglandin stimulation in cervical ripening, dilation, and/or membrane rupture. The intensity and duration of the insult, the gestational age at the time of insult, and the host response to the injury (e.g., relative cervical competence [see Chapter 40], nutritional status, immune function) all affect the likelihood of preterm birth. A single risk factor may be sufficient to initiate labor or rupture of membranes (e.g., extreme uterine distention in multiple pregnancy). Recurrent spontaneous premature birth appears to be a syndrome analogous to atherosclerotic cardiovascular disease in which the underlying pathology is complete or partial occlusion of a blood vessel caused by the combined influence of cholesterol, smoking, blood pressure, etc. In recurrent prematurity, the pathologic event is an ischemic and/or infectious injury to the fetoplacental unit sufficient to trigger labor or membrane rupture that is influenced by variables such as uterine volume and contraction frequency, microbial colonization of the lower and upper genital tract, hypoxic or hemorrhagic injury to the fetal-maternal interface, fetal paracrine signals for labor, and host factors such as cervical competence.

PREVENTION AND TREATMENT

Tertiary care–treatment after the diagnosis has been made–has no effect on the incidence of a disease but is aimed at reducing morbidity and mortality after an illness occurs. For spontaneous prematurity, tertiary care includes prompt diagnosis and referral to an appropriate care site, treatment of the primary diagnosis with appropriate medication (e.g., tocolytic drugs for preterm labor or antibiotics for amnionitis), and corticosteroids to reduce neonatal mortality and morbidity. Secondary care–selection of patients with increased risk for surveillance and/or prophylactic treatment–includes risk-scoring systems, early diagnosis programs, prophylactic medications (e.g., tocolytic drugs, progesterone supplementation, antibiotics), and reduced activity. Primary care–the elimination or reduction of risk in an entire population–is not yet possible for spontaneous preterm birth because effective interventions have not been demonstrated. A public health program to reduce prematurity will probably include prevention of smoking and sexually transmitted disease, fertility management to avoid higher order multifetal gestation, planned pregnancy, workforce policies that allow women to have variable work schedules, physical and sexual activity advice, and a cervical assessment at 20 to 26 weeks gestation.

TERTIARY CARE

Initial Evaluation

Women who will experience spontaneous preterm delivery may have diverse complaints, ranging from obvious ("I'm in labor" or "I think my bag of waters has broken") to seemingly minor symptoms such as increased pelvic pressure or vaginal discharge, occasional spotting, or an awareness of painless contractions. Any woman who reports persistent abdominal or pelvic symptoms between 18 and 35 weeks should be evaluated promptly for possible PTL or preterm PROM. The first step is determining whether membrane rupture has occurred, because both maternal and fetal risks of continuing the pregnancy are heavily influenced by the status of the membranes. The next concern is often an evaluation of fetal maturity. Pulmonary immaturity is the most frequent cause of serious newborn illness and death. Amniotic fluid studies of fetal pulmonary maturity are consequently an important part of the evaluation of the patient with impending preterm delivery. In patients with intact membranes, if the quality of obstetric dating is good and intrauterine fetal well-being is not compromised, the likelihood of neonatal RDS can often be satisfactorily estimated from the gestational age. Amniocentesis to assess fetal pulmonary maturity becomes important when dates are uncertain and/or when fetal jeopardy may occur by continuing the pregnancy (e.g., when membranes have ruptured, fetal heart patterns are nonreassuring, or growth restriction is suspected). Amniocentesis may also be indicated for fetal karyotype in cases of PTL complicated by polyhydramnios, or for culture, glucose, and gram stain when amnionitis is suspected. In contrast, amniocentesis should always be considered in women with preterm PROM, for whom the risks of infection and fetal compromise are greater.

Adjunctive Care

Despite the various treatments for PTL and preterm PROM, most women do not deliver at term. About 60% to 70% of women with PTL and more than 80% of those with preterm PROM will deliver before 37 weeks. Often the most important care these infants receive is provided by the obstetrician in the form of medications given to the mother *before birth* to reduce the infant's chances of RDS, IVH, and perinatal group B streptococcal infection, and in maternal transfer to a tertiary care hospital with appropriate facilities for complicated maternal and neonatal care. These simple steps are among the most effective in perinatal medicine to reduce perinatal mortality and morbidity. Administration of penicillin during labor (2 million units intravenously every 4 to 6 hours) or an equivalent antibiotic is effective to reduce the incidence of neonatal group B streptococcal sepsis. When administered 24 or more hours before preterm birth, corticosteroids (12 mg of Celestone, a combination of 6 mg each of betamethasone phosphate and acetate) can reduce the incidence and severity of RDS and

IVH, and thereby reduce as well the perinatal mortality rate in infants born before 34 weeks. Regionalization of perinatal care allows uncommon perinatal illnesses to be cared for by personnel who have a concentrated experience in centers that have appropriate facilities for these mothers and infants.

Diagnosis of Preterm Labor

The diagnosis of PTL is based on persistent uterine contractions and change in the dilation and/or effacement of the cervix by digital examination; however, the accuracy of these criteria is poor. Approximately 40% of subjects diagnosed by these criteria who are treated with placebo will deliver at term. This high rate of false positive diagnosis leads to unnecessary treatment of many women with persistent uterine activity who do not actually have PTL. False negative diagnosis is also a significant problem. Poor diagnostic accuracy occurs because the symptoms and signs of early PTL are common in normal healthy women, and because the digital examination of the cervix is imprecise. Symptoms of PTL are nonspecific (mild contractions that often are not terribly painful, pelvic pressure, an increase in vaginal discharge, and menstrual-like cramps) and are not necessarily those of labor at term. It is important to emphasize that contractions may be painful or painless and may be distinguished from the normal contractions of pregnancy (termed *Braxton-Hicks contractions*) only by their persistence. Contraction frequency often forms the basis of the diagnosis but can be misleading. There is wide variation in contraction frequency according to gestational age and time of day. Contractions normally occur more often at night and increase after 24 weeks. Uterine contraction frequency decreases after maternal rest and increases after coitus. Digital assessment of cervical dilation ≥3 cm is straightforward; however, in early labor, when accuracy is most important, the detection of small changes in dilation, effacement, and cervical consistency (soft or firm) are highly subjective and poorly reproducible.

A newly approved test, an assay for the presence of fetal fibronectin in cervicovaginal secretions, may lead to more accurate diagnosis of early PTL, with improvements in both specificity and sensitivity over traditional methods. Fibronectin is an extracellular matrix protein that functions as the "glue" that attaches fetal membranes to the maternal decidua. Its presence in cervicovaginal secretions after 22 weeks of pregnancy is uncommon and is associated with an increased risk of preterm birth for 14 days after a positive test. More importantly, a negative fibronectin test in a symptomatic patient with cervical dilation <3 cm carries a negative predictive value of 99.5% for delivery within 1 week. The test should help to avoid the common problems of overdiagnosis and treatment. A transvaginal ultrasound measurement of the cervix that indicates a length of 30 mm or more has also been found to have a high negative predictive value for preterm delivery in symptomatic women. In summary, diagnosis of premature labor is often uncertain, and treatment is not always benign. To increase the sensitivity of diagnosis without treating unnecessarily, it is best to be *liberal* in looking for PTL, but *conservative* in diagnosis and treatment. The goal of first contact with a patient who may have PTL should be sensitivity, whereas the goal of evaluation in labor and delivery should be specificity.

Treatment of Preterm Labor

The initial evaluation of preterm labor is focused on the risks and benefits of continuing the pregnancy. Contraindications to tocolysis are shown in Box 39-1.

Potential causes of PTL should be sought not only in the initial evaluation of the patient, but should also be reassessed during the course of treatment. A cause of labor may be found that is best treated by delivery (e.g., abruptio placentae or amnionitis), that may influence the choice of tocolytic (e.g., a degenerating myoma is best treated with a prostaglandin inhibitor), or that may require adjunctive treatment (e.g., antibiotic for pyelonephritis or a therapeutic amniocentesis for polyhydramnios).

Tocolytic drugs are reasonably safe when used according to published protocols for 24 to 48 hours. The most commonly used agents are drugs that antagonize the effects of calcium (magnesium sulfate and the calcium channel blocker nifedipine), the beta sympathomimetic drugs (ritodrine and terbutaline), and prostaglandin inhibitors (indomethacin) (Box 39-2).

Diagnosis of Preterm PROM

Preterm PROM should never be entirely excluded in any patient with either oligohydramnios or symptoms of persistent leakage. A history of passing

BOX 39-1
Contraindications to Tocolysis

MATERNAL

Significant hypertension (eclampsia, severe preeclampsia, chronic hypertension)
Antepartum hemorrhage
Cardiac disease
Any medical or obstetric condition that contraindicates prolongation of pregnancy
Hypersensitivity to a specific tocolytic agent

FETAL

Gestational age ≥37 weeks
Advanced dilation/effacement
Demise or lethal anomaly
Birth weight ≥2500 g
Chorioamnionitis
In utero fetal compromise
- Acute: Fetal distress
- Chronic: IUGR/substance abuse

BOX 39-2
Protocols for Tocolytic Drugs

MAGNESIUM SULFATE

1. Loading dose is 6 g magnesium sulfate in 10% to 20% solution over 15 minutes (60 ml of 10% magnesium sulfate in D5 0.9 normal saline).
2. Maintenance dose is 2 g/hr (40 g magnesium sulfate added to 1 L D5 0.9 normal saline or Ringer's lactate at 50 ml/hr). The infusion may be increased by 1 g/hr until the patient has one or no contractions per 10 minutes or maximum dose of 4 to 5 g/hr is reached. While patient is taking magnesium sulfate, check deep tendon reflexes and vital signs hourly, intake and output every 2 to 4 hours. Magnesium levels may be checked if the infusion is >4 g/hr or if there is clinical concern about toxicity.
3. When contractions are <4/hr, maintain magnesium sulfate for 12 to 24 hours, and then reduce the infusion by 1 g/hour each hour, discontinuing the infusion when the dose reaches 2 g/hr.
4. Maternal side effects include flushing, nausea, vomiting, headache, muscle weakness, diplopia, shortness of breath, and pulmonary edema. Neonatal complications are uncommon. Lethargy, hypotonia, and respiratory depression have been observed.

NIFEDIPINE

1. Administer 5 to 10 mg sublingually initially, then 10 mg every 15 to 20 minutes for as many as three additional doses, then 10 to 20 mg orally every 4 to 6 hours.
2. Maternal side effects include a decrease in blood pressure and increased heart rate rarely accompanied by significant hypotension, headache, flushing, dizziness, and nausea. Skeletal muscle blockade may occur when nifedipine is used in conjunction with magnesium sulfate.
3. Neonatal side effects are uncommon and are secondary to maternal hypotension.

BETA-SYMPATHOMIMETICS

Ritodrine

1. Begin intravenous infusion at 50 μg (0.05 mg)/minute, and increase by 50 μg every 20 minutes until contraction frequency is ≤6/hr, or a maximum dose of 350 μg/minute is reached.
2. When contractions are ≤4/hr, maintain the infusion for 1 hour, and then decrease the dose to the lowest rate that maintains contractions at <4/hr.
3. Continue this rate for 12 hours.

Terbutaline

Terbutaline may be given intravenously, but is more commonly administered subcutaneously.

1. A single dose of 250 μg (0.25 mg) via subcutaneous injection may be repeated every 3 to 4 hours for up to 3 doses.

BOX 39-2
Protocols for Tocolytic Drugs—cont'd

BETA-SYMPATHOMIMETICS—cont'd

Terbutaline—cont'd

2. A dose of subcutaneous terbutaline, 0.25 mg, may be given adjunctively with intravenous magnesium without increasing maternal or neonatal side effects. Continued treatment with more than one or two subcutaneous doses of terbutaline in combination with intravenous magnesium is associated with an unacceptable increase in side effects.

Side Effects of Beta-Sympathomimetics

1. Maternal side effects include tachycardia, hypotension, arrhythmia, hyperglycemia, hypokalemia, hypocalcemia, nausea and vomiting, chest pain, jitteriness, pruritis, and pulmonary edema. Maternal deaths have occurred when beta-sympathomimetics were given to patients with occult cardiac disease.
2. Most neonatal side effects are a consequence of the maternal side effects: tachycardia, neonatal hypotension, fetal hyperglycemia with subsequent neonatal hypoglycemia, and myocardial hypertrophy and ischemia.
3. There is preliminary evidence that beta-sympathomimetic tocolytics may increase the incidence of serious neonatal intraventricular hemorrhage.

INDOMETHACIN

1. Use only before 32 weeks gestation.
2. Loading dose of 100 mg rectally or 50 mg orally; may repeat in 1 hour if no decrease in contractions, followed by 25 to 50 mg every 4 to 6 hours for 48 hours.
3. Check amniotic fluid volume before initiation and at 48 to 72 hours.
4. Do not use the drug for longer than 48 consecutive hours.
5. Discontinue therapy promptly if delivery seems imminent.
6. Maternal side effects include nausea, heartburn, and vomiting. Rare but serious complications include gastrointestinal bleeding, alterations in coagulation, thrombocytopenia, asthma in aspirin-sensitive patients, and acute increases in blood pressure in hypertensive women. Prolonged treatment can lead to renal injury. Indomethacin may obscure a clinically significant fever. Maternal contraindications to indomethacin tocolysis include renal or hepatic disease, active peptic ulcer disease, poorly controlled hypertension, asthma, and coagulation disorders.
7. Three principal neonatal side effects have been reported, all of which occur rarely if at all when the duration of treatment is ≤48 hours: constriction of the ductus arteriosus, oligohydramnios caused by reduced urine production, and neonatal pulmonary hypertension. Fetal contraindications to indomethacin include growth restriction, renal anomalies, chorioamnionitis, oligohydramnios, ductal-dependent cardiac defects, and twin-twin transfusion syndrome.

fluid through the vagina should be evaluated by a sterile speculum examination to look for fluid pooled in the vagina or leaking from the cervix, to perform pH testing (Nitrazine test–a pH of 7 or more is consistent with amniotic fluid) of any fluid, and to obtain a swab of fluid on a slide for the "fern" test. In equivocal cases the fibronectin assay may be useful because it will be strongly positive in the presence of ruptured membranes. Digital examination should be avoided in women with preterm PROM because of the risk of introducing bacteria into the endocervix. Even a single digital examination may increase the risk of infection. Ultrasound assessment of amniotic fluid volume should also be performed; a finding of decreased or absent fluid supports a diagnosis of ruptured membranes. The patient should be monitored to evaluate fetal well-being and uterine contractions. Compression of the umbilical cord secondary to decreased amniotic fluid may cause variable decelerations.

The duration of pregnancy after PROM is inversely related to the gestational age at time of membrane rupture. Before 26 weeks gestation, 30% to 40% of patients will deliver more than 7 days after rupture; 20% may even gain 4 weeks or more before delivery. When PROM occurs between 28 to 36 weeks gestation, 70% to 80% of patients will deliver within the first week after PROM and more than half of these within the first 4 days. At term, 80% of women go into labor within the first 24 hours after rupture of the membranes. It is difficult to predict the clinical course of an individual patient after preterm PROM.

Intrauterine infection is a potentially serious complication of preterm PROM. Up to 25% to 30% of women with preterm PROM will have a positive amniotic fluid culture, but only about 10% of patients with preterm PROM will develop overt chorioamnionitis. Remarkably, a clinical diagnosis of amnionitis in the mother usually does not result in neonatal infection. Sepsis occurs in approximately 10% to 15% of babies born after preterm PROM, and although more common (up to 50%) after maternal chorioamnionitis, it is not limited to infants born to mothers with overt infection. The risk of neonatal infection can be reduced by antepartum treatment with antibiotics. The frequency of neonatal infection increases as the gestational age at presentation decreases. Serious noninfectious fetal complications of preterm PROM are shown in Box 39-3.

Management of Preterm PROM

Care of women with prematurely ruptured membranes is one of the most controversial subjects in obstetrics. The many opinions about management provide strong evidence that no one treatment is appropriate for every clinical situation. In conservative (expectant) management, the patient is hospitalized for surveillance for signs of fetal distress or infection; if either occurs, labor is allowed or induced if necessary. The advantages are that this approach provides maximum opportunity to prolong pregnancy and a low rate of cesarean delivery. Disadvantages are that it requires daily assessment of fetal well-being and infection and tests are not always accurate. In the immediate delivery approach, pregnancies beyond a certain gestational age (e.g., ≥32 weeks) or estimated fetal weight (e.g., ≥1500 to 1800 g) are delivered promptly. Advantages are that it avoids the need for daily

BOX 39-3
Noninfectious Risks of Preterm PROM

Cord compression and prolapse: more common in nonvertex presentations
Cesarean delivery for fetal distress/cord compression and for failure to progress
Abruption: 5% to 6% of preterm PROM; 25% abruption rate if bleeding after PROM
Pulmonary hypoplasia: risk correlates with gestational age at rupture
19 weeks: 50%
22 weeks: 25%
26 weeks: <10%

From Rotschild et al: *Am J Obstet Gynecol* 162:46-52, 1990.

surveillance for fetal well-being and infection. Outcomes are generally good for most infants after 32 weeks. Disadvantages are that it commits to delivery some women who might have continued the pregnancy long enough to allow additional fetal maturity before delivery. The rate of cesarean delivery for failed induction is high. In the delayed delivery with interventions approach, antibiotic treatment is used to reduce infection, corticosteroids are used to accelerate fetal lung maturation, and/or tocolytic drugs are used to delay delivery. Advantages are that this approach attempts to maximize fetal condition and avoid prolonged fetal surveillance. Benefits of steroids and antibiotics for group B streptococcus prevention have been endorsed by ACOG and NICHD. As a disadvantage, the magnitude of benefit remains controversial, especially for delayed delivery 48 hours or more after membranes rupture.

All three strategies are appropriate choices depending on the gestational age and individual and population-based assessments of the risk of infection and prematurity. For example, expectant management is often chosen for women who present before 26 to 28 weeks, immediate delivery for women after 32 to 34 weeks, with interventionist strategies employed between 26 and 32 weeks. Guidelines for the diagnosis of preterm labor are shown in Box 39-4.

KEY POINTS

1 Preterm birth is the leading cause of perinatal mortality and morbidity in nonanomalous infants.

2 Spontaneous preterm birth is a syndrome of clinical disorders that includes preterm labor, preterm PROM, amnionitis, and abnormal cervical competence.

3 Early diagnosis of preterm labor is difficult: false positive and false negative diagnoses are common. Fetal fibronectin in cervicovaginal secretions and transvaginal ultrasound measurement of cervical length improve preterm labor detection by reducing false positive diagnoses.

BOX 39-4
Guidelines for the Diagnosis of Preterm Labor

1. Patient presents with the following signs/symptoms suggesting PTL or preterm PROM: Persistent contractions (painful or painless); intermittent abdominal cramping, pelvic pressure, or backache; increase or change in vaginal discharge; vaginal spotting or bleeding.
2. Sterile speculum examination for pH, fern, pooled fluid, cultures for group B streptococcus (outer third of vagina and perineum), chlamydia (cervix), and *N. gonorrhoeae* (cervix); and fibronectin swab (external cervical os and posterior fornix, avoiding areas with bleeding).
3. Transabdominal ultrasound examination for placental location, amniotic fluid volume, estimated fetal weight and presentation, and fetal well-being.
4. Digital examination (if preterm PROM ruled out by above)
   Cervix ≥3 cm dilation: The diagnosis of PTL is confirmed; candidate for tocolysis.
   Cervix 2-3 cm dilation: The diagnosis of PTL likely but not established. Send fibronectin and monitor contraction frequency. Repeat digital examination in 30 to 60 minutes. Candidate for tocolysis if any cervical change, contractions increase in frequency, or if fibronectin is positive.
   Cervix <2 cm dilation: The diagnosis of PTL uncertain. Monitor contraction frequency, obtain fibronectin swab, and repeat digital examination in 1 to 2 hours. Candidate for tocolysis if there is a 1 cm change in cervical dilation or if fibronectin swab is positive.
5. Treatment of symptomatic positive fibronectin
   Parenteral tocolysis
   Maternal transfer
   Group B streptococcus prophylaxis
   Steroids
   Hospitalize for 3 to 7 days
6. Treatment of sympatomatic negative fibronectin
   Parenteral tocolysis begun (cervix ≥2 cm)
      Risk for delivery at ≤7 days is 1.7% to 3.5%
      Conclude course of tocolysis
   Reduce hospital stay
   Tocolysis not begun
      Risk for delivery at ≤7 days is up to 1.8%
      Observe in outpatient setting
   Cervical sonography should be considered in these patients to assess risk of spontaneous preterm delivery.

Note: Fibronectin has been approved by the FDA for use in the management of symptomatic women with questionable PTL. Use in asymptomatic subjects is not FDA approved.

4 The goal of treatment of PTL is to delay delivery.

5 There is no one best method of managing all patients with preterm PROM.

SUGGESTED READINGS

American College of Obstetricians and Gynecologists Committee on Obstetric Practice: *Antenatal corticosteroids therapy for fetal maturation,* clinical opinion 147, December 1994, ACOG.

Fanaroff AA et al: Very-low-birth-weight outcomes of the national Institute of Child Health and Human Development Neonatal Research Network (1991-1992), *Am J Obstet Gynecol* 173:1423-31, 1995.

Higby K, Xenakis EMJ, Pauerstein CJ: Do tocolytic agents stop preterm labor? A critical and comprehensive review of efficacy and safety, *Am J Obstet Gynecol* 168:1247-1259, 1993.

Iams JD, ed: Preterm labor, *Clin Obstet Gynecol* 38:673-810, 1995.

Iams JD: Preterm birth. In Gabbe SG, Niebyl J, Simpson JL: *Obstetrics: normal and problem pregnancies,* ed 3, New York, 1996, Churchill Livingstone.

40

Abnormal Cervical Competence

JAY D. IAMS

The ability of the cervix to retain the fetus until delivery at term is called *cervical competence,* a continuous variable in which the risk of spontaneous preterm birth *increases* as cervical competence *decreases.* Incompetence is simply the lowest end of a spectrum of clinical pathology for which the traditional clinical presentation remains the most clearly diagnostic.

DIAGNOSIS

In the first affected pregnancy, the diagnosis of abnormal cervical competence is very difficult. Painless dilation of the cervix, unaccompanied by contractions, bleeding, fluid leakage, or signs of infection, is the most distinctive presentation, but is uncommon. The most common presentation is a history of mild symptoms (pelvic pressure, an increase in vaginal discharge, or light spotting) between 16 and 26 weeks that were ignored by the patient, her family, and/or the health care team until a day or two later when overt preterm labor, PROM, bleeding, or amnionitis occurred.

When there is a history of a prior preterm delivery between 16 and 26 weeks of pregnancy, the possibility of abnormal cervical competence should be considered in the care of subsequent pregnancies. If the "classic" presentation of painless and passive dilation can be documented, the diagnosis is secure. When the prior history is not distinctive, frequent assessment of the cervix with both digital and transvaginal ultrasound examination is required to assess for premature cervical softening on digital examination and shortening or funneling of the cervix on ultrasound. When a patient with a nondiagnostic history has a cervical length less than 20 mm after 18 weeks, a presumptive diagnosis of abnormal competence may be made. The presence of a dynamic funnel at the internal os on ultrasound is not always seen, but is highly diagnostic if observed in a patient with a suggestive history. The clinical significance of funneling of the internal os in a patient without a history of delivery between 17 and 28 weeks is uncertain.

Recurrent preterm birth in the late second and early third trimester is typical for women with reduced cervical competence, with progressively earlier deliveries in successive pregnancies. An obstetric history in which a preterm delivery before 28 weeks is followed in the next pregnancy by a birth at term without treatment (e.g., cerclage, bedrest) or evidence of cervical shortening suggests an etiology other than abnormal competence. The clinical presentation of abnormal or reduced competence is distinguished primarily by a gestational age at presentation of less than 28 weeks and may include preterm labor, PROM, or amnionitis, in addition to the classical presentation. Cervical dilation may be disproportionate to the duration and/or intensity of the patient's symptoms. Previous labors may have been short (less than 8 hours), and there is often a history of advanced dilation at arrival at the hospital. When a birth at term is followed by a subsequent delivery before 28 weeks, the possibility of trauma to the cervix during a prior delivery must be considered. Possible risk factors associated with abnormal cervical competence are shown in Box 40-1.

BOX 40-1
Potential Risk Factors for Abnormal Cervical Competence

Repeated preterm deliveries before 26 to 28 weeks
Cone biopsy: cervix length may be short but functional; most will not need cerclage
DES exposure: sonography of cervix very helpful; most will not need cerclage
Elective abortion: second trimester, or multiple first trimester; most will not need cerclage
Short cervix by digital examination; most will not need cerclage
Prior cesarean delivery after long second stage labor; most will not need cerclage

MANAGEMENT

Cervical Cerclage

Cervical cerclage, a surgical reinforcement of the cervix with a purse-string suture, has been the standard albeit somewhat controversial treatment for abnormal cervical competence. If competence is viewed as a bell-shaped curve, then cerclage may be an essential but not necessarily sufficient treatment only for patients whose cervical competence is at the lowest end of the curve. Cerclage is not the "cure" for reduced or absent competence. Whether the effect of cerclage is purely the physical reinforcement of the cervix, as traditionally thought, or has other effects (e.g., maintenance of the cervical mucus barrier) is not clear, nor is the role of cerclage for patients whose competence is low but not absent. A guide to selection of candidates for cerclage is shown in Box 40-2.

Prophylactic Cerclage

Cerclage placement may be either prophylactic or emergent, depending on when the diagnosis is made. If there is a classic history of painless dilation in a prior pregnancy, then prophylactic placement of a cerclage at 10 to 15 weeks is customary. A prophylactic cerclage may also be appropriate for some women with a history of recurrent early preterm births before 26 weeks. When the history is uncertain, transvaginal cervical sonography every 1 to 2 weeks beginning at 16 to 18 weeks may be used to make the diagnosis. Prophylactic cerclage in doubtful cases is occasionally justified, but usually carries more risk than benefit. Cervical sononography performed before 16 weeks most commonly reveals a normal-appearing cervix, and is rarely useful to make a decision about placement of a cerclage at that time in pregnancy. After 16 weeks, the lower uterine segment and cervix have different sonographic textures, and sonographic images become more clinically useful. Digital exam will indicate cervical softening,

BOX 40-2

Selection of Patients for Cerclage

- History of second trimester delivery
  - Classic presentation (painless dilation without contractions): elective cerclage
  - Expanded presentation (see text)
    - Recurrent second trimester delivery: Elective cerclage or follow cervical sonography
    - Single: Follow with cervical sonography and digtal examinations every 1-2 weeks
    - Atypical: Follow with cervical sonography and digital examinations; place stitch if cervical length <25 mm with funnel or <20 mm
- Potential risk factors without a history of second trimester delivery
  - Follow with cervical sonography and digital examinations every 1-2 weeks

but dilation of the cervix typically occurs late, *after* ultrasound indicates a shortened or funneled cervix. A patient followed expectantly because of a suspect obstetric history should be offered a cerclage if the cervix shortens below 20 mm, or below 25 mm in the presence of a funnel. Measurement of the cervix shortens below 20 mm, or below 25 mm in the presence of a funnel. Measurement of the cervix with ultrasound can be difficult to standardize. The most consistently reproducible measurement is the distance between the apposed walls of the cervical canal, *exclusive of any funnel.* The length of the funnel can be measured separately, but is less useful because it can be evanescent over a matter of minutes, and because there can be substantial technical variation in the observance of a funnel. Zilianti et al have suggested a useful acronym to describe the process of effacement as seen by transvaginal sonography: **TYVU.** These letters form, in chronologic sequence, the sonographic appearance of the cervical canal and lower segment as it changes from the uneffaced **T** to the beginning funnel **Y,** with further shortening to **V,** and finally to a fully developed lower uterine segment, **U.** Dilation of the cervix typically occurs after effacement, thus explaining the well-known difficulty in detecting cervical incompetence with digital examination. The appropriate measurement is the vertical arm of the **T** or **Y,** and the thickness of the cervix at the bottom of the **V** or **U.**

The complications of prophylactic cerclage include bleeding, infection, and erosion or slippage of the cerclage down the cervix. A good cerclage candidate is therefore a nonsmoker (who does not cough), who has no history of sexually transmitted disease, and in whom the cervix is the only evident risk factor for preterm birth.

Management of women whose history suggests reduced but not absent cervical competence (a history of prior preterm birth between 24 and 32 weeks and a cervical length of 20 to 30 mm) focuses on evaluation of the role of risk factors such as physical and sexual activity; smoking; infection with bacterial vaginosis, trichomonas, chlamydia, or gonorrhea; and excessive uterine contractions. If these factors are controlled or excluded and the cervix continues to shorten below 20 mm, a cerclage may be considered in these patients, but is rarely required.

MANAGEMENT IN THE SECOND TRIMESTER

The acute presentation of previously unsuspected abnormal cervical competence is variable and may include spotting, pelvic pressure, preterm labor, amnionitis, or PROM. The immediate management is aimed at stabilizing the patient and preventing further cervical dilation while simultaneously excluding both amnionitis and ruptured membranes. It involves placing the patient in the Trendelenburg position, monitoring external fetal heart rate and contractions, obtaining vaginal cultures for group B streptococcus, *N. gonorrhoeae,* and chlamydia. Sterile speculum examination is performed to look for the amniotic sac at the cervix, pooled fluid, and ferning, and to test the pH level. Temperature, CBC, and differential are also routine. Transabdominal ultrasound is used to measure amniotic fluid volume, estimate fetal weight and biometry, assess fetal presentation, and evaluate fetal and uterine anomalies. Transvaginal ultrasound determines cervical length and funneling if the amniotic sac is not visible by speculum examination. Indications for prompt delivery include amnionitis or other maternal illness requiring delivery and a lethal fetal anomaly.

The blades of the vaginal speculum should be carefully placed into the anterior and posterior fornices under excellent light and while paying close attention to the possible presence of a bulging amniotic sac. If the sac is not visible, additional gentle pressure may be applied to the speculum blades to evert the external os, a step that may reveal the membranes just inside the external os. Confirmation of PROM is a contraindication to the placement of a cerclage. Bacterial colonization of the amniotic fluid occurs frequently when the membranes have been exposed to the vaginal flora. This observation leads most physicians to treat these patients with broad spectrum prophylactic antibiotics, and some to perform an amniocentesis to detect infection before placing a cerclage.

The presence of contractions does not exclude the diagnosis of abnormal competence. Labor may be either the result of inflammation occurring after the cervix has effaced and dilated, or may be the cause of the dilation or effacement. In patients presenting before 24 to 26 weeks, the former is more likely (see Chapter 39). Contractions must be easily suppressed before any consideration is given to placement of a cerclage. Persistent contractions despite modest doses of tocolytics in this setting are strongly suggestive of intrauterine infection that would contraindicate a stitch. Any tocolytic may be used, but indomethacin is a particularly good choice because it has few side effects and may prevent the local surge in prostaglandin production known to occur after cervical cerclage.

The decision to place a cerclage is influenced by the gestational age (rare after 24 weeks), cervical dilation (rare after 4 cm), the degree to which the sac has prolapsed through the cervix, and the likelihood of infection and/or membrane rupture. The emotional status of the parents is also important.

SURGICAL MANAGEMENT

Placement of a McDonald Cervical Cerclage

There are several satisfactory techniques for placement of a cervical cerclage. The McDonald purse-string technique is a straightforward procedure that may be used either prophylactically or emergently and has a high rate of success and a low rate of complications. Four or five "bites" as high on the cervix as possible are made, encircling the cervix with a permanent suture such as Ethibond or Mersilene, with the knot tied at either the 6 or 12 o'clock position. Preoperative and intraoperative care differs depending on whether the procedure is prophylactic or emergent, but adequate anesthesia and surgical assistance are required whenever the procedure is performed. The protocols for prophylactic and emergent cerclage are contrasted in Table 40-1.

Short-term risks of emergency cerclage include preterm labor, ruptured membranes, and amnionitis. The likelihood of complications rises as the cervical dilation and gestational age increase. Cervical injury at the time of

TABLE 40-1
Perioperative Care of Cervical Cerclage

	Prophylactic cerclage	Emergency cerclage
Gestational age	10 to 20 weeks	18 to 24 weeks
Status of the cervix	Closed, 1+ cm of length	Amniotic sac into vagina
Preoperative antibiotics	Pencillin for group B streptococcus	Broad spectrum ampicillin, gentamicin, clindamycin
Perioperative tocolytics	None	Indomethacin 50 mg rectally every 6-8 hr for 24-48 hr
Anesthesia	Conduction preferred	Conduction preferred
Technique to reduce the membranes	Not required	Foley balloon into the cervix; preoperative amniocentesis; fill maternal bladder
Postoperative care	Home same day, penicillin for 5 days, return visit 7-10 days	Hospitalize for bed rest; IV antibiotics, indomethacin for 5+ days, with cervical ultrasound to assess suture placement before discharge
Activity restrictions	No coitus; varies with sonographic localization of suture and cervical length: If cervix <25 mm, off work If cervix <20 mm, bed rest If sac protrudes beyond the cerclage, readmit to hospital	No coitus; home bed rest with bathroom privileges

delivery and scarring leading to delayed dilation may occur after both prophylactic and emergency cerclage. The outcome after prophylactic cerclage placement is reported to be good, with more than 80% to 90% of women delivering at term, although these data were reported before the use of ultrasound to make an accurate diagnosis. The outcomes for women treated with emergent second trimester cerclage are much better than generally appreciated. Regardless of when it is placed, the cerclage can be removed electively at 37 weeks gestation. If membrane rupture occurs before 37 weeks, the cerclage should be removed promptly. Removal is also advisable if preterm labor occurs that cannot be easily stopped with tocolytics.

KEY POINTS

1. Cervical competence is a continuum that correlates with the length of the cervix at 24 to 28 weeks gestation: the shorter the cervix, the greater the risk of preterm birth.
2. The diagnosis of abnormal cervical incompetence is made by an obstetric history of a preterm birth between 18 and 26 weeks that is either "classic" (passive and painless cervical dilation) or that is accompanied by sonographic documentation of cervical shortening and funneling.
3. Because cervical effacement begins from the internal os and proceeds caudad, cervical dilation will occur late in the clinical presentation of abnormal cervical competence.
4. Cervical cerclage is a surgical procedure that, while helpful in appropriately selected patients, does not provide a "cure" for abnormal cervical competence.

SUGGESTED READINGS

Aarts JM et al: Emergency cerclage: a review, *Obstet Gynecol Surv* 50:459-469, 1995.

Iams JD et al: Cervical competence as a continuum: a study of sonographic cervical length and obstetrical performance, *Am J Obstet Gynecol* 172:1097-1106, 1995.

Iams JD et al: The length of the cervix and the risk of spontaneous premature delivery, *N Engl J Med* 334:567-572, 1996.

MRC/RCOG Working Party on Cervical Cerclage: Final report of the Medical Research Council/Royal College of Obstetricians and Gynaecologists multicentre randomised trial of cervical cerclage, *Br J Obstet Gynecol* 100:516-523, 1993.

Zilianti M et al: Monitoring the effacement of the uterine cervix by transperineal sonography: a new perspective, *J Ultrasound Med* 14:719-24, 1995.

41

Third Trimester Bleeding

Rosemary E. Reiss

Depending on its etiology, bleeding in the third trimester may herald a major disaster or be of minimal concern. Because bleeding can quickly become fatal to mother or fetus, stabilization of the patient and evaluation of fetal well-being must not await determination of its cause (Fig. 41-1). Bleeding is most threatening to the fetus when it

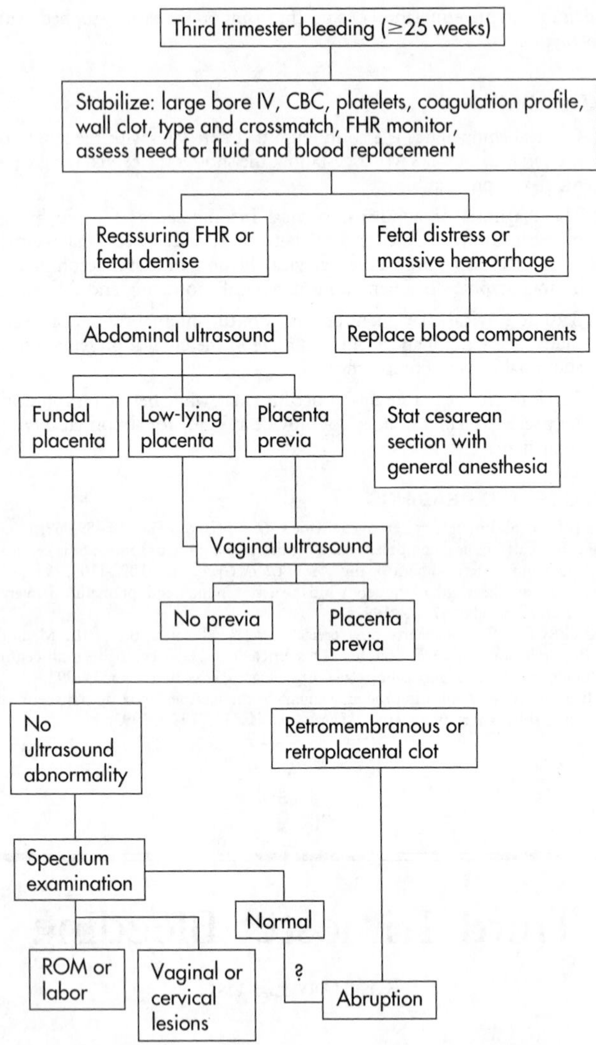

FIG. 41-1 Management of placental abruption.

is from the placenta or its bed (placenta or vasa previa or placental abruption). If these are not the source of blood loss, other sites in the genital tract, most commonly the cervix and the vagina, should be considered. In more than a third of patients a definite diagnosis may never be established; perinatal outcomes in this group of patients, though better than for patients with previa or abruption, are worse than in the general population.

PLACENTAL ABRUPTION

Pathophysiology

Separation of the placenta from the uterine wall is usually initiated by bleeding into the decidua basalis from small arteries in the placental bed. Less commonly, abruption can be caused by bleeding from lacerated fetoplacental vessels. Accumulating blood creates a hematoma that dissects within the decidua, extending the placental separation from the uterine wall. The extending clot can compress the intervillous space and destroy placental tissue. The hematoma may also extend between the membranes and the uterine wall or through the myometrium, leading to discoloration of the peritoneal surface **(Couvelaire uterus).** Extension of the abruption leads to loss of surface area for respiratory and nutrient exchange, placing the fetus at risk for asphyxia or sudden demise. The extravasated blood also stimulates contractions and in some cases uterine tetany. Vaginal bleeding accompanies abruption only when blood tracks behind the membranes and through the cervix. Vaginal blood loss may only represent a fraction of the total blood loss. Morbidity is higher with "concealed" abruptions, where most of the blood remains behind the placenta, leading to significant loss of exchange surface and damage of villi. Consumptive coagulopathy occurs in 10% of abruptions because of tissue thromboplastins released from the damaged placenta into the maternal circulation.

Incidence and Significance

Abruption occurs in about 1% of pregnancies and accounts for about 20% of third-trimester bleeding. Of all third-trimester stillbirths, approximately 12% are caused by abruption. The neonatal death rate after severe abruption is nearly 20%. In surviving infants, CNS injuries are approximately four times higher than in gestational age–matched controls. Recurrence risk in future pregnancies is 8% to 13% after one abruption and 25% after two.

Risk Factors

Pregnancy-induced or chronic hypertension is present in approximately 50% of abruptions associated with fetal demise. Hypertension is also a risk factor for milder abruption. Use of cocaine is associated with placental abruption. Cocaine use should be suspected, especially if there is associated transient maternal hypertension or if abruption occurs before 28 weeks gestation. Other risk factors include abdominal trauma, tobacco use, sudden decompression of the uterus (e.g., delivery of a first twin or rupture of the membranes when polyhydramnios is present), prolonged premature rupture of the membranes, uterine anomaly or leiomyomata, high parity, and prior abruption.

Diagnosis

The diagnosis is based on the history and physical findings. Classically, patients with placental abruption present with vaginal bleeding and abdominal or back pain. The absence of pain or bleeding by no means excludes abruption. Abdominal pain is present in only 50% of cases. Uterine contractions, hypertonus, and tetany are physical findings. Contractions may be hard to detect by external monitor if they have high frequency but low amplitude, or if there is continuous high uterine tone. Uterine palpation is important, but increased uterine tone may make palpation of the fetus difficult. Hypotension or tachycardia may be present if patient is hypovolemic. Symptoms of hypovolemia that cannot be accounted for by the amount of observed vaginal blood loss are suspicious for abruption. However, the degree of hypovolemia may be masked in the presence of chronic hypertension or preeclampsia. Similarly, volume depletion may obscure the diagnosis of underlying preeclampsia. Fetal demise or nonreassuring fetal heart rate tracing are other findings.

Laboratory testing may detect anemia, depending on the acuity of the abruption and the amount of blood loss. Coagulopathy is present in 10% of abruptions, and in almost 40% of abruptions is severe enough to produce fetal demise. Fibrin split products rise earliest; fibrinogen then falls and PT/PTT eventually become prolonged. Whole-blood clotting time (clot observation test, "wall clot") can be used as a screening test to detect severe coagulopathy quickly and allow prompt administration of blood replacement products. It does not replace the other coagulation assays. Serum is obtained and left undisturbed for 8 minutes. Formation of a firm clot indicates fibrinogen >100 mg/dl. Formation of a soft clot that dissolves easily suggests fibrinogen 50 to 100 mg/dl, and no clot formation suggests a fibrinogen <50 mg/dl.

On ultrasound, acute hemorrhage may have the same echodensity as the placenta. Thus a fresh placental separation may appear as an abnormally thick placenta. Older hematomas appear as hypoechoic areas behind the placenta or more commonly elevating the membranes from the uterine wall. Absence of ultrasound findings does not exclude placental abruption. Only in cases where blood remains contained behind the membranes or placenta can it be seen. Performance of ultrasound is nonetheless important in all patients with vaginal bleeding to exclude placenta previa.

Treatment

For stabilization use a large bore IV for fluid and blood replacement. Use a Foley catheter to assess hourly urine output. Obtain CBC with platelets, coagulation profile, and wall clot; crossmatch 4 units of blood. Begin continuous fetal heart monitoring and perform ultrasound to exclude previa, confirm fetal viability, and ascertain fetal lie. These procedures must be performed quickly. If DIC is present, maintain platelets >50,000 and raise fibrinogen >100 mg/dl with FFP or cryoprecipitate, especially if cesarean delivery is required. Each unit of FFP contains 1 g of fibrinogen and will raise the fibrinogen by 15 to 20 mg/dl. FFP is usually preferable to cryoprecipitate because it contains more clotting factors and confers less hepatitis risk. Once the placenta is delivered, DIC will stop and fibrinogen will rise.

The mode of delivery is next determined (Fig. 41-2). For a dead fetus vaginal delivery should be promoted by amniotomy and oxytocin augmentation if needed. With a live fetus and certain diagnosis (i.e., if coagulopathy is present or fetal heart rate tracing is worrisome), the fetus is in imminent danger of demise and cesarean delivery should be performed as soon as the mother has received appropriate blood component replacement. If coagulation is normal and fetal heart rate tracing is reassuring, vaginal delivery can be attempted. Amniotomy should be performed and internal monitoring begun as soon as possible. Ongoing evaluation of coagulation, hemoglobin, and urine output is required. Facilities and staff, including an anesthesiologist, must be continuously available for emergency cesarean delivery if fetal distress should occur. With a live fetus and uncertain diagnosis, delivery is usually indicated for term pregnancies. In preterm pregnancies, patients with contractions and unexplained bleeding are observed with close fetal monitoring. Tocolytics may be used, with $MgSO_4$ the best choice because it has the least hemodynamic effects and does not affect coagulation. If symptoms suggesting abruption continue, the patient should be delivered.

PLACENTA PREVIA

The central portion of the placenta **(total previa)** or the placental edge **(partial previa)** may cover the cervix. These terms originate from a time when the diagnosis of placenta previa could only be made when the cervix was dilated. Now that the diagnosis of placenta previa is made by ultrasound, the terms **central** and **lateral** placenta previa make more sense since the cervical canal before labor is only a few millimeters wide and is either covered by placenta or is not. The term **marginal placenta previa** is used for a placenta whose edge is beside the cervical canal.

Pathophysiology and Natural History

Placenta previa occurs when the blastocyst implants in the uterine isthmus instead of the thicker endometrium of the upper uterus. The frequency of lower implantation is increased by higher parity, previous cesarean delivery, and dilation and currettage. The relationship of the placenta to the cervix changes during the second trimester with the growth of the lower uterine segment and the restriction of villi to the chorion frondosum. Ultrasound in the second trimester finds 5% to 8% of placentas impinging on the cervix; 95% of these will **not** cross the cervix at term, and many will not even be low lying. Bleeding from placenta previa rarely occurs before the third trimester, and 90% of placenta previas bleed before 38 weeks. Placenta accreta, increta, and percreta are more common with low

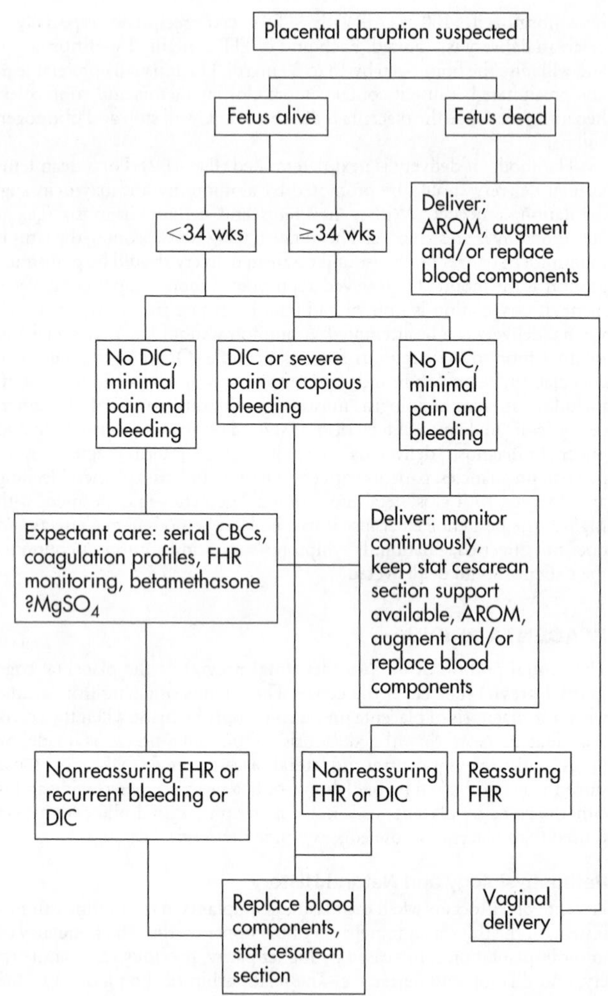

FIG. 41-2 Management of placenta previa.

placental implantation, especially with a history of cesarean delivery. The risk of placenta accreta is 10% after one prior cesarean, and up to 50% after two or more.

Incidence

The incidence of placenta previa is as follows: general population–0.4% to 0.6%, nulliparas–0.2%, multiparas–5%, and recurrence–4% to 8%.

Diagnosis

Painless vaginal bleeding is found in 70% to 80% of patients. The bleeding may be spontaneous or follow vaginal examination or coitus. Bleeding with contractions occurs in 20% of patients.

Physical findings include Leopold maneuvers showing breech or transverse lie increase suspicion for placenta previa. Tachycardia and postural hypotension may be present depending on the amount of blood loss. Ultrasound must *always* be performed before digital vaginal examination in patients with third-trimester bleeding. When ultrasound suggests placenta previa, digital examination should be avoided because sudden, massive hemorrhage often follows. In rare cases when delivery is thought to be imminent and placenta previa is thought to be marginal, vaginal examination may be performed but only under "double set-up" conditions (i.e., in an operating room with everything ready for an emergent cesarean delivery.) Transvaginal ultrasound renders this approach obsolete.

Transabdominal ultrasound can image the fetus and placenta as well as the cervix to determine fetal lie and look for retroplacental clots. No special probes are needed. However, localization of the placental edge is difficult when the placenta is posterior. In about one-third of patients, the cervical canal cannot be seen. The need to fill the bladder may impair accurate localization of the cervical canal. The negative predictive value (NPV) is only 80% (i.e., may miss 20% of previas), and the positive predictive value (PPV) is only 38% (i.e., may overdiagnose previa in 61% of patients). Transvaginal ultrasound has the advantage of proximity to the structures of interest and gives better resolution. The cervical canal can be seen and its relationship to the placenta precisely determined (NPV 100%, PPV 71%). A full bladder is not needed, and posterior and anterior placentae are equally well imaged. Though vaginal placement of an ultrasound probe theoretically could increase bleeding, clinical trials have not found this. The ultrasound probe is placed in the vaginal fornix, not through the cervix. Only in cases of advanced labor need transvaginal ultrasound be avoided.

Laboratory findings include anemia, depending on the amount and duration of blood loss, and coagulopathy is uncommon until there has been massive blood loss.

Treatment

Stabilization for placental abruption is performed. Monitoring for FHR is continuous. The ideal approach is to perform transabdominal ultrasound immediately after the patient's admission to the labor area. If the placenta is low-lying, transvaginal ultrasound should be performed when the patient is stable to determine if the placenta truly crosses the cervix. If lateral or marginal previa exists, rescan to reassess placental location before delivery. These steps must be performed quickly.

Timing of delivery is next determined (Fig. 41-3). Delivery must be accomplished promptly by cesarean section if bleeding is profuse or FHR tracing is not reassuring. If bleeding stops spontaneously and the patient is beyond 36 weeks gestation or pulmonary maturity is documented, delivery should be performed once the patient is stable, by cesarean section in most cases. If bleeding stops and the patient is preterm, the pregnancy may be continued with the patient on bed rest. Hospital bed rest is safest but costly. With careful selection criteria, some patients can be successfully managed at home. However, there are no prospective studies comparing home versus hospital management. If contractions are present and expectant management is planned, tocolysis with $MgSO_4$ may be considered to decrease bleeding. For cesarean delivery, general anesthesia is preferred because regional anesthesia prevents vasoconstriction and may increase hypotension. Since bleeding from the placental bed may be difficult to control, the patient should be counseled about the possible need for hysterectomy, and the surgeon should be prepared to perform uterine and hypogastric artery ligation and hysterectomy if necessary. Blood for transfusion should be available near the operating room. If bleeding is copious, hematocrit, platelets, PT, and aPTT should be checked intraoperatively, with blood replaced as needed.

VASA PREVIA

Fetal vessels may traverse the membranes in cases of velamentous cord insertion. Velamentous insertions are more common when multiple gestation or succenturiate placental lobes are present. If such vessels cross the cervix, they may rupture with labor or artificial rupture of the membranes. Though rare, ruptured vasa previa has neonatal mortality of 50% or more. Once vessels are torn, very rapid cesarean delivery may prevent fetal demise; however, since neonatal blood volume is small, even brief bleeding may cause exsanguination. If suspected, vasa previa may be identified with color Doppler before rupture so that elective cesarean delivery may be performed.

OTHER SOURCES OF BLEEDING

Labor or rupture of the membranes may present as bleeding ("bloody show"). Usually blood loss is minimal, but it may be greater with a low-lying placenta. Rupture of the membranes may lead to overestimation of blood loss, especially by the patient. Bleeding is most common at the onset of labor and is usually scant and mixed with mucus. Cervical polyps present as intermittent spotty bleeding, especially after coitus or cervical examination. Diagnosis is by visualization during speculum examination. As the frequency of cervical cancer in reproductive-age women is increasing, it should be considered in patients with bleeding from the cervix, especially if accompanied by watery discharge. If another cause of bleeding

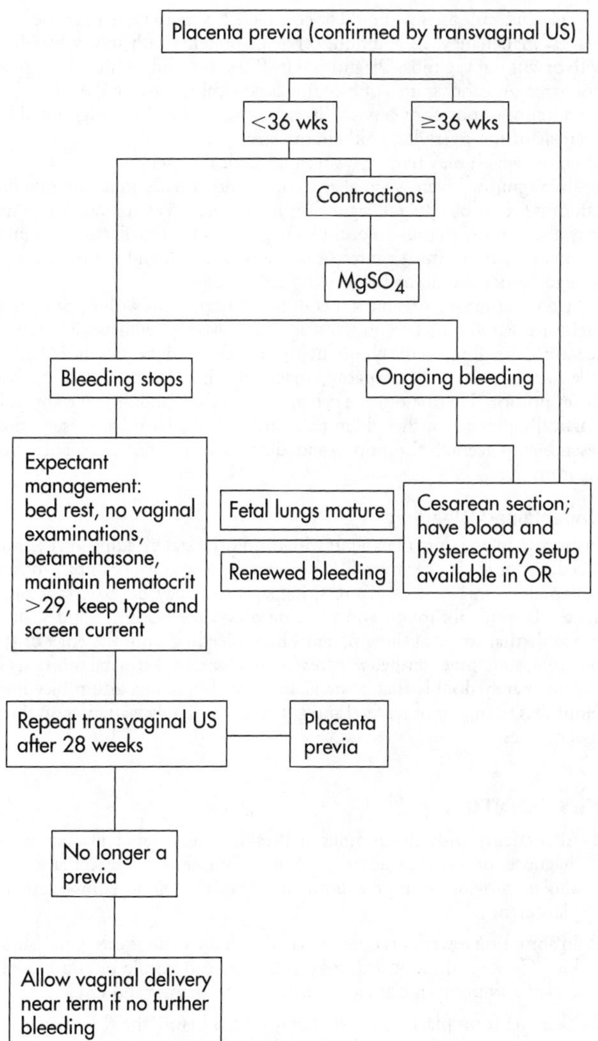

FIG. 41-3 Evaluation of third-trimester bleeding.

is not found, colposcopy should be considered even if a Pap smear does not suggest malignancy. In addition, cervicitis presents with spotty bleeding with or without vaginitis. Diagnosis is by Pap smear and wet prep of vaginal discharge. Another source of bleeding is cervical leiomyoma. A fibroid in the anterior or posterior cervical lip can cause profuse bleeding caused by necrosis of the overlying epithelium. Treatment is with local control of bleeding, which may require ligation of cervical vessels.

In vaginitis, severe vaginal infections with trichomonas or monilia can cause scant bleeding. Diagnosis is by wet prep. Vaginal varicose veins may also rupture to cause bleeding. Diagnosis is by visualization. Vaginal trauma may occur during intercourse. Sexual assault and the presence of foreign bodies should be suspected.

Uterine rupture is seen most commonly in patients with prior uterine incisions. Rupture occurs in 0.5% to 2% of women with prior cesarean section, depending on the type of uterine incision and the presence of other risk factors such as multiparity, oxytocin stimulation, and fetopelvic disproportion. Uterine rupture can also result from abdominal trauma. It classically presents with sudden pain and fetal bradycardia. Presentation resembles placental abruption, and diagnosis may not be made until laparotomy.

Unexplained Bleeding

In more than one third of patients with third-trimester bleeding, no definite bleeding source is ever found. If bleeding is slow and does not produce maternal anemia or fetal distress, management may be expectant once acute placental abruption and placenta previa have been excluded. It is probable that some of these patients have bleeding from the edge of the placenta, sometimes termed *marginal sinus separation*. Perinatal mortality is approximately double that of pregnancies without antepartum bleeding. Nonstress testing or other fetal surveillance is probably warranted in these pregnancies.

KEY POINTS

1 All patients with third-trimester bleeding need rapid evaluation to diagnose or exclude acute placental abruption or placenta previa and to provide prompt appropriate fluid and blood component replacement.

2 In abruption, severity is not correlated with the volume of vaginal blood loss. Concealed blood loss may greatly exceed visible bleeding. Concealed abruptions are at greater risk for fetal demise and DIC.

3 Bleeding from placenta previa rarely occurs before the third trimester, but develops by 38 weeks in about 90% of cases.

SUGGESTED READINGS

Benedetti TJ: Obstetric hemorrhage. In Gabbe SG, Niebyl JR, Simpson JL, eds: *Obstetrics: normal and problem pregnancies*, ed 2, New York, 1991, Churchill Livingstone.

Chamberlain G: Antepartum haemorrhage, *BMJ* 302:1526-1530, 1991.
Dommisse J, Tiltman AJ: Placental bed biopsies in placental abruption, *Br J Obstet Gynaecol* 99:651-654, 1992.
Droste S, Keil K: Expectant management of placenta previa: cost-benefit analysis of outpatient treatment, *Am J Obstet Gynecol* 170:1254-1257, 1994.
Farine D, Peisner DB, Timor-Tritsch IE: Placenta previa–is the traditional diagnostic approach satisfactory? *J Clin Ultrasound* 18:328-330, 1990.
Pritchard JA et al: On reducing the frequency of severe abruptio placentae, *Am J Obstet Gynecol* 165:1345-1351, 1991.
Spinillo A et al: Severity of abruptio placentae and neurodevelopmental outcome in low birthweight infants, *Early Hum Dev* 35:45-54, 1993.

42

Alloimmunization

RICHARD O'SHAUGHNESSY

Alloimmunization leads to destruction of fetal RBCs by maternal antibodies directed against them. The hemolytic process that results is called *erythroblastosis fetalis (EBF).* There are several types of RBC alloimmunization. ABO incompatibility is a very common but generally not severe, self-limited condition. EBF caused by Rh disease continues to affect approximately 11/10,000 live births. It is common and severe. Since the introduction of Rh immune globulin and the subsequent reduction in the number of cases of Rh disease, alloimmunization from antibodies other than anti-D has become increasingly apparent as a cause of EBF.

ETIOLOGY

Alloimmunization occurs because of maternal exposure to foreign RBCs, usually through blood transfusion or fetal-maternal hemorrhage (FMH). Blood transfusion is the most common cause of EBF caused by antibodies other than "D." This is an important reason for women in their reproductive years to avoid donor blood transfusions if at all possible.

Some FMH probably occurs in all pregnancies. The volume H and frequency of FMH increase as the pregnancy progresses. Nonetheless, the majority of FMHs are less than 1 cc.

Table 42-1 describes the risk of isoimmunization for the Rh negative woman who is pregnant with an Rh positive fetus. The table also indicates the protective effect of ABO incompatibility between mother and fetus in regards to the risk of alloimmunization to the Rh antigen.

TABLE 42-1
Frequency of Rh Alloimmunization (Rh Negative Mother/ Rh Positive Fetus)

	ABO compatible (80%)	ABO incompatible (20%)
Overall	16%	3%
Current pregnancy	2%	0.5%
Postpartum	14%	2.5%

It is important to screen for alloantibodies in every pregnant patient. Many antibodies other than anti-D are associated with EBF. The antibodies that cause EBF are IgG and can cross the placenta.

EFFECTS OF EBF

Alloantibodies attach to RBCs and lead to their destruction. Although most fetuses (approximately 80%) can compensate for the hemolytic anemia by making new RBCs, some (20%) cannot. The ability of the fetus to compensate depends on the antibody and fetal reserve. About 10% of those fetuses that can't compensate require delivery, and 10% require fetal transfusion.

Hydrops fetalis can develop after severe anemia ensues and is caused by diffuse tissue failure. This usually occurs when the fetal hemoglobin deficit is ≥7% (i.e., fetal hemoglobin ≤4%).

After birth, the bilirubin load may overwhelm the fetal liver's conjugating capacity and deposit in the brain causing kernicterus. Exchange transfusion is done to normalize hemoglobin and remove bilirubin and excess hemolytic antibody from the newborn. Phototherapy is a useful adjunct to photodeactivate bilirubin in the jaundiced newborn.

DIAGNOSIS

A blood type, Rh factor, and antibody screen should be done on *all* pregnant patients. Paternal blood type, Rh factor, and zygosity testing should be performed if maternal antibody is present. The likelihood that the fetus is affected must be determined. If paternity is not certain, it is best to assume that the fetus is affected.

Fetal blood typing should be considered if the father is heterozygous and there is a significant maternal antibody present or a history of prior affected newborns. There is then a 50% chance that the fetus is unaffected. Amniocentesis with PCR on amniocytes for genes encoding the Rh antigens can be performed. Laboratory advances will allow us to test for the genes encoding many other RBC antigens in the future. Cordocentesis can also be performed to measure the RBC specific antigens directly, but the risk of cordocentesis is significantly greater than amniocentesis.

MANAGEMENT

Samples of maternal serum, amniotic fluid, or fetal blood give a picture of the fetal condition at that moment. It is necessary to repeat samples at intervals of 1 to 4 weeks to monitor the fetal condition.

Serology

The value of antibody titers is very important in clinical management, especially in the first immunized pregnancy. The higher the titer, the more likely that EBF is severe. Using the Coombs' test (IgG) and saline (IgM) techniques, the laboratory will monitor the nature and concentration of the maternal antibody responses. No other tests are needed for monitoring if there is no history of prior affected newborns and the titer is $<1/32$. After $1/16$ ($\geq 1/32$), a critical titer is reached and is not sufficient to monitor EBF.

Amniocentesis

Amniocentesis should be performed if the titer is critical or greater in a first immunized pregnancy. If there is a history of prior affected newborns, the threshold is lowered for amniocentesis in subsequent pregnancies. Begin at 20 weeks and repeat at intervals. The delta OD 450 measures bilirubinoid pigments, an indirect indicator of fetal status. A trend is helpful when interpreting significance, especially in zone II.

Cordocentesis

Cordocentesis may be indicated if the delta OD 450 is in zone IIB or III. This test measures fetal hemoglobin and hemolytic indices directly. Cordocentesis is a more risky procedure, but gives direct analysis of fetal anemia. Transplacental cordocentesis (or amniocentesis) should be avoided since this will increase the intensity of the antibody response because of the resultant FMH. (See Figs. 42-1 and 42-2 for management algorithms.)

Management Aids

Ultrasound signs of alloimmunization and fetal anemia include the following: cardiomegaly, increased liver length, polyhydramnios, large umbilical vein, large placenta, and pericardial effusion. These signs may give evidence of worsening fetal condition, but can't be relied on exclusively as first-line monitoring. Other biophysical factors include BPS, daily fetal movement counting, Doppler scanning, and NST (sinusoidal). The severely anemic fetus may demonstrate a sinusoidal fetal heart tracing.

Intrauterine transfusion is performed if significant fetal anemia develops before 32 weeks gestation. Intraperitoneal transfusion involves absorption of RBCs occurring via peritoneal lymphatics. Absorption is limited if fetal hydrops is present. Intravascular transfusion is the definite choice when fetal hydrops is present. If the fetal hematocrit is <30%, transfuse to the desired hematocrit of 40% to 50%. Calculation of the transfusion volume is done by formula or nomogram. The hematocrit will drop about 1%/day after transfusion.

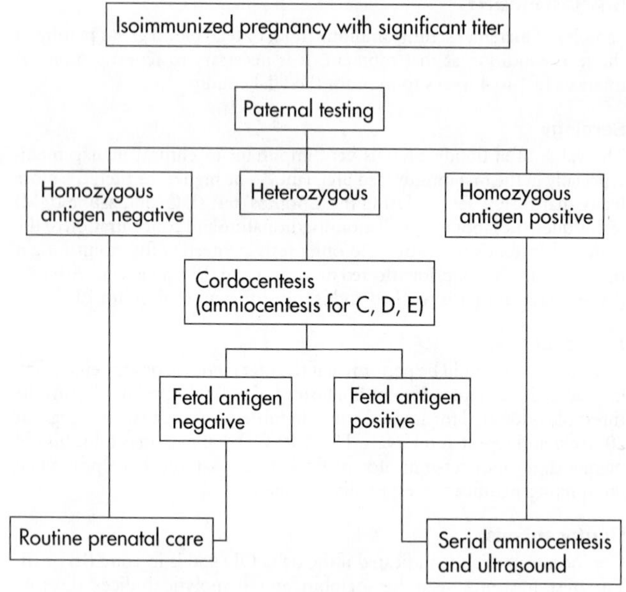

FIG. 42-1 Management of isoimmunized pregnancy with significant titer.

Other therapies that have been tried and found not to be helpful include plasmapheresis, oral antigen, promethazine, phenobarbital, corticosteroids, IV gamma globulin, and stem cell transplantation.

Rh IMMUNE GLOBULIN

Maternal alloimmunization can be directed against any of 400 different red cell antigens. The most common causes of hemolytic disease of the newborn (HDN) are ABO antibodies and anti-D. Although ABO-HDN is a relatively mild disease, anti-D causes moderate to severe disease.

In 1968 RhIg was licensed for postpartum use. The exact mechanism of action of RhIg remains unclear, but administration of appropriate doses at appropriate times can prevent the primary immune response of Rh-negative women bearing Rh-positive infants. The use of postpartum RhIG reduced the incidence of alloimmunization by 90%, from 12% to 16% for each pregnancy to 1.5% to 2%. The introduction of prophylactic antepartum use of RhIg at 28 weeks, as well as at delivery, should reduce the incidence of immunization from 1.5% to 2% to 0.2%.

Male volunteer studies established that 20 μg of purified anti-D was more than adequate to prevent immunization by 1 ml of Rh-positive RBCs

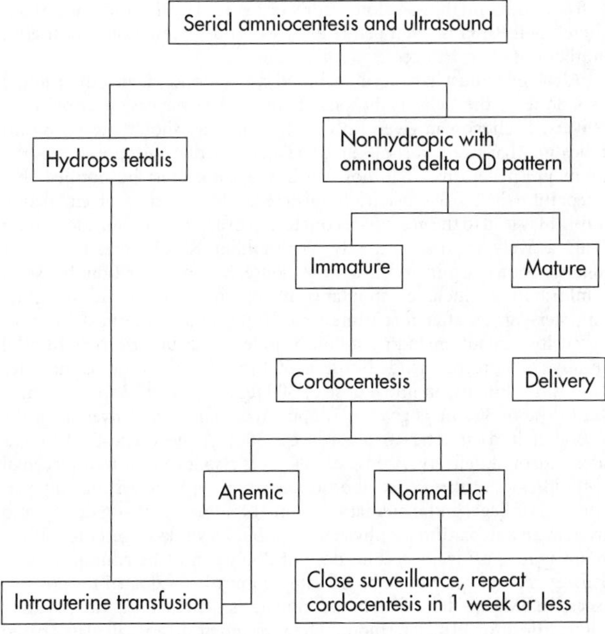

FIG. 42-2 Use of serial amniocentesis and ultrasound in EBF.

(not whole blood). Thus a 300-μg dose of RhIG will prevent immunization by 15 ml of RBCs or about 30 ml of whole blood. The volume of FMH during labor and delivery is usually much less than 15 ml, so most deliveries are adequately protected. For first-trimester abortions, a dose of 50 μg is adequate because the fetal blood volume is less than 5 cc whole blood. Other possible causes of transplacental hemorrhage include amniocentesis, external cephalic version, antepartum hemorrhage, and maternal abdominal trauma. Excessive hemorrhage (i.e., greater than 30 ml) can occur and must be recognized for adequate doses of RhIG to be administered. The most commonly used test to quantitate these bleeding episodes is the Kleihauer-Betke acid elution stain. The Rosette test is often used just to screen for excess hemorrhage.

The half-life of passively administered anti-D (RhIG) is approximately 25 days. The administration of a 300-μg dose should provide adequate protection in a normal pregnancy for about 12 weeks. If delivery does not occur by then, a second dose of RhIG should be given to prevent possible enhancement or augmentation of the immune response. When the level of anti-D is low, it is possible that a few fetal RBCs will be inadequately coated with antibody and thus be more readily recognized by the immune system. Therefore if RhIG is given before 28 weeks and/or gestation is postterm, another dose may be necessary antepartum.

All women must have accurate blood typing done. Having these initial tests done at the delivery hospital reduces the chances of errors after delivery. Each woman given RhIG before delivery should receive a card indicating that fact and should receive a postpartum injection unless the infant is Rh negative. The hospital blood bank must be notified that antepartum RhIG has been administered. The presence of circulating anti-D may lead to the inaccurate conclusion of active immunization rather than passively acquired antibody. Withholding RhIG carries the risk of augmentation of a primary immune response. Recommendations for RhIG administration include spontaneous or induced abortions (first trimester–50 μg, after first trimester–300 μg) and full term delivery of Rh-positive infant, including stillbirths unless fetus proved to be Rho(D) negative. The recommended dose is 300 μg. If amniocentesis indicates Rh-positive infants, an initial dose of 300 μg is repeated 12 weeks later. A third dose of 300 μg is given if Rh-positive infants are delivered. In the second or third trimester, an initial dose of 300 μg may be repeated 12 weeks later and/or at delivery. A dose of 300 μg is also given for transplacental FMH in cases of threatened abortion, external cephalic version, antepartum hemorrhage, and maternal abdominal trauma. A 300-μg dose is also given as an antepartum prophylactic at about 28 weeks of gestation. If the infant is Rh positive, a second dose of 300 μg must be administered at delivery. A maternal whole blood sample must be evaluated for possible excessive FMH (>30 ml fetal blood in maternal circulation), necessitating a 300 μg dose for 30 ml fetal blood. The appropriate dose is calculated based on the volume of fetal hemorrhage.

KEY POINTS

1. Alloimmunization leads to destruction of fetal RBCs by maternal antibodies directed against them.
2. The types of alloimmunization include ABO incompatibility, Rh disease, and alloimmunizations from antibodies other than anti-Ds.
3. Although approximately 80% of fetuses can compensate for hemolytic anemia by making new RBCs, 20% cannot.
4. A blood type, Rh factor, and antibody screen should be done on all pregnant patients; if paternity is not certain, it is best to assume the fetus is affected.

SUGGESTED READINGS

American Association of Blood Banking Committee Report, 1989, ACOG Technical Bulletins #147 and 148, October, 1990, ACOG.

Bennet et al: Use of amniocytes to test for fetal "D" typing, *N Engl J Med* 329:607, 1993.

Chavez GF, Mulinare J, Edmonds LD: Epidemiology of Rh hemolytic disease in the USA, *JAMA* 265:3270, 1991.

Moise K: Changing trends in the management of red blood cell alloimmunization in pregnancy, *Arch Pathol Lab Med* 118:421, 1994.
Queenan JT et al: Use of amniotic fluid optical density in evaluation of erythroblastosis fetalis, *Am J Obstet Gynecol* 168:1370, 1993.
Saade G et al: Fetal and neonatal hematologic parameters in red cell alloimmunization: predicting the need for late neonatal transfusion, *Fetal Diagn Ther* 8:161, 1993.
Weiner CP et al: Management of fetal hematolytic disease by cordocentesis, *Am J Obstet Gynecol* 165:546, 1991.
Witter FR et al: Post injection kinetics of antepartum RhIg, *Am J Obstet Gynecol* 163:784, 1990.

43

Thromboembolic Disease

JEFFREY G. BOYLE

Thromboembolic disease is a common cause of maternal morbidity and mortality during pregnancy. It accounts for 20% of all maternal deaths in the United States. Prevention, early diagnosis, and proper treatment can potentially improve the outcome of this disease.

INCIDENCE

The true incidence of thromboembolic disease in pregnancy is unknown. Deep venous thrombosis (DVT) and pulmonary embolism (PE) are relatively uncommon in the young, healthy, reproductive-age population. The overall pregnancy-related risk is 1/2000 to 1/2500. It is well known that a thromboembolism occurs three to five times more commonly after a cesarean delivery compared with a vaginal delivery. Moreover, the postpartum risk is up to 20 times higher than the antepartum risk.

When a DVT occurs during pregnancy, it most often affects the left lower extremity rather than the right and occurs with equal frequency in all three trimesters. In more than half of the cases, DVTs occur within 3 days post partum and can occur as late as 4 weeks after delivery. Perhaps most important is that the incidence of a PE depends on the diagnosis and treatment of a DVT. If a DVT goes untreated, 24% of patients will develop a PE, resulting in a 15% rate of maternal mortality. If treated, only 4.5% of patients with a DVT will develop a PE, resulting in a mortality rate below 1%.

PATHOPHYSIOLOGY

The increased risk of thromboembolism during pregnancy results from hypercoagulability, venous stasis, and vascular injury. The physiologic changes in pregnancy represent a hypercoagulable state. Fibrinogen and clotting factors V, VII, IX, X, and XII are increased during pregnancy, as are VW antigen, plasminogen, and antiplasmin. Fibrinolytic activity, factors XI and XIII, and protein S are decreased. Factors IX and V, protein C, and AT III are unchanged. Venous stasis occurs because of decreased venous tone, obstruction by the gravid uterus, and bed rest. Vascular injury can occur during labor and delivery with the use of stirrups or the lithotomy position and from tissue damage during a cesarean section. Risk factors for venous thrombosis include history of DVT or PE; inherited deficiencies in AT III, protein S, and protein C; antiphospholipid antibody syndrome; activated protein C resistance/factor C Leiden mutation; mechanical heart valve; myeloproliferative disorders; and cesarean delivery. Other risk factors are operative vaginal delivery, obesity, bed rest, advanced maternal age, infection, CHF, trauma, and multiparity.

DIAGNOSIS

Making an accurate and timely diagnosis is important during pregnancy because of the complications associated with treatment and the risks to the patient of an undiagnosed thrombus. The diagnosis also potentially commits a patient to chronic therapy as well as treatment during all subsequent pregnancies. Unfortunately, the clinical diagnosis of both DVT and PE is unreliable. The normal, physiologic changes of pregnancy can also make the diagnosis uncertain. Patients with a DVT may experience muscle pain, tenderness, swelling, and dilated superficial veins. They may also have a palpable deep linear cord, limb discoloration, or calf pain with passive dorsiflexion of the foot, referred to as *Homans' sign.* A carefully performed physical examination is necessary, however, to help exclude other diagnoses.

The clinical diagnosis of PE is also inaccurate. Dyspnea and tachypnea are the most common findings, but the differential diagnosis is extensive. Most PEs are asymptomatic. When small emboli obstruct distal flow, areas of infarction may develop, resulting in a cough, hemoptysis, pleuritic chest pain with splinting, and friction rub. A massive PE may be accompanied by signs of heart failure including hypotension, syncope, convulsion, right-sided heart failure, or jugular venous distention. Additional tests used in making the diagnosis of PE include LDH, bilirubin, fibrin split products, chest x-ray, ECG, and arterial blood gas. A pulmonary embolism can result in atelectasis, effusion, a pleural-based opacity, right axis shift, nonspecific T wave inversion, and hypoxemia.

Objective Studies

Objective studies include invasive and noninvasive techniques and some tests that involve limited radiation exposure to the fetus (Table 43-1). The risks of these procedures should be weighed against the risks of untreated venous thrombosis as well as the level of clinical suspicion. Techniques

TABLE 43-1
Radiation Exposure to the Fetus

Procedure	Radiation dose (rads)
Bilateral venography, no shield	0.628
Unilateral venography, no shield	0.314
Venography, shielded	<0.05
Pulmonary angiography, femoral vein	0.405
Pulmonary angiography, brachial vein	<0.05
Pefusion lung scan, Tc	0.006-0.018
Ventilation lung scan, Xe-133	0.004-0.019
Total V/Q scan	0.010-0.050
Chest x-ray	<0.001

Modified from Ginsberg JS et al: Risks to the fetus of radiologic procedures used in the diagnosis of maternal venous thromboembolic disease, *Thromb Haemost* 61:189, 1989.

used to minimize radiation exposure to the fetus include using the lowest doses possible, shielding the abdomen, and performing pulmonary angiography through a brachial rather than a femoral vein.

Venography

Venography is the most accurate (99%) test for diagnosing a DVT. Radiographic contrast dye is injected into a distal dorsal vein of the foot. The diagnosis is made by identifying a filling defect in multiple views. Although this is the standard diagnostic test, it is invasive, relatively expensive, and often difficult to interpret. This test is used to evaluate the lower extremity including the external and common iliac veins, but is not used for deep femoral or pelvic veins.

Doppler ultrasound

Doppler ultrasound is a noninvasive technique that is ideal for diagnosing proximal DVTs that include the popliteal, femoral, and iliac veins. It has a sensitivity of 90% to 95% but is insensitive for DVTs distal to the knee. Over half of small calf DVTs can be missed with this procedure because of collateral blood flow.

Impedance plethysmography

Impedance plethysmography (IPG) is a noninvasive technique that employs changes in electrical resistance after changes in limb blood volume. It is useful to diagnose proximal thromboses, and has a sensitivity of 95% and specificity of 98%. Compression of the inferior vena cava by the gravid uterus can cause a false positive result during the third trimester, and the test is not used to evaluate DVTs distal to the knee. Serial IPG may be an alternative to venography for diagnosing DVT.

Ventilation/perfusion scan

A ventilation/perfusion (V/Q) scan should be ordered for all patients in whom a PE is suspected. Technetium-99 microspheres are injected intravenously and are associated with a fetal radiation dose of 2 mrads. The test is 90% sensitive with false positives resulting from pneumonia, tumors, atelectasis, and effusion. The addition of a ventilation scan increases the specificity. A ventilation/perfusion mismatch is consistent with a PE.

Pulmonary angiography

Pulmonary angiography is the definitive test for diagnosing a pulmonary embolism. Radioactive contrast medium is injected into branches of the pulmonary artery for identification of filling defects consistent with a clot. There is a 4% to 5% morbidity rate associated with this procedure, which includes systemic hypersensitivity, acute tubular necrosis, pneumothorax, and arrhythmias. Angiography is indicated when the V/Q scan is indeterminate or does not correlate with the clinical presentation.

MANAGEMENT

When a DVT is diagnosed during pregnancy, the standard treatment is bed rest, although this measure may not prevent emboli from detaching. The affected extremity should be elevated by placing the patient in the Trendelenburg position rather than using pillows to prop up the extremity. The patient should ambulate as soon as symptoms abate. Moist heat and analgesic can also be used as needed. When a patient is diagnosed with a PE, oxygen should be administered to keep the PaO_2 above 70 mm Hg. Positive end-expiratory pressure (PEEP) may be necessary if pulmonary edema is present, and narcotics are used for pain and apprehension. The patient should be kept on bed rest for 5 to 7 days to allow time for initial clot organization. Antibiotics have not been shown to be effective.

Anticoagulation

Patients diagnosed with a thromboembolism should be treated with anticoagulant therapy to prevent spreading of the clot, to minimize the risks of recurrence, and in the case of a DVT, to prevent a PE. There are potential complications associated with the use of anticoagulants during pregnancy.

Heparin is considered the treatment of choice during pregnancy. Because of its large size and negative charge, heparin does not cross the placenta or appear in breast milk. It is a heterogeneous mucopolysaccharide with a molecular weight of 3000 to 40,000 daltons. Heparin acts by binding to and enhancing the activity of antithrombin-III, a potent inhibitor of thrombin and factors Xa, XIa, XIa, and XIIa. The half-life is 60 to 90 minutes, depending on the dose and thrombus size. Heparin does not stimulate fibrinolysis or directly lyse a clot. Anticoagulation can be reversed with protamine sulfate at a dose of 1 mg/100 U of heparin used. Most authors recommend 7 to 10 days of intravenous therapy for acute treatment. Because heparin does not interfere with diagnostic tests, it should be administered before studies are obtained in patients with a clinical presentation suspicious for a PE or DVT.

Patients should be closely followed with serial activated partial thromboplastin times (aPTTs). This is the most sensitive and widely available test. The goal of full anticoagulation should be to prolong the aPTT by 1.5 to 2.0 times control. Careful monitoring and proper adjustments in heparin dosing are important because subtherapeutic anticoagulation has been associated with a significant increase in recurrence risk. Weight-based dosing has been shown to be effective. The recommended loading dose is 80 U/kg followed by a maintenance dose of 18 U/kg/hr. Higher doses should be considered in cases of a massive PE or large proximal DVT because of the larger amount of thrombin present. The standard dosing regimen employs a 5000 to 10,000 U loading dose followed by a sufficient amount to maintain the aPTT at 1.5 to 2.0 times control.

Complications associated with the use of heparin include hemorrhage, osteoporosis, and thrombocytopenia. The most common complication is hemorrhage, which occurs in 5% to 10% of patients. Because platelets serve as a patient's hemostatic defense, drugs that affect platelet function (NSAIDs, dextran, aspirin) are contraindicated. Osteoporosis can occur with chronic heparin therapy at doses of at least 15,000 U daily for 3 or more months. This side effect is partially reversible and may be decreased by taking 1.5 g of supplemental calcium daily. Thrombocytopenia affects 2% to 3% of patients and is usually evident by 6 to 12 days after therapy is begun. A platelet count should be obtained after 1 week of treatment. Patients with thrombocytopenia are at an increased risk of thrombosis. There are no fetal complications associated with the use of heparin during pregnancy.

Low molecular weight heparin (LMWH), which consists of a smaller molecule that has a longer half-life and less variability, has been recently developed. It acts on ATIII to inhibit factor Xa, but does not affect thrombin directly. Advantages of this drug include less bleeding, less frequent administration, and fewer cases of thrombocytopenia. It does not cross the placenta and is safe in pregnancy. Currently, higher costs associated with this drug have prevented it from being used as first-line therapy.

Coumarin derivatives (warfarin) are oral anticoagulants that are contraindicated during pregnancy because of their teratogenic effects. The use of coumarin during the first trimester is associated with embryopathy in 10% to 25% of cases including nasal cartilage hypoplasia, bone stippling, and hypertelorism. During the second and third trimesters, coumarin has been associated with dorsal midline dysplasia, microcephaly, midline cerebellar atrophy, optic atrophy, and hemorrhage. In addition, there is an increased risk of spontaneous abortion and fetal demise. It is safe to use coumarin during breastfeeding because it is protein bound and is not found in breast milk in appreciable amounts. Coumarin should only be used during pregnancy for life-threatening circumstances in which heparin cannot be used.

Other options for management include fibrinolytic therapy and surgical intervention. Streptokinase and urokinase have been used for clot lysis in cases of massive DVT and PE. Surgical therapy (thrombectomy) may be necessary when anticoagulants are contraindicated or ineffective. A vena caval interruption or intracaval device can also be used when anticoagulation is contraindicated, in cases of recurrent PE despite coagulation, or after an embolectomy.

The subcutaneous pump has been tested during pregnancy with little success. The potential advantages of this method of treatment are continuous dosing and elimination of injections. However, there have been major bleeding complications and a PE associated with this therapy.

Acute Thromboembolism During Pregnancy

An acute DVT (proximal and calf) or PE during pregnancy should be treated with anticoagulation. After an initial loading dose of 80 U/kg or 5000 to 10,000 U, patients are placed on a maintenance dose of 15 to 20 U/kg/hr and adjusted as needed to achieve an aPTT of 1.5 times control. The intravenous therapy should continue for 7 to 10 days. The patients can then be switched to subcutaneous heparin in divided doses every 8 or 12 hours. The aPTT should be maintained at 1.5 times control and adjustments in heparin made to achieve this level. Full anticoagulation should continue for 3 months after the acute event. Prophylactic doses of 7500 to 10,000 U subcutaneously every 12 hours should be given for the remainder of the pregnancy if necessary.

Intrapartum and Postpartum Therapy

Patients at high risk for an initial venous thrombosis or recurrence should be managed with full anticoagulation during and after labor. Indications include a recent PE or iliofemoral DVT, mechanical heart valves, ATIII deficiency, and protein C and S deficiency. Patients should be switched to or continued on intravenous heparin so that an aPTT of 1.5 to 2 times control is maintained throughout labor and delivery. After delivery, patients should continue using heparin or coumarin therapy. Epidural and spinal anesthesia are contraindicated because of the risks of hematoma formation. Depending on the risks and indications of intrapartum therapy, another option is to use a prophylactic dose of heparin, 7500 U subcutaneously every 12 hours until delivery. This dose should also be used for patients at high risk who require a cesarean delivery. Patients being treated with prophylactic doses of heparin during pregnancy should restart the drug 2 to 6 hours post partum and continue for 4 to 6 weeks. Physicians must keep in mind that a thrombosis is most likely to occur in the postpartum period.

Antepartum Prophylaxis

Patients who have had a previous DVT or PE, except in cases of trauma, should be placed on prophylactic heparin therapy during pregnancy. Other indications for antepartum and postpartum prophylactic heparin therapy are antiphospholipid antibody syndrome, myeloproliferative disorders (thrombocythemia, polycythemia vera), paroxysmal nocturnal hemoglobinuria, paralysis (immobility), and a combination of risk factors such as bed rest, advanced maternal age, and obesity. Several studies have demonstrated that the risk of recurrence during pregnancy is approximately 10%. The amount of heparin required for adequate prophylaxis is greater in pregnancy because of the increased volume of distribution, decreased plasma albumin, and increase in factors VII, VIII, IX, X, and fibrinogen. Most of the recommendations for prophylactic therapy are based on studies in nonpregnant patients. For prophylactic therapy during pregnancy, an aPTT level is too insensitive to accurately monitor prophylactic therapy, heparin requirements increase with gestational age, and 5000 U subcutaneously every 12 hours is an insufficient dose for prophylaxis. Recommendations for adequate prophylactic therapy during pregnancy include 7500 U subcutaneously every 12 hours during the first and second trimesters and 10,000 U subcutaneously every 12 hours during the third trimester.

KEY POINTS

1 Thromboembolic disease accounts for 20% of maternal mortality in the United States with the true incidence of thromboembolic disease in pregnancy approximately 1/2000 to 1/2500.

2 The postpartum risk of a DVT or PE is 20 times higher than the antepartum risk, and a cesarean delivery is associated with a 3 to 5 times higher risk of embolism compared with a vaginal delivery.

3 Heparin requirements are increased in pregnancy.

4 Patients with inherited deficiencies of ATIII, protein S, and protein C should be anticoagulated during pregnancy and the intrapartum, and postpartum periods.

SUGGESTED READINGS

Barbour L et al: A prospective study of heparin-induced osteoporosis in pregnancy using bone densitometry, *Am J Obstet Gynecol* 170:862, 1994.

Barbour LA, Pickard J: Controversies in thromboembolic disease during pregnancy: a critical review, *Obstet Gynecol* 86:621, 1995.

Dahlman T, Lindvall N, Hellgren M: Osteopenia in pregnancy during long-term heparin treatment: a radiological study postpartum, *Br J Obstet Gynaecol* 97:221, 1990.

Dahlman RC, Sjoberg HE, Ringertz H: Bone mineral density during long-term prophylaxis with heparin in pregnancy, *Am J Obstet Gynecol* 170:1315, 1994.

Demers C, Ginsberg JS: Deep venous thrombosis and pulmonary embolism in pregnancy, *Clin Chest Med* 13:645, 1992.

Ginsberg JS, Hirsh J: Use of antithrombotic agents during pregnancy, *Chest* 102:385S, 1992.

Ginsberg JS et al: Venous thrombosis during pregnancy: leg and trimester of presentation, *Thromb Haemost* 67: 519, 1992.

Hirsh J, Fuster V: Guide to anticoagulation therapy, *Circulation* 89:1449, 1994.

Raschke RA, Reilly BM, Guidry JR: The weight-based heparin dosing nomogram compared with a standard care nomogram, *Ann Intern Med* 1119:874, 1993.

Rutherford SE, Phelan JP: Deep venous thrombosis and pulmonary embolism. In Clark SL et al, eds: *Critical care obstetrics,* ed 2, Boston, 1991, Blackwell Scientific Publications, pp 151.

Warkentin TE et al: Heparin-induced thrombocytopenia in patients treated with low-molecular-weight heparin or unfractionated heparin, *N Engl J Med* 332:1330-5, 1995.

44

Intrauterine Growth Restriction

Steven G. Gabbe

Intrauterine growth restriction (IUGR), defined as weight at birth at or below the 10th percentile for gestational age, accounts for approximately one third of all low-birth-weight infants (<2500 g). The term *intrauterine growth restriction* is preferred over the term *intrauterine growth retardation* because "restricted," while describing a pathologic process, is most often associated with a good perinatal outcome. "Retarded," on the other hand, may lead parents to believe their unborn child has already been found to be neurologically damaged. Not only is perinatal mortality increased in pregnancies complicated by IUGR, but short-term neonatal morbidity is as well, including hypoglycemia, hypothermia, meconium aspiration, hyperviscosity, and pulmonary alveolar hemorrhage. Finally, the fetus with IUGR has a significantly increased risk for long-term neurologic sequelae, including learning deficits.

Of all infants born with a weight below the 10th percentile, approximately 70% are normal, constitutionally small infants. They may have a mother of short stature and/or low body weight. Review of a patient's obstetric history will often reveal that her infants, although small at birth, have had a normal course in the nursery.

About half of all growth-restricted infants result from insults to the fetus occurring in the first trimester. Because fetal growth in the first third of pregnancy is characterized by hyperplasia or an increase in cell number, these pathologic processes result in an infant with too few cells in *all* organs (i.e., an infant that is symmetrically growth restricted). The symmetrically growth-restricted fetus may result from an infection with rubella, CMV, or toxoplasmosis; exposure to a teratogen such as Coumadin or isotretinoin; or a chromosomal abnormality, such as trisomy 21, 18, or 13. Because the insult to the fetus occurs so early in gestation, the prognosis for these infants is generally poor.

During the second half of pregnancy, processes broadly termed *uteroplacental insufficiency* restrict fetal growth primarily by reducing the size of fetal cells, or cellular hypertrophy. Approximately 15% of growth-restricted infants result from preeclampsia or underlying chronic hypertension, diabetes mellitus with vasculopathy, collagen vascular disease, or renal disease. Because these pregnancies are often complicated by intrauterine fetal death and have a high likelihood for nonreassuring fetal heart rate patterns during labor, antepartum fetal surveillance, careful intrapartum monitoring, and timely delivery can improve perinatal outcome. In contrast to symmetric growth restriction, pregnancies complicated by uteroplacental insufficiency result in asymmetric growth restriction, with preservation of brain growth at the expense of body fat and hepatic glycogen deposition.

DIAGNOSIS

Because detecting abnormal growth for gestational age is the cornerstone of identifying IUGR, precise knowledge of gestational age is essential. In patients at low risk for this process, gestational age should be established based on menstrual dating and an early pelvic examination. Ultrasound dating will be necessary in patients with uncertain menstrual histories. Serial fundal height measurements can then be used. Should the fundal height measure 4 cm less than the expected measurement for gestational age, an ultrasound study can be performed to assess fetal growth. In patients at high risk for IUGR, such as those with vascular disease, accurate gestational dating with ultrasound is again important. Serial fundal height measurements can be used to follow the patient, but in these cases, ultrasound studies should also be performed every 4 to 6 weeks to assess fetal growth.

The three most important ultrasound characteristics of IUGR are (1) reduced amniotic fluid volume; (2) an estimated fetal weight below the 10th percentile; and for asymmetric IUGR, (3) an elevated head circumference (HC)/abdominal circumference (AC) ratio. Decreased amniotic fluid volume, determined by measuring the amniotic fluid index (AFI), reflects decreased renal blood flow, a compensatory mechanism seen in the fetus with asymmetric IUGR. Amniotic fluid may be increased in symmetric IUGR, especially in cases of trisomy 18. An elevated HC/AC ratio, greater than the 95th percentile for gestational age, indicates preserved brain growth at the expense of decreased growth of the abdominal fat and the liver, a characteristic finding in asymmetric IUGR. With symmetric IUGR, the HC/AC ratio remains normal because both the HC and AC are reduced.

In general, decreased amniotic fluid volume is the first sign of asymmetric growth restriction, followed by a decreased AC and, late in the process, a decreased HC. Two ultrasound parameters, both of which do not require a precise knowledge of the patient's gestational age, may also be helpful in detecting asymmetric IUGR–placental grade and the femur length (FL)/AC ratio. Approximately one third of fetuses with advanced placental grade (a grade III placenta) will demonstrate IUGR. In the normally growing fetus, the FL/AC ratio remains constant at 22 from 21 to 40 weeks gestation. However, an elevated FL/AC ratio >23.5 suggests asymmetric IUGR, with reduced AC size but preserved FL growth.

Ultrasound can also be helpful in identifying the pregnancy with symmetric IUGR. As noted above, in such cases both HC and AC growth lag. The abnormalities are usually present before 20 weeks. In this setting, a comprehensive ultrasound study should be performed to detect fetal anomalies. In the presence of symmetric IUGR, especially if an anomaly and/or hydramnios are noted, a fetal karyotype should be obtained by amniocentesis or umbilical cord blood sampling. Because many fetuses with trisomy 18 demonstrate worrisome fetal heart rate patterns during labor that might lead to an emergency cesarean delivery, and these babies have such a poor prognosis, recognizing the fetus with trisomy 18 before labor could avoid an unnecessary cesarean delivery. Should the maternal history suggest a viral infection, ultrasound evidence such as hydrops or ventriculomegaly may be found. Appropriate maternal serologic titres or an amniotic fluid culture in the case of suspected CMV infection may be helpful in establishing the etiology.

In asymmetric IUGR and symmetric IUGR caused by chromosomal abnormalities, resistance to flow in the placenta is increased, and the diastolic component of the systolic-diastolic complex may be reduced. When used as a screening technique, studies of umbilical artery velocimetry have been disappointing, with a sensitivity and specificity of approximately 60% and 85%, respectively. However, once the pregnancy complicated by IUGR has been detected. Doppler flow studies may be used to assess fetal condition and assist in the timing of delivery. Absence of end diastolic flow or reversal of diastolic flow in the setting of asymmetric IUGR is an ominous finding and is associated with a high likelihood of perinatal morbidity and mortality.

TREATMENT

The prognosis for the fetus with significant symmetric growth restriction is generally poor. In such cases, counseling the patient and her partner can help them understand the etiology of the growth disorder, the prognosis for the fetus, and the likelihood for recurrence.

In cases complicated by asymmetric IUGR, efforts should be made to improve the intrauterine fetal environment and monitor fetal condition. The patient should be encouraged to increase bed rest, improve her diet, and stop smoking or substance abuse. Antepartum fetal surveillance may include maternal counting of fetal movement, twice weekly nonstress tests, and weekly assessment of amniotic fluid volume. Should fetal compromise be suspected on the basis of this testing protocol, a BPP or contraction stress test can be performed to help further clarify fetal status (Fig. 44-1). In this setting, Doppler velocimetry of the umbilical artery may also help define the timing of delivery. Certainly, delivery should be considered at 36 weeks gestation in all cases of documented IUGR, because it is beyond this gestational age that the intrauterine fetal death rate increases.

During labor, continuous electronic fetal heart rate monitoring is important to detect nonreassuring fetal heart rate patterns. An amnioinfusion may be used if meconium is detected or to reduce cord compression if oligohydramnios complicates the pregnancy. The timing of delivery should be coordinated with the neonatologist because these infants are at great risk for immediate neonatal morbidity.

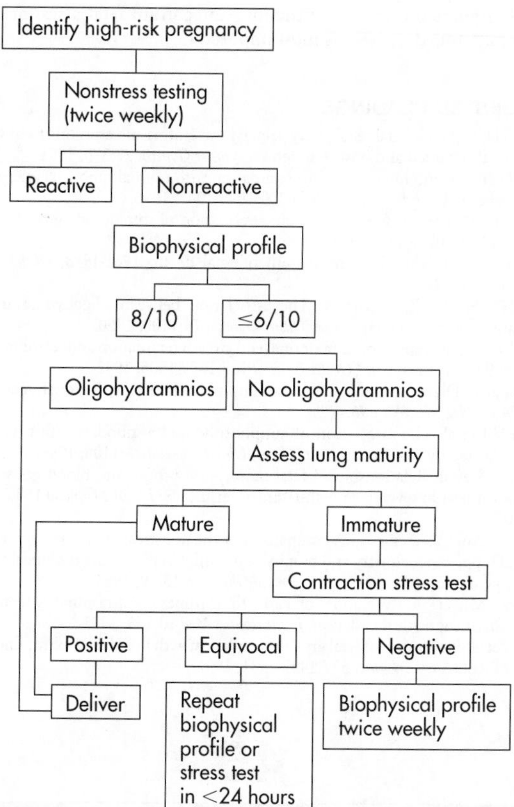

FIG. 44-1 Management of IUGR. (From Sonek J, Reiss RE, Gabbe SG: Antenatal assessment of the fetus. In Iams JD, Zuspan FP, Quilligan EJ, eds: *Manual of obstetrics and gynecology,* ed 2, St. Louis, 1990, Mosby, p 93.)

KEY POINTS

1 IUGR is associated with an increased rate of perinatal mortality as well as significant short-term and long-term neonatal morbidity.

2 The diagnosis of IUGR requires early and accurate dating of the pregnancy and serial assessments of fetal growth with ultrasound.

3 For the fetus suspected of suffering symmetric growth restriction, a thorough evaluation to determine the etiology is essential; for the fetus with asymmetric growth restriction, antepartum fetal assessment and carefully timed delivery is most important.

SUGGESTED READINGS

Arduini D, Rizzo G: Fetal renal artery velocity waveforms and amniotic fluid volume in growth-retarded and post-term fetuses, *Obstet Gynecol* 77:370, 1991.

Burke G et al: Is intrauterine growth retardation with normal umbilical artery blood flow a benign condition? *Br Med J* 300:1044-1045, 1990.

Doubilet PM, Benson CB: Sonographic evaluation of intrauterine growth retardation, *AJR* 164:709-717, 1995.

Fretts RC et al: The changing pattern of fetal death, 1961-1988, *Obstet Gynecol* 79:35-39, 1992.

Lin C-C, Sheikh Z, Lopata R: The association between oligohydramnios and intrauterine growth retardation, *Obstet Gynecol* 76:1100, 1990.

Low JA et al: Association of intrauterine fetal growth retardation and learning deficits at age 9 to 11 years, *Am J Obstet Gynecol* 167:1499-1505, 1992.

Pardi G et al: Diagnostic value of blood sampling in fetuses with growth retardation, *N Engl J Med* 328:692-696, 1993.

Polzin WJ et al: The association of antiphospholipid antibodies with pregnancies complicated by fetal growth restriction, *Obstet Gynecol* 78:1108, 1991.

Ribbert LS et al: Relationship of fetal biophysical profile and blood gas values at cordocentesis in severely growth-retarded fetsus, *Am J Obstet Gynecol* 164:569-571, 1990.

Shalev E, Zalel Y, Weiner E: A comparison of the nonstress test, oxytocin challenge test, Doppler velocimetry and biophysical profile in predicting umbilical vein pH in growth-retarded fetuses, *Int J Gynecol Obstet* 43:15-19, 1993.

Skovron ML et al: Evaluation of early third-trimester ultrasound screening for intrauterine growth retardation, *J Ultrasound Med* 10:153, 1991.

Uzan S et al: Prevention of fetal growth retardation with low-dose aspirin: findings of the EPREDA trial, *Lancet* 337:1427-1431, 1991.

45

Preeclampsia/Eclampsia

Frederick P. Zuspan

Preeclampsia is a syndrome of unknown etiology characterized by the sequential development of facial and hand edema, hypertension (BP>140/90), and proteinuria (2+ dipstick) after the 20th week of gestation. This patient may progress to a seizure-like state. She is then said to have eclampsia, which portends the possibility of death for either mother or fetus depending on multiple factors, the most significant of which are the gestational age of the pregnancy and location where the diseases occur.

Preeclampsia occurs in 6% to 8% of pregnancies and is principally a disease of the first pregnancy (85%). It occurs in 14% to 20% of multiple gestations and in 30% of patients with major uterine anomalies. It occurs in 25% to 30% of patients with chronic hypertension and/or chronic renal disease. Women who have repetitive severe disease during pregnancy most likely have the genetic tendency for a recessive gene.

The pathogenesis of preeclampsia is well understood even though the etiology remains obscure. The major goal of prenatal care is detecting the early onset of preeclampsia and to activate aggressive therapy to prevent severe complications for either the mother or the fetus. There currently are no specific forms of therapy to prevent the disease.

PATHOPHYSIOLOGY

The uteroplacental bed holds the key to the understanding of the cause and pathogenesis of preeclampsia. Fetal trophoblastic tissue migrates in two phases down the maternal spiral arteries, displacing the musculoelastic structure of these arteries. The migration is completed by 20 weeks of gestation and results in the dilation of the spiral arteries, which is associated with fetal health. The dilated spiral arteries are converted from a high-resistance system to a low-resistance system, which facilitates maximum interchange of nutrients and gases. The defect seen in preeclampsia is a lack of or an incomplete invasion of trophoblasts into the maternal spiral arteries. This is one of the basic lesions and begins at the time of implantation. Preeclampsia can be considered an acquired birth defect caused by abnormal implantation and is not preventable.

The adrenergic nerves, located at the base of the spiral artery, normally disappear or are denervated during pregnancy. If the patient is destined to develop preeclampsia, there is an incomplete denervation of the adrenergic nerves. Some immunologic mechanism does not permit the trophoblastic tissue to migrate in an appropriate manner to invade the spiral arteries, and concurrently the adrenergic nerves are incompletely denervated.

An imbalance exists in the arachidonic acid physiologic system that plays an important role in the development of pregnancy hypertension. This change in development within the spiral arteries establishes a mechanism whereby endothelial cell injury begins with the production of mitogens and the development of a decrease in prostacyclines and an increase in thromboxane A_2, a vasoconstrictor and platelet proaggregator. The placental production of prostacycline is significantly decreased, resulting in less dilation in the cardiovascular system with a relative greater balance of thromboxane, which probably contributes to generalized vasoconstriction. These gradual and subtle changes ultimately lead to an alteration in cardiovascular reactivity and the eventual development of hypertension.

The major end organ involvements are (1) the placenta, (2) the cardiovascular system, and the (3) kidney. When secondary organ involvement is superimposed on the primary organs, the patient is usually seriously ill. Secondary organ involvements are (1) the reticuloendothelial system, with platelet decrease and dysfunction; (2) the liver, with abnormal liver chemistries indicating severe liver impairment; and (3) the brain, with edema and/or hemorrhage.

DIAGNOSIS

Classification

International and American authorities do not agree on specific, objective ways to diagnose preeclampsia, nor on a common terminology. The American College of Obstetricians and Gynecologists (ACOG) 1972 classification differentiates preeclampsia/eclampsia, chronic hypertension, chronic hypertension with superimposed preeclampsia, and transient hypertension (now known as *gestational hypertension*). Objective parameters such as blood pressure reading and proteinuria are not consistent among different classification schemes.

DIFFERENTIAL DIAGNOSIS

The diagnosis of preeclampsia should be entertained in a first pregnancy (85% nullipara) after 20 weeks gestation if the patient's blood pressure remains >140/90 and urinary protein is >300 mg/L. Preeclampsia is categorized as mild or severe. Mild preeclampsia is diagnosed if criteria for severe preeclampsia are not present.

If the patient is multiparous, preeclampsia is observed only 15% of the time. Reevaluate the family history; if hypertension is present, the patient may also have chronic hypertension that is unmasked or worsened by pregnancy. Eclampsia is present when a patient who has preeclampsia develops generalized seizures.

The diagnosis of *severe preeclampsia* is significant if one or more of the following signs or symptoms are present: a persistent diastolic blood pressure of >110 mm Hg and systolic pressure >160; proteinuria of >5 g/L; platelets <100,000, especially if the trend is downward; an increase in liver enzymes or jaundice; oliguria of less than 400 ml/24 hours; and symptoms of epigastric pain and scotomata or some form of visual disturbances or severe headache. All patients who have severe preeclampsia should be hospitalized and evaluated.

TREATMENT AND MANAGEMENT

Assume that the severe preeclamptic/eclamptic patient constitutes a medical emergency and needs to be stabilized with the following regimen: intravenous magnesium sulfate, 4 to 6 g load given over 5 minutes, then 1 to 2 g/hour; control the blood pressure if the diastolic pressure is persistently >100 to 110 by using intravenous hydralazine in a 5 mg bolus; if blood pressure is not stabilized in 20 minutes, add 100 mg of hydralazine to 200 ml of normal saline and infuse by automated device. A Dinamap or similar blood pressure recording apparatus should be used to monitor the blood pressure between 80 and 100 diastolic. Other antihypertensive agents may be used, such as labetalol 10 to 20 mg intravenously, or a calcium channel blocker such as nifedipine 10 to 20 mg orally. A response should be noted within 20 minutes and drug dosage can then be altered (Fig. 45-1).

After appropriate laboratory data are obtained (CBC, platelets, electrolytes, liver battery, serum creatinine, BUN, uric acid) and results are evaluated, consider termination of the pregnancy if the patient does not improve. If gestation is less than 34 weeks, give betamethasone 12.5 mg every 12 hours for 2 doses, then wait 48 hours.

Fetal evaluation should include NST and BPP (ultrasound with fluid evaluation as minimal exam). The pregnancy can most likely be terminated by induction of labor with oxytocin, starting at 0.5 milliunits/minute. If cesarean delivery is utilized, general anesthesia is acceptable, but epidural anesthesia in selected patients is the method of choice. If magnesium sulfate is utilized, it should be continued for at least 24 hours after delivery.

If a magnesium sulfate overdose occurs, calcium chloride or gluconate (1 g) may be given intravenously. Once magnesium sulfate is administered, the patient presents as a bio-assay condition and monitoring can take place by assessing deep tendon reflexes. These should be hypoactive, but present, and should be checked on an hourly basis. Reflexes become absent if the serum magnesium concentration is >5 mmol/L. Respirations are

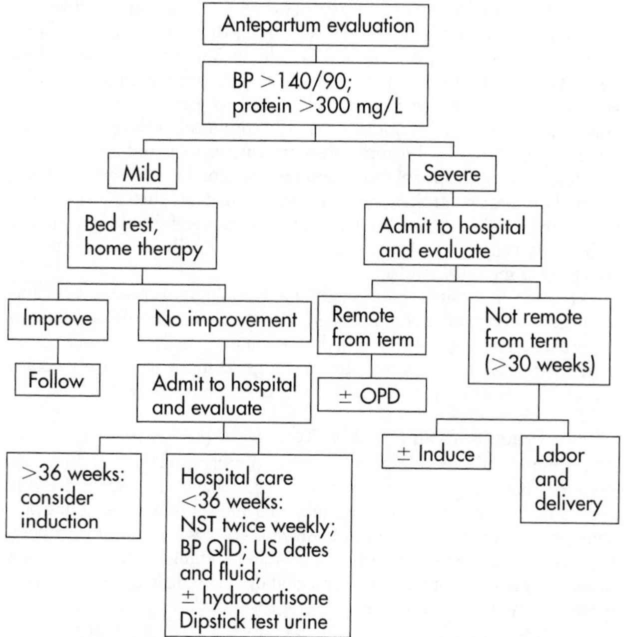

FIG. 45-1 Management of preeclampsia and eclampsia.

observed hourly and should exceed 12/hour. When the magnesium concentration exceeds 6.5 mmol, respirations may become obtunded; cardiac arrest may occur above 12 mmol/L. Urine output is monitored hourly utilizing a Foley catheter. At least 100 cc should be observed in a 4-hour period or approximately 25 cc/hour. If oliguria is present, the magnesium sulfate dosage may need to be decreased because the drug is excreted principally by the kidney. Serum magnesium levels may be obtained as a guidepost to therapy, but are usually not needed. Cord blood magnesium levels may be of help to the pediatrician because it takes approximately 48 hours for the newborn to excrete the magnesium. Magnesium cord levels and maternal levels are almost identical.

Decision for Delivery

Once the patient's seizure tendency and blood pressure are controlled, a decision can be made as to whether delivery should take place (Fig. 45-2). The decision is made on an individual basis and depends on gestational age, the condition of the patient and fetus, and the health care facilities. The more serious the condition of the patient, the greater the need to proceed to delivery. If the patient is <34 weeks gestation, she should be referred to a tertiary care center with a neonatal intensive care unit (NICU) available.

Delivery is the definitive care for preeclampsia/eclampsia. First, gestation is established by history, lung maturity, or ultrasound. Delivery is achieved as soon as possible in severe disease; laboratory tests should be evaluated before this decision and should include serum creatine and electrolyte levels and liver function tests to rule out impending HELLP syndrome. Selected patients may be allowed to prolong the pregnancy under intensive inpatient observation. The condition of the cervix can be evaluated; if a favorable Bishop score is present, oxytocin induction should be attempted. Appropriate monitoring of the fetus is necessary, utilizing external monitoring until membranes are ruptured and then a scalp clip. If labor is to be induced, an intrauterine pressure catheter should be inserted. If the fetus weighs <1500 g, cesarean delivery is usually considered unless the cervix is most favorable.

Magnesium sulfate is continued for at least 24 hours post partum and then the dose is gradually diminished. Blood pressure should continue to be controlled during this time, and the patient may need to continue taking antihypertensive medications after discharge. Diuresis most likely occurs within 72 hours post partum; if not, this is an ominous sign.

Severe Preeclampsia Remote From Term (<30 weeks)

As a generalization, patients with severe preeclampsia before 30 weeks gestation have a poor prognosis and many have chronic underlying hypertension. When considering maternal mortality and perinatal outcome, patients with mild preeclampsia and those with gestational hypertension (i.e., blood pressure 140/90, protein <300 mg/L), have outcomes similar to patients with a normal pregnancy. The challenge is to prevent severe disease from developing.

Bed rest is the only therapeutic modality that increases uterine blood flow and is protective to the fetus. Often this removes the patient from

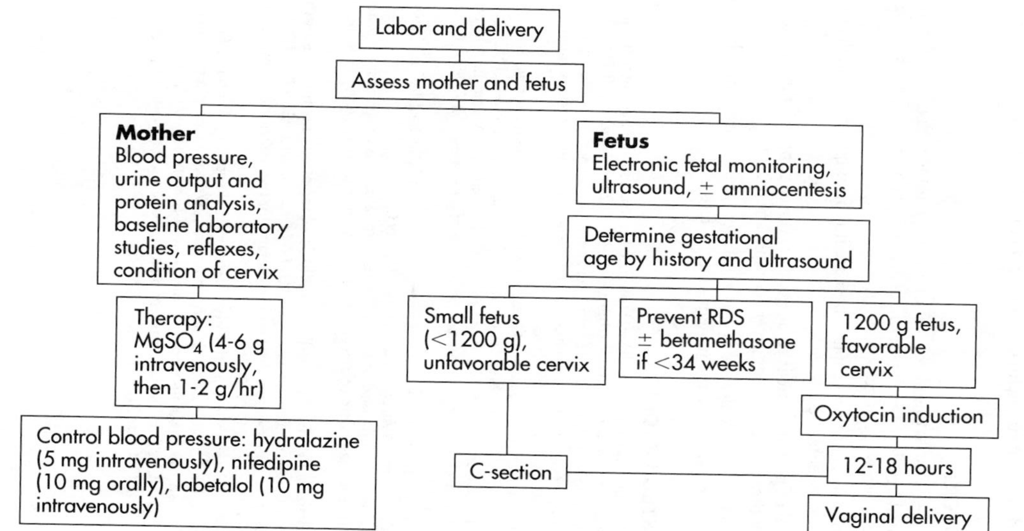

FIG. 45-2 Management of eclamptic patient during labor and delivery.

the environment in which she develops the disease and puts her into a hospital environment for closer observation. The gestational age of onset obviously dictates the outcome for the fetus. Studies involving low-dose aspirin and calcium supplementation are ongoing.

KEY POINTS

1 Preeclampsia is a syndrome of unknown etiology characterized by sequential development of facial edema, hypertension, and proteinuria after the 20th week of gestation.

2 Preeclampsia is not preventable because it is an implantation defect in the uteroplacental bed.

3 The goal of prenatal care is to detect early onset of preeclampsia and to activate therapy to prevent severe complications.

4 The decision for delivery is based on gestational age, health care facilities, and status of the patient and the fetus.

SUGGESTED READINGS

Barton JR, Stanziano GJ, Sibai BM: Monitored outpatient management of mild gestational hypertension remote from term, *Am J Obstet Gynecol* 170:765, 1994.

Chesley LC, Cooper DA: Genetics of hypertension in pregnancy: possible single gene control of preeclampsia and eclampsia in descendants of eclamptic women, *Br J Obstet Gynaecol* 93(9):898-908, 1986.

The Eclampsia Trial Collaborative Group: Which anticonvulsant for women with eclampsia? evidence from the collaborative eclampsia trial, *Lancet* 345:1455, 1995.

Pritchard JA, Cunningham FG, Pritchard SA: The Parkland Memorial Hospital protocol for treatment of eclampsia: evaluation of 245 cases, *Am J Obstet Gynecol* 148:951, 1984.

Sibai BM et al: Low-dose aspirin to prevent preeclampsia in healthy nulliparous pregnant women, *N Engl J Med,* October 21, 1993.

Sibai BM et al: A comparison of labetalol plus hospitalization versus hospitalization alone in the management of preeclampsia remote from term, *Obstet Gynecol* 70:323, 1987.

Villar J, Belizan JM, Fischer PJ: Epidemiologic observations on the relationship between calcium intake and eclampsia, *Int J Gynaecol Obstet* 21:271-278, 1983.

Walsh SW: Physiology of low-dose aspirin therapy for the prevention of preeclampsia, *Semin Perinatol* 14, 1990.

Zuspan FP et al (members of the Hypertension in Pregnancy Working Group): National High Blood Pressure Education Program Working Group report on high blood pressure in pregnancy, *Am J Obstet Gynecol* 163(5):1689-1712, 1990.

Zuspan FP, Samuels P: Editorial comment on low-dose aspirin trial during pregnancy, *N Eng J Med* October 21, 1993.

46

Postterm/Postdate Pregnancy

FREDERICK P. ZUSPAN

Postterm pregnancy is defined as the continuation of pregnancy beyond 295 days (term gestation is between 38 to 42 weeks duration). Approximately 5% to 7% of pregnancies go beyond 42 weeks gestation, but the true incidence of postterm pregnancy is unknown because of multiple factors. The most common reason for postterm pregnancy is unreliable dates.

Several related and unrelated factors are associated with pregnancies beyond 41 weeks gestation. The lowest perinatal morbidity and mortality is seen in deliveries between 39 to 41 weeks gestation. The majority of "diagnosed" postterm pregnancies are the result of factors such as inappropriate dating of the pregnancy or a prolonged follicular phase. The patient who has been taking her basal body temperature may be the only patient for whom the true EDC and actual postdate gestation can be accurately diagnosed. An early ultrasound before 12 weeks gestation should confirm the EDC by ±5 to 7 days. Prolonged gestation is also seen with congenital anomalies, absent pituitary as seen in anencephaly, hypoplastic fetal adrenal glands, placental sulphatase deficiency, and fetal osteogenesis imperfecta. Congenital anomalies are ruled out as part of the workup. The recurrence rate may be as high as 50%. Postterm pregnancy is seen more frequently in the primigravida, and a positive correlation exists with ethnicity (Australians, Greeks, and Italians).

PATHOPHYSIOLOGY

Two types of postterm gestation occur. One type is with a normal placenta (95% of cases), in which the fetus continues to grow and does not have any classic stigmata characteristically described as being seen in a fetus in a postterm pregnancy. The patient who has a normal placenta and goes beyond 295 days often will end up with a macrosomic fetus that may be associated with cephalopelvic disproportion (CPD); shoulder dystocia is not uncommon in these fetuses, and the incidence of cesarean section is higher because of CPD. In the second type of postterm pregnancies (5% of cases), the placenta is dysmature, and the fetal prognosis may be poor.

Placental function declines after 36 weeks gestation, and placental growth no longer continues. Placental aging may then begin, which may result in a dysmature placenta. The dysmature placenta has altered placenta function, a decrease in thickness, and an increase in infarction, fibrin, and calcium deposition, resulting in diminished placental reserve. Uterine sensitivity to oxytocin is often decreased, thus uterine inertia is seen more frequently. The cervix does not know when the fetus is to be delivered and frequently may be unfavorable with a low Bishop score. Amniotic fluid volume diminishes as gestation progresses. The estimated volume at 38 weeks is 1000 ml; at 42 weeks it is 300 to 400 ml and decreases further after 42 weeks gestation. Ultrasonography shows whether amniotic fluid volume is diminished; if so, it may be an ominous sign for the fetus and probably indicates a dysmature placenta. Low amniotic fluid volume is often associated with cord compression problems during labor and abnormal fetal heart rate tracings. Meconium staining of amniotic fluid may be present in 20% to 30% of cases in normal term gestation, but in postdate/postterm pregnancies the percentage of patients that have meconium staining is increased to as high as 50%. This may or may not be a sign of chronic placental aging. Importantly, the type and consistency of the meconium should be identified. The thicker the meconium, the worse the prognosis for the fetus and the more problems that will be encountered after delivery.

DIAGNOSIS

Pregnancy dating is the single most important issue when trying to diagnose postterm gestation. If the patient has been using the basal body temperature method for conception, it is the most reliable method of dating the pregnancy. Otherwise the LMP as reported by the patient can be used. Conducting an early pelvic examination before 12 weeks gestation in a nonobese patient is helpful because uterine size should equal gestational age in the absence of uterine leiomyomata. An ultrasonographic examination performed before the 12th week of gestation is accurate within a range of ±5 to 7 days. If an ultrasound examination is not done at 10 to 12 weeks gestation, one should be done at 16 to 20 weeks gestation to confirm the EDC. However, the EDC will be ±12 to 14 days. Quickening in the primigravida at ±18 weeks or in a multigravid patient at ±16 weeks is also helpful in dating the pregnancy. Uterine measurement from symphysis to uterine fundus by tape measure is most accurate when 28 cm equals 28 weeks gestation. If a discrepancy exists in the history, clinical examination, and uterine size, ultrasonographic examination should be done to firm up the EDC.

DIFFERENTIAL DIAGNOSIS

Fetal and Neonatal Findings

The diagnosis of postterm gestation usually affects only the fetus and not the mother. It is often made as an after-the-fact diagnosis in the nursery or in the delivery room. The newborn may exhibit the classic findings initially described in the fetus with a dysmature placenta:

1. First stage: long nails; skin with parchment-like wrinkling and peel-

ing; a long, thin infant who appears malnourished and lacks subcutaneous fat.

2. Second stage: identical to the first stage with the addition of meconium and amniotic fluid with staining of membranes, placenta, and fetal skin; there may or may not be meconium aspiration of the newborn.
3. Third stage: amniotic fluid, fetal skin, and membranes are markedly stained yellow; there may be a wrinkled, shriveled, "old-man" or "old-woman" appearance of the fetus who often may appear to be very apprehensive.

Problems for the newborn range from none to a stillbirth, with multiple problems between the two extremes. During the intrapartum period, the diminished amniotic fluid may result in variable cord sign decelerations of the fetal heart. If the placenta is too dysmature, late decelerations may also be seen. Once the baby is delivered, polycythemia and hypoglycemia may be present. If thick meconium is present, meconium aspiration may occur. A pediatrician should evaluate the newborn as soon as is practical. If a pediatrician is not present, the obstetrician may be obligated to put the baby in an incubator after using a DeLee suction trap when the baby's head first emerges from the perineum. Actual intubation may be necessary if a meconium plug is present in the trachea. A saline lavage may be necessary if thick, tenacious meconium exists.

THERAPY AND PREGNANCY MANAGEMENT

Fig. 46-1 is an algorithm on the management of postterm pregnancy. Three approaches to management of postterm pregnancy currently exist. The first approach prohibits labor induction, concluding the risk of induction may be greater than that of postterm pregnancy. The second involves routine induction. However, because the cervix is often unfavorable, the cesarean section rate will be higher than the current incidence of 20% to 25% for all pregnancies. The third approach is selective induction, which may be carried out when the cervix is favorable with confirmed pregnancy dates or when there is evidence of a failing fetoplacental unit.

Once a patient reaches 42 weeks gestation, one of these management methods can be instituted; fetal assessment programs are often helpful when the method of medical management is chosen. Sonography measures growth curves, fetal size, and most importantly, the amount of amniotic fluid, which is the single most important factor in decision making in induction of labor. Cardiotachometry is biophysical testing using nonstress testing or formal contraction stress testing with oxytocin. Testing should begin at the end of the 41st week of gestation and be done on a biweekly basis. This is done in conjunction with ultrasound, which is done on a weekly basis. The fetal activity score measures fetal movements. A BPP involves ultrasonography and a scoring system. It is the procedure of choice. The role of umbilical and uterine artery Doppler velocimetry is unclear.

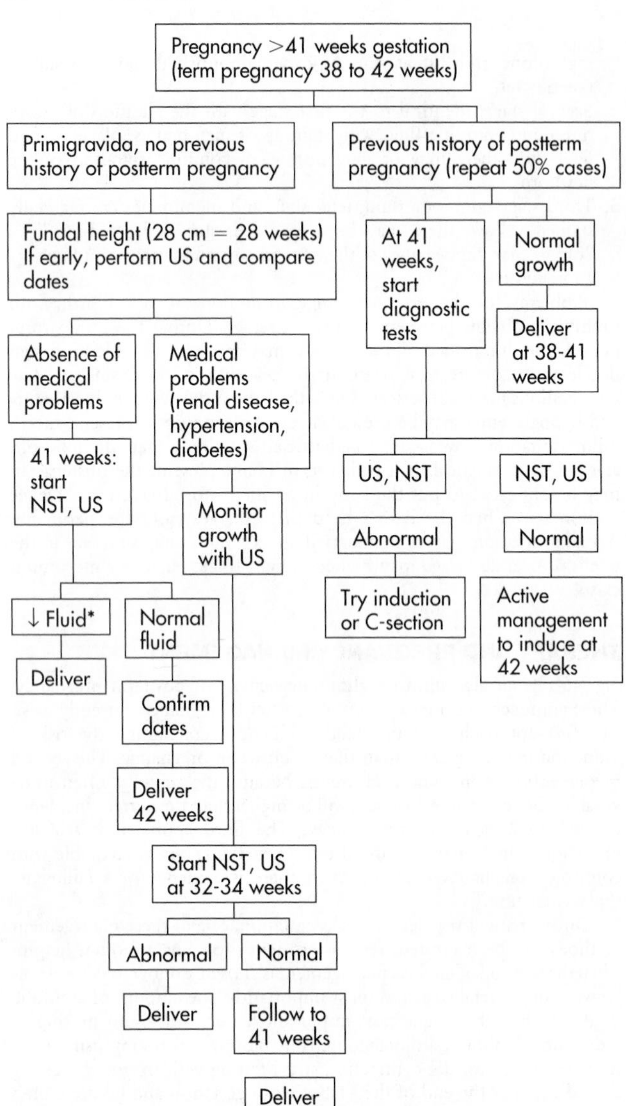

FIG. 46-1 Management of the postdate/postterm pregnancy. *Note: C-section rate increased over average of 20% in both mature and dysmature placenta. Mature placenta may see macrosomia, shoulder dystocia, CPD. Dysmature placenta may see meconium aspiration, abnormal fetal heart rate tracings. Send placenta to pathology for evaluation. *NST,* nonstress test; *US,* ultrasound.

Fetal Monitoring

If the patient has a postterm pregnancy, labor monitoring using direct fetal scalp monitoring is important. Thus rupture of membranes should be done early. This will also identify the presence of meconium. Scalp pH levels or scalp stimulation should be done if persistent abnormalities of the fetal heart rate are noted. Multiple variable decelerations as well as late decelerations may be present and should be considered as ominous for the fetus. Cervical ripening has been attempted with some degree of success using agents such as a Foley catheter, vaginal prostaglandins, intracervical laminaria, and intracervical vaginal prostaglandin gel. These agents are all used to convert an unfavorable cervix to a favorable cervix in an attempt to decrease the incidence of cesarean section. Many of these options have been very successful but the most common method is the insertion of a Foley catheter and the installation of saline with intact membranes. This is often used in conjunction with oxytocin induction.

The Delivery

If a dysmature placenta is not a consideration, CPD carries an increased incidence of macrosomia and shoulder dystocia. Shoulder dystocia may occur in 50% of patients who have a spontaneous vaginal delivery. The cesarean section rate with postterm gestations is increased and is most commonly the result of macrosomia and/or abnormal fetal heart patterns indicating some form of fetal distress. Adequate anesthesia must be available for possible complications. If available, a pediatrician should be present in the delivery room. Carefully inspect the placenta in the delivery room, record pertinent information, and then send the placenta to pathology for evaluation. A segment of the umbilical cord should also be sent to the laboratory for blood gas and pH determination if Apgar scores are less than 4.

KEY POINTS

1 The most common reason for postterm pregnancy is unreliable dates.

2 If the placenta is dysmature, a decrease in amniotic fluid volume may be present; this heralds a potential problem for the fetus during testing and in the intrapartum period.

3 The incidence of cesarean section is increased in patients who have both a dysmature placenta (decreased amniotic fluid, meconium, IUGR) and a mature placenta (CPD, shoulder dystocia, macrosomia).

4 A pediatrician or a person skilled in infant resuscitation should be present in the delivery room if thick meconium is encountered on rupture of the membranes. This may be a significant factor for the morbidity of the fetus.

SUGGESTED READINGS

Ballantyne JW: The problem of postmature infant, *J Obstet Gynaecol Br Emp* 2:36, 1902.

Freeman RK et al: Postdate utilization of the contraction stress test for primary fetal surveillance, *Am J Obstet Gynecol* 140:128, 1981.
Hannah ME et al: Induction of labor as compared with serial antenatal monitoring in post-term pregnancy: a randomized control trial, *N Engl J Med* 326:1587-1592, 1992.
NICHD: A clinical trial of induction of labor versus expectant management in postterm pregnancy, *Am J Obstet Gynecol* 170:716-723, 1994.

47

Medical Emergencies in Obstetrics

WAYNE C. TROUT

DIABETIC KETOACIDOSIS

Diabetic ketoacidosis (DKA) is a life-threatening complication. Although contemporary treatment has limited maternal mortality to less than 1%, fetal mortality is close to 50%. Common predisposing causes include skipping insulin injection coupled with some other stress such as an infection.

Diagnosis

Symptoms include polydipsia, polyuria, nausea, vomiting, headache, dry mouth, and abdominal pain. Physical findings include deep, rapid breathing (Kussmaul respiration); "fruity" acetone breath; hypotension; and change in mental status ranging from drowsiness to lethargy. Patients can become comatose if medical intervention is delayed. Laboratory findings include hyperglycemia, but glucose readings can be as low as 200 mg/dl. Ketones present in the blood will spill into the urine. Arterial pH is typically below 7.35, with an increase in the anion gap (Na – [Cl + HCO_3]) caused by the increase in ketoacids with a proportional decrease in serum bicarbonate, less than 15 mEq/L.

Pathophysiology

Decreased insulin combined with increased counterregulatory hormones (HPL, glucagon, cortisol) prevent the utilization of glucose and the clearance of ketones. Hyperglycemia promotes an osmotic diuresis. Dehydration occurs through renal losses of free water. Electrolyte imbalances occur through solute drag in the kidneys. The body can become potassium depleted without profound hypokalemia because the renal losses are compensated by a shift of intracellular potassium to the extracellular fluid in response to the acidemia (in fact, if the acidosis is severe enough, cellular shifts of K^+ may even result in hyperkalemia). The net effect is severe potassium depletion, and replacement is crucial.

Treatment

Admit the patient to an intensive care setting with continuous obstetric monitoring (Box 47-1). Establish intravenous access; typically two IV lines will be required. Insertion of an arterial line may be useful to facilitate frequent blood draws (every 1 to 2 hours) and to follow the arterial pH levels. The fluid deficit is typically 3 to 5 L. Isotonic saline should be given rapidly (1000 to 2000 ml) in the first hour. The hypernatremic patient should receive 0.45% saline. After the first hour, fluid administration should be decreased to 300 to 500 ml/hr.

Insulin is required to lower the blood glucose level; insulin is also vital in the metabolism of the ketoacids and to correct the acidosis. Initial intravenous administration of 10 to 20 units of regular insulin is required. Insulin should then be given as a continuous infusion of 10 U/hr. If there is no improvement in the pH over 3 hours or the serum glucose remains over 300 mg/dl, then higher infusion rates of insulin will be required. With continued insulin administration, dangerous hypoglycemia will develop unless exogenous glucose is given. Rapid shifts in the blood glucose will affect osmolarity; rapid shifts in osmolality may cause cerebral edema.

BOX 47-1

Management of Diabetic Ketoacidosis

- Admit to hospital
  - Establish lines
  - Monitor fetus
- Fluid resuscitation
  - 1-2 L in first hour, 300-500 ml/hr thereafter
- Insulin management
  - Bolus 10-20 units intravenously
  - Infuse 10 U/hr
  - Use higher infusion rates if no improvement in pH or glucose >300 after 3 hours
- Glucose management
  - When glucose drops to 200-250, change to D5 containing fluids, decrease insulin rate by 50%
- Electrolyte management
  - Monitor potassium levels; when K^+ returns to normal, replace with 10-20 mEq/hr
- Acid-base balance
  - If pH <7.10 or HCO_3 <5, add bicarbonate to fluids–1 amp/L 0.45% saline

Fluids containing 5% dextrose should be administered once the serum glucose reaches 200 to 250 mg/dl, and the insulin infusion should then be decreased by 50%, but not discontinued. Give insulin and glucose concurrently.

Initially hyperkalemia may be noted, but there is overall potassium depletion. Potassium replacement should be instituted once the serum levels return to normal (or low normal) at a rate of 10 to 20 mEq/hr.

If the arterial pH is <7.10 or serum bicarbonate is <5 mEq/l, additional bicarbonate should be given. Mixing 1 ampule (44mEq $NaHCO_3$) to 1 L of 0.45% saline will provide a nearly isotonic solution that will also buffer the pH.

THYROID STORM

Diagnosis

Thyrotoxicosis complicates 1/2000 pregnancies. Thyroid storm is a severe form of thyrotoxicosis that is a medical emergency and is associated with a 25% mortality. Patients in "storm" present with a multitude of clinical findings including the following:

Fever: Skin is warm and flushed with a temperature >100° F
Cardiac: Tachycardia, atrial fibrillation, and possibly CHF
Gastrointestinal: Nausea, vomiting, and diarrhea are common findings
CNS: Irritability, agitation, tremors, and even psychosis may be identified
Laboratory: Elevated T4 and T3, low TSH

Treatment

Admit patient to hospital, order laboratory studies (thyroid functions, electrolytes, CBC), and search for an underlying infection as a potential triggering event. Treat hyperthermia with acetaminophen, a cooling blanket, and adequate hydration. Control heart rate with beta-blockers; propranolol 40 mg every 6 hours has classically been used. Cardioselective agents or short-acting agents may also be utilized. Antithyroid medications to be given include propylthiouracil (PTU); PTU is the preferred therapy because it blocks conversion of T3 to T4. Methimazole may be given. Potassium iodide 1 g orally can be given to block the release of stored thyroid hormone.

ASTHMA

Asthma affects about 1% of women in the reproductive years. Acute exacerbations of air exchange as seen in asthma attacks are one of the more common medical problems encountered during pregnancy. Status asthmaticus is a life-threatening emergency.

Outpatient Management

Asthmatic patients should be encouraged to monitor their respiratory status with peak flow monitors and titration with inhaled bronchodilators at the first sign of diminished air flow.

During an acute asthma attack, an initial bronchospasm will result in hypoxemia. The normal physiologic response is to increase the respiratory rate; this hyperventilation will result in a lower Pco_2. The patient will note dyspnea, tachypnea, audible wheezing, and utilization of accessory muscles of respiration. Arterial hypoxia occurs next because the patient can no longer compensate by hyperventilation. This stage is then followed by ventilation/perfusion mismatch, carbon dioxide trapping, respiratory acidosis, and finally complete respiratory collapse. The physician must remember the physiologic alterations of pregnancy (decreased Pco_2 and increased pH) when interpreting ABG values because advanced disease may have "normal" lab values. Oxygenation should be monitored with cutaneous pulseoximetry. Initial therapy usually includes inhaled or nebulized β-agonists; effectiveness of therapy should be monitored by clinical signs of improved air exchange and objective improvements in peak airflow.

Diagnosis

A history of an asthma attack should note time of onset of disease and any predisposing factors. List current medications (including any recent steroid use) and recent hospitalizations or emergency room visits for asthma.

General symptoms include cough, wheezing, chest tightness, breathlessness, and diaphoresis. Physical findings include alterations in vital signs–respiratory rate >30 breaths/min, pulse >120 bpm, pulsus paradoxus ≥12 mm Hg (a fall in systolic BP with inspiration)–and pulmonary signs–wheezing (patients with severe disease may have no wheezing), decreased air movement, and use of accessory muscles of respiration. Laboratory findings include FEV_1 or PEFR <30% to 50% of baseline, Po_2 <60 mm Hg, O_2 saturation <90%, Pco_2 ≥40 mm Hg.

Treatment

Nebulized β-agonist is the preferred therapy for the initial treatment of acute, severe asthma (Box 47-2). β-agonists are given at 20-minute intervals for 3 to 4 doses; the use of a metered-dose inhaler with a spacer is able to achieve similar drug delivery. Monitoring with peak flow meters before and after a treatment will document response. Improvement of less than 10% is an indication of deteriorating condition. Subcutaneous β-agonists (such as terbutaline) may be used in the unresponsive patient, though the side effects (e.g., tachycardia) are greater.

Corticosteroids are an important therapeutic modality for refractory cases of asthma, and concurrent pregnancy should not preclude their use. Corticosteroids should be used early in very severe cases of asthma. Patients that do not respond after 1 hour of initial β-agonist therapy (i.e., 3 doses) should be given steroids. Early use of steroids is important because the onset to action is 6 to 12 hours; typically methylprednisolone 80 to 125 mg is used.

Oxygen should be given to the asthmatic gravida at 2 to 4 L/min. Titration to an O_2 saturation of 94% with a continuous pulse oximeter is necessary to provide adequate fetal oxygenation. Improvements in Po_2 do not correlate with improvements in peak flow, so this aspect of therapy should also be closely monitored.

BOX 47-2
Pharmacotherapy of Acute Asthma

Inhaled β-agonists
- Albuterol 2.5 mg (0.5 ml of a 0.5% solution)
- Metoproterenol 15 mg (0.3 ml of a 0.5% solution)
- Isoetharine 5 mg (0.5 ml of a 1% solution), dilute with 2-3 ml saline

Subcutaneous β-agonists
- Epinephrine 0.3 mg
- Terbutaline 0.25 mg

Corticosteroids
- Methylprednisolone 60-80 mg intravenously every 6-8 hours
- Hydrocortisone 2.0 mg/kg every 4 hours
- Oral methylprednisolone 60 mg initially followed by 60-120 mg daily in divided dosages, tapering over several days once the patient improves

Methylxanthines
- Aminophylline 6 mg/kg loading dose followed by 0.6 mg/kg/hr infusion
- Theophylline total daily amniophylline dose multiplied by 0.80 divided in one to two daily dosages of a sustained-release preparation

Antibiotics should not be routinely used because most URIs that precipitate an acute asthmatic exacerbation are viral. Antibiotics for a community-acquired pneumonia should be used when fever and purulent sputum are present. Methylxanthines do not significantly affect the initial emergency room course of acute asthma when frequent administration of a β-agonist is used. Long-term maintenance therapy with oral theophylline may allow decreased frequency of β-agonist therapy.

AMNIOTIC FLUID EMBOLISM

Amniotic fluid embolism (AFE) is a rare condition complicating 1/7000 to 300,000 deliveries. Although rare, the mortality rate is 80% and accounts for 10% of all maternal deaths. In most cases, AFE is marked by profound coagulopathy and respiratory and circulatory collapse, although it is possible that some women may be asymptomatic.

Diagnosis

The classic presentation of AFE is sudden hemorrhage and respiratory collapse in an older multipara having just completed a vigorous delivery. The diagnosis can be made when the hallmark complications are encountered but is best confirmed by identification of fetal material (squames, hair, vernix) in the lungs during postmortem examination or from a specimen of blood obtained from the right heart. The complications of AFE are biphasic.

Pulmonary phase

The sudden onset of dyspnea and hypotension mark the first phase. The patient will typically have evidence of pulmonary edema on chest x-ray, with hypoxemia and a mixed respiratory alkalosis/metabolic acidosis on ABGs. Approximately 10% to 20% will have seizures. Left-sided heart failure then follows, which exacerbates the pulmonary edema, and ARDS occurs. The mortality rate of the first phase is probably 50%, usually in the first hour after the embolism.

Hemorrhagic phase

Of those surviving the first phase, 40% to 50% will then demonstrate a profound coagulopathy. There will be bleeding from intravenous and venipuncture sites. There may be uterine hemorrhage unresponsive to uterotonics and the uterus may become atonic, accounting for even more blood loss.

Pathophysiology

Because AFE is rare, very little is understood about the mechanism by which it causes cardiorespiratory collapse.

Treatment

Supportive therapy is the mainstay of treatment; there are no set treatment protocols.

Respiratory support

Delivery of high concentrations of O_2 is important. Intubation and mechanical ventilation may be necessary for the unconscious patient. Positive end-expiratory pressure (PEEP) may be required for the treatment of pulmonary edema/ARDS.

Cardiac support

Therapy is best guided with a flow-directed pulmonary artery (Swan-Gantz) catheter. Hypotension is typically cardiogenic. Administration of fluids should be judicious to prevent worsening pulmonary edema. Cardiac ionotropes can be used to improve cardiac output.

Hematologic support

Fresh frozen plasma and packed RBCs should be given until bleeding caused by coagulopathy stops.

POSTPARTUM HEMORRHAGE

The normal blood loss after an uncomplicated vaginal delivery is less than 500 ml. The physiologic expansion of blood volume during pregnancy compensates for this loss. Tetanic contractions of the myometrium compress the spiral arteries that supply the blood to the uterus.

Treatment

Treatment of postpartum hemmorhage will depend on the underlying cause. The physician should have a systematic approach to patients with excessive bleeding after delivery (Box 47-3).

BOX 47-3
Postpartum Hemorrhage

Recognize excessive bleeding
Administer dilute oxytocin solution intravenously
Perform uterine massage via abdominal massage or bimanual compression
Inspect for vaginal or cervical trauma
Perform uterine exploration
- Ensure adequate analgesia
- Manually remove clot and placenta
- Access uterine scar if prior hysterotomy

Pharmacologic treatment of atony
- Methergine 0.2 mg intramuscularly
- Prostaglandin 15 methyl-$PGF_{2\alpha}$ 0.25 mg intramuscularly

Evaluate for surgical intervention
- Curettage for retained placenta
- Uterine packing (temporizing for definitive treatment)
- Uterine artery embolization
- Hypogastric artery ligation
- Hysterectomy

Uterine atony

Most cases of postpartum hemorrhage are the result of ineffective uterine contractions after delivery of the placenta. Predisposing factors are uterine infection, retained placental fragments, multiparity, overdistention of the uterus (twins, macrosomia, hydramnios), both precipitous and prolonged labors, inhalational anesthetics, and infusions of magnesium for preeclampsia. However, most cases will have no explanation.

Oxytocin. Infusion of dilute oxytocin 10 to 20 units/1000 ml at rates of 100 ml/hr immediately after the completion of the third stage of labor has become standard practice in many centers. This practice has prevented many cases of hemorrhage and eliminated the need for transfusion in many women. Oxytocin can also be given as an intramuscular injection in those patients who do not have intravenous access.

Uterine massage. Compression of the uterine fundus through the abdominal wall is often sufficient to stimulate uterine contractions in cases of uterine atony. Uterine massage can be facilitated by compression of the uterus from a hand in the vagina and the other hand on the abdomen.

Ergotamine. Refractory cases of atony may be treated with an ergot preparation such as Methergine 0.2 mg intramuscularly; intravascular injection can cause profound hypertension and should be avoided. Repeat administrations of Methergine can be given every 20 minutes for five doses. Treatment with ergotamines should be avoided in women with hypertensive conditions.

Prostaglandins. Pharmacologic preparations of prostaglandins are also able to induce contractions in cases of uterine atony. Dosages of $PGF_2\alpha$ 0.25 mg intramuscularly can be repeated at 20-minute intervals. Patients with reactive airway disease may experience bronchospasm with prostaglandin preparations; severe hypertension has also occurred in patients treated with prostaglandins.

Retained placenta

Fragments of placenta remaining in the uterine cavity can prevent efficient myometrial contractions. The placenta should be examined in all cases to ensure no fragments are left behind. Uterine exploration (providing that the patient has adequate analgesia) can be performed to remove placental fragments or large blood clots that may be present. Placenta accreta can be identified with uterine exploration and will often require hysterectomy.

Genital trauma

Lacerations of the vagina or cervix can occur. These areas should be systematically examined when hemorrhage is encountered in the presence of a well-contracted uterus. Women with prior cesarean deliveries can have uterine scar separation (dehiscence of the myometrium) or rupture (complete defect of the myometrium and peritoneum). Atony typically is present to some degree in these cases. The diagnosis is made by uterine exploration. Uterine rupture after abdominal trauma is usually an antepartum event that presents with fetal distress.

Uterine inversion

Traction on the umbilical cord or uterine massage before separation of the placenta can cause uterine inversion. The uterus may then become incarcerated when myometrial contraction occurs. Usually when inversion is identified, the uterus can be replaced vaginally. The incarcerated uterus will bleed profusely. Treatment with an inhalational anesthetic will relax the uterus enough to reduce the inversion by placing a hand within the uterine cavity. The hand should be left in the cavity while oxytocics are given and the uterus "firms up." In rare situations laparotomy will be required. Traction on the round ligaments will facilitate reestablishment of the normal configuration; when this fails, a relaxing incision in the posterior uterine wall can be made.

Surgical intervention may be required to arrest hemorrhage. Uterine packing has been advocated by some but has fallen out of favor. It is difficult to pack the uterus tightly enough to stop the bleeding and the packing may conceal ongoing bleeding. Radiographic embolization may be available in some centers and is effective. Curettage may be performed to remove retained placental fragments. Aggressive curettage, particularly in the presence of a uterine infection, can cause Asherman's syndrome with obliteration of the endometrial cavity. Laparotomy may be required to perform hypogastric ligation. Hysterectomy, typically for treatment of placenta accreta, may be needed as a last resort. The patient should be transfused with packed RBCs and fresh frozen plasma as guided by hemoglobin and coagulation parameters. An indwelling urinary catheter is vital to guide fluid resuscitation because oliguria is one of the first signs of hypovolemia.

KEY POINTS

1 Fetal mortality is close to 50% with maternal diabetic ketoacidosis.

2 Patients in thyroid "storm" often experience fever, cardiac abnormalities ranging from tachycardia to congestive heart failure, gastrointestinal disorders (e.g., nausea, vomiting, diarrhea), CNS-related symptoms (e.g., irritability, agitation, tremors, psychosis), and elevated T4 and T3 levels with decreased TSH levels.

3 Acute exacerbations of air exchange as seen in asthma attacks are one of the more common medical problems encountered during pregnancy. Status asthmaticus is a life-threatening emergency.

4 Although amniotic fluid embolism is rare, the mortality rate is 80% and accounts for 10% of all maternal deaths.

5 Most cases of postpartum hemorrhage are the result of ineffective uterine contractions after delivery of the placenta.

SELECTED READINGS

American College of Obstetrics and Gynecology: *Diagnosis and management of postpartum hemorrhage,* technical bulletin 143, July 1990, ACOG.

Clark SL, Phelan JP, Cotton DB, eds: *Critical care obstetrics,* Oradell, NJ, 1987, Medical Economics Books chapters 10-11, 16-17, and 19.

Hagay ZJ, Reece EA: Diabetes mellitus in pregnancy. In Reece EA, ed: *Medicine of the fetus & mother,* Philadelphia, 1992, JB Lippencott, pp 1001-1003.

National Asthma Education Program: *Guidelines for the diagnosis and management of asthma,* DHHS publication no. (NIH) 91-3042, Bethesda, Md, 1991; National Heart, Lung, and Blood Institute.

48

Malpresentation

Geri D. Hewitt

In the majority of pregnancies, the fetus lies with its spine parallel to the mother's spine and head down with its chin tucked onto its chest. Any deviation from this is called a *malpresentation* and occurs in approximately 5% of pregnancies at term. Risk factors for malpresentation include anything that may impair fetal mobility, such as multiple gestation, prematurity, hydramnios, hydrocephaly, increased parity, abnormal placentation, anecephaly, hydrocephaly, uterine malformations, pelvic tumors, and macrosomia.

Fetal lie is the alignment of the fetal spine in relation to the maternal spine. Types of fetal lie are longitudinal (or parallel), transverse (or perpendicular), or oblique (in between longitudinal and parallel). **Fetal presentation** is the fetal part that lies closest to the pelvic inlet. Types of fetal presentation include vertex, breech, or shoulder. **Fetal position** is the relationship between a designated fetal part and the vertical and horizontal planes of the birth canal. Each fetal presentation has a landmark that is used to describe the position of that fetal part in relation to the pelvis. Examples of fetal position are "left occiput anterior" or "right sacrum anterior."

BREECH PRESENTATION

The fetus in breech presentation is in a longitudinal lie with its lower extremities or buttocks presenting at the pelvic inlet. Like all malpresentations, breeches are more common preterm, with 25% of fetuses being breech at 28 weeks, 7% at 32 weeks, and 3% to 4% at term. Breeches are the most common type of malpresentation.

The three types of breech presentations are as follows (Fig. 48-1):

1. Frank breech, the most common, is seen in about 70% of breech fetuses. Here, the buttocks are lowest in the pelvis, the hips flexed, and the knees extended.
2. Complete breech occurs when the buttocks present in the pelvic inlet with the hips flexed and the knees flexed.
3. Incomplete or footling breech occurs when the fetus has one or both of the hips extended so that the fetal lower extremity is entering the pelvis before the fetal buttocks.

The diagnosis of a breech is commonly made with a combination of Leopold's maneuvers, vaginal examination, and ultrasound.

Breech fetuses face many risks. They have a perinatal mortality rate three to five times higher than that of vertex fetuses. This is at least partially caused by an increased risk of prematurity and congenital anomalies. The incidence of congenital anomalies in breech fetuses is about 6.3%, compared with about 2.4% for vertex fetuses. Breech fetuses are also at increased risk of antepartum, intrapartum, and postpartum complications, regardless of the mode of delivery. In particular, the risk of cord prolapse is increased. The risk is lowest for frank breech (0.5%) and highest for incomplete breech (15% to 18%). Complete breech has an intermediate risk (4.6%).

Great controversy exists in the obstetric community surrounding the optimal mode of delivery for breech fetuses (Fig. 48-2). Options include cesarean section, external cephalic version, and vaginal breech delivery. Although the majority of breech fetuses are now delivered by cesarean section, this trend has not shown a proportional drop in perinatal mortality. Cesarean deliveries increase maternal morbidity and mortality when compared with vaginal deliveries. Clear indications for cesarean delivery include preterm breech fetuses weighing ≤1500 g, breech fetuses with a hyperextended head, incomplete breeches, and any other obstetric contraindications to labor, such as placenta previa. Most breech fetuses at term can be delivered by a low transverse cesarean section, allowing the patient a trial of labor with subsequent pregnancies. Preterm breeches with a poorly

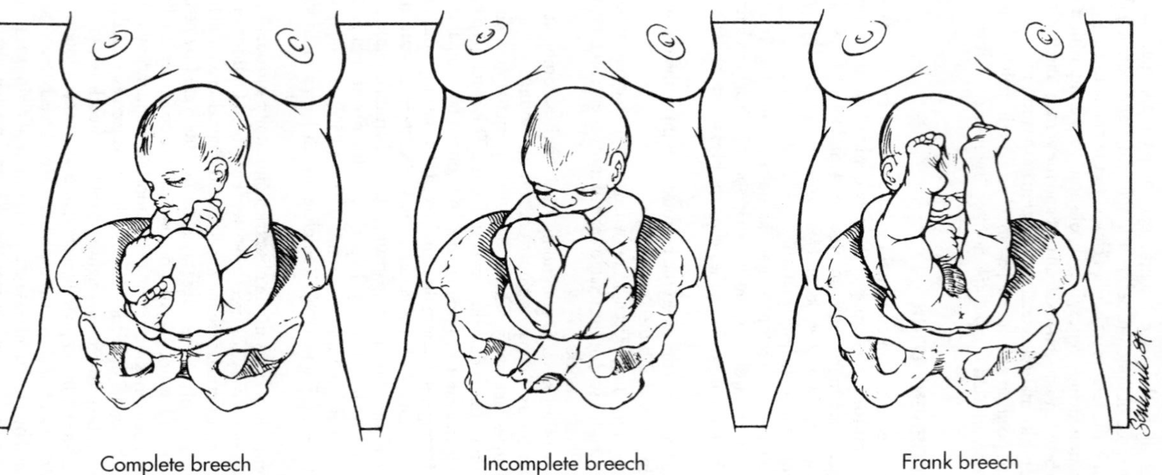

FIG. 48-1 Three possible breech presentations: the complete breech, the incomplete breech, and the frank breech. (From Gabbe SG, Niebyl JR, Simpson JL: *Normal and problem pregnancies,* ed 2, New York, 1991, Churchill-Livingstone.)

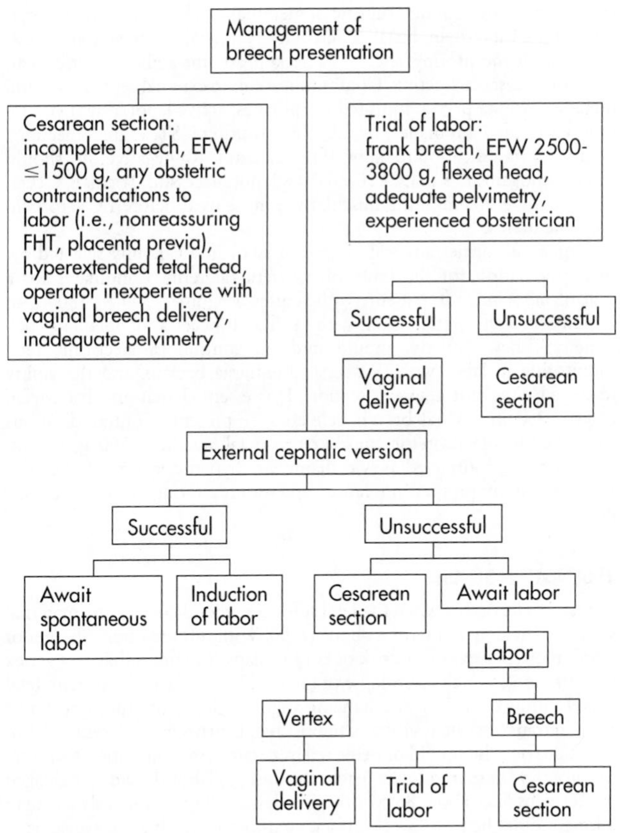

FIG. 48-2 Management of breech presentation. *EFW*, estimated fetal weight; *FHT*, fetal heart tones.

developed lower uterine segment may require a low vertical or classical cesarean section.

External cephalic version (ECV) involves manually rotating the fetus from breech to vertex by manipulating fetal parts palpated through the maternal abdomen under sonographic guidance. Once the fetus is in vertex presentation, the patient can either wait for spontaneous labor or undergo an induction of labor. ECV has a success rate of about 60% to 70%. Factors that decrease the success rate include maternal obesity, engagement of the breech, and oligohydramnios. Because the risks of ECV include fetal heart rate tracing abnormalities, rupture of membranes, abruption, and labor, it is performed at term in the labor and delivery unit with intravenous access, sonographic monitoring, anesthesia backup, and the ability to perform an immediate cesarean section. Contraindications to external cephalic version include placenta previa, ruptured membranes, active labor, oligohydramnios, congenital anomalies, IUGR, nonreassuring NST, vaginal bleeding, or any contraindication to labor. If the patient is Rh negative, she should receive Rhogam after an ECV, even if it was not successful. Tocolytics, such as terbutaline 0.25mg intramuscularly, can be used before ECV to help relax the uterus.

Some authorities advocate a trial of labor in a carefully selected patient population for the frank breech fetus at term. Candidates for a trial of labor include patients with fetuses weighing 2500 to 3800 g in a frank breech presentation with a flexed head and adequate pelvimetry. These patients should undergo continuous electronic fetal monitoring in labor with IV access, anesthesia backup, and the ability to do an emergent cesarean section. It is essential that an obstetrician experienced in vaginal breech deliveries be present. Contraindications to labor include obstetric inexperience, fetal weight ≤1500 g, incomplete breech, contracted pelvic diameters, hyperextension of the fetal head, arrest of progress in labor, and nonreassuring fetal heart tone patterns.

TRANSVERSE LIE

Transverse lie occurs when the fetal spine is perpendicular to the maternal spine. Its incidence at term is about 1/300. With rupture of membranes or labor, there is a significant risk of cord prolapse (20 times that of a vertex presentation), as well as prolapse of the fetal hand or arm because no fetal head is filling the pelvis. Spontaneous vaginal delivery of a fully developed fetus in transverse lie is virtually impossible. Patients who present in labor with transverse lie should be delivered by cesarean section. Patients who are diagnosed with transverse lie before the onset of labor should be managed expectantly since about 85% of these patients will spontaneously rotate to a longitudinal lie by 39 weeks. If a patient persists with a transverse lie at 39 weeks, she can be offered an ECV. If ECV is unsuccessful, the patient may then undergo cesarean section or wait to see the fetal presentation at the time of labor. The patient should be given strict labor precautions because of the increased risk of prolapse of the umbilical cord or fetal small parts.

Oblique lie is considered a transitory presentation that usually converts either to a longitudinal or transverse lie in labor and should be managed according to the presenting part at the time of labor.

Many patients undergoing cesarean section for a transverse lie require a vertical incision on the uterus, particularly if the lower uterine segment is poorly developed. In about 25% of cases when a low transverse incision is made on the uterus, a second vertical incision must be made to deliver an entrapped head (Fig. 48-3).

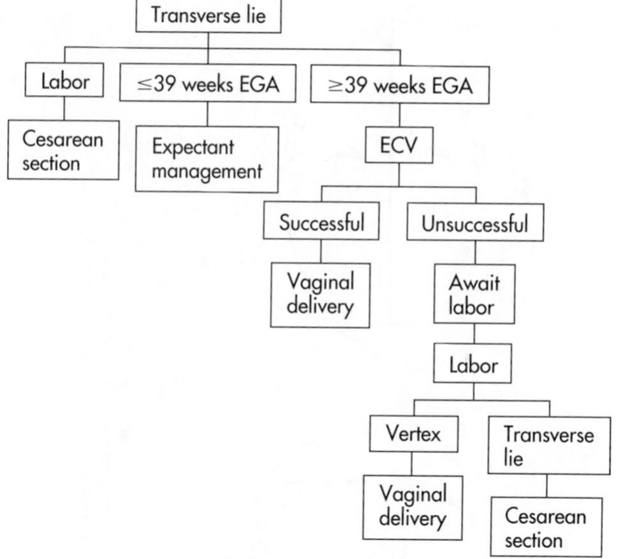

FIG. 48-3 Management of transverse lie. *EGA,* estimated gestational age; *ECV,* external cephalic version.

FACE AND BROW PRESENTATION

In the face presentation, the fetus is in a longitudinal lie with the fetal vertex extended on the fetal spine with the occiput against its upper back. Face presentations occur in about 1/500 births.

The fetal chin, or mentum, is used to designate the position of a face presentation (Fig. 48-4). In the most common position for a face presentation, the fetal chin is pointing toward the symphysis pubis, known as the *mentum anterior position.* Face presentations are most commonly diagnosed by vaginal examination with confirmation by ultrasound. Only approximately 50% of face presentations are diagnosed before the second stage of labor. Fetuses with face presentations are at increased risk for prolonged labor and fetal heart rate tracing abnormalities, and they should have continuous electronic fetal monitoring throughout labor. When necessary, internal monitoring should be used, with great care to avoid damage to the fetal eyes.

Approximately 70% to 80% of fetuses in face presentation will deliver vaginally (Fig. 48-5). For labor and delivery to be successful, the fetal vertex must rotate to the mentum anterior position and then flex the head to deliver under the symphysis. Approximately 10% to 15% of fetuses with face presentation will be in a mentum transverse position, with the

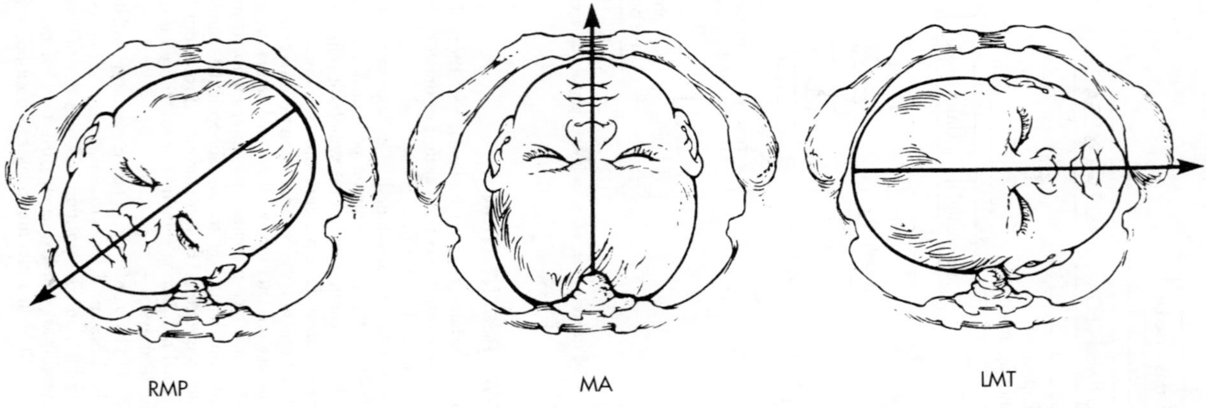

FIG. 48-4 Three pelvic views of the fetus demonstrating the various positions the fetus might occupy in a face presentation. The point of designation is the fetal chin or mentum. *RMP,* Right mentum posterior; *MA,* mentum anterior; *LMT,* left mentum transverse. (From Gabbe SG, Niebyl JR, Simpson JL: *Normal and problem pregnancies,* ed 2, New York, 1991, Churchill-Livingstone.)

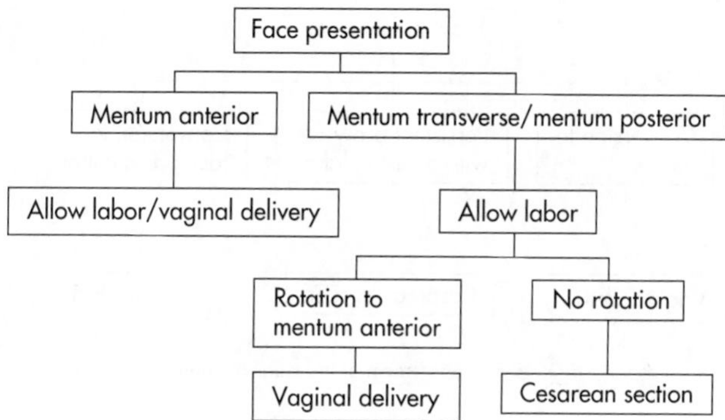

FIG. 48-5 Management of face presentation.

majority rotating to the mentum anterior position and delivering vaginally. Approximately 20% to 25% of fetuses with face presentation will present in mentum posterior position, and only one third will successfully achieve rotation to mentum anterior position and vaginal delivery. The remainder require cesarean section for delivery. Manual attempts to convert a face presentation to a flexed attitude, to rotate the mentum from posterior to anterior, or attempts at internal cephalic version and breech extraction are all contraindicated.

Brow presentations occur in about 1/1500 deliveries and are considered an unstable presentation that usually converts either to a face or vertex presentation and then can be managed according to the final presentation. The brow presentation is midway between a vertex and face presentation with the position of the fetal head between the orbital ridge and the anterior fontanel presenting at the pelvic inlet. The frontal bones are the point of designation in determining fetal position. Frontum anterior is the most common position.

Like the face presentation, the brow presentation is most commonly diagnosed by vaginal examination, and only about 50% are diagnosed before the second stage of labor (Fig. 48-6). Brow presentations in labor can be managed expectantly in the presence of reassuring fetal heart tones and adequate progress in labor while hoping for a change to a more favorable presentation. Brow presentations are at increased risk for prolonged labor and arrest disorders. In the term fetus, a persistent brow presentation with an arrest disorder in labor should be delivered by cesarean section. Manipulation either manually or with forceps is contraindicated.

COMPOUND PRESENTATION

Compound presentation occurs when an extremity is found prolapsing beside the presenting part. It is typically seen in premature fetuses with the

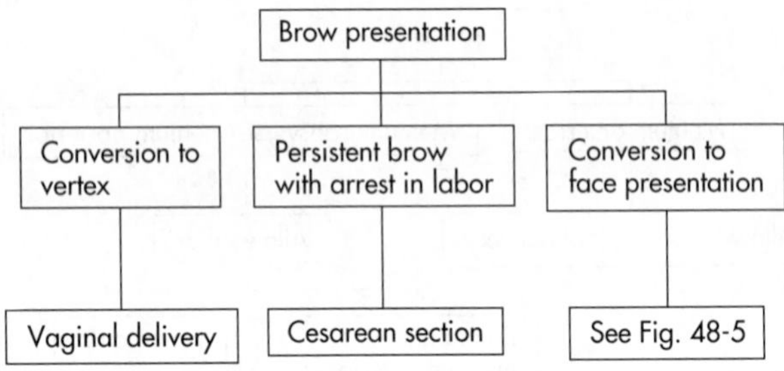

FIG. 48-6 Management of brow presentation.

upper extremity prolapsed beside the vertex. It is usually diagnosed by vaginal examination with about half of the diagnoses made during the second stage of labor.

Birth trauma and cord prolapse are the greatest fetal risks in compound presentation and occur in up to 20% of cases. A trial of labor is indicated in compound presentations because as the presenting part descends, the extremity usually retracts spontaneously. During labor the prolapsed extremity should not be manipulated, and continuous electronic fetal monitoring should be used because of the risk of cord prolapse. Cesarean section should be performed for cord prolapse or an arrest disorder in labor.

KEY POINTS

1 Malpresentation occurs in approximately 5% of pregnancies at term.

2 Etiologic factors include multiple gestation, prematurity, oligohydramnios, uterine abnormalities, congenital anomalies, multiparity, pelvic tumors, macrosomia, and abnormal placentation.

3 Breech presentation is the most common malpresentation, occurring in 3% to 4% of pregnancies at term.

SUGGESTED READINGS

Gabbe SG, Niebyl JR, Simpson JL: Obstetrics–normal and problem pregnancies, ed 2, New York, 1991, Churchill Livingstone.

Phalen JP et al: The nonlaboring transverse lie, *J Reprod Med* 31:184, 1986.

Pritchard JA, MacDonald PC: Williams obstetrics, ed 19, New York, 1993, Appleton and Lange.

Van Dorsten JP, Schifrin BS, Wallace RC: Randomized control trial of external cephalic version with tocolysis late in pregnancy, *Am J Obstet Gynecol* 141:417, 1981.

49

Multiple Gestations

Jeffrey G. Boyle

Multiple gestations occur in approximately 1% of all live births in the United States but account for 12% of all perinatal mortality. Compared with singletons, patients with multiple pregnancies are at an increased risk of both maternal and fetal complications. Prenatal care is an important factor in minimizing the risks and improving perinatal outcome. These patients require frequent follow-up and close monitoring throughout pregnancy, as well as special consideration at the time of delivery. The increased perinatal mortality results primarily from prematurity, IUGR, congenital anomalies, and placental vascular abnormalities. Prematurity is the leading cause of death in twin pregnancies.

Multiple gestations are described as either monozygotic or dizygotic, depending on the number of ova involved. Monozygotic twinning occurs at a fairly constant rate worldwide (4/1000 live births), whereas the rate of dizygotic twinning is related to advanced maternal age, race, maternal obesity, parity, ovulation induction, and family history. A monozygotic twin gestation is a single fertilized ovum that divides into separate fetuses. As a result, these fetuses are genetically identical. Dizygotic pregnancies arise from the fertilization of two separate ova and therefore are genetically dissimilar. Two out of three twin pregnancies are dizygotic.

The true cause of multifetal gestations is unknown. Ovulation induction agents are associated with a higher rate of dizygotic twinning. These drugs act by increasing serum levels of follicle-stimulating hormone (FSH) and luteinizing hormone (LH). The frequency of twinning with clomiphene citrate (Clomid) is 10%, and with Pergonal is 30% to 50%. There is greater uncertainty surrounding the etiology of monozygotic twinning. Hypotheses involving exposure to teratogens during embryonic development have been proposed based on findings of studies using animal models.

Determining chorionicity and understanding its relationship to zygosity are essential in the proper management of multiple gestations. Zygosity is directly related to perinatal outcome. Dizygotic twinning consists of two placentas that can be separate or fused depending on where the blastocysts implant. Dizygotic gestations are always dichorionic/diamniotic (67% incidence of all multiple gestations). Each fetus is separated by two amnion and two chorion layers. These pregnancies have the best prognosis of all types of twinning.

In monozygotic pregnancies, placentation is determined by the timing of the blastocyst division (Fig. 49-1). If division occurs within 3 days of

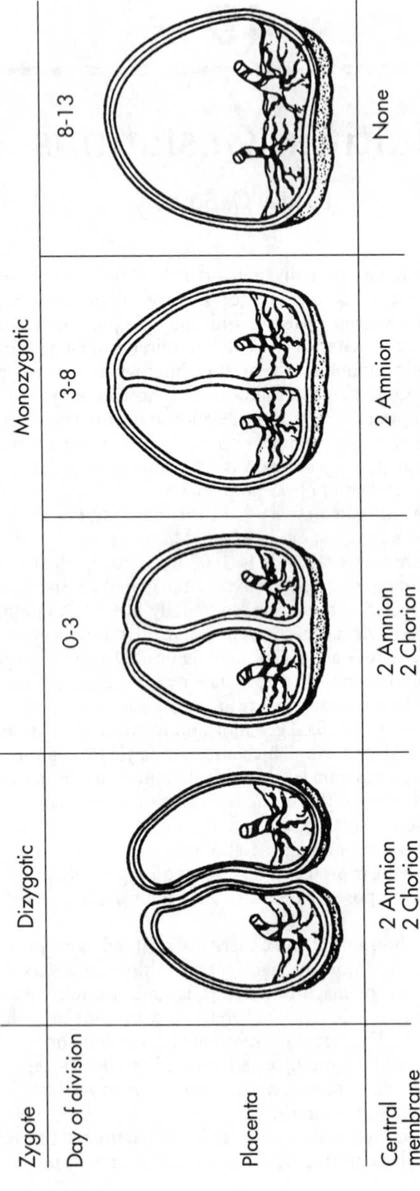

FIG. 49-1 Placentation in monozygotic and dizygotic pregnancies. (From Spellacy WN: Multiple pregnancies. In Scott JR, Hammond CB, Spellacy WN, eds: *Danforth's obstetrics and gynecology*, ed 7, Philadelphia, 1994, JB Lippincott.)

conception, each embryo will develop within its own amnion and chorion and the pregnancy will be dichorionic/diamniotic (11% incidence rate). This type of placentation is identical to that of dizygotic twins. Division occurring between 4 and 8 days after conception leads to a monochorionic/diamniotic placenta, the most common type of monozygotic twin pregnancy (22% incidence rate). If the division occurs between 8 and 13 days after conception, after the amnion has differentiated, a monochorionic/monoamniotic gestation (1% incidence rate) results, which is associated with significantly higher morbidity and mortality than other types of placentation. Division occurring even later, 13 days or more after conception, will result in conjoined twins.

Monochorionic placentas are always monozygotic. In the United States, approximately 22% of all twin pregnancies are monochorionic. Monochorionic pregnancies are associated with the most morbidity and mortality of all twin gestations. Complications include twin-twin transfusion syndrome, acardia, cord entanglement, conjoining, fetal demise, and growth abnormalities. Vascular communication between fetuses is common. Management decisions regarding one twin with fetal demise or a lethal malformation depend on the correct identification of chorionicity.

DETERMINING MONOZYGOSITY VERSUS DIZYGOSITY

The easiest way to establish zygosity is to determine fetal sex by ultrasonography. If the twins are of opposite sex, the pregnancy is dichorionic (dizygotic). If the twins are the same sex, other diagnostic measures must be used. Of all twin pregnancies, 35% are opposite sex. If two separate placentas are identified, the pregnancy is most likely (90%) dichorionic (dizygotic). If fetuses are the same sex with a single placenta, the dividing membrane thickness can be used to predict chorionicity. The best time to determine chorionicity by evaluating membrane thickness is between 16 and 24 weeks gestation. Monochorionic-diamniotic membranes are typically <2 mm and have a thin, hairlike or wispy appearance. Membranes that are over 2 mm in thickness are more likely dichorionic. All placentas should be carefully examined at the time of delivery to confirm chorionicity and to look for evidence of vascular anastomoses. A complete evaluation should include gross and histologic studies. Genetic studies including blood, HLA typing, or skin graft testing may be required in some same sex, dichorionic pregnancies to determine zygosity.

DIAGNOSIS

Because of the increased risk of complications, early diagnosis of multiple gestations is important. Maternal complications include hyperemesis, preterm labor, preeclampsia, cholestasis, anemia, and placental abruption. Placenta previa, vasa previa, postpartum hemorrhage, polyhydramnios, and UTIs are other complications. Fetal complications include congenital anomalies, prematurity, growth abnormalities, cord entanglement, twin-twin transfusion syndrome, and perinatal mortality. With the widespread use of ultrasound in obstetrics, the diagnosis is known in more than

90% of twin pregnancies before delivery. Compelling reasons for offering routine ultrasound examinations to all pregnant patients include diagnosing multiple gestations early and establishing frequent follow-up.

A patient's chance of having twins is increased if she has previously had dizygotic twins or if her first degree relatives have had twins. Paternal family history has no affect on a patient's chances of having twins. Consider the diagnosis in pregnancies where infertility drugs or IVF are used. Also consider the diagnosis of multiple gestations if a patient's uterine size is greater than expected or if multiple heart tones are auscultated. Multiple pregnancies can cause elevated levels of MSAFP. Look for congenital anomalies if values exceed 4 MoM. Ultrasound is 98% sensitive in making the diagnosis. Remember that false positive and false negative results are possible, especially in obese patients. A systematic approach is recommended and should include fetal sex, number of placentas, and membrane thickness. Transvaginal ultrasound may be useful in early gestation. A yolk sac can be confused with a separate pregnancy. Look for separate fetal cardiac activity to confirm the diagnosis.

MANAGEMENT

Antepartum

Early ultrasound provides early diagnosis and accurate dating, which is essential for the proper management of multifetal pregnancies (Fig. 49-2). Approximately 20% of multiple pregnancies diagnosed by early ultrasound are lost before 14 weeks gestation. This loss, called *vanishing twin*, occurs by resorption of the gestational sac and results in a blighted ovum or fetus papyraceous. Most patients are asymptomatic, but up to 25% can experience vaginal bleeding. A normal prognosis can be expected for the remaining fetus.

Because perinatal morbidity and mortality are increased with multiple pregnancies, selective reduction has been used in certain circumstances to improve perinatal outcome for the remaining fetuses. To date, this procedure only improves outcomes for pregnancies of four or more gestations. Reduction is also an option when one fetus is affected by a chromosome abnormality or a major congenital anomaly. After appropriate counseling, these patients should be referred to centers with extensive experience with this procedure. Pregnancy outcome after this technique depends on the clinical indications and the number of pregnancies involved.

Early cervical examinations and frequent follow-up are essential. Routine bed rest beginning at 24 weeks gestation is controversial. Consider bed rest and limited activity for patients with cervical change or a significant number of risk factors. A cerclage should be used only in patients diagnosed with incompetent cervix. Prophylactic tocolysis is of no benefit.

There are insufficient data to allow interpretation of biochemical markers (MSAFP, HCG, uE3) for determining risks of aneuploidy in multiple gestations. Aneuploidy risks should be based on maternal age and the results of a comprehensive ultrasound examination. MSAFP should be ordered only to determine risks of NTDs. MSAFP values of >4 MoM are considered increased.

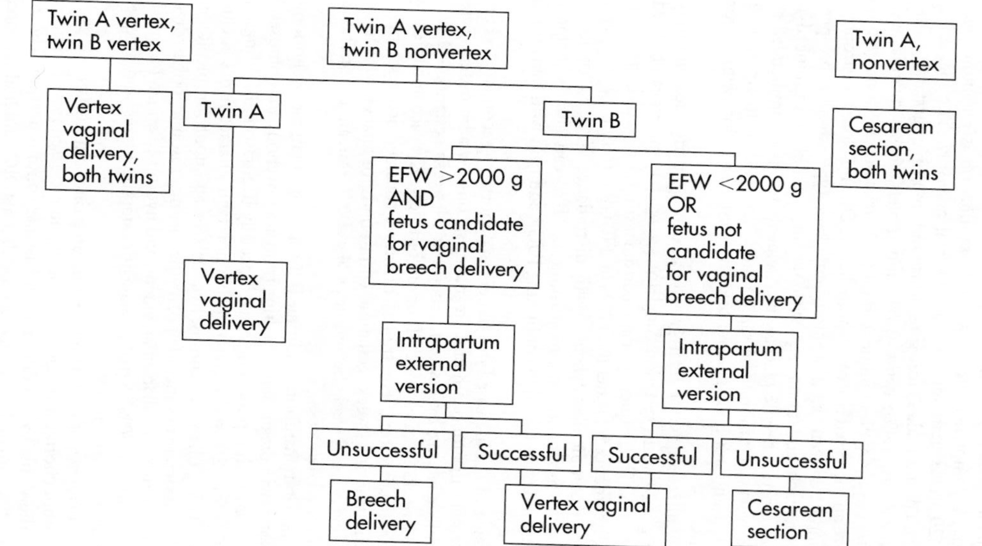

FIG. 49-2 Intrapartum management of twin gestations (From Chervenak FA et al: *Obstet Gynecol* 65:119, 1985.)

Daily folic acid (1 mg) and elemental iron (60 mg) supplements are recommended. Glucocorticoids should be considered to enhance fetal lung maturity when the probability of preterm delivery exists.

Anomalies occur up to three times more frequently in twins than in singletons. A comprehensive ultrasound examination is recommended at 18 to 20 weeks gestation to evaluate fetal anatomy. The incidence of congenital anomalies for singletons and multiple gestations includes singletons, 1.4%; twins, 2.7%; and triplets, 6.1%. Acardia and conjoining are anomalies unique to multifetal pregnancies. Monozygotic twins have an increased risk of sirenomelia, NTDs, and cloacal exstrophy. When indicated, an amniocentesis for karyotype should be performed on each gestational sac with the use of indigo carmine dye to confirm correct needle placement. A glucola test is recommended at 24 to 28 weeks gestation. The same criteria are used in interpreting a glucola test and a 3-hour glucose tolerance test (GTT) for twins as for singletons.

Serial ultrasounds for fetal growth should be performed monthly beginning at 24 weeks gestation. Singleton growth parameters can be used until 32 weeks. The frequency of antepartum testing should be increased if growth discordance is greater than 25% or if IUGR is found. Twice weekly NSTs are recommended when growth discordance is >25% or if the pregnancy is monochorionic-monoamniotic. BPP can also be helpful. Doppler studies are useful in confirming IUGR and twin-twin transfusion syndrome.

Because of the increased risk of perinatal mortality secondary to cord entanglement in monoamniotic pregnancies, consider administering steroids and delivering by cesarean section at 34 weeks gestation. Deliver before 34 weeks in cases of IUGR or discordance >25% accompanied by abnormal fetal testing. For triplets or more, consider bed rest and/or hospitalization at 24 weeks gestation. Ultrasounds for fetal growth should be done every 2 to 3 weeks beginning at 24 weeks. Cesarean section should be used for all deliveries.

Twin-twin transfusion syndrome is most common in monochorionic-diamniotic twin pregnancies resulting from arteriovenous anastomoses. It is associated with a poor prognosis, especially if ultrasound findings are present before 26 weeks gestation. Donor twin characteristics include anemic, IUGR, oligohydramnios, hypotensive, and nonhydropic. Recipient twin characteristics include polycythemic, macrosomic, polyhydramnios, hypertensive, cardiac enlargement, and hydrops. Perinatal mortality occurs in up to 70%. Serial therapeutic amniocenteses and frequent follow-up are recommended.

The incidence of fetal demise of one pregnancy among twins is 2% to 7%. In monochorionic pregnancies, there is an increased risk of embolization to the viable twin resulting from vascular communication. This can result in disseminated intravascular coagulation (DIC) and multiple organ damage. Expectant management is recommended until pulmonary maturity or evidence of DIC. Weekly coagulation studies, platelet counts, and fibrinogen should be obtained. Serial ultrasounds for fetal growth and twice weekly NSTs are recommended.

Delivery

The route of delivery for patients with multiple gestations depends on gestational age, estimated fetal weights, and fetal presentations. The incidence of vertex/vertex presentation is 40%, vertex/breech is 26%, breech/vertex is 10%, breech/breech is 10%, vertex/transverse is 8%, and other combinations make up 6%. Continuous electronic fetal monitoring should be used throughout labor. There is no recommended maximum time before twin B should be delivered as long as fetal well-being is assured by monitoring. An ultrasound should be available for use during delivery of twin B to evaluate fetal position.

A vaginal delivery is recommended regardless of gestational age or estimated fetal weights when both twins are presenting vertex. When appropriate, a vaginal birth after cesarean (VBAC) and oxytocin augmentation are acceptable.

Route of delivery with vertex/nonvertex presentation depends on fetal weight. If estimated fetal weight is >2000 g, twin A is delivered vaginally and twin B by total breech extraction or external version. If estimated fetal weight is <2000 g, cesarean delivery is recommended. For nonvertex/either presentations, delivery is by cesarean regardless of gestational age and/or estimated fetal weight. With three or more fetuses present, cesarean section is used.

Postpartum Hemorrhage

Patients delivering multiple gestations are at increased risk of uterine atony and postpartum hemorrhage. Prolonged monitoring for 2 to 3 hours after delivery, adequate use of oxytocics, and intravenous access are recommended.

KEY POINTS

1 Multiple pregnancies represent approximately 1% of all live births but account for 12% of the perinatal mortality.

2 Neither prophylactic tocolytics nor cercalges are of benefit in managing multiple gestations.

3 The most common presentation for twins at the time of labor is vertex-vertex.

4 Route of delivery for twins depends on gestational age, estimated fetal weight, and fetal presentation.

SUGGESTED READINGS

American College of Obstetricians and Gynecologists: Committee opinion no. 141, August, 1994.

Brown JE, Schloesser PT: Pregnancy weight status, prenatal weight gain, and the outcome of term twin gestation, *Am J Obstet Gynecol* 162:182, 1990.

Davison L et al: Breech extraction of low-birth weight second twins: can cesarean section be justified? *Am J Obstet Gynecol* 166:497, 1992.

Fusi L, Gordon H: Twin pregnancy complicated by single intrauterine death, *Br J Obstet Gynaecol* 97:511, 1990.

Johnson JM et al: Maternal serum alpha fetoprotein in twin pregnancy, *Am J Obstet Gynecol* 162:1020, 1990.
Saunders NJ, Snijders RJM, Nicolaides KH: Therapeutic amniocentesis in twin-twin transfusion syndrome appearing the second trimester of pregnancy, *Am J Obstet Gynecol* 166:820, 1992.
Rodis JF et al: Intrauterine fetal growth in discordant twin gestations, *J Ultrasound Med* 9:443, 1990.
Vergani P et al: Prenatal management of twin gestation–experience with a new protocol, *J Reprod Med* 36:667, 1991.

50

Fetal Heart Rate Monitoring

EDWARD J. QUILLIGAN

MONITORING METHODS

Intermittent auscultation has been suggested as an alternative method of fetal evaluation for those patients who have a totally uncomplicated labor and pregnancy. With this method, a fetoscope is placed on the maternal abdomen (usually over the anterior fetal shoulder), the fetal heart is then located, and the heart rate is counted for a period of at least 30 seconds. This should be performed in the latter half of the uterine contraction so that the count actually continues into the uterine relaxation period. The heart rate should be counted at least every 30 minutes during the first stage of labor and every 15 minutes during the second stage; it is preferable to count the rate every 15 minutes in the first stage and every 5 minutes in the second stage. The fetal heart rate should be counted after every contraction or at least every 5 minutes in the delivery room. Every counted heart rate must be recorded on the patient's chart. A fetal heart rate that persistently stays below 100 beats/min or decreases to values of less than 100 beats/min at the conclusion of each contraction indicates fetal distress and should be treated with discontinuance of any oxytocin infusion, administration of 100% oxygen to the mother by mask, and turning the mother on her left side. If there is any decrease in blood pressure, that should be corrected by proper fluid administration. If these measures fail to correct the heart rate, delivery of the fetus by the most expeditious means is indicated.

When continuous fetal heart rate monitoring is used, each heartbeat is picked up using either an ultrasound transducer on the maternal abdomen or a scalp electrode placed directly into the fetal scalp. The heartbeat is counted, converted to an analog rate, and recorded on a strip chart recorder along with the uterine activity, which is determined by using either an abdominal transducer or a catheter placed into the amniotic cavity and connected to a strain gage. The monitoring of both the instantaneous fetal heart rate and uterine activity allows the nurse or physician to evaluate not only the fetal heart rate on a moment-by-moment basis but also the relationship of the heart rate to the uterine activity.

FETAL EVALUATION

The upper line on the strip chart recorder is the fetal heart rate. Baseline heart rate is the resting heart rate or heart rate between uterine contractions (Fig. 50-1). The normal limits are 120 to 160 beats/min. A change in baseline rate requires 15 minutes at the new rate. A heart rate of <120 beats/min is defined as *bradycardia* and must be differentiated from a prolonged deceleration, which is usually a sudden drop in heart rate with absent variability in a prolonged deceleration. Bradycardia of 120 to 100 beats/min is usually of no consequence; however, baseline heart rates of <100 bpm may indicate severe fetal distress or a fetal heart block, which has a high incidence of congenital malformations and is frequently associated with lupus erythematosus in the mother. Fetal tachycardia may also indicate fetal hypoxia and can be caused by maternal fever, amnionitis, fetal anemia, maternal hyperthyroidism, and maternal use of drugs such as atropine. There is a severe form of fetal tachycardia, paroxysmal fetal tachycardia, that can be lethal if prolonged because the heart rate is frequently above 200 to 250 beats/min. It can occasionally be corrected by maternal use of digitalis.

Heart rate variability is the constant change present in the heart rate of a normal person. Heart rate variability has been characterized as short-term, beat-to-beat variability, and long-term 4 to 6 cycles/min. A decrease below 5 beats/min, particularly in association with an abnormal periodic change in heart rate, increases the possibility that the fetus is distressed rather than stressed. Significantly reduced or absent variability may also be present in the severely brain damaged, congenitally anomalous, or the heavily medicated fetus.

The periodic changes in heart rate include accelerations and three types of decelerations. Accelerations may occur at any time but are usually in association with contractions or fetal movement. An acceleration is an increase in heart rate of 15 beats/min or more, lasting 15 seconds or longer. The presence of acceleration of the heart rate, either spontaneous or induced by scalp or vibroacoustic stimulation, is a good indication that the fetus is not acidotic. The periodic decelerations are early, late, and variable, and are named in relation to their onset in the uterine contraction. Early decelerations are caused by compression of the fetal head. The deceleration begins early in the contraction, usually correlated with the onset of the contraction, and the heart rate seldom drops below 80 to 100 beats/min. This deceleration is not associated with fetal stress or distress. The etiology of late decelerations is diminished oxygen delivery to the fetal side of the placenta, the most common reasons being a reduced maternal intervillous blood flow because of excessive uterine activity or maternal hypotension and diminished placental surface, placental edema, and maternal hypoxia. Variable decelerations can begin at any time during the uterine contraction and are distinguished from early and late decelerations by their rapid deceleration in contrast to the gradual deceleration of the early and late. Usually the return of the heart rate to baseline is equally rapid, but if the

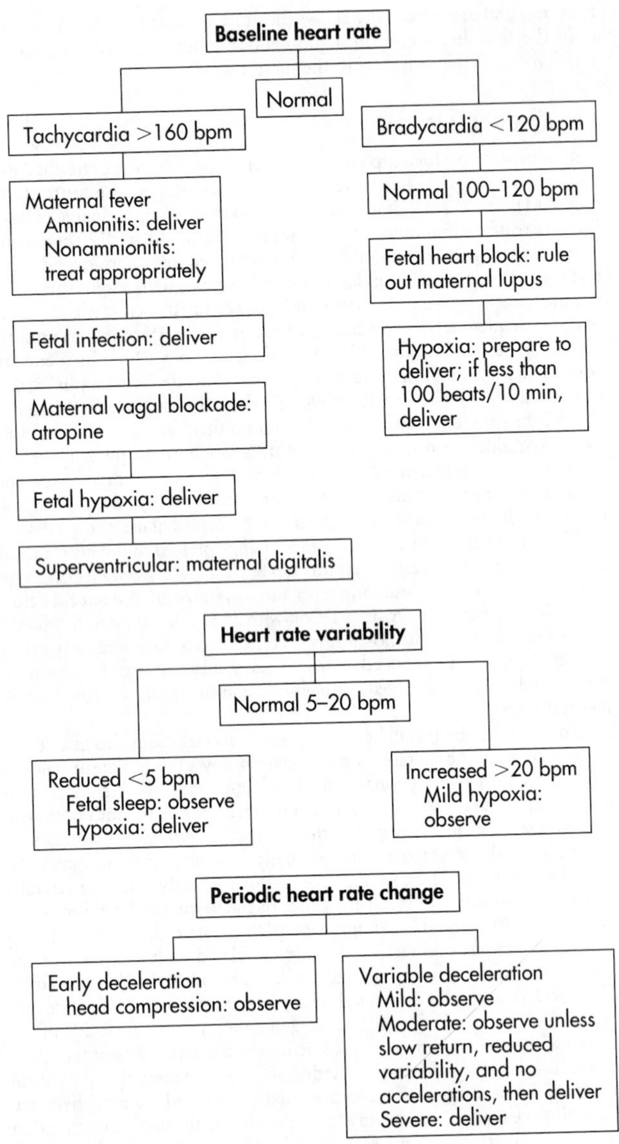

FIG. 50-1 Technique for evaluating electronic fetal heart rate monitoring.

fetus is more hypoxic there may be a more gradual return to the baseline. Baseline tachycardia and loss of variability are again very important in the assessment of whether the fetus is distressed. The etiology of variable decelerations is compression of the umbilical cord.

Unusual fetal heart rate changes include the sinusoidal pattern. This is a continuous sign wave that has a magnitude of at least 10 beats/min. The pattern is associated with severe fetal distress, severe fetal anemia, and some drugs such as Nisentil. An intermittent sinusoidal pattern is innocuous, except in the rhesus-sensitized patient where it signifies mild anemia. Occasionally one sees premature ventricular contractions. These are usually insignificant.

TREATMENT

The treatment of abnormal fetal heart rate patterns begins with determining if there are conditions present that can correct the abnormal pattern and if not, whether the fetus is suffering sufficient oxygen deficiency to cause either death or damage. Discontinuance of oxytocin, maternal administration of 100% oxygen by mask, and maternal position change should be automatic. If there is maternal hypotension, correction by fluid administration is essential. When oligohydramnios is accompanied by variable decelerations, amnioinfusion will frequently correct the problem. There are other changes in the FHR that will assist in making the determination of fetal acidosis. When there are accelerations present, the fetus is almost never seriously acidotic. On the other hand, absence of accelerations coupled with late or moderate to severe variable decelerations, diminished variability (<5 bpm), and baseline tachycardia has a very high yield of acidotic fetuses. When the diagnosis of protracted oxygen deficiency is made, the only therapy is expeditious delivery. The delivery must be extremely rapid (within 10 minutes) if the fetus is receiving no oxygen (i.e., complete placental separation or sudden maternal death); however, in most situations the physician will have at least 30 minutes and probably more of relative fetal oxygen deficiency before damage may occur. When the fetal heart rate is reduced for 5 minutes, one must move toward delivery. If the heart rate returns suddenly to normal, which it frequently does, a cesarean section may be aborted and the patient closely observed. When this type of change has happened more than once, delivery is indicated because although the fetus is usually normal at birth, there is an increased frequency of fetal demise with this pattern.

KEY POINTS

1 In the low-risk patient, intermittent auscultation is done every 30 minutes during the first stage, and every 15 minutes during the second stage. It is equivalent to continuous electronic fetal heart rate monitoring in the results obtained.

2 With electronic fetal heart rate monitoring there is a high false positive rate; therefore additional methods are necessary before cesarean delivery is performed. Additional methods of evaluation (e.g., acoustic stimulation) are necessary before emergency delivery is performed.

3 The periodic decelerations, variable and late, tend to occur with a hypoxic fetus before loss of heart rate variability. A combination of the two is an indication that the fetus is in distress.

4 Fetal heart rate variability can be altered by sleep state. It is usually reduced when the fetus is in quiet sleep and increased when the fetus is in REM sleep or awake. The sleep periods seldom last more than 40 minutes. Thus a marked decrease in variability lasting more than 40 minutes is probably not related to a sleep state.

SUGGESTED READINGS

Freeman RK, Garite TJ, Nageotte MP: *Fetal heart rate monitoring,* ed 2, Baltimore, 1991, Williams and Wilkins.

Hon EH: Observations on pathologic bradycardia, *Am J Obstet Gynecol* 77:1084, 1959.

Hon EH, Quilligan EJ: The classification of fetal heart rate, *Conn Med* 31:779-784, 1967.

Morrison JC et al: Intrapartum fetal heart rate assessment: monitoring by auscultation or electronic means, *Am J Obstet Gynecol* 168:63, 1993.

Vintzileos AM et al: A randomized trial of intrapartum electronic fetal heart rate monitoring versus intermittent auscultation, *Obstet Gynecol* 81:899, 1993.

51

Obstetric Anesthesia

KATHRYN ZUSPAN

Obstetric anesthesia involves anesthesia given to the pregnant patient. These patients are managed differently because the pregnant woman's physiology alters her response to anesthesia. For example, the respiratory mucosa is more vascular and edematous, which can obscure the airway and make intubation more difficult. The pregnant patient has a lower functional residual capacity, increased oxygen consumption, and is more likely to hyperventilate. This increases the risk of maternal and fetal hypoxia, especially in cases of difficult intubation. In addition, the increased size and weight of the pregnant uterus increases the risk of aortocaval compression for pregnant patients in the supine position. This leads to maternal hypotension and decreased ureteroplacental blood flow to the neonate. Therefore left lateral uterine displacement using a wedge under the right hip is necessary when the patient is supine. Finally, gastrointestinal changes of pregnancy place the patient at significant risk for vomiting and aspiration. Aspiration accounts for one third of all maternal deaths caused by obstetric anesthesia. Steps to prevent or lessen aspiration risk include giving a clear antacid by mouth and an H_2-antagonist before anesthetic procedures, intubating all patients under general anesthesia, and limiting oral intake during labor. Patients in labor should receive nothing by mouth except for small sips of water or ice chips.

ANESTHESIA FOR LABOR

Lamaze stresses education in ways to deal with pain. The patient and her support person concentrate on breathing techniques that distract the patient so she doesn't concentrate on the pain. Intravenous medications used to relieve labor pain all cross the placenta and can potentially affect the fetus. Sedatives and tranquilizers are used to decrease anxiety, promote sleep, and potentiate narcotics. The most common ones are promethazine (Phenergan) and hydroxyzine (Vistaril). Opioids are used to relieve labor pain. Undesirable maternal side effects include postural hypotension, itching, nausea and vomiting, and respiratory depression. Neonatal side effects involve neurobehavioral changes and respiratory depression. The most commonly used opioids are meperidine (Demerol), butorphanol (Stadol), nalbuphine (Nubain), fentanyl (Sublimaze), and morphine. The opioid antagonist of choice in obstetrics is naloxone (Narcan). The paracervical block involves injecting local anesthetic at points around the cervix. Once popular, this technique is now relatively contraindicated in obstetrics because of the high incidence (1% to 30%) of associated fetal bradycardia.

Spinal anesthesia for labor, also called *intrathecal narcotics or opioids,* is used three different ways. The single injection technique is best for patients in active labor, anticipating a spontaneous vaginal delivery within 3 hours. The typical drug combinations used are fentanyl or sufentanil combined with bupivacaine or morphine. Onset is almost immediate. The duration of action is 2 to 3 hours. Additional doses are rare. The continuous infusion technique involves continuously dosing through a 27-gauge or smaller spinal catheter. This technique has only been used via study protocols since May 1992. In the combined spinal-epidural technique, the epidural needle is placed in the epidural space. A longer spinal needle is inserted through the epidural needle into the subarachnoid space. A subarachnoid dose is given through the spinal needle, which is then removed. An epidural catheter is then threaded via the epidural needle into the epidural space. This technique is useful for patients in early labor, when delivery is expected in more than 3 hours. The patient gets labor pain relief and can usually still ambulate. Later when the spinal dose has worn off or in the event that an instrumented delivery is needed, an additional dose can be supplied through the epidural catheter.

Possible side effects of spinal anesthesia for labor include itching (common), nausea and vomiting (common), hypotension, urinary retention, drowsiness or dizziness, spinal headache, motor function weakness, fetal heart rate changes, and maternal respiratory depression (rare). Patients require a 200 to 500 cc bolus preload of a non–glucose-containing solution. Continuous fetal heart rate monitoring is appropriate. Maternal blood pressure should be monitored at bedside for at least 20 minutes after the subarachnoid injection. Maternal respirations should be monitored for the period dictated by the drugs used (e.g., morphine 18 to 24 hours, fentanyl 2 to 4 hours).

Epidural anesthesia for labor involves placing a small catheter via an epidural needle into the epidural space. Once secured, this catheter is maintained through delivery. The epidural is dosed with local anesthetics with or without opioids. After the initial dose, further doses can be given at intervals based on block regression or duration of the drug used. Another option is to continuously infuse a small amount of a dilute concentration of the epidural drug. This technique is best for patients in labor with or without pitocin augmentation. Possible complications include failure to relieve pain, a one-sided block, hypotension, and intravascular placement of the catheter, which if unrecognized could lead to possible seizures or cardiovascular collapse. A subarachnoid placement of the catheter is also possible, which could result in a spinal headache. If unrecognized and the epidural dose is given, this subarachnoid placement could lead to a "high spinal" and possible respiratory and cardiovascular compromise. Prerequisites for a labor epidural include continuous fetal heart rate monitoring and prehydration with a 500 to 1000 cc intravenous bolus of a non–glucose-containing solution. Maternal blood pressure is appropriately monitored at bedside for at least 20 minutes after the total dose is injected.

Labor epidural benefits include reducing labor pain and maternal stress, thus maintaining the fetal acid-base status. Epidurals have little direct effect on uteroplacental blood flow and tone as long as maternal blood pressure is maintained. They may actually accelerate the first stage of labor in patients with dysfunctional labor. Patients with epidurals are more controlled during "pushing" in the second stage of labor. These patients also have an anesthetic method in place in case of need for a semiemergent cesarean section. Labor epidurals most likely do not prolong the second stage. They do not increase the incidence of dystocia, fetal malrotation, operative delivery, or prolonged postpartum back pain. Spinal and epidural anesthesia is contraindicated in parturients with infection at the insertion site, hypovolemia, coagulopathy, or patient refusal.

ANESTHESIA FOR VAGINAL DELIVERY

Local infiltration is used for spontaneous deliveries requiring episiotomy. Pudendal blocks are used for spontaneous and instrumented vaginal deliveries. The pudendal block anesthetizes the internal pudendal and perineal nerves to relax the perineal muscles and anesthetize the perineal skin. The drug of choice is typically 1% lidocaine. Complications are rare. There is the possibility of maternal seizures if there is an unintentional intravascular injection of drug.

Useful for spontaneous or instrumented vaginal delivery, the epidural block placed during labor is then extended to include the sacral nerves. This "perineal," "sit-up," or "top-up" dose is given when the fetal head is "crowning." The patient is placed in a sitting position and dosed with a larger volume and stronger concentration of local anesthetic than was used earlier in labor. For instrumented vaginal deliveries, the epidural can be placed and dosed in a similar fashion before placement of the forceps or vacuum device. Complications are similar to those for labor epidurals.

The spinal or "saddle block" is used for instrumented vaginal delivery. It is called a *saddle block* because anesthesia is maximized in the anatomic areas that would touch a saddle if the patient were riding a horse. This technique uses different drug combinations than the spinals used for labor. The traditional spinal technique is used, and a small dose of hyperbaric local anesthetic is given to the patient in the sitting position, resulting in sacral anesthesia. Possible complications include inadequate block, spinal headache, "high-spinal" anesthesia, infection, and hypotension.

Inhalation analgesia combined with local infiltration of the perineum or pudendal block is now rarely used for spontaneous or instrumented vaginal delivery. The inhalation agents commonly used are nitrous oxide, methoxyflurane, and enflurane in low concentrations. Possible complications include neonatal depression as well as the significant risk of maternal respiratory depression, loss of consciousness, and aspiration.

ANESTHESIA FOR CESAREAN SECTION

Guidelines dictate the use of preoperative aspiration pneumonitis prophylaxis with a clear, nonparticulate antacid. Left lateral uterine displacement is required intraoperatively. Typically, regional anesthesia (spinal or epidural) is safer than general anesthesia for cesarean delivery for several reasons. There is less risk of aspiration or difficult intubation. There is less risk of neonatal depression caused by drug exposure or to a prolonged abdominal incision to delivery time. There is also less blood loss.

Epidural anesthesia for cesarean section requires a greater preload of intravenous lactated Ringer's solution; 1500 to 2000 ml is appropriate. A stronger concentration and larger volume of local anesthetic is used for cesarean section versus labor. The level of the block is extended to T4-6. The epidural catheter may be redosed at appropriate intervals during the cesarean section to maintain the surgical level of anesthesia. Possible complications are similar to those with a labor epidural.

Spinal anesthesia for cesarean section requires an intravenous preload of fluids similar to that used for epidurals. Hyperbaric local anesthetic in a dose larger than that used for vaginal delivery produces an anesthetic level to T4-6. Possible complications are similar to those for a spinal for vaginal delivery.

Local infiltration and block of the anterior abdominal wall (essentially a cesarean section under "local anesthesia") is rarely used but of major importance to the obstetrician. This technique is appropriate for an emergency cesarean section when an IV line cannot be placed or when no one trained in anesthesia is available. Gentle handling of the patient's tissues and the instruments is critical. Typically, procaine or lidocaine are diluted and injected before cutting each layer. Large volumes of any local anesthetic can lead to toxic reactions such as seizures and should be used cautiously. The maximum safe dose must be known and observed.

The general anesthesia used for cesarean section ideally utilizes fewer drugs in smaller quantities than used in general surgical cases. This is done to minimize fetal exposure to drugs and allow for safe recovery from anesthesia. The patient feels no pain, but a few may experience some recall of conversations from the operating room.

All pregnant patients receiving general anesthesia require intubation. A cuffed endotracheal tube is placed after a rapid sequence induction. With this induction, cricoid pressure must be given. Positive pressure ventilation before muscle paralysis for intubation is avoided. Extubation is carried out when the patient is awake and in control of her gag reflex. These steps help prevent aspiration of gastric contents.

KEY POINTS

1. Alterations in physiology secondary to pregnancy increase the patient's risk of hypoxia, aspiration, difficult intubation, and supine hypotension.
2. Laboring patients should receive nothing by mouth except for small sips of water or a few ice chips.
3. Standard of practice guidelines recommend use of a clear, nonparticulate antacid by mouth for all pregnant patients before receiving anesthesia.
4. To avoid supine hypotension, all patients should have left lateral uterine displacement.
5. As a general rule, regional anesthesia (spinal or epidural) is safer than general anesthesia for instrumented vaginal or cesarean delivery.

SUGGESTED READINGS

American Academy of Pediatrics & American College of Obstetricians and Gynecologists: *Guidelines for perinatal care,* ed 3, Washington, DC, 1992, The Academy and the College.

Chestnut DH: *Obstetric anesthesia principles and practice,* St. Louis, 1994, Mosby.

Datta S: *Anesthetic and obstetric management of high-risk pregnancy,* St. Louis, 1991, Mosby.

Norris MC: *Obstetric anesthesia,* Philadelphia, 1993, JB Lippincott.

Shnider SM, Levinson G: *Anesthesia for obstetrics,* ed 3, Baltimore, 1993, Williams & Wilkins.

52

Breastfeeding

Chris Harter

The Surgeon General issued a charge for health care providers to promote breastfeeding to achieve the Healthy People 2000 goal of having a 75% breastfeeding rate in the hospital and a 50% rate at 6 months post partum. Information given should be current and accurate to meet this goal.

PRENATAL EDUCATION

The advantages of breastfeeding for baby and mother are well documented but need to be shared with mothers prenatally. A breast assessment of the pregnant woman should be performed at 32 to 36 weeks gestation to determine nipple type and integrity for breastfeeding (Fig. 52-1). If nipples are flat or inverted, devices such as breast shells may be prescribed. Mothers are no longer told to roughen or toughen nipples before delivery by rubbing with a towel or washcloth.

A detailed patient history should be obtained that includes information about previous breastfeeding experience, breast surgeries, and disease conditions such as severe depression, thyroid disorders, and diabetes. Breastfeeding management of problems associated with these conditions should include a collaborative effort with other health care providers, including a lactation consultant. Most conditions would not justify discouragement from breastfeeding. The decision to breastfeed is a very deep, emotional commitment and should be supported as much as possible. Reassurance that assistance will be available early in the hospital and after discharge should be given.

Mothers should be encouraged to attend breastfeeding classes and written information and/or videos should be made available as resources. The more information mothers have to help them, the more likely breastfeeding will be successful.

PRACTICAL INFORMATION

Basic information about breastfeeding should include the breast structures involved in milk production and transfer (nipple and areola), correct positioning of baby's mouth over the nipple and areola, hormonal regulation of milk production and delivery, and synthesis of human milk at the cellular level. Supply and demand is regulated by frequent nursing. Explain how the bottle-suck and breast *suckling* differ. Maternal nutrition also plays a key role in breastfeeding, since the mother's energy levels can be quickly depleted. She needs more protein, vitamins, and fluids. Babies' growth needs are highest in the first few months of life, so frequent nursing is the norm. Growth spurts occur at 3 weeks, 6 weeks, 2 months, and 6 months.

Medical problems in the mother and/or baby also impact lactation (i.e., cleft lip/cleft palate, Down syndrome, prematurity). Diabetic mothers or mothers with chronic illnesses need more intense help and follow-up with breastfeeding. Mothers also need to know the following:

1. Early nursing in the labor/delivery/recovery area is essential to elevate prolactin levels so milk supply won't be delayed or compromised. If mother and baby are separated, mother should use an electric breast pump within the first 6 to 8 hours after delivery.
2. Baby and mother should room-in as much as possible so baby can be nursed often, at least 8 times a day. Frequent removal of milk is essential in regulating milk supply.

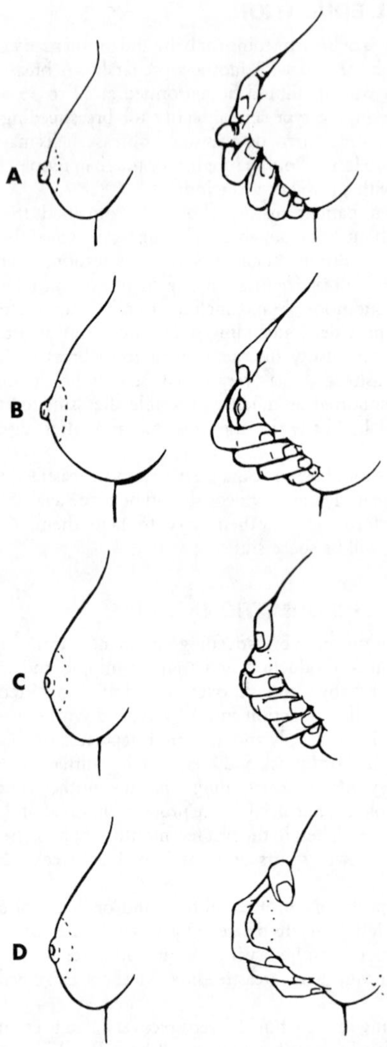

FIG. 52-1 A, Protracting normal nipple. **B,** Moderate to severe retraction. **C,** Inverted-appearing nipple when compressed using pinch test will either invert further inward or protract forward *(upper right).* **D,** True inversion; nipple inverts further *(lower right).* (From Auerbach K, Riordan J: *Breastfeeding and human lactation,* 1993, Jones and Bartlett.)

3. Wake baby for feedings during the day, every 2 to 3 hours, and allow baby to suckle 10 to 20 minutes on each breast at each feeding. Feed on baby's demand after midnight.
4. Bottle feedings should not be offered unless there is a medical need and a physician order for it. Pacifiers, nipple shields, and other artificial nipples should not be encouraged.
5. Assistance at the bedside should be available on request to ensure the baby is positioned and latched on correctly. Baby's suck should be assessed to be sure it is effective and efficient in removing milk from the breast. If breastfeeding hurts, more assessment is needed and follow-up after discharge should be a priority.
6. Wet diapers, bowel movements, and weight gain are yardsticks to use to determine if baby is getting enough nourishment. Most babies want to nurse 8 to 10 times a day, and families perceive this to mean that baby isn't getting enough. Reassure families that frequent feeds are normal and needed. Each day after birth, the number of wet diapers and bowel movements increases by one to two each day. Don't expect six wet diapers or yellow, seedy stools until the sixth to seventh day. Mature milk is present after 2 weeks, and bowel habits may change. Some older, breastfed babies may only have a bowel movement every 4 to 8 days.
7. Available help by phone or early follow-up by a lactation consultant or professional care giver should be offered. Breastfed babies should be seen within 5 to 7 days after discharge to assess weight gain and the general health status of baby and mother.

The World Health Organization (WHO) and UNICEF have authorized the use of *10 Steps to Successful Breastfeeding* as part of the "Baby Friendly Hospital Initiative" to promote breastfeeding worldwide. Copies of these 10 steps can be obtained from local lactation consultants or by contacting WHO/UNICEF.

GETTING STARTED

1. Position mother and baby comfortably. Baby should be tummy to tummy with mother; baby's ear, shoulder, and hip should be in a straight line. Pillows help to support mother's arm and back, and help keep baby at the right height with mother's nipple.
2. Mother should tickle baby's lips with nipple, wait for baby's mouth to open wide like a yawn, then pull baby onto breast.
3. Baby's lower and upper lip may need to be everted to flange out around nipple to make a proper seal.
4. Every 2 to 3 hours during the day, let baby nurse 10 to 20 minutes on each breast. Feed on baby's demand after midnight. Some babies need to be awakened for some feedings in the early weeks.
5. Generally, babies need to gain 5 to 7 oz/week. Early weight checks can be very reassuring for parents.
6. If weight gain is inadequate, supplemental bottle feedings of expressed breast milk or formula may be used for a short time until feedings get back on track. Mothers should not fear "nipple confusion" so much that baby is denied needed calories and fluids. Other feeding devices may

also be used as needed, such as droppers, oral syringes, a spoon, or a supplemental nursing system (Lact-Aid), if bottles are so feared. Breastfeeding support should continue.

7. Most mothers' milk appears in more copious amounts between the third and fifth day after delivery. Most babies begin to breastfeed with more vigor and success at this time. Birth weight may not be regained until the third week for breastfed infants.
8. Mothers need practical advice about continuing to nurse when they return to work. Planning ahead is essential. A sample plan might be to nurse baby before leaving for work/school, nurse or pump on lunch break, nurse when mother gets home, nurse again after the evening meal, once again before bedtime, and once at night if baby wakes for a feeding. Child care workers should support and value breastfeeding.

DIAGNOSIS/TREATMENT

Common difficulties are as follows (Fig. 52-2):

Engorgement

The mother may complain of swollen, tender breasts. A history of breastfeeding may reveal infrequent emptying of the breast or inadequate amounts of milk removed to soften the breast at feedings. Frequent nursing for 10 to 20 minutes or long enough to soften the breast is essential. An electric breast pump may need to be used to remove milk if baby is not doing an adequate job of it. Ice packs under the arm and along the side of the breast will help relieve swelling. Regular milk removal at 3- to 4-hour intervals prevents later engorgement. Massage the breasts to get milk flowing, then remove milk with a nursing baby or a breast pump. Ice packs, ibuprofen, or acetaminophen can be used to relieve fever and discomfort.

Sore Nipples

The mother may complain that her nipples are red, cracked, or raw. A history reveals that baby has had difficulty latching on. Be sure that baby is being positioned correctly for latch-on. Getting as much of the nipple and areola deep into baby's mouth is necessary to reduce friction on the nipple. Baby's tongue should cup under the nipple to cushion it from the gums. Baby's lower jaw should glide deep and wide while suckling. Limited use of USP modified lanolin before nursing may offer some relief. Air dry breast milk on the nipple after feedings to aid healing.

Plugged Ducts

The mother may complain of a tender lump in the breast that persists after nursing or pumping; she has no fever and feels well, but the lump worries her. Frequent, regular removal of milk from the breast can prevent or treat ducts clogged with unremoved milk. Tender lumps can be gently massaged, then let baby nurse or pump and remove milk every 2 to 3 hours until lumps go away. Restrictive clothing and underwire bras can contribute to the problem.

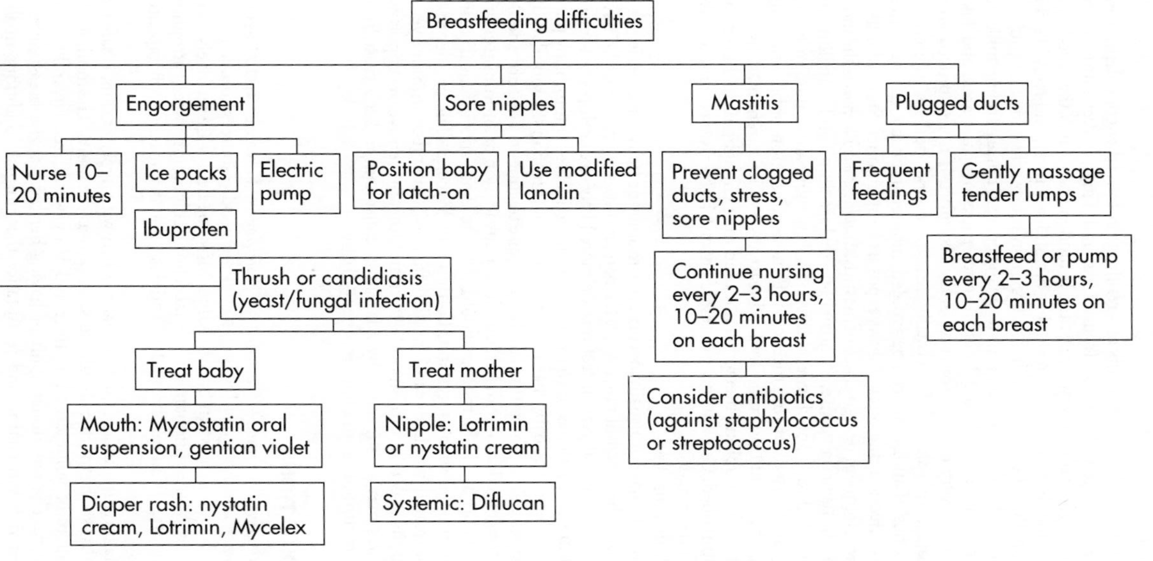

FIG. 52-2 Management of breastfeeding difficulties.

Mastitis

Mothers may develop mastitis as a result of prolonged engorgement, sore nipples, plugged ducts, or from stress and fatigue. Preventing these conditions usually prevents mastitis. If mother complains that she has a red, wedge-shaped, tender area in her breast, has a fever, and feels like she has the flu, she probably has a breast infection. The first avenue of treatment should be to have mother go to bed, rest, nurse or pump milk out of her breast every 2 to 3 hours, use ice packs over the area, and take ibuprofen every 6 hours for fever and discomfort. If not improved after 24 hours, she should be visually reassessed and perhaps prescribed antibiotics. If antibiotics can be avoided, mother and baby may be spared a yeast infection that often follows exposure to antibiotics. Stasis of milk is the most frequent benign cause of mastitis. *Staphylococcus aureus* is the most common bacterial cause. Amoxicillin, dicloxacillin, and nafcillin are usually used for staphylococcal infection. Penicillin, ampicillin, or erythromycin are used for streptococcal infections. Cessation of breastfeeding during this condition could lead to breast abscess. Recurrent mastitis may occur when antibiotic therapy is not used long enough; 10 to 14 days is recommended. One authority states that thrush is the most common cause of recurrent mastitis.

Thrush mastitis

Thrush mastitis usually occurs after mother or baby have undergone antibiotic therapy, but not always. Diabetic mothers or mothers who have a history of vaginal yeast infections are more likely to develop yeast breast infections and also pass it to their babies via vaginal secretions or by poor hand hygiene. The baby may have symptoms of thrush in the mouth or in the diaper area. Both mother and baby require treatment. The baby should be treated by a doctor with Mycostatin oral suspension or antifungal cream in the diaper area. The mother should be treated with an antifungal cream for her nipples such as nystatin, Lotrimin, or Mycelex. The mother may also be treated with Diflucan, if needed, for persistent infection. Some yeast infections may take 1 to 2 months to clear. Other preventive or supportive measures may be suggested by a lactation consultant to keep yeast from being reintroduced to either mother or baby.

MEDICATIONS

Breastfeeding: A Guide for the Medical Profession by Lawrence and *Drugs in Pregnancy and Lactation* by Briggs et al are good resources to determine drugs that are safe when breastfeeding. Most medicines are relatively safe. Exceptions are sulfonamides, tetracycline, chloramphenicol, atropine, cimetidine, lithium, bromides, iodides, and radioactive therapeutic agents.

Magnesium sulfate, used to treat mothers with hypertension, is safe for the baby, so the mother should nurse as early as she wants. The mother has a small milk volume at this time and baby would receive only scant amounts. The emotional uplift of having her baby at the breast gives a mother rich satisfaction and reassurance that normal conditions finally exist. One authority has written that a baby would get more magnesium from special care formula than from a mother who nurses after magnesium sulfate therapy.

Mothers taking heparin or Coumadin may nurse if the baby is healthy and not scheduled for major surgery.

Smoking and alcohol use should be kept to a minimum. Smoking may decrease a mother's milk supply, and the secondary smoke harms the baby.

Birth Control

Barrier methods are probably the contraceptives of choice, including the diaphragm, condom, and foam. Other safe alternatives are Depo-Provera, Norplant, and the progestin-only mini-pill. Using these methods, the mother may nurse early, and there is no need to delay using the medication if nursing. However, estrogen and progestin combination pills can dramatically decrease the mother's breast milk supply and may cause irreversible lactopoetic effects.

BREAST PUMPS

Breast pumps manufactured by breast pump companies are preferred. Medela* or Ameda/Egnel offer the classic breast pumps used by most hospitals and are available for rent or purchase. Other manual, battery-powered, or small electric breast pumps are available at retail stores, but vary widely in their ability to remove milk comfortably.

Pumping and Storing Breast Milk

Breast milk should be collected with clean hands into clean containers. Collect in 2- to 4-oz portions. Breast milk can be stored in the refrigerator for 72 hours, or in a large freezer compartment for 5 to 6 months. Breast milk may be thawed in hot tap water. It should never be boiled or microwaved. Never refreeze thawed breast milk. Breast milk not used during a feeding should be discarded.

WEANING

Weaning may occur when mother or baby wants to stop. Breastfeeding is preferred for 6 to 12 months if possible. Abrupt weaning should be avoided to prevent engorgement, plugged ducts, and/or mastitis. Gradual weaning is easier on mother and baby. Dropping off one feeding every 2 to 3 days helps keep everyone more comfortable. A supportive bra should be worn, and ice packs may be used to relieve any swelling.

KEY POINTS

1 Breastfeeding is regarded as the ideal feeding method for babies for the first 6 to 12 months of life.

---

* 1-800-TELL-YOU, Medela, Inc.; P.O. Box 660; McHenry, IL 60051

2 Basic breastfeeding support and assistance should include early frequent nursing, nutritional guides for mother, latch-on assistance, and prevention and/or relief of common difficulties.

3 Mothers or infants with medical problems that may impact lactation need more intense help and follow-up to ensure successful breastfeeding.

4 Most medications are relatively safe during lactation, but a mother should consult professional lactation experts and her physician. Barrier methods of birth control are usually preferred.

5 Weaning should be done gradually when mother and baby are ready. Dropping off one feeding every 2 to 3 days helps prevent problems such as engorgement and mastitis.

SUGGESTED READINGS

Auerbach K, Riordan J: *Breastfeeding and human lactation,* Boston, 1993, Jones and Bartlett.

Gabbe S, Neibyl J, Simpson J, eds: *Obstetrics: normal and problem pregnancies,* 1991, Churchill Livingstone, pp 175-176.

Iams J, Zuspan F, eds: *Zuspan & Quilligan's manual of obstetrics and gynecology,* ed 2, St. Louis, 1990, Mosby, pp 259-261.

Lawrence R: *Breastfeeding: a guide for the medical profession,* St. Louis, 1994, Mosby, pp 207-208, 511.

Sears W, Sears M: *The baby book,* 1993, Little, Brown & Co, Boston, pp 131, 147, 183-84, 165-69, 161-62.

Shrago L, Bocar D: The infant's contribution to breastfeeding, *J Obstet Gynecol Neonatal Nurs* 19:3, 1990.

Spisak S, Gross S: *Second follow-up report: the Surgeon General's workshop on breastfeeding and human lactation,* National Center for Education in Maternal and Child Health, Washington, DC, 1991.

53

Adolescent Pregnancy

Geri D. Hewitt

Teen pregnancy is common in all social, economic, and racial groups in the United States. The United States has the highest teen pregnancy rate of all developed countries, with approximately 1 million American teens becoming pregnant each year. Of these pregnancies, 35% will end in termination, 15% will end with a spontaneous abortion or ectopic pregnancy, and 50% will be delivered. Approximately 90% of the babies delivered will remain with the mother, and approximately 10% will be adopted. The best estimates are that 80% of teen pregnancies are unintended. The majority of teens conceive within the first 6 months of initiating sexual activity while not using any means of contraception.

PSYCHOSOCIAL DEVELOPMENT

Adolescence is a time for rapid change in physical, emotional, and cognitive development. The "tasks" of an adolescent are to develop an identity unique from her family, to develop intimate physical and social relationships, and to begin to develop her life's work. Peer group identity and influences commonly take precedence over her family. Adolescents often participate in risk-taking behavior because they are unable to accept the consequences of their actions because they are just beginning to develop abstract thinking. This combination of peer pressure, risk-taking behavior, and an emerging sexuality often leads to sexual activity that is not protected from STDs and pregnancy. Some studies indicate that 20% of girls are sexually active by age 15 and 50% are sexually active by age 17. Approximately 12 million cases of STDs are diagnosed in the United States each year; 3 million, or 25%, of these will be contracted by adolescents.

PREGNANCY RISKS

Teens who are pregnant are often at increased risk for low socioeconomic status, poor health before pregnancy, limited job skills, poor education, limited access to health care, inadequate parenting skills, STDs, substance abuse, smoking, and poor nutrition. In addition, risk of preeclampsia, low-birth-weight infants (from preterm deliveries or IUGR), complications of substance abuse, and anemia increases.

PRENATAL CARE

Often teens delay entry into prenatal care because of denial, fear of parental anger, or ignorance of the signs and symptoms of pregnancy. Only 59% of teens begin care in the first trimester, and 10% will receive either no prenatal care or begin care in the third trimester. The younger the patient, the more likely she will delay entry into prenatal care. Patients are best served by a "team approach" that includes physicians, midwives, nurses, dieticians, social workers, and psychologists. Prenatal care for teens should include information on reproductive biology, physiologic changes in pregnancy, signs and symptoms of disease, nutrition, childbirth, child care, lactation, and government and community services.

NUTRITION

Pregnant adolescents have special dietary needs because the pregnancy competes with the developing adolescent for nutritional support. Approximately 25% of pregnant adolescents are thought to be nutritionally deficient during pregnancy. Pregnant adolescents should be consuming 2700 to 3000 kcal/day of a nutritionally sound, balanced diet. Weight gain should represent at least a 20% increase above the 50th percentile weight for height for that patient. For an obese adolescent, a weight gain of at least 20 lbs is recommended.

REPEAT PREGNANCIES

Approximately 25% of adolescent births in 1992 were not first-time births. Studies show that within 1 year of delivering, 20% to 25% of teens will be pregnant again and within 2 years the rate increases to 30% to 40%. Younger maternal age (<16 years old) correlates directly with an increased incidence of short pregnancy intervals. Teen multiparous patients are at increased risk for low-birth-weight infants and perinatal deaths. Risk factors for repeat teen pregnancy include younger maternal age (<16 years old), school failure, low socioeconomic status, and poor familial support.

KEY POINTS

1. One million teens in the United States become pregnant each year; 3 million American teens contract an STD each year.
2. Pregnant teens may be at increased risk for preeclampsia, low-birth-weight infants, poor nutrition, STDs, anemia, and substance abuse.
3. Only 59% of teens begin prenatal care in the first trimester; 10% receive no prenatal care or prenatal care only in the third trimester.
4. Pregnant adolescents have special nutritional needs; 25% of adolescents are thought to be nutritionally deficient during pregnancy.
5. Approximately 20% to 25% of teens will become pregnant again within 1 year of delivery.

SUGGESTED READINGS

American College of Obstetricians and Gynecologists: *The adolescent obstetric-gynecologic patient,* ACOG technical bulletin 145, Washington, DC, 1990, ACOG.

Brown HL, Fan YD, Gonsowlin WJ: Obstetric complications in young teenagers, *South Med J* 84:46-48, 1991.

Centers for Disease Control and Prevention: Sexual behavior among high school students: United States, 1990, *MMWR* 40:886, 1992.

Centers for Disease Control and Prevention: Teenage pregnancy and birth rates–United States, 1990, *MMWR* 42:773-737, 1993.

Henshaw SK: Teenage abortion, birth, and pregnancy statistics by state, 1988, *Fam Plann Perspect* 25:122-126, 1993.

Pritchard JA, MacDonald PC: *Williams obstetrics,* ed 19, New York, 1993, Appleton and Lange.

Reece EA et al: Medicine of the fetus and mother, Philadelphia, 1992, JB Lippincott Co.

Turner RJ, Grindstaff CF, Phillips N: Social support and outcome in teenage pregnancy, *J Health Soc Behav* 31:43-57, 1990.

54

Substance Abuse in Pregnancy

Phillip Shubert

Substance abuse can have a profound effect on a developing fetus or neonate. The increased incidence of birth defects, spontaneous miscarriages, preterm labor, IUGR, abruption, and maternal morbidity among substance abusers has been well described. Thus the obstetrician must have a clear understanding of the complex management issues these patients present (Fig. 54-1).

DIAGNOSIS

The most important aspect of screening for substance abuse is taking a thorough history. Substance abuse is suspected with repeated injuries, frequent emergency room visits, missed appointments, domestic violence, psychiatric history, and premature delivery.

Two screening tools frequently employed are the CAGE and TACE questionnaires. CAGE questions include the following:

C: Have you ever felt a need to *cut down* on your drinking?

A: Have you ever been *annoyed* at criticism of your drug use?

G: Have you ever felt *guilty* about something you've done when you've been using drugs?

E: Have you ever had a morning *eye-opener?*

One positive response indicates problem use; two positives indicate an even greater likelihood of dependence.

The TACE questionnaire was established to specifically deal with alcohol-abusing pregnant patients. The **T** in TACE addresses the issue of *t*olerance, asking "how many drinks does it take to make you feel high?" An answer of two or more drinks is considered positive.

Few tests are available for the screening and diagnosis of substance abuse. Fortunately, a number of drugs can be detected in urine toxicology specimens. However, many drugs may not be detected because of their relatively short half-life. Amphetamines and cocaine can be detected anywhere from 12 to 48 hours after the last dose. Opiates can be detected between 2 to 4 days later. Some drugs are not detectable in urine (i.e., inhalants, alcohol). Thus it is very important to look for sequelae of prior abuse. In essence, a good history and physical examination remain important aspects of any evaluation for substance abuse.

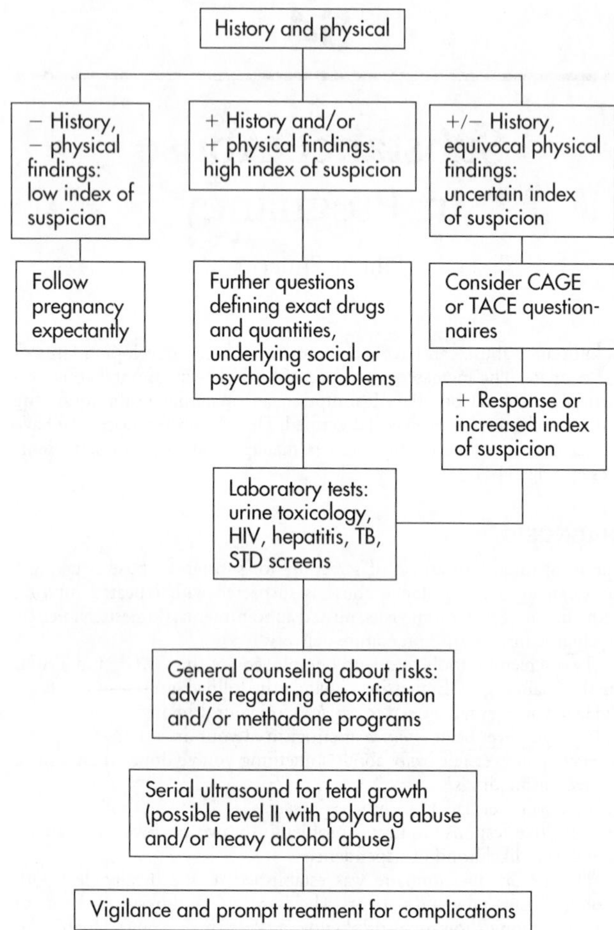

FIG. 54-1 Screening for and detection of substance abuse.

DIFFERENTIAL DIAGNOSIS

In caring for the pregnant substance abuser, one must understand the close association of underlying social and psychologic pathology. About 50% of pregnant substance abusers are involved in abusive (psychologic, physical, and sexual) relationships. A large number engage in prostitution to support their drug habits. Finally, addressing underlying depression and/or personality disorders is critical.

TREATMENT

The incidence of alcohol abuse during pregnancy varies, but ranges between 1% and 2% of all pregnant women in the United States. The incidence of fetal alcohol syndrome (FAS) ranges between 1/300 and 1/2000. Alcohol is the leading preventable cause of mental retardation. Approximately 10% to 20% of all mental deficiency (IQ 50 to 80) in children is attributed to maternal alcohol use.

No "safe" threshold for alcohol intake during pregnancy has been established. One to two drinks/day is associated with an increased incidence of IUGR and doubles the risk of spontaneous abortion. Perinatal mortality is approximately 17% with chronic alcohol abuse. Thus once problem drinkers have been identified, immediate attention should be made to withdraw them from alcohol. If medications are required for withdrawal, a short-acting barbiturate (i.e., pentobarbital) can be used. Benzodiazepines should be avoided.

In addition to the detoxification of the patient, emphasis should be placed on adequate dietary intake. Poor nutrition can have a significant impact on the mother and fetus. Decreased thiamine levels predispose to Wernicke's encephalopathy. Thus patients with a history of alcohol abuse should be given liberal thiamine replacement and prenatal vitamins early in pregnancy.

Treatment of the pregnant alcoholic does not end with delivery of the fetus. In the event that medications are required for withdrawal, the patient should be maintained on the medication for approximately 1 week after delivery. However, the most important aspect of postpartum care is to encourage the patient to continue counseling and to participate in self-help programs.

Approximately 9000 births/year occur in narcotic-addicted women in the United States. Opiates have been clearly associated with fetal loss and growth restriction. In addition, there appears to be a propensity toward prematurity and low-birth-weight infants in heroin-addicted mothers. Opiate use does not result in an increased risk of teratogenicity. However, additional teratogenetic risk may be caused by contaminants of the street drugs (e.g., strychnine, quinine, Coumadin).

Once the diagnosis of opioid addiction is established, attempts should be made to alter the patient's drug dependence as soon as possible in the pregnancy. One of the approaches is to place the patient on an alternative drug. Methadone is an orally-acting agent that relates a high degree of cross-tolerance to other opioids, reducing the euphoria associated with heroin. The long half-life of methadone also makes once-daily dosing possible.

Methadone maintenance during pregnancy may result in more prenatal care, decreased use of illegal narcotics, and babies with more normal birth weight. The disadvantage of methadone maintenance during pregnancy appears in the infant of the methadone-addicted mother. Moderate to severe withdrawal symptoms occur in 50% to 75% of these infants. A target goal of 20 mg/day of methadone should be attempted during the pregnancy. When the methadone dose at delivery is no greater than 20 mg/day, only 18% of newborns develop withdrawal symptoms. If methadone detoxification/maintenance is to be performed, it should be done only during the second trimester by reducing the dose approximately 2 to 5 mg/week.

Finally, if methadone detoxification is not desirable, clonidine may be used as an alternative. Clonidine decreases the adrenergic symptoms of opiate withdrawal (i.e., tremors, tachycardia, and hypertension). Patients undergoing withdrawal may be given 0.1 to 0.2 mg sublingually every hour for up to 0.8 mg if signs of withdrawal persist.

Cocaine can be detected in urine or blood for 6 to 12 hours after exposure. However, its metabolites (benzoylecgonine, legonine methylester, and norecgonine) can be present for up to 6 days. Chronic cocaine use has many adverse effects on pregnancy. Preterm labor and birth, low birth weight, reduced head circumference, and placental abruption have been reported. Cocaine has also been implicated as a teratogenic agent. A possible association with intrauterine cerebrovascular accident (CVA) and genitourinary malformation has been reported. Cocaine poses numerous risks to the mother because of excessive CNS stimulation. Agitation, paranoia, sleeplessness, and even frank psychosis can result from excessive use. Cocaine intoxication can result in tachycardia, hypertension, arrhythmias, myocardial infarction, and CVA.

Signs of cocaine withdrawal include depression, irritability, and appetite and sleep dysfunction. These withdrawal symptoms are caused by depletion of dopamine reserves in the brain. Thus without cocaine, the addict develops an intense desire for it and enters into high-risk behavior (e.g., prostitution) to obtain cocaine.

Marijuana is the most commonly used illicit drug among women of childbearing age (approximately 20% in peripartum). Chronic marijuana users may have positive urine toxicology screening for up to 4 weeks after use. To date, there is no clear evidence to suggest an increased incidence of IUGR or shortened pregnancy with marijuana use.

Amphetamines have been used medicinally to treat narcolepsy and as an appetite suppressant. The major abuse potential has focused on their illicit use. Recently, "ice," a smokable type of methamphetamine similar to crack cocaine, has become popular. Illicit use has resulted in increased risks of preterm labor, IUGR, and abruption. No consistent abnormalities are associated with amphetamine use.

There continues to be a high incidence of barbiturate abuse in therapeutic and nontherapeutic settings. Prolonged maternal consumption of barbiturates may result in tolerance and dependence in both the mother and fetus. If this occurs, abrupt withdrawal can occur in both the mother and fetus that resembles the narcotic withdrawal syndrome. No clear evidence exists to support a teratogenic potential in this class of drugs.

LSD (lysergic acid diethylamide) and PCP (phencyclidine) are two of the more common and notorious hallucinogens in use. Neither have been positively linked to birth defects or chromosomal damage in the fetus. Both have raised concerns regarding possible withdrawal syndromes (i.e., flashbacks, emotional lability).

KEY POINTS

1 Screening and patient education are critical aspects of identifying the pregnant substance abuser. An in-depth history is the most important aspect of screening.

2 There is a high incidence of underlying social and psychologic pathology.

SUGGESTED READINGS

Chasnoff I: Cocaine and pregnancy: clinical and methodologic issues, *Clin Perinatol* 18(1):113-123, 1991.

Evans AT, Gillogley K: Drug use in pregnancy: obstetric perspectives, *Clin Perinatol* 18(1), 1991.

Haegerman G, Schnoll S: Narcotic use in pregnancy, *Clin Perinatol* 18(1):51-76, 1991.

MacGregor SN, Keith LG: Drug abuse during pregnancy. In Rayburn WF, Zuspan FP, eds: *Drug therapy in obstetrics and gynecology,* ed 3, 1993, St. Louis, Mosby, p 181.

Shubert P, Savage B: Smoking, alcohol and drug abuse. In James DK, Steer PJ, Weiner CP, Gonik B, eds: *High risk pregnancy: management options,* London, 1994, WB Saunders.

Zuspan FP: *Detoxification and medical management of the pregnant drug abuser.* Presented at the First National Conference of the OSAP National Resource Center for the Prevention of Perinatal Abuse of Alcohol and Other Drugs, July, 1992.

55

Resuscitation of the Newborn

LEANDRO CORDERO AND RANDY R. MILLER

Every year 280,000 of the 4 million infants born in the United States require some form of assistance, such as blow-by oxygen and/or face mask ventilation, to transition successfully from intrauterine to extrauterine life. Another 80,000 infants require major interventions such as endotracheal intubation, epinephrine administration, and chest compression. About 10,000 live-born infants per year die before leaving the delivery room. Furthermore, failure to successfully treat neonatal depression (incorrectly termed *asphyxia*) either initiates (transient tachypnea of the newborn, persistent pulmonary hypertension of the newborn [PPHNB]) or worsens other underlying conditions (neonatal sepsis, hyaline membrane disease). On the positive side, 60% of infants apparently stillborn (Apgar 0 at one minute) will leave the delivery room alive; one third of these infants will survive with minimal or no detectable neurologic problems.

Approximately half of the infants described above would have been identified as at risk for neonatal depression during the antepartum or intrapartum period (biophysical, biochemical, or clinical signs of acute or chronic fetal distress). The other half would only be recognized at delivery or shortly thereafter.

ADAPTATION TO EXTRAUTERINE LIFE

Regardless of gestational age, infants should transition from fetal to neonatal life in the course of a few minutes, occasionally a few hours. Adjustments in many areas (especially respiratory and cardiovascular) should occur promptly and in synchrony.

With the clamping of the umbilical cord and the inflation of the lungs (onset of breathing), major hemodynamic changes occur in the infant. As the lungs inflate, pulmonary vascular resistance (PVR) dramatically falls, allowing pulmonary blood flow and venous return to the left atrium to increase, resulting in the functional closure of the foramen ovale. The fall of PVR reverses the pressure gradient between the pulmonary artery and the aorta, thereby eliminating the right to left shunt through the ductus arteriosus. At that moment, neonatal circulation resembles that of an adult, except for the anatomic patency of the foramen ovale and ductus arteriousus. Failure to inflate the lungs prevents the fall of PVR, reverting the whole circulation to the fetal arrangement but without the benefits of the placenta.

CLINICAL PRESENTATION

The classic presentation of a severely depressed newborn is that of a pale (or cyanotic), hypotonic, bradycardic infant with weak (if any) respiratory efforts. Yet despite appearing vigorous at birth, other neonates may develop respiratory distress or become apneic and bradycardic. Assigning points (0 to 2) to each of five clinical signs (heart rate, respiration, tone, reflex activity, and color) allows objective assessment of the infant's condition at birth and is called the *Apgar score.* Very likely, most infants whose Apgar scores at 1 minute are ≤3 will require full resuscitation, whereas those ≥7 will do well with minimal assistance. However, 5-minute scores reflect the severity of the neonatal condition (i.e., 0 and 1 at 1 and 5 minutes, respectively, after a full resuscitation). Evaluation of the newborn's condition should be prompt; resuscitation efforts are usually underway before the first minute of life.

ROUTINE DELIVERY ROOM CARE

Considering the high incidence of unsuspected neonatal depression, one or two health professionals experienced in neonatal resuscitation should be present at all deliveries. Birthing rooms, delivery rooms, and operating

BOX 55-1

Necessary Supplies for Delivery Room Resuscitation

Radiant warmer
Suction devices: meconium aspirator, bulb syringe, catheters
Resuscitation bag with manometer
Face masks (premature and full-term sizes)
Endotracheal tubes (2.5, 3.0, 3.5, 4.0 mm)
Endotracheal tube stylets
Laryngoscope
Laryngoscope blades (No. 0 and 1)
Adhesive tape
Logan bow
Tincture of benzoin
8 French feeding tube
Umbilical catheters (3.5 and 5 French)
Three-way stopcocks
Syringes (1,3, and 10 ml)
Medications
Epinephrine 1 : 10,000: .1-.3 ml/kg via endotracheal tube
Dextrose 10%: 2-3 ml/kg via IV
Sodium bicarbonate 4.2% (1 mEg/ml): 2 mEg/kg via IV
Saline .9N: 10 ml/kg via IV
5% Albumin: 0.1 mg/kg via IV
Naloxone 0.4 or 1 mg/ml: 0.1 mg/kg via ET, IV

suites should always have resuscitation equipment that is conveniently located and frequently checked (Box 55-1).

Drying the infant after delivery decreases heat loss while providing abundant tactile stimulation. Except for gentle tapping of the soles, all other forms of physical stimulation should be discouraged. Infants should be placed on their backs with their heads slightly extended (sniffing position). Unless thick meconium is present, suction of the oropharynx should be brief and gentle. Deep blind suctioning with a catheter may trigger untoward vagal responses with ensuing bradycardia and apnea.

Most infants are vigorous and require minimal assistance. For them, identification, eye prophylaxis, umbilical cord care, and mother-infant interaction should proceed according to preestablished protocol. Prevention of heat loss and continuous observation should be maintained throughout the entire delivery room experience.

BASIC ASSISTANCE

For about 7% of all newborns, some added assistance will be needed to ensure a successful transition to extrauterine life (Fig. 55-1). Infants who are

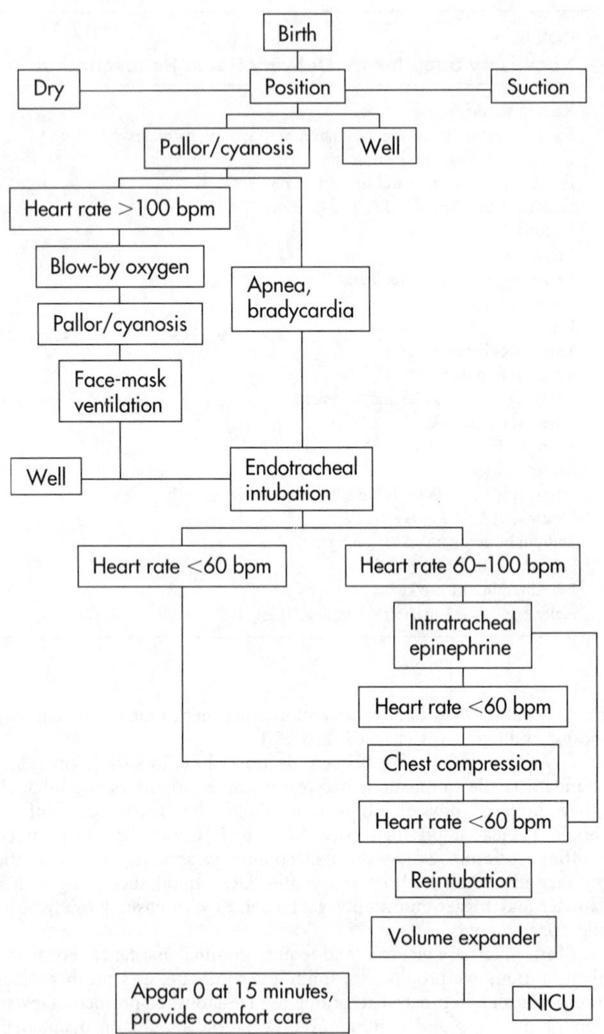

FIG. 55-1 Management of neonatal resuscitation.

not vigorous at birth (i.e., weak respiratory efforts, pale/dusky, fair muscular tone, and some reflex irritability) should receive blow-by oxygen through a mask connected to a pediatric anesthesia bag. Although warm, humidified oxygen is preferable, it is not available in most delivery rooms. A physical examination should take place while drying (stimulating) efforts and oropharyngeal suctioning are performed.

Infants who do not respond should receive face-mask ventilation with a pediatric anesthesia bag connected to an oxygen source, a pressure gauge, and a mask. Flow of oxygen should be sufficient to maintain the bag inflation while providing 40 to 50 breaths/minute with peak inflation pressures (PIP) up to 40 cm H_2O and positive end expiratory pressure (PEEP) of 4 to 6 cm H_2O. Infants should remain in the "sniffing" position while the mask is firmly applied to the face with one hand. To obtain adequate opening lung pressure, 35 cm H_2O of PIP is often necessary. The success of face-mask resuscitation rests on the establishment of an adequate functional residual capacity and also to the triggering of Head's paradoxic reflex (inspiratory efforts made in response to lung inflation). To avoid a hyperinflation reflex (which unnecessarily prolongs apnea), it is advisable to bag 8 to 10 times and then stop. If face-mask ventilation is not successful in two or three trials, preparations for endotracheal intubation should be initiated. Successful face-mask ventilation usually results in improvement in heart rate, tone, and color before improvements in respiratory effort are apparent.

ENDOTRACHEAL INTUBATION

The most common factors interfering with a successful resuscitation are inappropriate positioning of the infant's head, gripping too tight or levering the laryngoscope, and applying excessive cricoid pressure. Prolonged intubation attempts without periods of intermittent face-mask ventilation and endless suctioning of the airways are unnecessary and dangerous. Pulmonary fluid will continue to seep through the larynx until either strong inspiratory efforts or positive pressure ventilation force it into the lymphatic circulation of the lung. Commonly observed errors among those assisting the resuscitation are improperly holding the infant, not reporting heart rate, and bending or displacing the endotracheal (ET) tube while bagging. Taping the ET tube to the infant's face is common, but the use of a metal arch (Logan bow) provides more stability while maintaining easier access to the mouth.

OTHER RESUSCITATIVE MEASURES

If the heart rate remains between 60 and 100 bpm after ET intubation and adequate bagging, 0.1 to 0.3 ml of epinephrine 1:10,000 should be administered intratracheally. Heart rates below 60 bpm should prompt the initiation of chest compression according to standard technique. If the patient does not improve and the heart rate remains below 60 bpm, it is prudent to reintubate. In addition to malposition of the ET tube, the most common reason for a failed resuscitation is insufficient PIP. As soon as a clinical response is obtained, it is advisable to decrease PIP progressively to about 18 cm H_2O at a rate of 30 to 40 times/minute. The incidence of lung rupture (pneumothorax, pneumomediastinum, pulmonary interstitial emphysema) is related (among other factors) to the magnitude of the PIP used and to the duration of positive pressure ventilation.

In spite of a successful ET intubation and adequate lung inflation, some infants (especially premature infants), remain unstable (hypotension, metabolic acidosis, hypoglycemia) and unresponsive. A slow infusion of 10 ml/kg saline followed by 1 to 2 mEq/kg of sodium bicarbonate is used. Intravenous epinephrine can also be administered. To correct hypoglycemia, 2 to 3 ml/kg of D10W can be safely given. For a more permanent correction of hypotension, 10 cc/kg of plasmanate can be used over 20 minutes and occasionally an infusion of 10 to 15 μg/kg/min of dopamine. The administration of Narcan is indicated only in cases of suspected neonatal depression caused by the administration of Demerol, morphine, or other narcotics to the mother.

Ending resuscitative efforts is a complex decision. The coexistence of fatal or severe congenital malformations or evidence of extreme prematurity are important factors. Resuscitation options should be discussed with the parents. Severely depressed newborns (Apgar 0-1 at 1 and 5 minutes) who are still unresponsive (Apgar 0 at 10 to 15 minutes) seldom survive and therefore justify the cessation of resuscitative efforts.

SPECIAL CLINICAL SITUATIONS

Elective ET intubation should be used in all cases of immune or nonimmune hydrops fetalis, diaphragmatic hernias, gastroschisis, major omphaloceles, pleural effusions, and all infants under 26 weeks of gestational age or those with birth weights <800 g.

MECONIUM ASPIRATION

Approximately 10% of all deliveries are characterized by the presence of meconium in the amniotic fluid and/or on the newborn (Fig. 55-2). In most cases, the event is clinically insignificant. Characterization of meconium is important because it is often the only information available to the resuscitator on arrival at the delivery room. *Thin* describes a small amount of meconium diluted by amniotic fluid or a large amount that has been in the amniotic cavity for several hours or days. *Thick* denotes abundance and recent passage. *Late* does not refer to amount or consistency, only to the moment in labor when it occurs. From the standpoint of the newborn, problems related to untimely meconium passage fall into two categories: the magnitude of any accompanying fetal distress and the presence of meconium in the airways. Profound, prolonged fetal distress often leads to severe neonatal depression. Typically, a postmature, bradycardic, hypotonic, pale, apneic infant, covered with thick meconium is presented to the resuscitator. The absence of gasping/breathing facilitates suction of the

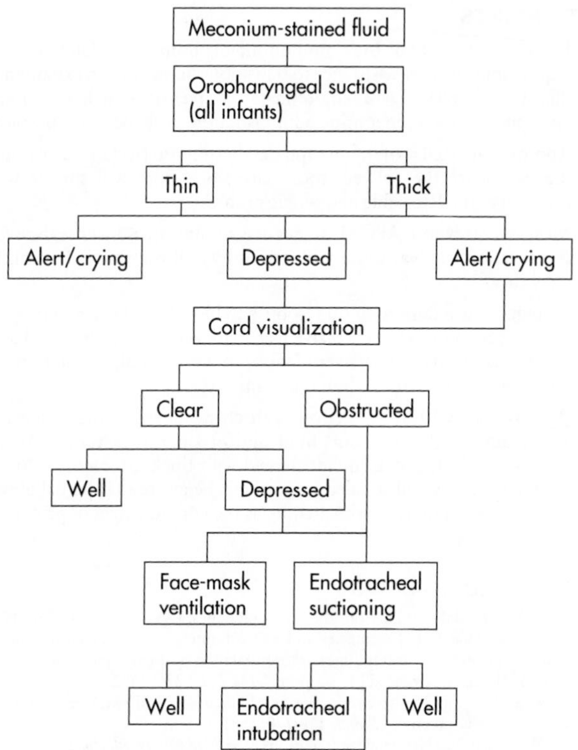

FIG. 55-2 Management of the meconium-stained infant.

oropharynx and the airways. An infant stained with thick meconium should always be intubated and suctioned. Even if suctioning has to be repeated, the initiation of positive pressure ventilation should not be delayed longer than 1 or 2 minutes. Thick meconium may plug the ET tube, prompting removal and replacement. Do not expect to remove all inhaled meconium; be aware that airway obstruction is not as life threatening as the consequences of prolonged hypoxia. PPHNB is the feared component of the meconium aspiration syndrome.

Airway obstruction created by thick meconium may lead to localized or diffuse atelectasis, pneumonitis (meconium aspiration pneumonia), and lung rupture (pneumothorax, pneumomediastinum). Enthusiastic suctioning of the trachea under direct vision is not necessary in the presence of thin meconium with an active, vigorous, crying infant.

KEY POINTS

1 Every year 280,000 of the 4 million infants born in the United States require some form of assistance to transition successfully to extrauterine life. Another 80,000 will require major interventions such as endotracheal intubation, epinephrine administration, and chest compression.

2 Approximately 60% of infants apparently stillborn (APGAR 0 at 1 minute) will leave the delivery room alive; one third will survive with minimal or no detectable neurologic problems.

3 Most infants whose APGAR scores at 1 minute are ≤3 will require full resuscitation whereas those with scores ≥7 will do well with minimal assistance.

4 Nonvigorous infants with no response to blow-by oxygen and oropharyngeal suctioning should receive face-mask ventilation with a pediatric anesthesia bag. If face-mask ventilation is not successful, preparations for endotracheal intubation should be initiated.

5 Approximately 10% of all deliveries are characterized by the presence of meconium in the amniotic fluid and/or on the newborn. Always intubate and suction an infant stained with thick meconium. Do not expect to remove all inhaled meconium; be aware that partial airway obstruction is not as life threatening as the consequences of prolonged hypoxia.

SUGGESTED READINGS

Elliot RD: Neonatal resuscitation: the NRP guidelines, *Can J Anaesth* 41:742, 1994.

Emergency Cardiac Care Committee and Subcommittees, American Heart Association: Guidelines for cardiopulmonary resuscitation and emergency cardiac care. Part VI: Neonatal advanced life support, *JAMA* 268-276, 1992.

Jain L et al: Cardiopulmonary resuscitation of apparently stillborn infants: survival and long-term outcome, *J Pediatr* 118:778, 1991.

Khan NS, Luten RC: Neonatal resuscitation, *Emer Med Clin North Am* 12:239, 1994.

Perlman JM, Risser R: Cardiopulmonary resuscitation in the delivery room: associated clinical events, *Arch Pediatr Adolesc Med* 149:20, 1995.

Troutman MS: Neonatal resuscitation: be prepared, *Contemp Pediatr* 12:101-113, 1995.

Wimmer JE Jr: Neonatal resuscitation, *Pediatr Rev* 15:255, 1994.

PART III

Primary Care

Edward J. Quilligan, Editor

56

AIDS

David A. Wininger

Attention to acquired immunodeficiency syndrome (AIDS) in women has been steadily increasing since AIDS was first recognized in homosexual and bisexual men in the early 1980s. Of American adult/adolescent AIDS cases in 1995, 19% were women; of those, 38% acquired HIV via injected drug use and 38% via sexual contact with an at-risk male. In 1994 AIDS was the third leading cause of death among women ages 25 to 44.

Infection by HIV (HIV-1 worldwide and HIV-2 primarily in western Africa) destroys the immune system and predisposes patients to the opportunistic infections and malignancies that characterize AIDS. HIV enters the body primarily via direct introduction into the bloodstream or through sexual contact and targets CD4+ T lymphocytes as well as the monocyte/macrophage system. The retrovirus integrates into the patient's DNA and rapidly replicates, achieving peak serum viral levels before the development of the primary immune response. During this period of primary infection, an associated syndrome similar to mononucleosis (may include fever, rash, pharyngitis, lymphadenopathy, arthralgias, headache, aseptic meningitis, and other constitutional symptoms) occurs in an ill-defined proportion of patients. Infection by HIV can directly contribute to chronic fatigue, wasting, diarrhea, and dementia.

DIAGNOSIS

Analysis for HIV by ELISA with confirmatory Western blots provides sensitivities and specificities greater than 99%. Infection by the virus can usually be detected serologically within 3 months, although repeat testing 6 months after the last high-risk exposure can further exclude the possibility of a false negative result occurring during seroconversion. (Management of the HIV-infected patient is outlined in Fig. 56-1).

Testing during pregnancy is advised given the substantial potential for reducing vertical transmission with the use of peripartum zidovudin. Diagnosis of another sexually transmitted disease warrants a recommendation for HIV testing. Manifestations of possible HIV infection (such as recurrent oral or vaginal candidiasis, profound weight loss, prolonged fever, herpes zoster infection, and generalized lymphadenopathy) without a reasonable alternative explanation should also prompt testing for HIV.

Contirm the diagnosis ot HIV intection
- ELISA + Western Blot

Assess disease stage
- History and physical examination for signs of opportunistic infections
- CD4 lymphocyte count
- Serum HIV RNA quantitation

Screen for chronic, latent, or occult infections/illnesses
- PPD
- Toxoplasma IgG
- RPR
- Hepatitis B +/− Hepatitis A and Hepatitis C serologies
- CMV IgG
- Pap smear with colposcopic biopsy if indicated

Prophylactic Antimicrobials

PCP	If CD4 <200, history of thrush or PCP
Toxoplasmosis	If CD4 <100 and Toxoplasma IgG positive
MAC	Consider if CD4 <75 if no active mycobacterial disease
CMV retinitis	Consider if CD4 <50, balancing cost-benefit

Consider initiation of antiretroviral agents
- All patients with symptomatic AIDS
- Most patients with <350-500 CD4 lymphocytes
- Most patients with "high" serum HIV RNA regardless of CD4 cell count
- Pregnancy

Monitor for end organ injury from HIV, opportunistic pathogens, or medications
- Cell blood counts with platelets
- Liver enzymes
- Amylase levels
- Urinalysis; BUN/creatinine and electrolyte levels
- Creatinine kinase (if signs of myopathy)

Reducing perinatal transmission of HIV

At 14 or more weeks gestation	AZT 100 mg orally 5 times daily
During labor	AZT 2 mg/kg load over 1 hour, then 1 mg/kg/hr infusion
Newborn, beginning at 8-12 hours	AZT 2 mg/kg orally every 6 hours for 6 weeks

FIG. 56-1 Managing the newly diagnosed HIV-infected patient.

The CDC case definition of AIDS is met in HIV-infected patients who develop any one of a long list of opportunistic infections, a specifically defined wasting syndrome, HIV encephalopathy, or certain malignancies such as Kaposi's sarcoma, primary CNS lymphoma, or non-Hodgkins lymphoma. Some diseases are so distinctive of AIDS (e.g., *Pneumocystis carinii* pneumonia) that they can define a case in the absence of confirmed HIV infection as long as no other cause of immunodeficiency is present. The AIDS definition was expanded in 1993 to include patients with established HIV infection who had CD4 lymphocyte counts <200 cells/ml or pulmonary tuberculosis, recurrent bacterial pneumonias, or invasive cervical carcinoma.

The CD4 lymphocyte count has been a reasonable surrogate marker of disease progression, with certain opportunistic conditions tending to manifest when this count falls within certain ranges. Although the lower limits of normal are loosely defined, most patients with normal immune systems have CD4 lymphocyte counts ranging from 600 to 1900/ml. During the early years of HIV infection, generalized lymphadenopathy and cutaneous manifestations such as tinea pedis, folliculitis, and localized herpes zoster can be noted. As counts reach 500 cells/ml, recurrent sinusitis, vaginal candidiasis, and oral thrush may manifest. With additional decline, recurrent bacterial pneumonias, especially *Streptococcus pneumoniae,* are more common. *Pneumocystis carinii* pneumonia can be observed as CD4 lymphocytes fall below 200/ml, whereas cytomegaloviral retinitis or gastrointestinal disease and disseminated *Mycobacterium avium* complex (MAC) disease are generally not seen until counts have dropped below 50 to 100/ml.

TREATMENT

The history and physical examination should suggest the extent of disease and can uncover active opportunistic infections that require acute management. Patients require education about the nature of HIV/AIDS and transmission prevention. Sexual or needle-sharing partners and state health departments may need to be notified.

Baseline laboratory studies should be obtained for future reference. The CD4 lymphocyte count has been the primary marker of disease stage, but sensitive measures of HIV RNA in serum are a superior indicator of long-term prognosis. CBCs, liver enzymes, and BUN/creatinine levels can screen for abnormalities attributable to HIV, opportunistic conditions, and medications. Screening for prior or latent infections should include an RPR, Toxoplasma IgG, CMV IgG (so that CMV-negative patients can be designated to receive only leukocyte-filtered blood products), PPD (followed by a chest x-ray if positive), and hepatitis A and B serologies (if vaccinations for these viruses are being considered).

Even though immunizations have an acute negative effect on HIV load, most authorities continue to advise the use of annual influenza vaccines and the multivalent pneumococcal vaccine (every 5 years) in all HIV-infected patients. Hepatitis A and B vaccines should be offered to high-risk patients who lack serologic evidence of prior exposure.

Gynecologic Primary Care

According to the CDC, all newly diagnosed HIV-infected women should have a Pap smear, and if it is normal, it should be repeated in 6 months. After the second normal examination, annual Pap smears are recommended. Colposcopic examination is recommended for squamous intraepithelial lesions and atypical squamous cells. The Pap smear should be repeated in 3 months if there is severe inflammation with reactive squamous cellular changes. In addition to the increased frequency and aggressiveness of cervical neoplasia in HIV-infected women, these patients have a high incidence of condyloma from HPV infection. Effective treatment for ulcerative genital infections in the patient and her partners has heightened importance because the associated lesions can serve as a cofactor in HIV transmission.

Prophylaxis for Opportunistic Infections

Prophylaxis for certain opportunistic processes are initiated based on the patient's CD4 lymphocyte count and history of opportunistic infections. Patients with a prior history of PCP, oral thrush, or a CD4 lymphocyte count <200/ml should be placed on prophylaxis for PCP indefinitely. Trimethoprim/sulfamethoxazole (TMP/SMX) (generally one double-strength tablet daily) is the optimal prophylactic regimen, with dapsone (100 mg orally once daily) the preferred second choice (outside of pregnancy). Although previously popular, inhaled pentamidine can fail to adequately penetrate certain segments of the lung and provides no protection from extrapulmonary pneumocystosis. TMP/SMX is a more reasonable choice after the first trimester of pregnancy because of its superior efficacy.

For Toxoplasma IgG–positive patients, TMP/SMX (or dapsone plus pyrimethamine) provides the added benefit of prophylaxis against toxoplasmosis reactivation in addition to PCP; it is recommended by the CDC for patients with CD4 lymphocyte counts <100/ml. Toxoplasma IgG–negative patients should avoid contact with cat litter and eating undercooked meat to prevent acute primary toxoplasmosis–especially if pregnant.

PPD-positive patients with no evidence of active tuberculosis should receive isoniazid and pyridoxine for 12 months if they have not previously done so.

The CDC recommends that prophylaxis for disseminated MAC disease be considered for patients with <75 cells/ml, taking into consideration the following factors:

1. Prophylaxis can delay the onset of mycobacteremia and associated fever and anemia but does not prolong survival.
2. Active infection with *M. tuberculosis* and MAC must be ruled out before initiation of prophylaxis.
3. Prophylaxis may promote the development of antimicrobial resistance.
4. Significant drug-drug interactions and intolerance are associated with prophylactic medications. Rifabutin was the original agent approved for MAC prophylaxis, but more recent data support consideration of clarithromycin and azithromycin.

The use of prophylaxis for CMV retinitis in patients with extremely low CD4 lymphocyte counts is controversial. Although approved by the FDA, not all studies support the use of high-dose oral ganciclovir in this setting. Expense and potential hematologic side effects have caused many physicians to rely on regular (e.g., every 6 months) screening to enhance early detection of retinitis rather than employing primary prophylaxis.

Primary prophylaxis for fungal infections is not generally recommended. Frequent recurrent candidiasis can respond to intermittent or chronic therapy with topical antifungals or oral triazoles, although resistance to these agents is a growing concern. Lifelong secondary prophylaxis after primary infection with histoplasmosis, cryptococcosis, or coccidiodomycosis is always indicated because of the substantial risk for relapse in HIV-infected patients.

Patients with frequent recurrences of anogenital herpes simplex virus (HSV) infection may benefit from suppressive acyclovir or possibly one of the newer pro-drugs, famciclovir or valacyclovir. Acyclovirresistant HSV may respond to more intensive acyclovir dosing, but alternatives such as foscarnet or topical trifluridine are sometimes required.

Antiretroviral Therapy

Options for directly attacking HIV have greatly expanded since zidovudine (AZT, ZDV, Retrovir) was introduced. The initial class of antiretrovirals inhibits reverse transcriptase (RT), the enzyme necessary for deriving HIV DNA from RNA for incorporation into the host cell genome. AZT, didanosine (DDI, Videx), zalcitabine (DDC, Hivid), stavudine (D4T, Zerit), and lamivudine (3TC, Epivir) are all nucleoside RT inhibitors approved for use by the FDA. RT inhibitors that are nonnucleoside analogues (e.g., delavirdine and nevirapine) are being studied in ongoing clinical trials.

Early trials of AZT monotherapy demonstrated a survival advantage, and there was a delay in progression to AIDS-defining illnesses in patients who started AZT "early" (CD4 lymphocyte counts 200 to 500 cells/ml) compared with patients who waited until CD4 lymphocyte counts were lower (<200 cells/ml). In subsequent studies, the lack of a survival advantage in patients given early AZT compared with delayed treatment was attributed in part to the development of AZT-resistant virus.

More recent studies have focused on combination therapies and the introduction of the newer RT inhibitors. Combinations such as AZT + DDI and AZT + DDC as well as DDI monotherapy are superior to AZT monotherapy even in AZT-naive patients. Recent data suggest that AZT + lamivudine may be a another superior RT-inhibitor combination.

Protease inhibitors are the newest class of antiretroviral agents and provide the theoretical advantage of attacking the virus at an alternative site in its life cycle closer to final viral particle assembly. Of the three FDA-approved agents, ritonavir (Norvir) and indinavir (Crixivan) appear more efficacious in clinical trials than saquinavir (Invirase), possibly because of differences in bioavailability. Data from short-term clinical trials of these agents in combination with AZT in patients in an advanced stage demonstrated dramatically improved viral burdens and CD4 lymphocyte counts compared with AZT monotherapy. Correlation with long-term clinical outcome is pending.

Patients need to be monitored both for response to therapy (general well-being, weight gain, CD4 lymphocyte counts, and probably viral burden) and side effects (neurosensory examination, cell blood counts, liver enzymes, amylase levels, etc). Drug intolerance or evidence of progressive disease are the most common indications for altering the antiviral regimen. Nausea, vomiting, headache, and skin changes are side effects common to several of the agents. AZT and 3TC can suppress the bone marrow, whereas neuropathy and pancreatitis are more commonly associated with DDI, DDC, and D4T. The protease inhibitors can cause nausea and diarrhea, and alter levels of hepatically metabolized medications; indinavir is associated with nephrolithiasis. Preexisting conditions such as neuropathy or pancytopenia often preclude the use of certain agents and help to focus treatment options.

Formal clinical guidelines for the use of antiretroviral therapy rapidly become obsolete as new data and new agents become available. The timing of initiation of therapy as well as subsequent regimen modification is controversial. Such decisions are guided by changes in the patient's CD4 lymphocyte count, general sense of well-being, evidence of new opportunistic infections, side effect tolerance, and (more recently) measures of serum viral RNA burden.

Special Considerations During Pregnancy

Vertical transmission of HIV can occur antepartum and peripartum, and data suggest that infants that acquire infection in utero may have a more rapidly progressing disease course. Prolonged rupture of membranes has been associated with an increased risk of transmission. The use of cesarean section to attempt to preclude the peripartum transmission is controversial. Breastfeeding is contraindicated because of the risk of maternal-infant transmission. One of the major breakthroughs since the beginning of the AIDS epidemic was the demonstration that AZT could reduce the rate of vertical transmission from 26% to 8% when given orally to HIV-infected, AZT-naive mothers with CD4 lymphocyte counts >200/ml from the beginning of the second trimester and intravenously through labor. The newborns were also given AZT for 6 weeks. Currently AZT is recommended in a similar treatment strategy for HIV-infected pregnant women of all stages of disease and their newborns, although the risk/benefit is unknown for women with a history of prior AZT use or more advanced disease. Alternative antiretroviral agents are being studied in this setting, but it is unknown whether the dramatic reduction in serum viral load noted with the use of protease inhibitors and/or combination therapy will translate into reduced rates of vertical transmission. A complete listing of the fetal safety of medications commonly used in HIV care is beyond the scope of this book. Such risks will have to be balanced against the potential benefits to the mother and her baby. Likewise, it is unclear what effect the introduction of antiretrovirals during pregnancy will have on the mother's overall disease course.

KEY POINTS

1 HIV overwhelms the immune system by continuous destruction of CD4+ infection-fighting cells in the blood, lymph nodes, and other tissues.

2 The incidence of specific opportunistic infections increases as the HIV-infected patient's CD4 lymphocyte count falls below certain thresholds.

3 Primary care for HIV-infected women includes initial Pap smears every 6 months to either establish a normal baseline or to diagnose prevalent cervical dysplasia, neoplasia, and condyloma accuminata.

4 Pregnant HIV-infected women need to be informed of the significant potential benefits and possible risks of using antepartum and peripartum AZT to prevent perinatal transmission of HIV.

SUGGESTED READINGS

Carpenter CCJ et al for the International AIDS Society-USA: Antiretroviral therapy for HIV infection in 1996, *JAMA* 276:146-154, 1996.

CDC: *HIV/AIDS surveillance report* 7(No. 2), 1995.

CDC: 1993 revised classification system for HIV infection and expanded surveillance case definition for AIDS among adolescents and adults, *MMWR* 41(No. RR-17), 1992.

CDC: 1993 sexually transmitted diseases treatment guidelines, *MMWR* 42(No. RR-14):88-91, 1993.

CDC: Recommendations of the U.S. Public Health Service Task Force on the use of zidovudine to reduce perinatal transmission of HIV, *MMWR* 43(No. RR-11), 1994.

CDC: Update: AIDS among women–United States, 1994, *MMWR* 44(5):81-84, 1995.

CDC: USPHS/IDSA guidelines for the prevention of opportunistic infections in persons infected with human immundeficiency virus: a summary, *MMWR* 44(No. RR-8), 1995.

CDC: U.S. Public Health Service recommendations for human immunodeficiency virus counseling and voluntary testing for pregnant women, *MMWR* 44(No. RR-7), 1995.

Conner EM et al: Reduction of maternal-infant transmission of human immunodeficiency virus type 1 with zidovudine treatment, *N Engl J Med* 331:1173-1180, 1994.

Fauci AS et al: Immunopathogenic mechanisms of HIV infection, *Ann Intern Med* 124:654-663, 1996.

Fleming PL et al: Gender differences in reported AIDS-indicative diagnoses, *J Infect Dis* 168:61-67, 1993.

Landesman SH et al: Obstetrical factors and the transmission of Human Immunodeficiency Virus Type I from mother to child, *N Engl J Med* 334:1617-1623, 1996.

57

The Annual Examination

VICKI C. DARROW AND F. ALLAN HUBBELL

The annual examination is undoubtedly one of the most important mechanisms that obstetricians and gynecologists have to prevent disease and promote health. Traditionally, obstetricians and gynecologists have been at the forefront of prevention of disease as exemplified by the decrease in the incidence of cervical cancer through the recommendation of the annual Pap smear and the early identification of preeclampsia with the advent of prenatal care. The opportunity to perform evaluations on an annual basis allows obstetricians and gynecologists to continue as primary health care providers for the prevention of disease in women.

PREVENTION FOCUS

One of the primary goals of the annual examination is to prevent acute and chronic disability and premature death. To do so, it is important to be aware of the leading causes of morbidity and mortality in women. Boxes 57-1 and 57-2 list the age-related leading causes of death and morbidity.

PRINCIPLES OF SCREENING

Screening programs are most successful when certain criteria are followed:

1. The disease must have a significant effect on the quality or length of life.
2. There must be effective treatment available for the disease.
3. There must be an asymptomatic period during which detection and treatment of the disease decreases morbidity and mortality.
4. Treatment in the asymptomatic phase must produce better outcomes than treatment after symptoms develop.
5. The test must be sensitive enough to detect disease during the asymptomatic period.
6. The test must be specific enough to produce a low false positive rate.
7. The test must be acceptable to the patient.
8. The population screened must have sufficiently high disease prevalence to justify the cost.
9. The population must be accessible for testing.

Once these criteria have been met, a judgment must be made about whether the cost-effectiveness of the screening program compares favorably with other uses of health care resources.

BOX 57-1
Leading Causes of Death

Ages 13-18: Motor vehicle accidents, homicide, suicide, leukemia
Ages 19-39: Motor vehicle accidents, cardiovascular disease, homicide, AIDS, breast cancer, coronary artery disease, cerebrovascular disease, uterine cancer
Ages 40-64: Cardiovascular disease, coronary artery disease, breast cancer, lung cancer, cerebrovascular disease, colorectal cancer, obstructive pulmonary disease, ovarian cancer
Over age 65: Cardiovascular disease, coronary artery disease, cerebrovascular disease, pneumonia/influenza, obstructive lung disease, colorectal cancer, breast cancer, lung cancer, accidents

BOX 57-2
Leading Causes of Morbidity

Ages 13-39: Upper respiratory and ear infections; viral, bacterial, and parasitic infections; sexual abuse; injuries; acute urinary conditions
Age 40 and older: Upper respiratory infections, hypertension, heart disease, back pain, injuries, osteoporosis, arthritis, urinary incontinence, hearing and vision impairments

COMPONENTS OF THE ANNUAL EXAMINATION

The annual examination offers the physician an opportunity to obtain a clear and complete history from the patient that includes her personal medical history, her family history, and her psychosocial history (Fig. 57-1). A thorough, complete physical examination should be performed at the time of the annual examination, regardless of the complaint. Appropriate laboratory analysis should be ordered and should be targeted to age-based risks, history provided by the patient, and findings on physical examination.

Patient/Physician Relationship

It is crucial when obtaining a history from a patient that the physician listen carefully in a nonjudgmental way. It is often helpful to interview the patient when she is fully dressed and in a comfortable and private setting and then move to the examination room for the physical examination. While interviewing the patient, it is important to sit in a chair, maintain eye contact, and appear relaxed and receptive.

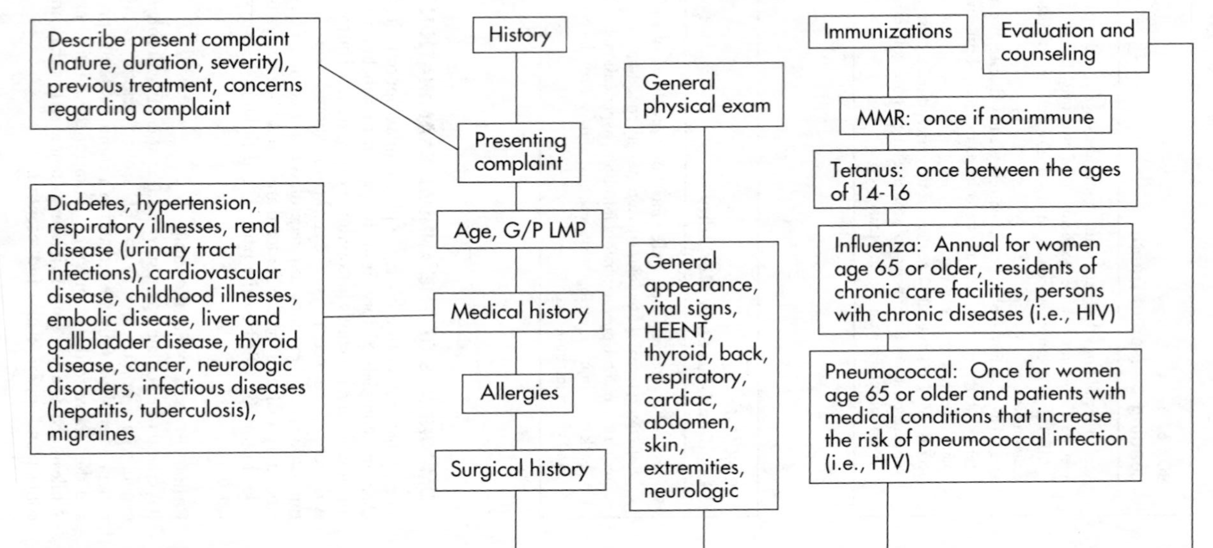
Describe present complaint (nature, duration, severity), previous treatment, concerns regarding complaint
Diabetes, hypertension, respiratory illnesses, renal disease (urinary tract infections), cardiovascular disease, childhood illnesses, embolic disease, liver and gallbladder disease, thyroid disease, cancer, neurologic disorders, infectious diseases (hepatitis, tuberculosis), migraines
History
Presenting complaint
Age, G/P LMP
Medical history
Allergies
Surgical history
General physical exam
General appearance, vital signs, HEENT, thyroid, back, respiratory, cardiac, abdomen, skin, extremities, neurologic
Immunizations
MMR: once if nonimmune
Tetanus: once between the ages of 14-16
Influenza: Annual for women age 65 or older, residents of chronic care facilities, persons with chronic diseases (i.e., HIV)
Pneumococcal: Once for women age 65 or older and patients with medical conditions that increase the risk of pneumococcal infection (i.e., HIV)
Evaluation and counseling

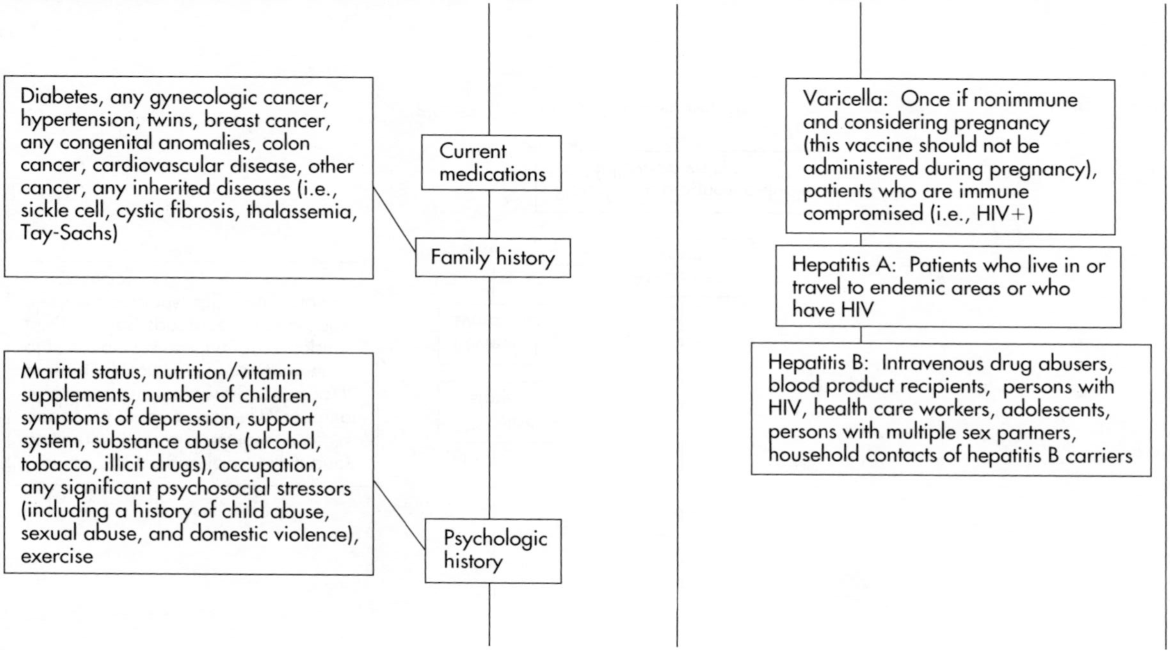

Current medications

Family history

Diabetes, any gynecologic cancer, hypertension, twins, breast cancer, any congenital anomalies, colon cancer, cardiovascular disease, other cancer, any inherited diseases (i.e., sickle cell, cystic fibrosis, thalassemia, Tay-Sachs)

Psychologic history

Marital status, nutrition/vitamin supplements, number of children, symptoms of depression, support system, substance abuse (alcohol, tobacco, illicit drugs), occupation, any significant psychosocial stressors (including a history of child abuse, sexual abuse, and domestic violence), exercise

Varicella: Once if nonimmune and considering pregnancy (this vaccine should not be administered during pregnancy), patients who are immune compromised (i.e., HIV+)

Hepatitis A: Patients who live in or travel to endemic areas or who have HIV

Hepatitis B: Intravenous drug abusers, blood product recipients, persons with HIV, health care workers, adolescents, persons with multiple sex partners, household contacts of hepatitis B carriers

FIG. 57-1 Annual examination, Part I.

Continued

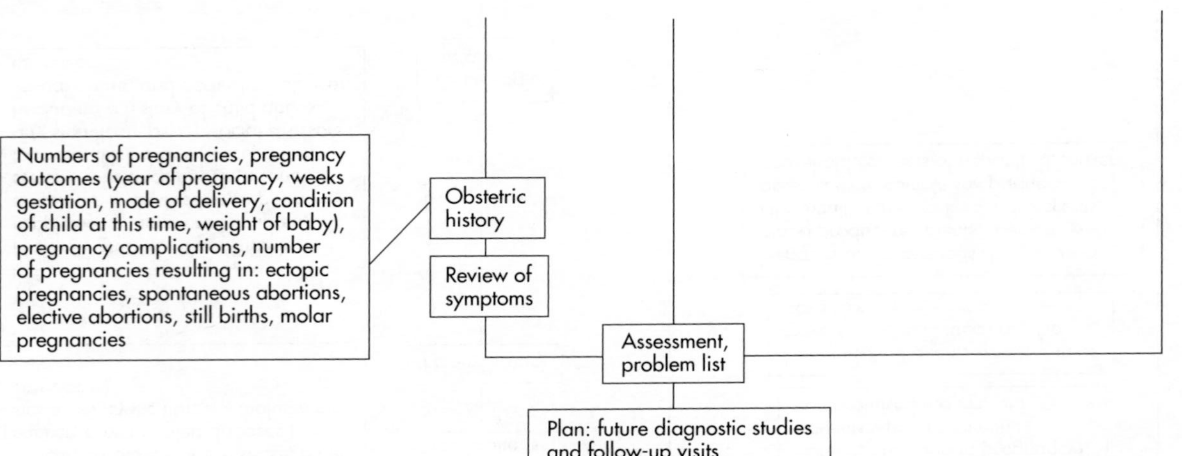

FIG. 57-1, cont'd For legend see page 509.

Patient History

The intent of obtaining a complete medical history from the patient is to investigate any illnesses that she may have had in her life that may affect her functioning at this point or effect any future health issues.

Physical Examination

A physical examination is needed for women who are young and who present for contraceptive counseling requesting only an annual Pap smear as well as for postmenopausal women requesting gynecologic care for hormone replacement (Fig. 57-2). It is recommended that a female assistant always accompany the health care provider during the physical examination. In addition to performing a complete physical examination, it is also important to document all aspects of the examination.

The breast examination

A complete breast examination should be performed. Initially the patient should be sitting in the upright position, and both breasts should be inspected visually for any abnormalities in contour or skin retraction. It is sometimes helpful to have the patient place her hands on her hips and compress so that any changes in the contour of the breasts are evident. After this inspection the patient is asked to lie on the examination table in the supine position. The patient should be draped so that each breast is examined individually while the other is covered. It is often easier to examine the breast with the patient's arm above her head. The key to an adequate breast examination is to thoroughly palpate all of the breast tissue in all quadrants, including the axillary tail. Approximately 50% of all breast cancers are found in the upper outer quadrant of the breast, which includes the tail. There are many different methods for examining the breast, all of which are acceptable. One method commonly used is to move the fingertips in a circular motion throughout the breast tissue and then to palpate the nipples, noting any discharge. In addition, the patient's axillary, supraclavicular, and suprastemal lymph nodes should be palpated. During this examination, it is important to reinforce the monthly breast self-examination. Approximately 85% of breast cancers are found by the patient.

The pelvic examination

The patient should be placed on the examining table in the dorsal lithotomy position with her head elevated to allow appropriate eye contact. The patient should empty her bladder before this examination. In addition, it is important to drape the patient appropriately so she is comfortable with the examination.

Visually inspect the entire area of the external genitalia including the vulva, labia majora and minora, clitoris, urethral meatus, and fourchette, noting evidence of lesions. Palpation should be performed along the glandular areas, including the Bartholin's and Skene's glands.

Observe the appearance of the vagina. Inspect for masses or lesions. Note any hypoestrogenic effects such as atrophy, erosions, or the presence or absence of a vaginal discharge. If the patient has any signs of vaginal vault prolapse, it is important to have her perform a Valsalva maneuver at this

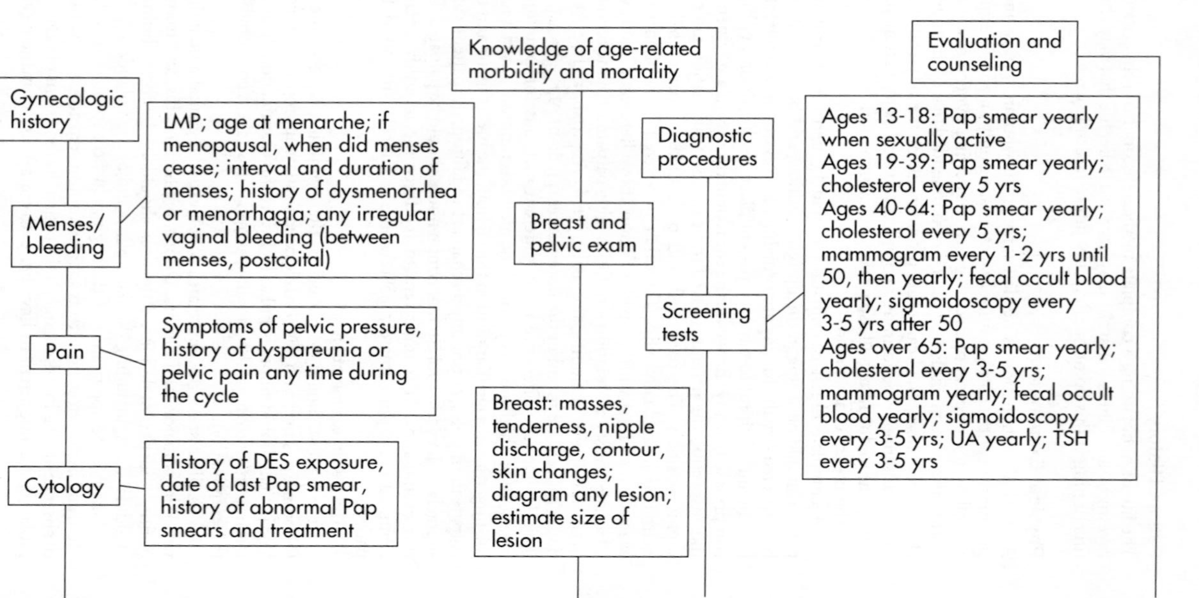
Gynecologic history
Menses/ bleeding
LMP; age at menarche; if menopausal, when did menses cease; interval and duration of menses; history of dysmenorrhea or menorrhagia; any irregular vaginal bleeding (between menses, postcoital)
Pain
Symptoms of pelvic pressure, history of dyspareunia or pelvic pain any time during the cycle
Cytology
History of DES exposure, date of last Pap smear, history of abnormal Pap smears and treatment
Knowledge of age-related morbidity and mortality
Breast and pelvic exam
Breast: masses, tenderness, nipple discharge, contour, skin changes; diagram any lesion; estimate size of lesion
Diagnostic procedures
Screening tests
Ages 13-18: Pap smear yearly when sexually active
Ages 19-39: Pap smear yearly; cholesterol every 5 yrs
Ages 40-64: Pap smear yearly; cholesterol every 5 yrs; mammogram every 1-2 yrs until 50, then yearly; fecal occult blood yearly; sigmoidoscopy every 3-5 yrs after 50
Ages over 65: Pap smear yearly; cholesterol every 3-5 yrs; mammogram yearly; fecal occult blood yearly; sigmoidoscopy every 3-5 yrs; UA yearly; TSH every 3-5 yrs
Evaluation and counseling

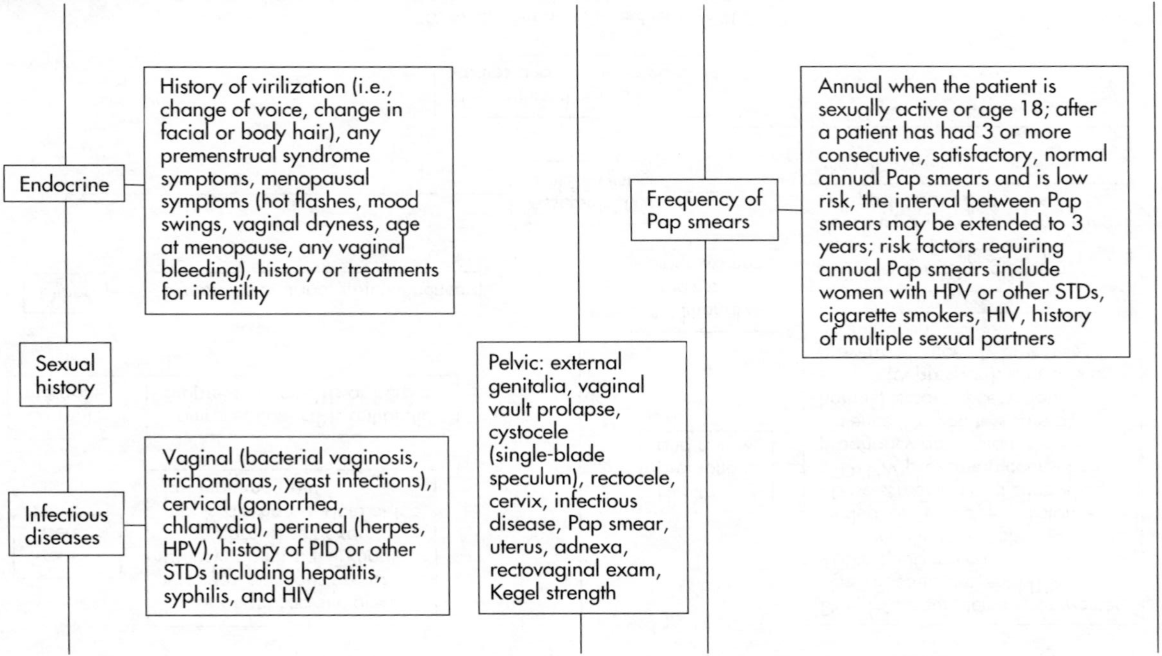

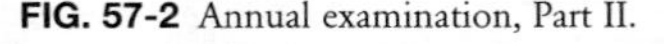

Endocrine

History of virilization (i.e., change of voice, change in facial or body hair), any premenstrual syndrome symptoms, menopausal symptoms (hot flashes, mood swings, vaginal dryness, age at menopause, any vaginal bleeding), history or treatments for infertility

Sexual history

Infectious diseases

Vaginal (bacterial vaginosis, trichomonas, yeast infections), cervical (gonorrhea, chlamydia), perineal (herpes, HPV), history of PID or other STDs including hepatitis, syphilis, and HIV

Pelvic: external genitalia, vaginal vault prolapse, cystocele (single-blade speculum), rectocele, cervix, infectious disease, Pap smear, uterus, adnexa, rectovaginal exam, Kegel strength

Frequency of Pap smears

Annual when the patient is sexually active or age 18; after a patient has had 3 or more consecutive, satisfactory, normal annual Pap smears and is low risk, the interval between Pap smears may be extended to 3 years; risk factors requiring annual Pap smears include women with HPV or other STDs, cigarette smokers, HIV, history of multiple sexual partners

FIG. 57-2 Annual examination, Part II.

Continued

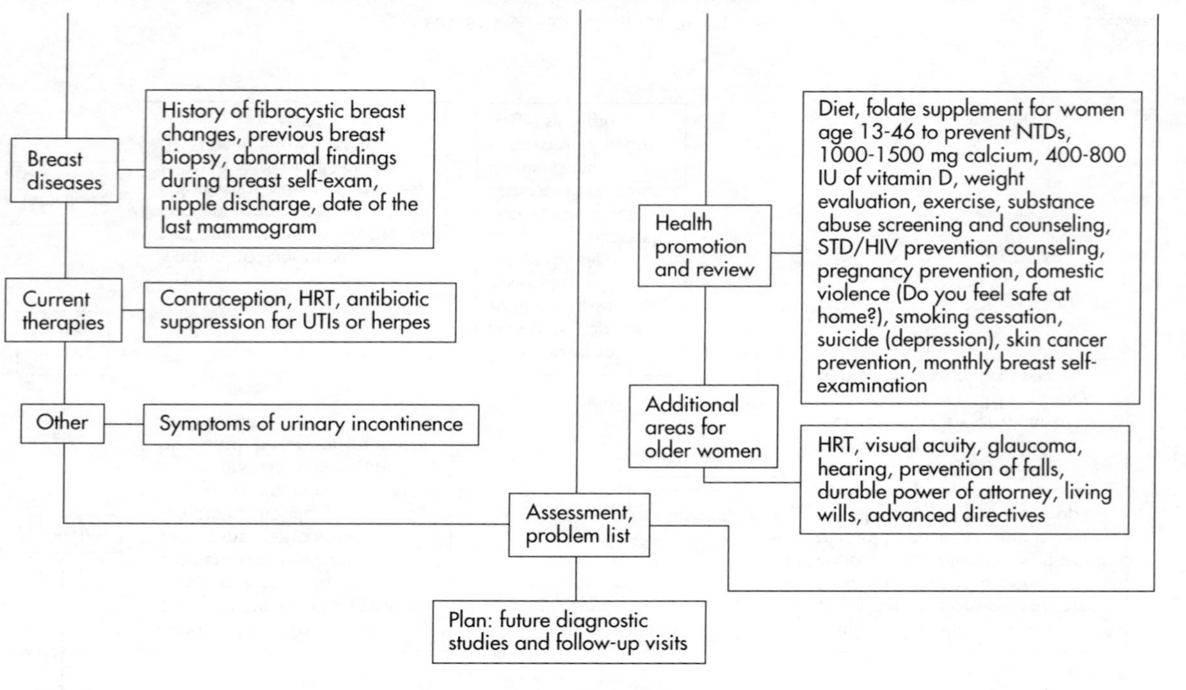

FIG. 57-2, cont'd For legend see page 513.

point to evaluate for rectocele, enterocele, and cystocele. A warm speculum is then gently inserted into the vagina. It is perfectly acceptable to lubricate the speculum with water or a small amount of lubricant. The walls of the vagina are inspected as the speculum is inserted, and then the cervix is viewed. Visually inspect the cervix for state of parity and any abnormalities, including lesions, polyps, discharge, or bleeding. If the patient has any concerns about a vaginal discharge or any sexually transmitted disease or pelvic pain, it is important to obtain a wet mount specimen and cultures.

Bacterial vaginosis, trichomonas, or vaginal yeast infection are best diagnosed by wet mount rather than by culture. To perform a wet mount, place a cotton-tip applicator inside the vagina and remove some of the discharge. Apply the cotton-tip applicator to two glass slides, one of which has saline and the other KOH. KOH is used to perform the Whiff test for bacterial vaginosis and to examine under the microscope for the presence or absence of candida.

Perform cultures for chlamydia and gonorrhea in the endocervical area. Since chlamydia is an obligate intracellular organism, it is imperative to obtain endocervical cells for diagnosis by placing a dacron-tipped applicator inside the endocervix. Since 50% of women diagnosed with chlamydia are asymptomatic, it is important to have a high index of suspicion and to screen frequently. Prevalence of chlamydia does vary according to populations, and routine screening should be considered in areas with high prevalence.

To perform the Pap smear, the ectocervical area that includes the entire portion and transformation zone is sampled with a wooden spatula in a 360° fashion. The cytobrush is then gently inserted into the endocervix, rotated 360°, and then removed and wiped on a cytology slide. It is important to spray the slide immediately with a fixative to reduce the incidence of drying artifact. The speculum is then gently removed.

A single-blade speculum examination is needed with any evidence of prolapse or any history of urinary incontinence. The speculum is split in half, and the single blade of the speculum is then replaced into the vagina. Initially this is placed in the posterior area of the vagina, the patient is asked to perform the Valsalva maneuver, and the degree of prolapse is noted. The single blade is moved circumferentially around the vagina. In addition, the patient is asked to cough to see if there is any demonstration of stress incontinence. In addition to this examination in the supine position, it is also important to repeat the single-blade speculum examination in the upright position to further determine the degree of prolapse and any additional evidence of incontinence (see Chapter 23).

To do a bimanual examination, place a small amount of lubricant on your examination fingers and gently place your fingers inside the patient's vaginal vault, moving very slowly and gently to the cervix. Note the consistency, size, and mobility of the cervix. Place your other hand on the patient's abdomen to palpate the uterus and adnexal structures. Note the size, shape, consistency, position, and mobility of the uterus and the presence or absence of tenderness. The examination should include palpation of the uterosacral ligaments and posterior cul-de-sac. When examining the adnexa, note the size, position, and mobility of the ovaries and the presence or absence of masses and tenderness. It is important to confirm your bimanual exam with a rectovaginal exam. In addition, for women over the age of 40, a stool sample should be obtained and tested for fecal occult blood.

It is important to instruct all women in the proper use of Kegel exercises. These exercises build pelvic floor support, which prevents or improves symptoms of urinary incontinence. At the conclusion of the bimanual examination and before the rectovaginal examination, place one or two fingers in the patient's vagina. Ask her to tighten her vagina around your fingers. These exercises are most effective when the pubococcygeus muscle is contracted in isolation from other surrounding muscles so that the abdominal and gluteal muscles remain relaxed. Symmetry of the contraction, strength, and duration should be noted. A woman with good perineal strength can usually hold the contraction for 6 seconds or more. Instruct the patient to perform these exercises by squeezing 3 to 10 seconds and then relaxing for 3 to 10 seconds in sets of 6 to 10, 4 to 5 times per day. She should not do a larger quantity at one time because this may cause muscle fiber fatigue.

In addition, do not instruct the patient to perform Kegel exercises while urinating. During micturition the detrusor muscle of the bladder is contracting while the urethra is relaxing. If you override this process by repetitively contracting the muscles to stop urine, this may cause long-term nerve damage to the system.

Health promotion screening and review

It is useful to evaluate the patient for any age-related risk factors and then to counsel her with the appropriate recommendations. For the older woman, counseling may address hormone replacement therapy, visual acuity, glaucoma, hearing, environmental control and prevention of falls, durable power of attorney, living will, and advanced directives.

Cardiovascular risk factors

It is important to evaluate and counsel the patient regarding cardiovascular risk factors including family history, hypertension, hyperlipidemia, obesity, diabetes, and lifestyle.

Sexual history and STD/HIV prevention

It is important to assess high-risk behaviors and to discuss frankly the importance of barrier methods to protect against STDs, which include HIV, hepatitis, syphilis, gonorrhea, and chlamydia. Counseling regarding sexual function and contraceptive options is also important.

Diagnostic Procedures

Diagnostic procedures should be geared toward age-related and high-risk circumstances that pertain to a particular patient. Screening tests are intended to reduce morbidity and mortality in a group at a reasonable cost. Criteria for appropriate screening tests include (1) the disease is significant in terms of prevalence, morbidity, and mortality, (2) screening, and thus early detection, can reduce the morbidity or mortality, and, (3) the screening test is safe, reasonably priced, sensitive, and specific (Table 57-1).

With all diagnostic procedures, it is imperative that appropriate

TABLE 57-1
Risk Factors as Indications for Screening Tests

Test	Risk factor
Varicella and rubella titer	Women of child-bearing age lacking evidence of immunity
PPD test	Close contact with a person with TB, HIV-infected patients, health care workers, patient resided in country or institution of high prevalence
Lipid profile	Elevated cholesterol, history of parent or sibling with high cholesterol or premature coronary artery disease, diabetes mellitus, smoking
Mammogram	35 years or older, family history of premenopausally diagnosed breast cancer in a first-degree relative (or 10 years before the age at diagnosis of family member's breast cancer)
Fasting glucose every 3-5 yrs	Family history of diabetes, history of gestational diabetes, obese
Thyroid-stimulating hormone	Family history of thyroid disease, other autoimmune disease
Colonoscopy	History of inflammatory bowel disease or polyps; family history of polyps, colorectal cancer
Bacteriuria testing	Persons with diabetes mellitus
HIV testing	Persons with STDs, intravenous drug abusers, history of multiple partners, reside in area of high prevalence, blood transfusion 1978-1985, abnormal cervical cytology, pregnancy
STD testing	Multiple sexual partners, partner with multiple contacts, history of repeated episodes
Hemoglobin	Persons of Caribbean, Latin American, Asian, Mediterranean, African heritage, excessive menstrual flow

follow-up be obtained so that any abnormalities in the diagnostic tests will be acted on expeditiously.

CONCLUSION OF THE ANNUAL EXAM

At the conclusion of the annual exam, it is important to discuss your findings, normal and abnormal, with the patient. She may have questions provoked by the history and physical examination process and these should be answered. And finally, you should discuss your recommendations for continued prevention of disease and health promotion and your recommendation for follow-up. It is often helpful to develop a problem list. List current problems, any past problems of significance to the patient's current status, further diagnostic workup planned for each problem, treatment planned, date of identification and resolution for each problem, medications, drug allergies, and plans for health maintenance (i.e., date of Pap smear, mammogram, PPD test).

KEY POINTS

1. The annual examination is the primary mechanism for the prevention of disease and promotion of health. Be aware of the leading causes of morbidity and mortality in women and evaluate women based on age-related risks.
2. During every annual examination, a complete medical and psychosocial history should be obtained from the patient, irrespective of her presenting complaint. In addition, all aspects of the presenting complaint should be evaluated historically.
3. A complete physical examination should be performed.
4. Age- and risk-related screening diagnostic procedures should be performed in addition to diagnostic studies for any abnormalities noted on the patient's history and physical examination. Appropriate immunizations should also be performed.

SUGGESTED READINGS

ACOG Task Force on Primary and Preventive Health Care: *The obstetrician-gynecologist and primary-preventive health care,* 1993, ACOG.

ACOG: *Health maintenance for perimenopausal women,* technical bulletin no. 210, August 1995, ACOG.

ACOG: *Cervical cytology: evaluation and management of abnormalities,* technical bulletin. No 183, August 1993, ACOG.

Carlson KJ et al: *Primary care of women,* St. Louis, 1995, Mosby.

Herbst AL et al: *Comprehensive gynecology,* ed 2, St. Louis, 1992, Mosby.

Lemcke DP et al: *Primary care of women,* Norwalk, 1995, Appleton and Lange.

Nichols DH, Sweeney PJ: *Ambulatory gynecology,* ed 2, Philadelphia, 1995, JB Lippincott.

Scott JR et al: *Danforth's obstetrics and gynecology,* ed 7, Philadelphia, 1995, JB Lippincott.

Seltzer VL, Pearse WH: *Women's primary health care office practice and procedures,* New York, 1995, McGraw-Hill.

Urinary Incontinence Guideline Panel: *Urinary incontinence in adults: clinical practice guideline,* AHCPR Pub No. 92-0038, Rockville, Md, Agency for Health Care Policy and Research, Public Health Services, US Dept Health and Human Services, March 1992.

58

Anxiety Reaction

CHRISTOPHER M. DEGROOT

Women's primary care physicians have a major role in the diagnosis and treatment of anxiety disorders. These physicians are often the first and many times the only health care provider for anxious women. Of the most common psychiatric illnesses in the general population, woman may be three times more likely to suffer an anxiety disorder than men. Although there are different types of anxiety disorders, several generalizations can be made: somatic symptoms are often prominent, anxiety symptoms have specific characteristics, and effective treatment modalities exist (Fig. 58-1). The anxiety disorders reviewed in this chapter are included in the *Diagnostic and Statistical Manual of Mental Disorders,* fourth edition (DSM-IV).

OBSESSIVE-COMPULSIVE DISORDER

Obsessive-compulsive disorder (OCD) is characterized by recurrent unwanted obsessions or compulsions that cause marked distress and significantly interfere with normal, routine functioning or relationships. Previously thought to be a rare disorder, current data suggest OCD is quite common, with a 1-month prevalence of 1.3% and a lifetime rate of 2.5%. The age of onset is between 10 and 25 years for more than 70% of patients.

Description

Obsessions are recurrent, persistent thoughts or impulses typically experienced as intrusive and inappropriate. These thoughts cause significant anxiety, and the person tries to ignore, suppress, or neutralize them. Common obsessions include contamination fears, unbidden violent images, fears of harming oneself or others, forbidden sexual thoughts, and impulses toward symmetry or exactness.

Compulsions are repetitive behaviors or mental acts performed in response to an obsession or to prevent or reduce a dreaded situation. Common compulsions include checking, cleaning or washing, counting, repeating, ordering, and collecting or hoarding. Mental compulsions are also common. For example, patients may systematically repeat particular words or sentences to ward off evil or feared catastrophic occurrences. In most clinical samples, multiple obsessions and compulsions are present.

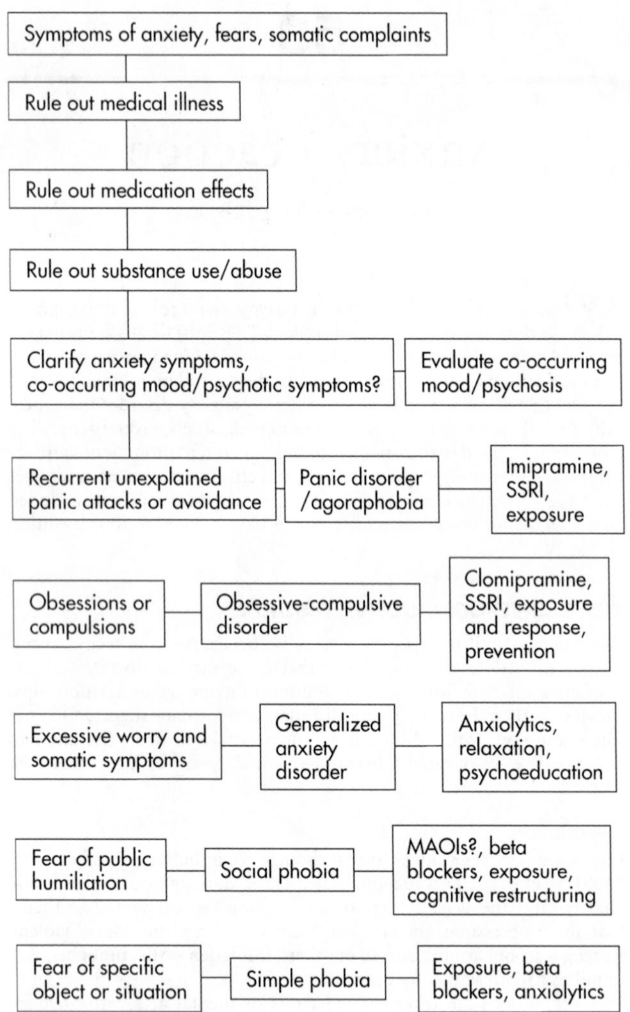

FIG. 58-1 Management of anxiety reactions.

Differential Diagnosis

The symptoms of OCD must be differentiated from schizophrenia, major depression, simple phobias, Tourette's syndrome, amphetamine intoxication, and obsessive-compulsive personality disorder. In contrast to schizophrenia, bizarre behavior is limited to execution of compulsive rituals. Irrational convictions are limited to obsessional ideation. Depressive ruminations can be similar to obsessions, but tend to have a clear depressive or guilty quality and resolve with mood resolution. Compulsive behavior associated with amphetamine or cocaine intoxication is mechanical and without the obsessional quality and intent of OCD.

Etiology

The neurobiologic hypothesis of OCD posits dysfunction of brain serotonin (5-hydroxytryptamine) neurotransmitter systems. Evidence rests on the efficacy of serotonergic reuptake inhibitors in reducing symptoms, indirect measures of abnormal CNS serotonin levels, and induction of OC symptoms with serotonin agonists. Cognitive theories suggest a defect in cognitive information processing with a mismatch between beliefs and sensory data. For example, patients believe their hands remain dirty because they do not "feel" clean. Behavioral theorists invoke a two-stage classical instrumental conditioning model. Spontaneous anxiety is conditioned to otherwise neutral environmental stimuli. Initially unrelated compulsive rituals decrease anxiety and are thus reinforced. Successful avoidance and anxiety reduction through ritual performance preserves behaviors.

Treatment

The mainstay of nonpharmacologic treatment of OCD is behavioral therapy through exposure and response prevention. Exposure to feared objects or situations will decrease anxiety through habituation. Response prevention aims to decrease compulsive rituals. Briefly, patients are instructed to expose themselves to feared situations and to avoid anxiety-reducing rituals or compulsions.

The tricyclic antidepressant (TCA) clomipramine (CMI) is the best studied medication that is effective in the pharmacologic treatment of OCD. It is believed that CMI's prominent serotonergic effects are responsible for the reduction of OCD symptoms. CMI, like other TCAs, has many unfortunate anticholinergic side effects that may warrant consideration of a selective serotonin reuptake inhibitor (SSRI). Fluoxetine, sertraline, fluvoxamine, and paroxetine reduce OCD symptoms, and because of their fewer side effects may be advantageous first choices.

Once a diagnosis of OCD is made, an SSRI can be started with the expectation of improvement over 8 to 12 weeks. Dosages somewhat higher than those used for antidepressant effects may be required. Failure of improvement in 2 to 3 months warrants a change in medication to CMI, another SSRI, or psychiatric consultation.

PANIC DISORDER WITH OR WITHOUT AGORAPHOBIA

Panic disorder is common and often disabling. Lifetime prevalence in the general population is 1.5%. Females may be at greater risk than males. Panic attacks occur in other anxiety disorders, including social phobia, special phobia, and posttraumatic stress disorder. Although patients may fear "going crazy," psychotic illness is not an outcome of panic disorder. The significance of the association of panic disorder and mitral valve prolapse (MVP) is controversial.

Description

Panic disorder is subdivided into panic disorder with or without agoraphobia. Panic attacks are characterized as periods of discrete, circumscribed, intense fear or discomfort with physical/psychologic symptoms that typically reach a peak within 10 minutes and are largely resolved within 30 minutes. Somatic symptoms include palpitations, paresthesias, sweating, feelings of choking, nausea, dizziness, and trembling. Psychologic symptoms include a sense of impending doom, derealization, or depersonalization. Some patients experience panic that awakens them from sleep. Agoraphobia consists of excessive fear and usually avoidance of situations in which escape would be difficult or help unavailable were an attack to occur. Agoraphobic avoidance may become the most debilitating symptom.

Etiologies

Biologic theories implicate specific neurotransmitter abnormalities of the adrenergic, serotonergic, benzodiazepine, and opiate neurotransmitter systems. Behavior theorists hypothesize that the random pairing of events (contiguity learning) leads to agoraphobia. For example, the spontaneous onset of a panic attack may be linked with driving on the freeway. Subsequently, instrumental learning or operant conditioning (modification of behavior to avoid future negative events) results in phobic avoidance (fear of driving). Alternatively, phobic avoidance is thought to be a learned adaptive (decreased anxiety) response to internal rather than external stimuli. Patients associate somatic sensation with perceived threats, anxiety, and fear and seek ways of diminishing or avoiding overwhelming anxiety.

Differential Diagnosis

Panic disorder may mimic a variety of serious medical illnesses, including disturbances of the gastrointestinal, neurologic, endocrinologic, or cardiovascular systems. Nevertheless, a careful history and clinical evaluation should clarify the diagnostic impression. A common case presentation is of subjective feelings that a catastrophic cardiovascular or neurologic event has occurred, yet no objective signs or symptoms arise to substantiate such an occurrence.

Along with the consideration of a medical etiology, the possibility of alcohol or other substance-induced anxiety should be considered. A careful review of all medications may uncover use of anxiogenic drugs (e.g., pseudoephedrine).

Panic disorder is often associated with other psychiatric disorders, including major depression, other anxiety disorders (specific phobia), and substance use. Patients suffering from depression often manifest signs of anxiety and agitation and may have frank panic attacks. Patients with panic disorder alone generally do not demonstrate the full range of vegetative symptoms that are seen in depression. Most anxious patients do not lose the capacity to enjoy things or to be cheered up as endogenously depressed patients do. Panic disorder differs from generalized anxiety disorder in that true panic attacks are distinguished by discrete intense episodes of anxiety.

Treatment

The most established medication for the treatment of panic disorder with or without agoraphobia is the TCA imipramine hydrochloride. Other TCAs may also be effective. Monoamine oxidase inhibitors (MAOIs) are also very effective; however, the strict low-tyramine diet required is often not tolerated. Preliminary data suggest that the SSRIs, including sertraline, fluvoxamine, fluoxetine, and paroxetine, may also be effective. Trazodone and bupropion appear to be less effective. Short-term use of a long half-life benzodiazepine is often helpful, particularly while waiting for the full anxiolytic effect of an antidepressant (6 to 8 weeks).

Prolonged exposure in vivo is the most effective nonpharmacologic approach. Patients are exposed to least-feared situations and gradually exposed to more severe stressors. Cognitive therapy may have a role in the reduction of irrational beliefs and the introduction of positive thoughts or relaxation techniques. Psychoeducation has an important role in reassuring patients who may believe they have a life-threatening condition. A combination of behavioral therapy and pharmacologic intervention is most often employed.

GENERALIZED ANXIETY DISORDER

Generalized anxiety disorder (GAD) is characterized by excessive worry about multiple life circumstances, accompanied by symptoms of tension, restlessness, fatigue, difficulty with sleep, and irritability. The experienced anxiety should be unrelated to panic disorder, phobias, obsessions, substance use, or medical illness. The 1-month prevalence rate is estimated at 2.5%. The age of onset is typically in the second or third decade; however, GAD may begin in childhood as over-anxious disorder. The course of GAD is usually chronic.

Description

Excessive anxiety or worry needs to have been present for more than six months. Patients will report having a difficult time controlling the extent of their worries, resulting in significant distress or functional impairment. Associated symptoms include restlessness, fatigue, muscular tension, sleep disturbance, poor concentration, or gastrointestinal complaints.

Treatment

Nonpharmacologic interventions include behavioral treatment with progressive muscle relaxation and anxiety management. Other forms of psychotherapy have had only partial success. The most common pharmacologic intervention is the use of benzodiazepine anxiolytics such as diazepam, alprazolam, lorazepam, and clonazepam. The disadvantages of anxiolytics include sedation and abuse potential. An alternative choice is the azaspirone anxiolytic buspirone. Some evidence exists that the TCAs and SSRIs are also effective in treating GAD and are useful alternatives in patients with histories of alcohol or substance use. In contrast to the rapid anxiolytic effects of benzodiazepines, a therapeutic response to antidepressants may require several weeks.

POSTTRAUMATIC STRESS DISORDER

Posttraumatic stress disorder (PTSD) is characterized by the delayed development of specific debilitating symptoms after personal exposure to a catastrophic event. Examples of traumas include combat, natural disasters (flood, earthquake), physical assault (rape, mugging), or witnessing a death. A latent period of months or years may intervene between the trauma and the onset of symptoms.

Description

The affected individual must have seen or experienced a serious or traumatic event. This event is persistently or periodically reexperienced by recollections, dreams, or flashbacks. The affected person avoids stimuli that symbolizes or cues the experienced trauma. In addition, patients have symptoms of marked arousal including hypervigilance, irritability, and poor concentration. Mood disturbance is a typically prominent characteristic. These symptoms cause significant distress and social or occupational impairment. High rates of alcohol and substance abuse problems occur with PTSD.

Treatment

Early intervention may minimize subsequent symptoms. Usually a combination of pharmacologic and psychologic treatment is optimal. Medications should be targeted to specific symptoms (e.g., antidepressants for depressed mood). Nonpharmacologic interventions include both individual and group supportive therapies. Group therapy may be particularly helpful for those with shared traumatic experiences (e.g., combat or surviving a plane crash). There are few controlled trials for the treatment of PTSD. Phenelzine and imipramine reduce intrusion (reexperiencing) but have little affect on avoidant behaviors. Clonidine and propranolol relieve explosiveness, nightmares, and intrusive reexperiencing in some patients.

ACUTE STRESS DISORDER

Victims of disasters such as fire and earthquake are often at risk for the development of PTSD-like symptoms. The likelihood of developing

PTSD-like symptoms is highly correlated with the severity of the initial traumatic exposure. The diagnosis is made when the level of personal or occupational distress becomes clinically significant. In most cases the course is self limiting, and medication is not necessarily indicated. If the duration of symptoms is greater than 1 month, the diagnosis of PTSD may be considered.

SOCIAL PHOBIA

Commonly seen in otherwise healthy persons, a persistent and overwhelming fear of social or occupational dysfunction may indicate social phobia. Estimates of the 6-month prevalence are 1.2% to 2.2%. The distribution appears to be even across age spans. Typically, the onset of social phobia is between 15 and 20 years, and the course is most often chronic. Complications include associated alcohol use and comorbid depression.

Description

Patients suffer persistent and exaggerated fears of embarrassment in social situations. Examples include speaking in public, being unable to urinate in public, or the inability to have a conversation in public. Exposure to the feared social situation inevitably invokes severe anxiety. The affected person recognizes that their fear is excessive; nevertheless, feared situations are avoided.

Differential Diagnosis

The principal differential diagnostic dilemma is between social phobia and normal performance anxiety. Normal performance anxiety tends to diminish with exposure, whereas phobic social interaction does not attenuate. In contrast to panic disorder, social phobics experience situational panic resulting from exposure to social situations. Panic disorder and social phobia may coexist. The avoidant behavior associated with major depression resolves with remission of the depressive episode.

Treatment

Low-dose beta blockers will attenuate the prominent sympathetic component to social phobia. There is also evidence that the MAOI phenelzine may prove useful. Nonpharmacologic interventions include repeated exposure to feared social conditions, relaxation training, and cognitive restructuring. The combination of exposure and cognitive restructuring techniques appear to be superior to either treatment alone.

SPECIFIC PHOBIA

Previously named *simple phobia,* specific phobia refers to the development of phobic anxiety or avoidance of circumscribed objects or places (blood/injections/injury), situations (elevators, planes), or the natural environment (water, insects). Social phobia is thought to have a 6-month prevalence rate of 5% to 11%, with a higher rate for females than males. The age of onset varies with specific phobias (e.g., blood phobia in adolescence and animal phobia in childhood).

Description
Specific phobia presents as marked and persistent fears that are cued by a specific object or situation. Exposure to the feared object or situation immediately elicits an anxiety response. The patient recognizes the phobic anxiety, and fear is excessive. Blood phobia is the most common example.

Differential Diagnosis
Unlike social phobia, fears do not involve fear of scrutiny or embarrassment, and unlike agoraphobia the fear is not of being trapped or of having a panic attack. Isolated fears are common in the population, thus a diagnosis of specific phobia is reserved for situations causing marked distress and impairment.

Treatment
The standard treatment is exposure to the feared object or situation to achieve habitation or extinction of the anxious response. When exposure to phobic stimulus is infrequent and predictable, benzodiazepines on an as-needed basis may be appropriate.

KEY POINTS

1 Assessment of female anxious patients should include a comprehensive evaluation of potential pharmacologic and medical etiologies of anxious symptoms with particular attention to medical disorders that occur more commonly in women (e.g., systemic lupus erythematosus, thyroid dysfunction, and anemia).

2 Treatment of anxiety disorders usually includes a combination of pharmacologic and psychosocial interventions specific to the anxiety disorder.

3 Pharmacologic treatment in pregnant women presents particular challenges. Tricyclic antidepressants are the best studied; however, all psychotropics have a potential for teratogenic effects. Consultation with psychiatric physicians may be helpful.

4 The differing pharmacokinetics and pharmacodynamics between men and women is not well understood; thus careful monitoring of medication plasma levels is recommended. Additionally, dosage adjustment may be warranted during menstrual periods, pregnancy, the postpartum period, and menopause.

SUGGESTED READINGS

American Psychiatric Association: *Diagnostic and statistical manual of mental disorders*, ed 4, 1994, the Association, pp 393-444.

Hollander E, Simeon D, Gorman JM: Anxiety disorders. In Hales RE, Yudofsky SC, Talbott JA, eds: *Textbook of psychiatry*, ed 2, 1994, American Psychiatric Press.

59

Arthritis and Related Musculoskeletal Disorders

PAMELA E. PRETE

OSTEOARTHRITIS

Osteoarthritis (OA), or degenerative joint disease (DJD), is the most common arthritic disease. It is confined to the joints and results from a progressive loss of articular cartilage, with new bone formation in the subchondral trabeculae and at the joint margins (osteophytes). Approximately 80% of those 75 or older are affected; women are about twice as likely as men to be affected. Obesity is associated with a higher incidence, especially in the knee. OA is classified into idiopathic (primary) and secondary forms.

Pathophysiology

Major trauma and repetitive use are implicated as causes of OA. Genetic factors suggest an autosomal dominant transmission in women and recessive inheritance in men. Recent studies uncovering a point mutation in the cDNA cloning for type II collagen in several generations of a family demonstrate that an osteoarthritic disorder can develop in association with a generalized genetic defect in the matrix of articular cartilage. Cartilage loss results from destruction of matrix collagen from increases in collagenases and loss of proteoglycans and hyaluronan content.

Clinical Features

Symptoms of pain occur after joint use and are relieved by rest in OA. Signs are usually localized tenderness over various components of the joint and pain on passive or active motion. Osteoarthritic changes in weight-bearing joints are suggested by a limp or loss of motion. Spinal osteoarthritis results from involvement of the intervertebral discs, vertebral bodies, and/or posterior apophyseal articulations. OA can occur in joints generally considered protected from OA (i.e., elbows, shoulders, interphalangeal joints of toes) if trauma or repetitive overuse is present. Primary generalized (nodal) osteoarthritis involves the distal and proximal interphalangeal joints of the hands. Heberden's nodes (bone spurs formed at the dorsolateral and medial aspects of the distal interphalangeal joints) are characteristic; similar changes at the proximal interphalangeal joints are called *Bouchard's nodes.* The first carpometacarpal joint, knees, hips, and metatarsophalangeal joints are also affected. Synovial fluid appears normal, with the cell count <1000/mm^3. Plain roentgenograms are insensitive and CT, MRI, and ultrasonographic techniques rule out soft tissue lesions or internal joint structure derangements (i.e., torn menisci) but provide little additional information.

Management and Treatment

Key is the protection of joints from overuse, which includes orthotic or assistive devices such as canes, and weight loss or lifestyle adjustments. Analgesic agents such as acetaminophen, administered 2 or 3 tablets every 4 to 6 hours, are very effective for OA pain. Other analgesic agents include aspirin and nonsteroidal antiinflammatory drugs (NSAIDs). Oral or parenteral therapy with adrenal corticosteroids is never indicated, but intraarticular injections of corticosteroids may be beneficial (not more frequently than once every 3 to 4 months). Hip and knee replacement produce striking pain relief and improved range of motion in disabled OA patients. Physical therapy is useful, and arthroscopic irrigation is controversial. Osteoarthritis of the first carpometacarpal joint responds to intraarticular steroids and splinting. Spinal symptoms can benefit from support, such as a cervical collar or lumbosacral corset.

RHEUMATOID ARTHRITIS

Rheumatoid arthritis (RA) is an autoimmune disorder characterized by a symmetric and erosive synovitis of peripheral joints and multisystem involvement. Nonarticular manifestations include subcutaneous nodules, vasculitis, pericarditis, pulmonary nodules, interstitial lung fibrosis, mononeuritis multiplex, episcleritis, Sjögren's and Felty's syndromes. It is estimated between 1% and 2% of the adult population is affected with definite or classic RA, with a 2.5 to 1, female to male ratio. Oral contraceptives decrease the risk of RA, and symptom onset during menopause is common.

Pathophysiology

The cause of RA is unknown. A majority of patients with RA have the class II MHC alleles DR4, or share epitopes or conformationally equivalent structures in the DR beta chains. Rheumatoid factor is found in the serum of 85% of patients. There is a synovial fluid leucocytosis (WBC >2000/mm^3), histologic presence of a chronic proliferative synovitis, and radiologic evidence of characteristic marginal joint erosions. Erythrocyte sedimentation rate (ESR) and other acute phase reactants, such as C-reactive protein, are elevated and are used to measure activity of the disease.

Clinical Features

Clinical features include morning stiffness, often lasting more than 1 hour, and erythematous effusions in multiple tender joints. Although RA spares the spine, cervical involvement is frequent, with significant C1-C2 instability producing myelopathy. Small joints of the hand and wrist are affected in 75% of patients, with sparing of the distal interphalangeal (DIP) joints. Classic deformities include ulnar drift at the metacarpophalangeal (MCP) joints, radial deviation at the wrists, swan-neck deformities (hyperextension at the proximal interphalangeal (PIP joints; flexion at the DIP joints), and boutonniere deformities (flexion at the PIP joints, hyperextension at the DIP joints). Major weight-bearing joints and the feet are similarly affected. A diagnosis of RA is confirmed when four out of the following seven criteria are present for 6 weeks or more: (1) morning stiffness, (2) arthritis in three or more joints, (3) arthritis in hands or wrists, (4) symmetric arthritis, (5) RA nodules, (6) RF factor, and (7) x-ray changes.

RA is a systemic disease. Rheumatoid nodules are characteristic, subcutaneous, rubbery lumps, usually located at the olecranon or along the Achilles' tendon. Small-vessel vasculitis in RA presents as digital infarcts. Sicca syndrome (dry eye, dry mouth) and secondary Sjögren's syndrome can appear as well as scleritis, with significant eye damage and visual loss called *scleromalacia perforans.* The mortality from pulmonary disease in RA is twice that of the general population. It can present as interstitial fibrosis, bronchiolitis obliterans, or solitary and multiple nodules. Pleuritis and small pleural effusions are often seen on chest x-rays with disease activity. Characteristically, the pleural fluid has a very low glucose level. Pericardial abnormalities or an effusion are also seen. Glomerular disease is absent or rare in RA. If proteinuria develops, it is usually either related to a drug therapy toxicity (gold or penicillamine) or secondary to amyloidosis. Neurologic complications are usually myelopathies related to cervical spine instability or entrapment neuropathies (carpal or tarsal tunnel syndromes) or ischemic neuropathies caused by complicating small-vessel vasculitis. Anemia of chronic disease is an almost universal accompaniment of active RA. Felty's syndrome is a combination of longstanding RA, with splenomegaly, leucopenia, and leg ulcers.

Management and Treatment

Prognosis of RA is uncertain because of its prolonged, inherently variable, and chronic natural course, and the difficulty in detecting subclinical forms of the disease. Basic treatment consists of patient education, balance between rest and exercise (often with physical and occupational therapy), and use of aspirin (ASA) or other NSAIDs in adequate doses to maintain a therapeutic serum level. However, aspirin is not tolerated in therapeutic doses in a number of patients. Rare hypersensitivity reactions such as asthma, nasal polyps, angioedema, and urticaria can be seen, but the most common side effects are tinnitus or gastropathy (gastritis, gastric ulceration, and bleeding). Misoprostol, an oral prostaglandin analogue, may be indicated in high-risk patients on aspirin or NSAIDs to reduce the risk of gastric ulceration (H-2 blockers only protect against duodenal symptoms). Nonacetylated or buffered salicylates induce fewer gastric symptoms. Specific NSAIDs (indomethacin and tolmetin) produce headache, dizziness, and confusion. Toxic amblyopia and aseptic meningitis have been reported with ibuprofen use. Glucocorticoids do not have disease modification potential but are indicated when vasculitis complicates the RA course. Intraarticular steroids may be helpful when one or two joints flare out of proportion.

Patients who do not respond are referred for second-line therapy (disease-modifying antirheumatic drugs, [DMARDS]). Gold salts have been used in the treatment of RA for about 60 years. Methotrexate is the second-line treatment of choice and an excellent remittive agent. A folic acid antagonist, methotrexate can be given orally or by injection, and the usual starting dose is 7.5 mg/week, with a clinical response seen in 6 to 8 weeks. A liver biopsy is suggested after 1.5 to 2 g of cumulative methotrexate or every 2 to 3 years. Penicillamine (a chelator of heavy metals) is also useful. Penicillamine is initiated in a dose of 250 mg/day and slowly increased until the usual maintenance dose of 750 mg/day is reached. Sulfasalazine can be used at doses of 2 to 3 g/day. Other remittive agents include azathioprine, a purine analogue that is usually used at a dose of 1.25 to 1.5 mg/kg/day; cyclophosphamide, an alkylating agent used at a dose of 75 to 100 mg/day; or cyclosporin, an experimental drug whose use may be limited by its severe nephrotoxicity. Surgical intervention is necessary for intractable pain, destroyed joints, or progressive neurologic disease from cervical spine involvement.

GOUT

Gout is a disease in which tissue deposition of monosodium urate crystals occurs from supersaturated extracellular fluids. This process results in (1) recurrent attacks of severe acute or chronic articular and periarticular inflammation called *gouty arthritis;* (2) accumulation of articular, osseous, soft tissue, and cartilaginous crystalline deposits called *tophi;* (3) renal impairment, referred to as *gouty nephropathy;* and (4) uric acid calculi in the urinary tract, called *nephrolithiasis.* Asymptomatic hyperuricemia in the absence of gout is not a disease state. Gout rarely occurs in men before adolescence or in women before menopause. Gout is familial. Overproduction of uric acid (10% of cases) occurs with a variety of acquired and genetic disorders characterized by excessive rates of cell (nucleic acid) turnover. Appearance of gout in a young woman suggests a myeloproliferative or lymphoproliferative disorder. The majority of patients (up to 90%) show a deficit in the renal excretion of uric acid. Diuretics, cyclosporine, low-dose salicylates, lactic acid, and lead intoxication alter renal tubular function and contribute to underexcretion.

Pathophysiology

Changes in the level of serum uric acid (up or down) trigger gouty attacks. Monosodium urate crystals must be identified inside a white cell for diagnosis of acute gout. Crystals are typically needle-shaped, and are usually visible with a light microscope. A polarizing microscope will reveal the crystal to be birefringent and bright yellow when parallel to the axis of slow vibration as marked on the polarizing microscope compensator (negative elongation). The synovial fluid contains 20,000 to 100,000 cells/mm^3, predominantly neutrophils. Since infection can coexist with urate crystals, joint fluid cultures should always be obtained.

Clinical Features

The metatarsophalangeal (MTP) joint of the first toe (podagra) is most often involved, followed by the ankle, tarsal area, and the knee. The inflammation is abrupt, marked, and especially painful. Attacks subside spontaneously over 3 to 10 days even without treatment. Subcutaneous monosodium urate crystal–containing tophi usually occur in advanced gout, although microtophi can be detected in the synovial membrane early. Bony erosions with a sclerotic margin or a thin, overhanging edge of displaced bone characterizing the erosion as a "gull wing" may be intraarticular or periarticular.

Management and Treatment

Colchicine is not effective when used after the first 24 hours of an attack. When used for acute gout, a single intravenous colchicine dose (diluted in 20 ml of 5% dextrose in water and administered over 10 to 20 minutes through a secured intravenous line to avoid thrombophlebitis or extravasation) should never exceed 2 mg, and the total cumulative dose for an attack should not exceed 4 mg in a 24-hour period. Then no more colchicine should be given by any route for 7 days. Colchicine can also be administered as 0.5 mg tablets taken hourly until one of three endpoints is reached: significant joint improvement, gastrointestinal toxicity, or a maximum total dose of 8 mg is ingested. Antiinflammatory doses of NSAIDs are probably used more often than colchicine for acute gout and are effective at any stage of the gouty episode. Corticosteroids and adrenocorticotrophic hormone (ACTH) have traditionally been used when colchicine and NSAIDs were contraindicated or ineffective. Oral doses of 20 to 40 mg of prednisone administered daily for 3 to 4 days, then gradually tapered over 1 to 2 weeks are effective. Intraarticular depot steroid injection is a useful alternative. Daily oral prophylactic colchicine, 0.5 mg tablet once or twice daily, or low-dose NSAIDs may be given to prevent attacks. Hyperuricemia alone is not a reason for treatment. Uricosuric drugs or xanthine oxidase inhibitors are selected according to patient need. Allopurinol is the preferred drug in patients with any renal insufficiency. However, a papular rash occurs in 3% to 10% of those receiving allopurinol, and rarely a severe hypersensitivity with mortality occurs.

CALCIUM PYROPHOSPHATE DISEASE

Specific identification of calcium pyrophosphate dihydrate (CPPD) crystals in synovial fluid permits differentiation of this crystal deposition disease from other inflammatory and degenerative arthritis. The inflammatory arthritis associated with CPPD crystal deposition can be classified as hereditary, sporadic (idiopathic), or associated with various metabolic diseases such as hyperparathyroidism, familial hypocalciuric hypercalcemia, hemochromatosis, hemosiderosis, hypothyroidism, gout, hypomagnesemia, hypophosphatasia, and amyloidosis or trauma.

Pathophysiology

Phagocytosis of the CPPD crystals by neutrophilic phagocytes results in release of lysosomal enzymes and cell-derived chemotactic factors.

Clinical Features

CPPD can present in a number of clinical patterns; an acute monoarthritis termed *pseudogout* is probably most common. The knee is the usual site in almost half of all attacks. The radiographic appearance of punctuate and linear densities in fibrocartilaginous tissues called *chondrocalcinosis* is diagnostically helpful. Acute attacks can be treated similarly to gout.

SPONDYLOARTHROPATHIES

The seronegative spondyloarthropathies are a group of multisystem inflammatory disorders that affect the spine, peripheral joints, and periarticular structures, with variable expression of characteristic extraarticular manifestations that typically predominate in males. The extraarticular manifestations include gastrointestinal or genitourinary inflammation, skin and nail lesions, aortic and pulmonary involvement, and increased prevalence of the HLA-B27 gene. Recognized clinical disease entities within the spondyloarthropathies are ankylosing spondylitis, reactive arthritis, Reiter's syndrome, arthritis associated with psoriasis or inflammatory bowel disease, and juvenile onset spondyloarthropathy.

Pathophysiology

Sacroiliitis and inflammation at sites of tendinous or ligamentous attachment are hallmarks of joint pathology and are more common than synovitis. Inflammation at peripheral sites, such as the calcaneal attachment of the Achilles' tendon is called *enthesopathy.* The inflammatory lesion in the outer annular fibers of the intervertebral disk forms a characteristic bony bridge seen in x-rays and is called a *syndesmophyte.*

Clinical Features

Ankylosing spondylitis (AS) is the prototypic seronegative spondyloarthropathy that affects the axial skeleton with sacroiliac joint involvement (sacroiliitis). It is the one spondyloarthropathy most strongly associated with HLA-B27 (>90%). Manifestations begin in late adolescence, and onset after age 40 is uncommon. The characteristic and earliest presentation is chronic low back pain with early morning back stiffness, which improves with physical activity. Inflammation at tendon insertions (enthesopathy) results in tenderness of costosternal junctions, spinous processes, scapulae, iliac crests, trochanters, ischial tuberosities, tibial tubercles, and heels. Slowly, limitation of forward flexion of the lumbar spine develops. Spinal ankylosis develops at a variable rate and pattern. Neurologic involvement from the spinal disease may occur related to spinal fracture and/or dislocation, atlantoaxial subluxations, or cauda equina syndrome.

The most common extraskeletal manifestation in ankylosing spondylitis is acute anterior uveitis. Cardiovascular involvement, although rare, affects the ascending aorta, resulting in aortitis, aortic valve incompetence, and conduction abnormalities. Lung involvement includes a slowly progressive fibrosis.

Reiter's syndrome develops after an infection by bacteria, *Chlamydia trachomatis* in the genitourinary tract or *Salmonella, Shigella, Yersinia,* or *Campylobacter* in the gastrointestinal tract. Reiter's syndrome is a reactive arthritis, accompanied by extraarticular involvement such as uveitis, dermatitis, bowel inflammation, urethritis, and carditis. Incidence is 3.5/100,000 in males under the age of 50. The male-to-female ratio is more like 5 : 1.

The arthritis (usually a uniformly swollen sausage digit) appears within 1 to 3 weeks after urethritis or diarrhea characteristic of this arthritis. Reiter's syndrome has been recognized in association with HIV. It is now important to look for chlamydia and HIV in every case of Reiter's syndrome.

There is an increased prevalence of inflammatory arthritis in association with psoriasis. Approximately 95% of patients with psoriatic arthritis have peripheral joint involvement. Others have pauciarticular asymmetric arthritis or exclusive DIP involvement. About 5% have exclusive spinal involvement. The arthritis can antedate the psoriasis rash. Eye inflammation occurs in 30% of patients. Radiographic features include erosion in DIP joints and tufts, and "pencil-in-the-cup" deformities.

Enteropathic arthritis includes arthritis associated with inflammatory bowel diseases (ulcerative colitis and Crohn's disease), the reactive arthritis triggered by enterogenic bacteriae, Whipple's disease, arthritis after intestinal bypass surgery, and arthritis associated with celiac disease.

Management and Treatment

Patient education is crucial because there is no cure. Appropriate use of NSAIDs and regular therapeutic exercise prevent deformity and disability. Acute anterior uveitis can be managed with corticosteroid eye drops. Splints, braces, and corsets are not helpful and may hasten loss of mobility. Aggressive and unremitting Reiter's may benefit from immunosuppressive drugs if associated HIV has been ruled out. Methotrexate has been recognized as an effective treatment for advanced psoriatic arthritis for 35 years and is the drug of choice.

INFECTIOUS OR SEPTIC ARTHRITIS

Acute bacterial infection in a joint (infectious or septic arthritis) produces pain, tenderness, and loss of function. Most septic arthritis affects a single joint (monoarthritis). Joints commonly involved are the knee (50% of cases), hip, shoulder, wrist, ankle, elbow, and the small joints of the hand or foot.

Comorbidity factors important in septic arthritis include age extremes (children and the elderly), coexistent systemic diseases, especially diabetes and malignancy, prosthetic joints, previous arthrocentesis, and intravenous drug use. Most infections are due to *Staphlococcus aureus (S. aureus),* which is often methicillin resistant, followed by streptococci or gram-negative organisms. Joint infections after animal bites are usually related to

S. aureus or *Pasteurella multocida;* joint infections after human bites are caused by gram-negative bacillus or oral anaerobes. Infection is the most devastating complication of prosthetic joint surgery because it leads to prosthesis loosening, failure, and sepsis. *Neisseria gonorrhoeae* (GC), a gram-negative intracellular diplococcus, most often produces septic arthritis in young, sexually active adults, especially in the small joints of the hands, wrists, elbows, knees, and ankles.

Clinical Features

Fever, shaking chills, multiple skin lesions (petechiae, papules, pustules, hemorrhagic bullae, or necrotic lesions), fleeting migratory polyarthralgias, and tenosynovitis in the fingers, toes, and ankles that evolves into a persistent mono or oligoarthritis is a common presentation, especially in GC septic arthritis. Positive gram stain and culture of the synovial fluid are the fundamental criteria for diagnosis of septic arthritis. Blood cultures can be positive in 50% of the cases. Synovial fluid analysis of the white blood cell count (WBC) is intensely inflammatory (>50,000/mm^3) in 50% of the cases. A plain radiograph should be obtained at the time of diagnosis to search for a contiguous focus of osteomyelitis and to provide a baseline to monitor adequacy of treatment.

Management and Treatment

Initial antibiotic selection for bacterial arthritis is directed by clinical setting, including age, antecedent history, extraarticular foci of infection, and comorbidity factors, together with synovial fluid gram stain findings. Parenteral administration should generally be initiated for 1 to 2 weeks, followed by oral antibiotics for 1 to 2 weeks. Duration of antibiotic therapy is determined by the clinical response but usually requires 2 weeks. Adequate drainage is usually accomplished by daily needle aspiration. Surgical arthrotomy is required for drainage and debridement of septic hips or septic joints with coexistent osteomyelitis, and joint infections that are not controlled within 5 to 7 days by needle or arthroscopic drainage.

NONBACTERIAL ARTHRITIS

The occurrence of acute inflammatory arthritis in some viral infections has long been recognized. Infection with human parvovirus B19 may be responsible for polyarthralgia or polyarthritis. Hepatitis B infection may cause an immune complex–mediated arthritis with hand and knee involvement. Rubella infection leads to a high incidence of joint complaints in adults, especially in women. Several musculoskeletal syndromes have been described in HIV-infected patients; two of these syndromes are clinically indistinguishable from psoriatic arthritis and Reiter's disease. Other infections that can rarely result in arthritis include syphilis, tuberculosis, leprosy, brucellosis, and fungal arthritis.

Lyme disease is an important complex multisystem illness caused by the tick-borne organism *Borrelia burgdorferi.* The Lyme disease organism is transmitted primarily by certain ixodid ticks that are a part of the *Ixodes ricinus* complex. After an incubation of 3 to 32 days, erythema migrans, a slowly enlarging annular lesion, occurs at the site of the tick bite in about 80% of patients. Neck stiffness, fever, chills, myalgias, arthralgias, and profound malaise and fatigue are common in the prodrome. Early in the illness, patients develop migratory joint pain. Months later, 60% of untreated patients develop frank arthritis. Chronic neurologic manifestations may develop. Within several weeks after the onset of illness, about 8% of untreated patients develop cardiac involvement. Serologic testing for the antibodies to *Borrelia burgdorferi* is currently the only laboratory test for Lyme disease. Lyme disease can usually be treated successfully with early oral antibiotic (amoxicillin or doxycycline for 10 days) therapy. Objective neurologic and late-onset cardiac abnormalities are less responsive to antibiotic therapy.

Fibromyalgia is a disorder of diffuse muscle or soft tissue pain in the absence of (1) demonstrable inflammation; (2) damage to any organ system, including joints; and (3) laboratory abnormality. Typical patients are young to middle-aged, asthenic females with anxiety and sleep disturbances. The physical examination is notable only for diffuse and focal tenderness described as "tender points." Tender points can function as "trigger" points if they trigger pain at a distance. The American College of Rheumatology defines fibromyalgia as a history of widespread diffuse pain and pain in 11 of 18 tender points or sites on digital palpation. No specific therapy except reassurance, mild exercise, and nonnarcotic analgesia is recommended. Sedating tranquilizers to induce restful sleep and injection of trigger points are also helpful.

OTHER COMMON REGIONAL MUSCULOSKELETAL DISORDERS

Neck pain is a regional musculoskeletal complaint that results in painful, restricted motion of the neck. Persistent cervical pain must be evaluated to rule out anginal equivalent, cerebrovascular accident, neurologic compromise, or aortic aneurysm dissection.

Regional musculoskeletal disease of the shoulder includes diseases of the glenohumeral, acromioclavicular, and sternoclavicular joints as well as surrounding periarticular tissues such as supraspinatus tendonitis and subacromial bursitis. Most regional musculoskeletal diseases respond to analgesics, NSAIDs, and judicious muscle strengthening and range of motion exercises. Intraarticular injections of steroids are sometimes useful in selected shoulder disorders.

KEY POINTS

1 Osteoarthritis consists of primary and secondary forms. Multiple factors contribute to the development of the secondary form.

2 Rheumatoid arthritis (RA) is a systemic disease with synovitis, serositis, nodules, and vasculitis. RA requires antiinflammatory doses of ASA or NSAIDs and sometimes second-line therapy such as methotrexate or gold.

3 Seronegative spondyloarthropathies are a group of inflammatory arthopathies that affect the axial spine and peripheral joints, are rheumatoid factor negative, and share variable expression of a number of extraarticular manifestations.

4 Fibromyalgia, a pain syndrome, is a diagnosis of exclusion (of other arthritic diseases) characterized by diffuse pain (not confined to the joints) with 11 of 18 tender points identified.

SUGGESTED READINGS

Altman RD: Criteria for classification of clinical osteoarthritis, *J Rheumatol* 18:10-12, 1991.

Esterhai JL Jr, Gelb I: Adult septic arthritis, *Orthop Clin North Am* 22:503-514, 1991.

Kent DL et al: Diagnosis of lumbar spinal stenosis in adults: a metaanalysis of the accuracy of CT, MR, and myelography, *Am J Roentgenol* 158:1135-1144, 1992.

Khan MA, van der Linden SM: A wider spectrum of spondyloarthropathies, *Semin Arthritis Rheum* 20:107-113, 1990.

Wolfe F, Hawley DJ, Cathey MA: Termination of slow acting antirheumatic therapy in rheumatoid arthritis: a 14-year prospective evaluation of 1017 starts, *J Rheumatol* 17:994-1002, 1990.

Wolfe F et al: The American College of Rheumatology 1990 Criteria for the Classification of Fibromyalgia: report of the Multicenter Criteria Committee, *Arthritis Rheum* 33:160-172, 1990.

60

Backache

VANCE O. GARDNER

The lumbar disc, the nerve root, the facet joint, and sacroiliac joint create the predominant amount of lower back pain in adult life and are therefore called *primary pain generators.* Secondary pain generators can be myofascial, ligamentous, and muscular and are less easily defined. Whether primary or secondary, the pain and dysfunction are usually self-limiting except in certain severe cases, when they can be chronic and disabling.

DIAGNOSIS

A specific mechanism of injury is unusual in spinal pain. Because most spinal pain is degenerative in nature, there is more commonly a series of events leading up to the present complaint.

The intensity and duration of the patient's pain is extremely important.

Pain associated with upright activities such as bending, lifting, standing, sitting, or walking is usually associated with the pain generators previously mentioned. This is mechanical pain and is considered benign. Unremitting constant pain that wakes one from sleep is a more ominous history and should be investigated more aggressively. *This type of pain may be associated with either infectious or neoplastic conditions and the patient should be closely followed.* Retroperitoneal structures such aortic aneurysm, pancreas, duodenal ulcer, and even direct extension from endometrial carcinoma can be the source of back pain. Metastatic disease to the vertebral body is quite frequent in the older population with cancer (especially breast cancer), and unremitting back pain can be the initial presentation.

Leg pain in addition to back pain is also a separate condition and usually denotes nerve root impingement. A younger patient will usually develop severe leg pain because of a herniated disc. This leg pain is acute and usually in the distribution of one specific nerve root. The patient can barely stand and has severe spasm. This "nerve tension" is an uncommon presentation in the elderly with "spinal stenosis" or narrowing of the spinal canal caused by years of degenerative changes. The older population will develop lower extremity symptoms of aching or weakness predominantly with walking (neurogenic claudication). It can be differentiated (by history) from vascular claudication. Usually the patient with spinal stenosis can ride a stationary bike but cannot walk long distances. The pain is relieved with sitting or lying. Patients with vascular claudication have trouble performing any physical exercise with their lower extremities, and the symptoms can persist after the activity ceases.

PHYSICAL EXAMINATION

Inspection

Inspecting for lumbar spasm in the form of a "list," lateral angulation, or loss of normal lumbar lordosis can be helpful. The ability to walk on the heels and toes is an important method to screen out neurologic dysfunction. Inability to heel walk indicates a foot drop (L5 nerve root). Inability to perform a heel raise at least 10 times on one leg is indicative of S1 nerve root dysfunction.

Range of Motion

Examining the patient from the side, have the patient flex until her fingers reach the maximum point. Record the depth of flexion as either to the knees, proximal calves, midcalves, ankles, or the ground. Extension is estimated in degrees (20, 30, 40 degrees). Both of these exams are best used by comparison to earlier values rather than as absolute static values.

Chest Expansion

Measurement of chest expansion is important if the examiner is suspicious that an occult spondyloarthropathy or inflammatory arthritis of the spine is present. These patients have involved costovertebral joints as the first clinical sign of the disease. The examiner simply wraps a tape measure around the patient at nipple level and measures the chest expansion. An expansion less than 2 cm is considered abnormal and should be investigated with appropriate lab and radiographic studies.

Straight Leg Raise

Straight leg raise maneuvers are performed for patients with leg pain. This is to elicit the sensation of pain in the leg and therefore it is performed gently; nerve tension is better elicited with the *bowstring* test with the hip and knee flexed. Slight pressure is placed in the popliteal fossa, causing sciatic nerve compression and therefore eliciting nerve tension of the affected L4, L5, or S1 nerve root. This usually indicates a herniated disc.

Neurologic Examination

Examination of the reflexes can be performed with the patient sitting or supine. If the patient has acute back pain, the supine examination is usually more comfortable and is performed by flexing the knee over the examiner's free arm for the patellar reflex (L3 or L4 nerve roots) and flexing the knee 30 degrees and rotating the hip externally for the Achilles reflex (S1 nerve root).

Sensation is tested with a sharp point or "pin prick" and is recorded as absent, impaired, or present within the various nerve root distributions. Motor strength is tested by manual motor testing. Ankle dorsiflexion tests the anterior tibialis function (L5 nerve root), plantar flexion the gastrocnemis muscle (S1 nerve root), and knee extension the quadriceps (L3 and L4 nerve roots).

Sacroiliac and Hip Joints

The sacroiliac joint is tested by manipulating it and therefore reproducing the patient's pain and isolating it to the joint. The pelvis is first "fixed" by flexing the contralateral hip to maximum and having the patient hold the hip in this position. The affected hip is then extended, thus rotating the SI joint and reproducing pain in a pathologic joint. The hip joint is rotated and compared with the other side. Flexion, abduction, and external rotation is diminished in diseased hip joints and may masquerade as lumbar disc disease unless tested.

LABORATORY TESTS

For the patient with "typical" pain of degenerative lumbar disc disease, an initial evaluation rarely requires laboratory studies. Patients with constant, unremitting pain of more than 1 month duration should be investigated with baseline laboratory tests such as a CBC (looking for an occult anemia that could be the initial presentation of multiple myeloma), panel 18 (liver function, kidney function, and electrolytes), and urinalysis. An ESR is very sensitive for detecting inflammatory or neoplastic etiologies of back pain.

If back pain persists and continues to be "atypical" and certain historic and/or physical examination findings lead one to suspect a spondyloarthropathy, an HLA-B27 antigen study should be ordered. Even though this disorder is rare in females, the diagnosis is missed in most patients for quite some time before the disease becomes obvious. This delay in diagnosis can lead to a number of unnecessary procedures.

IMAGING STUDIES

Plain X-rays

If the patient's back pain persists beyond 4 weeks, an experienced spine or bone and joint radiologist or clinical spine specialist should read well-performed lumbar spine x-rays. Classically, these have been performed as an A-P, lateral, and L5-S1 spot views. These simple views can provide a significant amount of information. The A-P view is best for evaluating the quality of the lumbar pedicles where metastatic tumors can be detected before they're seen in the vertebral body. In addition, spinal deformity, sacroiliac joint pathology, and congenital anomalies can be detected. The lateral view provides important information regarding the lumbar intervertebral discs and vertebral bodies. Abnormal spinal alignment (hyperlordosis or kyphosis) or translation (spondylolisthesis) can be a factor in lumbar pain and are diagnosed by a simple lateral lumbar x-ray. In addition, the soft tissue paravertebral shadows such as the aorta or other retroperitoneal structures are sometimes visible if enlarged or calcified. Finally, oblique lumbar spine views for facet joint and spondylolysis pathology and an A-P pelvis x-ray for hip or pelvic pathology should be ordered if these entities are suspected.

Nuclear Medicine

Occasionally, bone scanning of the vertebral column is needed because of suspicion of abnormal periarticular bone resorption "inflammatory arthritis," vertebral body destruction, tumor or infection, or abnormal bone formation that can be seen in primary bone tumors such as the benign osteoid osteoma or the malignant osteosarcoma. In addition, gallium and/or white cell scans are occasionally needed to investigate the possibility of osteomyelitis. However, with the development of sensitive MRI software, infectious processes can be imaged anatomically and qualitatively with one study, therefore decreasing the indications for nuclear scanning.

Myelography

The instillation of contrast material into the intrathecal space was the only method that could demonstrate intracanal soft tissue pathology until the advent of cross-sectional imaging techniques such as CT and MRI scanning. Today, myelography is rarely combined with CT in some special conditions or presurgical patients.

MRI

The hallmark of spinal imaging for most common pathologies and even rare manifestations of spinal disease is a *well-performed* MRI scan with at least a 1.5 tesla magnet. MRI has enabled the physician to evaluate not only the anatomic abnormality but also the quality of the tissue through the signal characteristics of the lesion. For example, a large mass impinging a nerve root on CT scan would almost always be described as a disc herniation, but this same mass could be shown to be an epidural hematoma on MRI scan, resulting in the prevention of unnecessary surgery. Obviously the cost-benefit ratio should be analyzed on every patient in this era of cost-effectiveness in medicine. However, multiple nondiagnostic but cost-effective studies are useless and can be demoralizing to the patient. If an advanced spinal imaging study is contemplated by the primary care physician, referral to a spinal specialist for consultation and the appropriate study will most often prove to be the most cost-effective clinical path.

TREATMENT

Nonoperative Care

Acute low back pain is an extremely common disorder. At least 70% of the population has experienced an episode of low back pain, but only 15% have pain that lasts more than 2 weeks. Most often, rest, NSAIDs, and early return to usual activities is sufficient for the successful resolution of symptoms (Fig. 60-1). Low back pain accompanied by sciatica is a more ominous sign, but is fortunately more rare. In those patients reporting low back pain for longer than 2 weeks, 16% reported sciatica. Of these patients, 50% will still have symptoms after 6 weeks. Of those patients with symptoms that resolve between 2 and 6 weeks, 60% to 85% suffer a recurrence within 2 years. Benign low back pain recurrence can be modified by a change in lifestyle with reduction of risk factors such as smoking and poor body mechanics along with a program that emphasizes nutritional awareness and exercise techniques. A 30-minute/day light aerobic workout, 3 days/week coupled with a lumbar range of motion and strengthening program is extremely effective in minimizing further attacks. This first "back attack" is analogous to the patient with early coronary artery disease that is urged to modify certain aspects of his/her lifestyle to prevent advancement of the disease and minimize recurrent "attacks." Persistent back pain requires a more comprehensive "spinal restoration program" that is designed to strengthen and "stabilize" the lumbar spine once the acute spasm diminishes. This program can require 6 to 12 weeks depending on the degree of muscle atrophy and deactivation.

Patients with persistent sciatica are taught a series of exercises designed to passively extend the lumbar spine and consequently increase the nutrition of the disc with increased diffusion and extension range of motion. As the patient performs this simple "half push-up," the symptoms should "centralize" or progressively change from leg pain to back pain over a few weeks. Patients with persistent leg pain may be additionally treated with a series of epidural steroid injections coupled with the progressive spinal restoration program. Approximately 50% to 70% of patients with persistent sciatica will resolve their symptoms with these techniques. However, for many patients with large contained or extruded disc herniations, the symptoms will persist or neurologic dysfunction will worsen, requiring operative intervention.

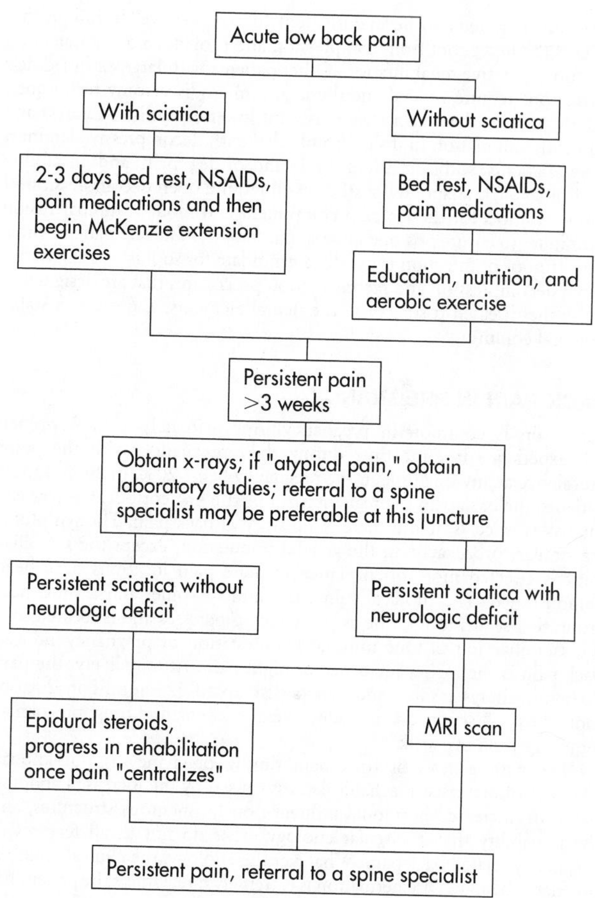

FIG. 60-1 Management of low back pain.

Operative Treatment

The surgical care of lumbar disc pathology requires detailed preoperative analysis and a patient that is failing appropriate nonoperative care. The goal is to improve neurologic function and relieve pain by performing the least invasive but predictably most effective procedure. For some patients with contained disc herniations that have failed a trial of spinal restoration, the procedure required may be an outpatient "decompressive" technique that relieves the nerve root from compression and provides a quick transition into postoperative rehabilitation. Other patients with large extruded disc herniations require general anesthesia and microdiscectomy techniques. Elderly patients that experience persistent lower extremity weakness and pain with ambulation find significant relief with decompressive laminectomy. Patients with persistent back and/or leg pain and instability syndromes such as spondylolisthesis will require open decompression of the nerve roots for the leg pain component and modern lumbar fusion techniques to ensure postoperative spinal stability. The rare patient with a spinal tumor or infection is usually a candidate for sophisticated anterior spinal decompression and reconstruction procedures that are designed to excise the diseased tissue, spare the neural elements, and create a stable vertebral column.

BACK PAIN IN PREGNANCY

Back pain is common in pregnancy. Approximately 1 in 2 women will experience it some time during their pregnancy, with the point prevalence at any one time in the pregnancy being 20%. In 20% of these patients, the back pain in pregnancy can be the first episode. Conversely, the risk is twice as high if there is a history of back pain. The symptoms are similar to backache in the general population, except the sacroiliac joint is effected more often. Three separate pain locations have been demonstrated. The thoracic spine, the lumbar spine, and a third pain group that seems to increase as pregnancy progresses and is located over the sacroiliac joints. One unusual manifestation of pregnancy-induced back pain is the higher incidence of night pain. After delivery, the pain does not always resolve and can persist up to 12 months in 20% of individuals. Risk factors include severe back pain during pregnancy, requiring time off work.

The pathogenesis of back pain during pregnancy is not known. Theories of increased mechanical stress caused by the increased abdominal girth, increased hormonal influence on ligamentous structures, and the possibility that a vascular etiology exists do not fit all features of pregnancy-related back pain. Whatever the etiology, the clinical course is invariably benign. Disc herniation is extremely rare. Unless the patient has an advancing neurologic deficit such as a cauda equina syndrome, the patient should be treated with light stretching exercises and abdominal "crunches" until the abdominal girth creates difficulty with rehabilitation. Walking as a preventive exercise decreases the rate of back pain in the general population and should be employed as a general conditioning program, especially in the high-risk patient with back pain symptoms preceding pregnancy.

KEY POINTS

1 The lumbar disc and facet joints are the primary pain generators of back pain.

2 Neurogenic leg pain is usually the consequence of compression of a nerve root by a herniated disc or spinal stenosis.

3 Constant, unremitting back pain unassociated with position or movement is "atypical" and should arouse suspicion of an inflammatory, neoplastic, or infectious etiology.

4 "Nerve tension" is an important physical finding in patients with acute neurogenic leg pain and is best demonstrated with the "bowstring test."

5 The MRI scan is the most useful imaging modality in the workup for low back pain.

6 Most complaints of back pain can be managed with an active nonoperative treatment program.

7 Low back pain in pregnancy is a common complaint, but is usually self-limiting.

SUGGESTED READINGS

Deyo RA, Diehl AK, Rosenthal M: How many days bed rest for acute low back pain? a randomized clinical trial. *N Engl J Med* 315:1064-1070, 1986.

Deyo RA, Bass JE: Lifestyle and low back pain: the influence of smoking, exercise and obesity, *Clin Res* 35:577A, 1987.

Oegema TR: Biochemistry of the intervertebral disc, *Clin Sports Med* 12:419-439, 1993.

Ostagaard HC, Andersson GBJ, Karlsson K: Prevalence of back pain in pregnancy, *Spine* 16:549-552, 1991.

Saal JA, Saal JS, Herzog RJ: The natural history of lumbar intervertebral disc extrusions treated nonoperatively, *Spine* 15:683-686, 1990.

Spengler DM: Lumbar discectomy: results with limited disc excision and selective foraminotomy, *Spine* 7:604-607, 1982.

61

Cholecystitis

GREGOR J. KOOBATIAN AND JOHN C. HOEFS

Gallstone disease (cholecystitis) can be asymptomatic or symptomatic. Symptomatic disease can be further subdivided into chronic and acute cholecystitis.

Epidemiologic studies show that cholesterol gallstones occur two to three times more commonly in women than in men. The increase in prevalence starts at puberty and continues throughout the years. The difference decreases to a two times higher incidence in females over the age of 60 than in males of the same age group. Women of lower socioeconomic status have a greater risk of gallstones. The majority of patients with acute cholecystitis have gallstones, but the majority of patients with gallstones do not develop acute cholecystitis. Women of childbearing age have an increased incidence of cholecystitis. In addition, approximately 1 in 10,000 pregnancies is complicated by cholecystitis. Pregnancy in and of itself is not a known risk for cholecystitis, but changes in biliary physiology during pregnancy may increase the tendency toward gallbladder disease.

PATHOPHYSIOLOGY

Bile stasis is a major factor in gallstone formation. Increases in the bile acid pool size and decreased bile salt excretion cause bile to become saturated with cholesterol. Decreased numbers of enterohepatic cycles and changes in the various types of bile acids, along with the above mentioned saturation of bile salts, contribute to stone formation.

Factors that affect the nidus of stone formation are lipoprotein A and mucous. More than 80% of gallstones are composed of greater than 50% cholesterol. The incidence of gallstones is increased with obesity, rapid weight loss, patients with high triglyceride levels, use of birth control pills, use of lipid-lowering drugs, and certain ethnic groups such as the Pima Indians. Women on estrogen replacement therapy also have a two to three times greater incidence of gallstones. Pregnancy causes decreased motility and increased gallbladder residual volume and as a result, bile stasis occurs.

DIAGNOSIS

Diagnosis of biliary colic or chronic or acute cholecystitis consists of clinical findings included in the history and physical as well as laboratory tests and imaging studies (Fig. 61-1). In asymptomatic gallstones, the finding is usually made incidentally during a workup for another medical problem. Primary considerations in the patient's history are right upper quadrant pain and previous episodes of biliary pain.

Biliary colic is the usual complaint in most symptomatic patients with gallstones. Biliary colic is a visceral pain that comes from transient obstruction of the cystic duct by a gallstone. Acute inflammation is usually not present except in patients with acute cholecystitis. There usually is no identifiable precipitating cause for a patient's symptoms. Biliary colic is described as a steady pain that gradually increases over 15 minutes to 1 hour and stays at a plateau for more than 1 hour and then slowly decreases.

In acute cholecystitis, the symptoms of pain usually last for more than 5 hours. Intolerance to fatty food is not more common in patients with gallstones than in those without gallstones. Continuous pain, nausea, vomiting, and fever along with an increase in WBC count suggests the development of acute cholecystitis. Disease activity tends to remain about the same over long periods. If the patient has been experiencing frequent attacks, she will usually continue to have episodes at the same frequency.

Physical examination often demonstrates right upper quadrant tenderness and pain radiating to the back or right shoulder or with palpation

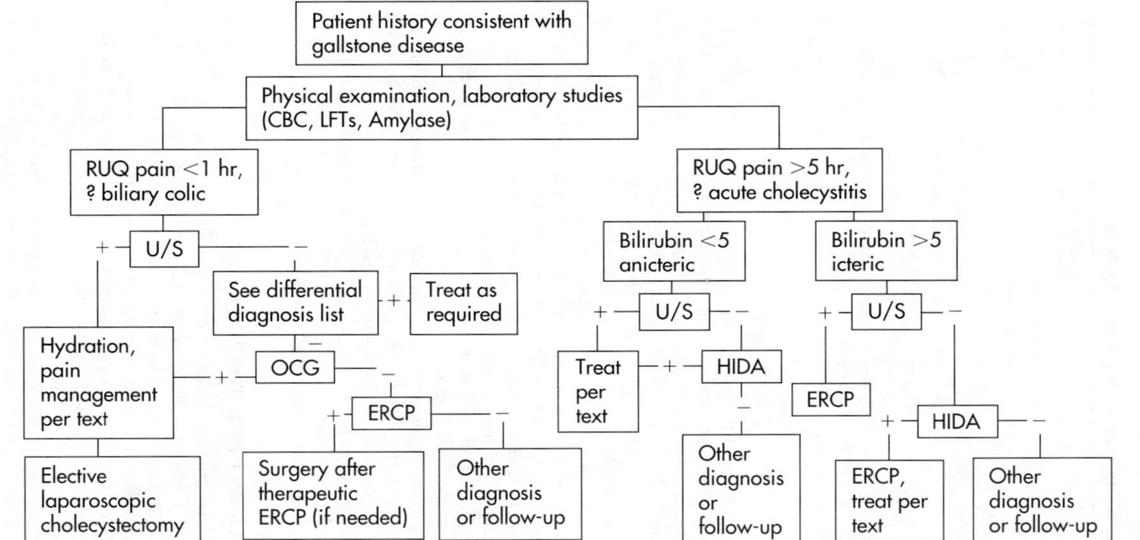

FIG. 61-1 Management of cholecystitis. *RUQ,* Right upper quadrant; *US,* ultrasound to diagnose gallstones in the gallbladder or common bile duct (CBD) as well as diagnose CBD dilation or pancreatitis; *ERCP,* endoscopic retrograde cholangiopancreatography to diagnose and possibly treat CBD stones or pancreatic disease; *OCG,* oral cholecystogram to diagnose CBD stone; *HIDA,* hepatoiminodiacetic acid scan to diagnose acute cholecystitis.

TABLE 61-1
Differential Diagnoses for Cholecystitis

Origin	Differential diagnoses
Cardiac	Myocardial infarction
Pulmonary	Right lower lobe pneumonia, pleurisy, pneumonitis, pulmonary embolus
Gastrointestinal	Peptic ulcer, acute pancreatitis, acute appendicitis
Hepatic	Acute hepatitis—viral or alcoholic, hepatic tumors
Renal	Renal disease/pyelonephritis
Infectious	Gonococcal perihepatitis (Fitz-Hugh–Curtis syndrome)
Pregnancy	Acute fatty liver of pregnancy, preeclampsia, HELLP syndrome

under the right costal margin on deep inspiration, called *Murphy's sign*. Occasionally an enlarged and tender gallbladder can be appreciated. Only 20% of patients develop jaundice or increased bilirubin. Laboratory tests results include an elevated WBC count with left shift and/or elevated transaminases and increased bilirubin. A bilirubin >5 mg/dl may be caused by common bile duct stones or inflammation of the liver. Other less common causes of increased bilirubin (usually <9 mg/dl) include sepsis and cystic duct stones. An amylase >1000 u/dl suggests gallstones in the distal common bile duct resulting in obstruction of pancreatic duct outflow. Ultrasound imaging of the right upper quadrant will usually identify gallstones if present in the gallbladder, but is not very effective in detecting common bile duct stones. ERCP is usually required to diagnose and treat common bile duct stones.

Findings of acute cholecystitis on ultrasound include gallbladder wall thickening and/or fluid around the gallbladder. If a right upper quadrant ultrasound is inconclusive, a hetapoiminodiacetic acid (HIDA) scan would be the next diagnostic test to obtain. HIDA scan has little risk to the fetus if it is done late in pregnancy.

For differential diagnoses, see Table 61-1.

MANAGEMENT AND THERAPY

The incidental finding of asymptomatic gallstones does not require intervention. Decision analysis has shown that prophylactic cholecystectomy decreases survival and is more costly compared with expectant management. The risk of prophylactic cholecystectomy outweighs the benefits, especially in pregnancy. Presentation of disease and medical therapy is the same in the pregnant patient as it is in the nonpregnant patient.

For symptomatic gallstones, the mainstay of management is conservative medical therapy with antibiotics, hydration, and analgesics. This is recommended for both biliary colic and acute cholecystitis. In the majority of cases, this will constitute the necessary therapy for the acute period. Healthy nonpregnant individuals with symptomatic gallstones should have a laparoscopic cholecystectomy. In the case of possible common bile duct stones (increased bilirubin, a dilated common bile duct by ultrasound), ERCP can be performed before laparoscopic cholecystectomy to remove the stones.

If a patient has minimal symptoms and does not want surgery, oral dissolution therapy with bile acids can be considered. The most successful use of bile acids in gallstone dissolution is in the symptomatic patient with floating cholesterol gallstones less than 5 mm in diameter in a functioning gallbladder. However, this therapy requires over 1 year of oral medication, and approximately 50% of the patients will have a recurrence in 5 years. If the symptoms are severe and risk of surgery is high, contact dissolution therapy with volatile acid directly instilled into the gallbladder can be considered. Open cholecystectomy remains the standard therapy with which the effectiveness of all other modalities is compared.

KEY POINTS

1. Asymptomatic gallstones do not require intervention.
2. If acute cholecystitis develops, do not delay medical therapy.
3. The presentation of cholecystitis is the same in pregnant as in nonpregnant patients.
4. Therapy is usually achieved with medical intervention with antibiotics, analgesics, nasogastric suction, and hydration.

SUGGESTED READINGS

Baillie J et al: Endoscopic management of choledocholithiasis during pregnancy, *Surg Gynecol Obstet* 171:1, 1990.

Cooper AD: Epidemiology, pathogenesis, natural history, and medical therapy of gallstones. In Slesenger MH, Fordtran JS, eds: *Gastrointestinal disease,* ed 5, Philadelphia, 1993, WB Saunders, p 1788.

Iafrati MD, Yarnell R, Schwaitzberg SD: Gasless laparoscopic cholecystectomy in pregnancy, *J Laparoendosc Surg* 5:2:127-130, 1995.

Morrell DG, Mullins JR, Harrison PB: Laparoscopic cholecystectomy during pregnancy in symptomatic patients, *Surgery* 112:5:856-859, 1992.

NIH Consensus Conference: Gallstones and laparoscopic cholecystectomy, *JAMA* 269:1018-1024, 1993.

Scott LD: Gallstone disease and pancreatitis in pregnancy, *Gastroenterol Clin North Am* 21:4:803-815, 1992.

Somberg KA, Lawrence WW, Sleisenger MH: Complications of gallstone disease. In Sleisinger MH, Fordtran JS, eds: *Gastrointestinal disease,* ed 5, Philadelphia, 1993, WB Saunders, p 1805.

62

Connective Tissue Diseases

Pamela E. Prete

SYSTEMIC LUPUS ERYTHEMATOSUS

Systemic lupus erythematosus (SLE) is the prototypic autoimmune disease characterized by the production of antibodies to components of the cell nucleus with diverse clinical manifestations caused by inflammation, vasculopathy, vasculitis, and immune complex deposition. Primarily a disease of young women, its incidence peaks between the ages of 15 and 40, with a female to male ratio of 5:1. SLE may coexist with other autoimmune conditions such as hemolytic anemia, thyroiditis, and idiopathic thrombocytopenia purpura (ITP).

Pathophysiology

The immunologic disturbance is the production of autoantibodies that bind nuclear proteins, DNA, RNA, and protein-nucleic acid complexes. Only two antibodies, one to double-stranded DNA and one to an RNA-protein complex termed *Sm* (marker antibodies) are in SLE criteria. Other autoantibodies associated with disease manifestations include antibodies to ribosomal P proteins (anti-P) with neuropsychiatric disease; antibodies to Ro (SS-A) with the neonatal lupus and subacute cutaneous lupus syndromes (SCLE); antibodies to phospholipids with vascular thrombosis, thrombocytopenia, and recurrent abortion; and antibodies to RBCs and WBCs. Genetic factors such as (HLA) DR2 and DR3 (and recently defined subspecificities), as well as exogenous and environmental factors, are implicated in the etiology.

Clinical Features

In SLE, sensitivity to the sun is associated with inflammation and degeneration at the dermal-epidermal junction; most common is the malar or facial "butterfly" rash that is precipitated by sun exposure and spares the nasolabial folds. SCLE also commonly occurs in sun-exposed areas; it may be generalized and may evolve further into the papulosquamous variant that mimics psoriasis or lichen planus. Discoid lupus consists of chronic erythematous papules or plaques with central atrophy, which occur in the absence of any systemic SLE manifestations.

Arthralgias and arthritis constitute the most common presenting complaint, confusing the diagnosis with rheumatoid arthritis. Kidney symptoms are not perceived by the patient until there is advanced nephrotic syndrome or renal failure. Nephritis is a serious cause of SLE morbidity and mortality, and kidney biopsy is necessary to see the extent and location of proliferative changes within glomeruli and in the basement membrane, as well as to make treatment decisions. Neuropsychiatric manifestations include intractable headaches, chorea, seizures, cerebrovascular accidents, cranial neuropathies, Guillain-Barré syndrome, transverse myelitis, frank psychosis, and organic brain syndrome. Most patients with neuropsychiatric involvement and half of those without involvement demonstrate significant cognitive impairment. Cerebrospinal fluid may show a mild pleocytosis. Multiple electroencephalogram (EEG) abnormalities are common, but brain scans and MRI are inconclusive. Serositis in SLE may present as pleurisy, pericarditis, or peritonitis. Gastrointestinal symptoms are manifested by diffuse abdominal pain, anorexia, nausea, and occasionally vomiting. Acute pancreatitis occurs in some patients with SLE. Hepatomegaly occurs commonly in SLE, but overt clinical liver disease is rare. Pulmonary involvement ranges from exudative pleural effusion to pneumonitis, pulmonary hemorrhage, pulmonary embolism, pulmonary hypertension, and shrinking lung syndrome. Cardiac involvement may consist of pericarditis, myocarditis, endocarditis, or coronary artery disease. Nonbacterial verrucous vegetations occurring on heart valves as classically described by Libman and Sacks are now much less common than they were in the presteroid era. Coronary vasculitis is rare. Lymphadenopathy in single or multiple sites is a nonspecific feature, and splenomegaly is common. Cytopenias include anemia, leukopenia, lymphopenia, and thrombocytopenia. Anemia is usually secondary to chronic inflammatory disease, renal insufficiency, blood loss, or drugs. Autoimmune hemolytic anemia caused by antibodies directed against RBC antigens is associated with a positive Coombs' test. Leukopenia is associated with active disease with WBC counts between 2500/mm^3 and 4000/mm^3. Two distinct subsets of thrombocytopenia have been identified in SLE. In one, thrombocytopenia follows the course of acute SLE and its response to treatment; the second persists around 50,000/mm^3 and does not respond or need to be treated. Clotting abnormalities occur, the most frequent being the SLE anticoagulant. A prolonged partial thromboplastin occurs with anticardiolipin antibody that crossreacts with the VDRL test for syphilis. A false positive test for syphilis is a positive VDRL with a negative TPI or an FTA-ABS test. Serum complement levels are low in patients with active SLE. A diagnosis of SLE is confirmed by the presence of four of the following 11 established criteria: (1) malar rash; (2) discoid rash; (3) photosensitivity; (4) oral ulcers; (5) arthritis; (6) serositis; (7) renal, (8) neurologic, (9) hematologic, or (10) immunologic disorders; and (11) antinuclear antibody (ANA).

Disorders Related to SLE

The antiphospholipid syndrome (APL) associated with SLE or as a primary form is the association of arterial and venous thrombosis, recurrent fetal loss, and immune thrombocytopenia with a variety of antibodies directed against cellular membrane phospholipid components that crossreact with clotting factors. Other hypercoagulable states should be ruled out and include protein C, protein S, or antithrombin III deficiency; dysfibrinogenemias; abnormalities of fibrinolysis; the nephrotic syndrome; malignancies; polycythemia vera; Behcet's syndrome; and paroxysmal nocturnal hemoglobinuria.

Drug-induced lupus may be diagnosed in a patient with no prior history suggestive of SLE, in whom the clinical and serologic manifestations of SLE appear while on the drug, and in whom improvement in clinical symptoms occurs quickly on stopping the drug with a more gradual resolution of serologic abnormalities. The features of drug-induced lupus are fever, rash, and arthritis, as well as a positive ANA in over 90% of cases because of antihistone antibodies.

Management and Treatment

The short-term prognosis for SLE has improved, but long-term mortality and morbidity have not and manifest the consequences of immunosuppressive treatment. Deaths occurring late are often related to myocardial infarction and atherosclerosis. Osteonecrosis causes disability, especially in the hip. Cortical atrophy (evident on CT scanning) and shrinking lung syndrome are seen in late disease. The chances of carrying a pregnancy to term with SLE are reduced (see Chapter 36).

Decisions regarding SLE treatment are guided by disease activity and severity. SLE patients must avoid sun exposure. Infections are common, and evaluation of fever is always necessary, especially in patients with renal failure, ulcerative skin lesions, cardiac valvular abnormalities, or primary complement deficiencies. NSAIDs are useful for treatment of arthritis, serositis, fever, and fatigue, but the possibility of NSAID-induced nephropathy or CNS symptoms exists and should be ruled out before the assumption of active lupus nephritis or CNS SLE. Ibuprofen can cause an aseptic meningitis syndrome. Intravenous methylprednisolone ("bolus therapy") is an alternative to high-dose oral corticosteroids. Antimalarial compounds are used to treat milder cutaneous, musculoskeletal, and constitutional features of SLE. Azathioprine and cyclophosphamide, low-dose oral (1 to 4 mg/kg daily) and high-dose intravenous (0.5 to 1.0 g/m^2) are used widely in the management of serious lupus manifestations as steroid-sparing agents. Cyclophosphamide retards lupus nephritis progression, but the toxicities are substantial and include nausea, vomiting, alopecia, hemorrhagic cystitis, and increased risk for infections.

SYSTEMIC SCLEROSIS

Systemic sclerosis (SSc, scleroderma, diffuse sclerosis) is a connective tissue disease of unknown etiology characterized by fibrosis of the skin and visceral organs and accompanied by relatively specific antinuclear antibodies and microvascular disturbances. Incidence peaks in the fifth and sixth decades of life; the female to male ratio is 2 to 1. Occupational exposure to silica, vinyl chloride, or various organic solvents may give rise to scleroderma-like conditions. The toxic oil syndrome that occurred in Spain from the ingestion of adulterated rapeseed oil and the eosinophilia-myalgia syndrome caused by ingesting chemically contaminated batches of L-tryptophan are conditions similar to diffuse scleroderma.

Pathophysiology

Fibrosis of the skin and other organs, including the blood vessels, as well as increased collagen in the dermis and thinning of the epidermis are seen. Specific autoantibodies include antibodies to the centromere, several RNA synthetases, and topoisomerase I (Scl-70). Patients with rapidly progressive, diffuse skin thickening (diffuse cutaneous involvement) are at greater risk to develop early, serious visceral involvement. Limited cutaneous involvement, also called the CREST syndrome, includes the following features: calcinosis, Raynaud's phenomenon, esophageal dysmotility, sclerodactyly, and telangiectasia.

Clinical Features

Raynaud's phenomenon, swelling and puffiness of the fingers, polyarthralgias, and polyarthritis are early features. Distal esophageal motor dysfunction is the most common manifestation of internal involvement. Other gastrointestinal complaints include reflux, stricture, and intestinal malabsorption, with characteristic wide-mouthed diverticula. Colonic hypomotility may result in obstipation. The most frequent pulmonary function abnormality is reduced diffusing capacity for carbon monoxide, followed by a restrictive lung disease. Pulmonary arterial hypertension develops in patients with limited cutaneous involvement (CREST). Myocardial involvement appears in patients with diffuse scleroderma. Renal involvement usually slowly reduces creatinine clearance, but also can present acutely as scleroderma renal crisis. Sjögren's syndrome has been confirmed in 20% or more of SSc patients because of lymphocytic infiltration or glandular fibrosis.

Related Syndromes

Eosinophilic fasciitis is a disorder characterized by the appearance over days or weeks of tender swelling of the arms and legs sparing the hands and feet. Deep biopsy of an involved area including tissue from the epidermis down to skeletal muscle shows a characteristic cellular (commonly eosinophiles) infiltrate surrounding the fascia. Eosinophilic fasciitis usually responds to low doses of corticosteroids.

Undifferentiated connective tissue syndromes are designations that have grown from the recognition that the systemic rheumatic diseases have several properties that may make a specific diagnosis difficult. An example is mixed connective tissue disease (MCTD) in which there may be the presence of features of SLE, dermatomyositis (DM), rheumatoid arthritis (RA), and systemic sclerosis in various combinations and in association with high titers of autoantibodies to the nRNP or U_1RNP antigen.

Management and Treatment

The 10-year cumulative survival rate is 65%. Death is caused by pulmonary or renal disease. Since the use of angiotensin converting enzyme inhibitors that reverse underlying hyperreninemia and control hypertension, the outcome of scleroderma renal crisis has greatly improved. Pulmonary hypertension and intestinal malabsorption are causes of mortality in the limited cutaneous variant. D-penicillamine, an immunomodulating agent that also interferes with cross-linking of collagen, is the most widely used drug treatment. Raynaud's phenomenon is aggressively treated by abstaining from smoking, avoiding cold exposure, and keeping the entire body warm; biofeedback training and calcium channel blockers prevent vasospasm of arteries in visceral organs, which slows the disease. Esophageal dysmotility therapy includes histamine blockade. Delayed bowel transit allows bacterial overgrowth; broad-spectrum antibiotics such as ampicillin, tetracycline, and metronidazole given in tandem in 2-week courses are helpful. Corticosteroids have little success altering the progression of the disease. A single or double lung transplant may be necessary because of advanced pulmonary fibrosis.

IDIOPATHIC INFLAMMATORY MYOPATHIES

Polymyositis (PM) and dermatomyositis (DM) are idiopathic inflammatory myopathies that cause symmetric proximal limb and neck weakness and muscle tenderness. The annual incidence is 5 to 10 cases/million, with women most frequently affected.

Pathophysiology

Focal muscle necrosis, regeneration, and inflammation are characteristic pathologic findings. CD8+ cytotoxic T lymphocytes are the predominant cells surrounding or invading muscle cells in affected tissue. Muscle biopsy establishes the diagnosis. Autoantibodies associated with myositis patients include antibodies to transfer RNAs, anti-Jo-1, anti-PL-7, anti-PL-12, anti-Mi-2, and anti-SRP. Routine tests are normal, but diagnostic elevations of muscle enzymes, serum creatine kinase, aldolase, lactic dehydrogenase, and the transaminases occur, along with a characteristic pattern on electromyography (EMG). EMG helps establish the diagnosis and exclude muscle diseases that result from denervation. The myositis EMG shows small-amplitude, short-duration, polyphasic motor-unit potentials with spontaneous fibrillations, positive sharp waves, and increased irritability. Inclusion body myositis (IBM) is an underrecognized disease within the idiopathic inflammatory myopathies. The diagnostic clue to IBM is based on the presence of characteristic cytoplasmic vacuoles in skeletal muscle biopsy in this disease.

Clinical Features

PM or DM patients first complain of difficulty climbing stairs or getting into or out of a car. In DM, cutaneous manifestations can precede, follow, or develop concomitantly with muscle involvement. The pathognomonic skin findings are Gottron's papules (violaceous, flat-topped papules overlying the dorsal surface of the hand joints), erythematous smooth or scaly patches over extensor surfaces and in the V area of the neck (the so-called *V sign*) in DM. The heliotrope rash is dusky purple and occurs over the often-edematous upper eyelids. The nailbeds frequently show cuticular overgrowth, periungual erythema, and telangiectasis. Subcutaneous calcification, more common in childhood dermatomyositis, also occurs in the adult myositis syndromes. Nearly half of patients have dysrhythmia, CHF, or ECG evidence of conduction defects, ventricular hypertrophy, or pericarditis. Disease can result in sudden paralysis of muscles of respiration, intrinsic lung pathology, or aspiration. Malignancy is found in a higher than expected rate in patients with PM and DM (relative risk, 1.8 for men and 1.7 for women with PM, and 2.4 for men and 3.4 for women with DM).

Management and Treatment

Daily high-dose oral corticosteroid therapy is the usual initial treatment for DM and PM. Methotrexate, effective orally and parenterally, is added if patients fail to respond to steroids alone.

SJÖGREN'S SYNDROME

Sjögren's syndrome (SS) is a chronic, slowly progressive, inflammatory autoimmune exocrinopathy of unknown etiology. Sicca and xerostomia are caused by diminished lacrimal and salivary gland function. A systemic (extraglandular) disorder affecting lungs, kidneys, blood vessels, and muscles, as well as development of B cell lymphoproliferative disorders are serious consequences of the disease. When no other connective tissue disease is associated, the syndrome is known as *primary Sjögren's syndrome.* Sjögren's syndrome is the second most common autoimmune rheumatic disorder after rheumatoid arthritis. Approximately 90% occurs in middle-aged women.

Pathophysiology and Clinical Features

Minor salivary gland biopsy is diagnostic for clusters of lymphocytic infiltrates with acinar atrophy and hypertrophy of ductal epithelial and myoepithelial cells. Antinuclear antibodies (ANA) are positive in 90% of patients, especially to SS-A (Ro) and SS-B (La) (Fig. 62-1). Features considered for diagnosis include ocular and oral symptoms and signs, salivary gland involvement with classic histopathology, and autoantibodies anti-Ro/SS-A and anti-La/SS-B. HIV infection also appears to produce a similar picture, but lacks the circulating antibodies. About half of the patients with primary SS present with extraglandular organ involvement including the lungs with diffuse interstitial disease, kidneys, blood vessels with palpable purpura, muscles, the reticuloendothelial system, and subclinical thyroid disease. Renal involvement includes interstitial nephritis, hyposthenuria, and renal tubular dysfunction with or without renal tubular acidosis. About half of Sjögren's patients have subclinical thyroid disease. Lymphomatous involvement with malignant lymphoma and Waldenström's macroglobulinemia occur in SS. Extraglandular processes are rare in secondary Sjögren's.

Management and Treatment

SS is treated symptomatically. Bromhexine given orally at high doses improves sicca manifestations. Treatment of malignant lymphomas or extraglandular involvement depends on the location, histology, and extent of disease and should include chemotherapy or radiotherapy.

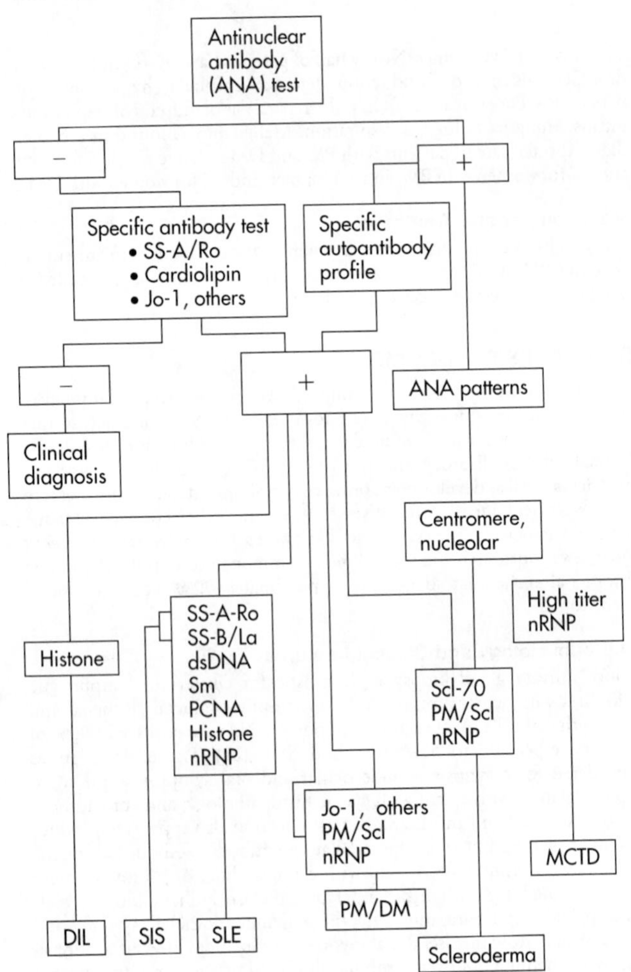

FIG. 62-1 If a characteristic pattern is seen on screening ANA, it may directly suggest a connective tissue disease. However, if the ANA is negative, certain autoantibodies (cell surface or very soluble one such as SS-A, SS-B, cardiolipin, or the myositis-associated antibodies anti Jo-1 or MI-2) may be missed by the screening ANA. Such autoantibodies can then be detected by specific autoantibody tests if suspected. *DIL,* Drug-induced lupus; SS, Sjögren's disease; SLE, systemic lupus erythematosus; PM/DM, polymyositis/dermatomyositis; PM/Scl, polymyositis-scleroderma overlap; MCTD, mixed connective tissue disease; *SS-A,* anti-Ro; *SS-B,* anti-La; *dsDNA,* double-stranded DNA antibody; *Sm,* Helen Smith antibody; *PCNA,* proliferating cell nucleus antibody; *Scl-70,* anti-topoisomerase; *nRNP,* high titer ribonucleoprotein; *anti Jo-1,* anti-histidyl-transferase RNA synthetase.

THE VASCULITIDES

The vasculitides are a heterogenous group of clinical syndromes characterized by inflammation of blood vessels.

Pathophysiology

Antineutrophil cytoplasmic autoantibodies (ANCA) are present in patients with systemic necrotizing vasculitis, including Wegener's granulomatosis and polyarteritis nodosa. The C-ANCA refers to antibodies demonstrated to bind to a serine proteinase (proteinase 3) found in the primary granules in the cytoplasm of the neutrophil. The C-ANCA is a useful diagnostic tool. Pathophysiologies are many and differ in each clinical syndrome.

Clinical Features

The clinical features in benign or fatal forms of vasculitis overlap. When a patient does not easily fit into one vasculitis disease, involvement should be defined and treatment decided accordingly.

Takayasu's arteritis, a chronic vasculitis of the aorta and its branches, is most common in young women of Asian descent and seldom appears after the age of 40. A history of a systemic inflammatory illness, altered arterial pulses, or bruits over large arteries should suggest the diagnosis. Vasculitis lesions similar to erythema nodosum may appear on the legs, with cool extremities, headaches, dizziness, amaurosis or diplopia, and angina. Biopsies are rarely obtained because the largest vessels are affected. The differential diagnosis includes carotid artery dissection, early arteriosclerosis in the setting of high-risk factors, heritable connective tissue disorders such as Ehlers-Danlos syndrome, and giant cell arteritis.

Giant cell arteritis, known as *temporal arteritis* or *cranial arteritis* because of its predilection for these vessels, affects exclusively individuals over 50 years of age and is more common in women. Its onset is often abrupt and flulike, with symptoms such as malaise, fatigue, fever (sometimes as high as 40° C), weight loss, and polymyalgia rheumatica (proximal muscle aching with no myositis). Manifestations of vessel involvement include headaches, scalp sensitivity, tender temporal arteries, jaw claudication (fatigue and discomfort in the masseter muscles of mastication during prolonged chewing or talking), visual loss, diplopia, aortic arch syndrome, and cough or sore throat. Visual loss occurs in about 15% of cases and may be a sudden early symptom. The ESR is much higher than in other vasculitides, ranging from 80 to 100 mm/hr (Westergren method). In a third of the cases, a thickened or tender temporal artery and a new onset of carotid, axillary, or brachial artery bruit appears. Biopsy of the most abnormal segment of the temporal arteries should be performed to confirm the diagnosis even when manifestations seem relatively typical.

Polyarteritis nodosa (PAN) should be suspected in middle-aged males with unexplained fever, weight loss, fatigue, and multisystem findings. Lung involvement is rare. The Churg-Strauss syndrome is an uncommon vasculitis with predominant involvement of the lungs with history of allergy and asthma. Cutaneous manifestations in PAN may include palpable purpura, infarctive ulcers of varying sizes, and livido reticularis. Multiple mononeuropathies are the most typical and occur in half or more of all cases. Segmental necrotizing glomerulonephritis usually causes renovascular hypertension. Gastrointestinal ischemia from mesenteric arteritis results in profound abdominal pain. Hepatitis B surface antigen and antibody have been found in 15% or more of patients; hepatitis C and A also have been identified. Diagnosis is made by biopsy of clinically involved tissues. An abnormal urinary sediment almost always suggests renal involvement. Mesenteric arteriograms with classic changes that include multiple arterial microaneurysms and tapered or narrowed arterial irregularities may suggest the diagnosis when abdominal pain or elevated hepatic enzymes are present and a biopsy site cannot be readily identified. Before the use of corticosteroids, the 5-year survival rate of polyarteritis was less than 15%.

Wegener's granulomatosis occurs in young or middle-aged adults and is more common in men. It consists of a triad of necrotizing granulomatous vasculitis of the upper respiratory tract, the lower respiratory tract, and focal segmental glomerulonephritis. Nasal or oral mucosal ulcerations, tracheal lesions, episcleritis, uveitis, proptosis, orbital granulomas, and otitis media are frequent manifestations. Approximately 80% of patients with Wegener's granulomatosis have positive C-ANCAs. Biopsy (usually nasal mucosa or lung) should be performed for diagnosis because septic processes, angiocentric T cell lymphomas, and other connective tissue diseases can produce similar lesions.

Hypersensitivity vasculitis is the most common vasculitis and is defined as vasculitis of very small vessels, especially arterioles and venules, secondary to an immune response to exogenous substances. Drug reactions are the most common cause. Clinical manifestations in hypersensitivity vasculitis are not distinctive, and similar clinical pictures may be associated with a variety of other disorders.

Cryoglobulinemia is a dysproteinemia caused by immunoglobulins that have the unique property of precipitating in cold temperatures. Type I cryoglobulins are a single, monoclonal protein and are associated with multiple myeloma, macroglobulinemia, and other neoplastic cell proliferations. Type II cryoglobulins are more than one class of immunoglobulin, have all the properties of an immune complex disease, and result in vasculitis through complement-mediated inflammation. Palpable purpura, urticaria, and ulcers and sudden onset of Raynaud's phenomenon are the most common presenting complaints, and progressive glomerulonephritis is the most serious. Cold-insoluble proteins can be determined by isolating the cryoglobulin and measuring the amount of precipitate formed (cryocrit) and should be assessed in all vasculitis.

Management and Treatment

The cornerstone for successful treatment of vasculitis is making an accurate diagnosis as quickly as possible. Corticosteroids continue to be the most effective therapy. Aggressive combination therapy with prednisone and daily cyclophosphamide have improved survival in Wegener's granulomatosis. When hypersensitivity vasculitis is mild, the likely causative agent should be discontinued. If ischemia or glomerulonephritis are present, daily corticosteroids should be added. Treatment of cryoglobulinemia depends on the type of cryoglobulin and the disease severity; progressive renal disease or neuropathy may require high-dose corticosteroids, immunosuppressive agents, and plasmapheresis.

KEY POINTS

1. Autoimmune diseases are a spectrum of clinical manifestations caused by altered immune responses sometimes associated with specific autoantibodies.
2. In addition to antinuclear antibodies in SLE, newer antibodies to cell membrane and cytoplasm components (ANCA) have been described.
3. Overlap can occur in the features of autoimmune diseases so that precise diagnosis cannot be achieved. Therefore treatment is always based on organ involvement and severity.
4. Vasculitides should be suspected in patients with profound multisystem disease and unexplained fever.
5. Although treatment can be as simple as removing the offending drug (as in hypersensitivity vasculitis), the mainstay of treatment of autoimmune disease is corticosteroids, sometimes with the addition of other immunosuppressive drugs.

SUGGESTED READINGS

Altman RD et al: Predictors of survival in systemic sclerosis (scleroderma), *Arthritis Rheum* 34:403-413, 1991.

Asherson RA, Cervera R: The antiphospholipid syndrome: a syndrome in evolution, *Ann Rheum Dis* 51:147-150, 1992.

Conn DL: *Vasculitis syndromes, Rheum Dis Clin North Am* 16:251-490, 1990.

Dalakas MC: Polymyositis, dermatomyositis, and inclusion-body myositis, *N Engl J Med* 325:1487-1498, 1991.

Leavitt RY et al: The American College of Rheumatology 1990 criteria for the classification of Wegener's granulomatosis, *Arthritis Rheum* 33:1101-1107, 1990.

McCurley TL, Collins RD, Ball E: Nodal and extranodal lymphoproliferative disorders in Sjögren's syndrome: a clinical and immunopathologic study, *Hum Pathol* 21:482-492, 1990.

63

Cystitis and Pyelonephritis

SANDRA R. VALAITIS

Urinary tract infections, a source of substantial morbidity in both pregnant and nonpregnant females, are responsible for approximately 7 million office visits and 1 million hospital admissions annually. Asymptomatic or covert bacteriuria is defined as the presence of more than 10^5 colony-forming units (cfu)/ml of voided urine in a patient without urinary complaints. Any bacterial count is abnormal in a catheterized specimen, and in some instances repeat counts of $<10^5$ cfu/ml may be significant in a woman with histories of relapsing symptomatic infections. Cystitis is defined as bacteriuria associated with inflammation of bladder mucosa causing symptoms of urinary frequency, urgency, and occasionally incontinence or irritative voiding symptoms. The number of colony-forming units may be $<10^5$/ml. *Acute pyelonephritis* is traditionally defined as bacteriuria associated with fever, chills, and flank pain. However, in many cases the pain may be atypical, absent, or even referred, for instance, to the abdomen.

PATHOPHYSIOLOGY

UTIs are far more frequent in women than men. These infections may be related to various anatomic, microbiologic, and physiologic factors and often progress from a stage of subclinical asymptomatic bacteriuria to frank pyelonephritis.

Anatomic

The female bladder and urethra lie in close proximity to the vagina and rectum. It is estimated that 10^8 to 10^9 bacteria reside in 1 ml of vaginal secretions. Also, the female urethra is short, approximately 3 to 4 cm in length. Thus it is not surprising that there is a sixtyfold increase in the risk of the development of a UTI within 48 hours of coitus. Use of contraceptive diaphragms increases the risk of UTI. This may be caused by mechanical friction and relative obstruction of the urethra. Also, the diaphragm must be retained for 8 hours to achieve full contraceptive effectiveness.

Individuals conditioned to void infrequently are at greater risk of infection. Such habits promote urinary stasis and provide bacteria with the milieu and time to multiply. Ureteral obstruction by a stone, tumor, or a foreign body in the bladder, such as a suture, also foster the growth of bacteria. Congenitally acquired urinary tract malformations such as duplicated or ectopic ureters or urethral diverticuli may lead to incomplete evacuation of urine, urinary stasis, and the development of UTIs.

Microbiologic

Approximately 80% of urine specimens isolated from patients with UTIs are colonized by *Eschericia coli*. This is not surprising given the close proximity of the urethra and bladder to the vagina and rectum. Other organisms are isolated in lesser frequency (*Staphylococcus saprophyticus* in 10%, *Klebsiella pneumoniae* in 5%, *Enterobacter sp.* in 2%, and *Proteus sp.* in 2%).

A loss of the protective proteoglycan layer within the bladder mucosa presumably allows for an increase in bacterial adherence. This disruption may occur with catheterization, surgical instrumentation, or the development of nephrolithiasis and the formation of a bladder stone. Incomplete eradication of a previous infection, either by an unfinished course of antibiotics or the use of an inappropriate antibiotic to which the isolated organism is resistant, may lead to recurrent infection. Inadequate hygiene and fecal soiling may increase the number of bacteria colonizing the perineal area and predispose the patient to developing a UTI.

Physiologic

The incidence of UTI varies with age. There is an increased incidence in the elderly possibly because of hormonal effects. For instance, a decrease in circulating estrogen results in reduced vascularity and collagen content within both the bladder and the urethra and subsequent atrophy of these tissues. This may be followed by vaginal prolapse (in the form of a cystocele), which, if significant, may impair complete elimination of urine and favor urinary stasis and infection. The presence of other chronic illnesses, especially those that impair immunity (i.e., diabetes), predispose the patient to a higher incidence of any infection.

DIAGNOSIS

In diagnosing a UTI, the physician must keep in mind that many women present in a manner atypical to that described in classic texts. A high index of suspicion and a readiness to perform a urinalysis will increase a physician's diagnostic acumen.

Patients with cystitis complain of frequency, hesitancy, dysuria, nocturia, suprapubic pain, hematuria, or urge or stress incontinence. Fever and chills are less common. Suprapubic or urethral tenderness may be present on physical examination. Pyelonephritis, however, can manifest with fever, chills, and back or flank pain, as well as irritative urinary symptoms and malaise. Costovertebral angle tenderness is frequently elicited and may occasionally be accompanied by abdominal pain and tenderness.

Laboratory Studies

Although the treatment of uncomplicated acute cystitis may be initiated based on symptoms alone, one should always verify the infection by obtaining a urine culture in cases of recurrent UTIs or when involvement of the upper urinary tract is suspected. A clean catch or midstream urine sample may be obtained in the physician's office and sent for urinalysis and culture. It is important to instruct the patient carefully in the appropriate technique for providing the sample to avoid contamination of the specimen. The urine may be grossly inspected for clarity and odor. A cloudy specimen may be the initial indication of pyuria. In the nonpregnant population, a positive leukocyte esterase dipstick result has a sensitivity of 75% to 96% in detecting pyuria associated with infection. Certain bacteria will convert urinary nitrates to nitrites that can also be detected with a dipstick. Quantitative proteinuria may also be an indication of a UTI, but this finding alone has a poor sensitivity (4.3%) and positive predictive value (20%). Microscopic examination of an unspun urine sample may reveal bacteria and red and white blood cells. A large number of squamous cells in the specimen is likely caused by vulvar or vaginal contamination of the sample.

Culture remains the gold standard for the diagnosis of recurrent or persistent infection after a course of antibiotics, in evaluation of upper UTI, or in hospital-acquired infections. The cost-effectiveness of cultures has been debated.

DIFFERENTIAL DIAGNOSIS

A number of other disorders may clinically mimic the symptoms of UTI. These include vulvovaginitis, interstitial cystitis, urethral syndrome, detrusor instability, nephrolithiasis, HSV infection, PID, and obstructive uropathy.

TREATMENT

Conservative methods such as rest, hydration, and acidification of urine by the intake of cranberry juice may aid in relieving some symptoms associated with uncomplicated lower UTIs. However, the gold standard of treatment remains antibiotic therapy (Fig. 63-1). The type of antibiotic chosen and the duration of its use depend on the severity and onset of the infection.

Uncomplicated cystitis can be treated with a 7- to 10-day course of antibiotics. Short-course treatment is more effective than single-dose therapy, which, although less expensive, has been associated with higher rates of recurrence and lower cure rates. Recurrent infections or pyelonephritis should be treated with a 10 to 14-day regimen of antibiotics. The inciting organism should be identified by culture, and its susceptibility to the chosen antibiotic should be documented.

Of the antibiotics available, trimethoprim-sulfamethoxazole has good cure rates and adequate effectiveness in the treatment of most UTIs (Table 63-1). Sensitivity to the drug in terms of gastrointestinal upset or rash is not uncommon. Nitrofurantoin is also commonly used. The generic form has reportedly greater rates of gastrointestinal upset than the macrocrystalline form (Macrodantin). Cephalosporins may also be used in patients who have no known allergies to these medications, but may be associated with

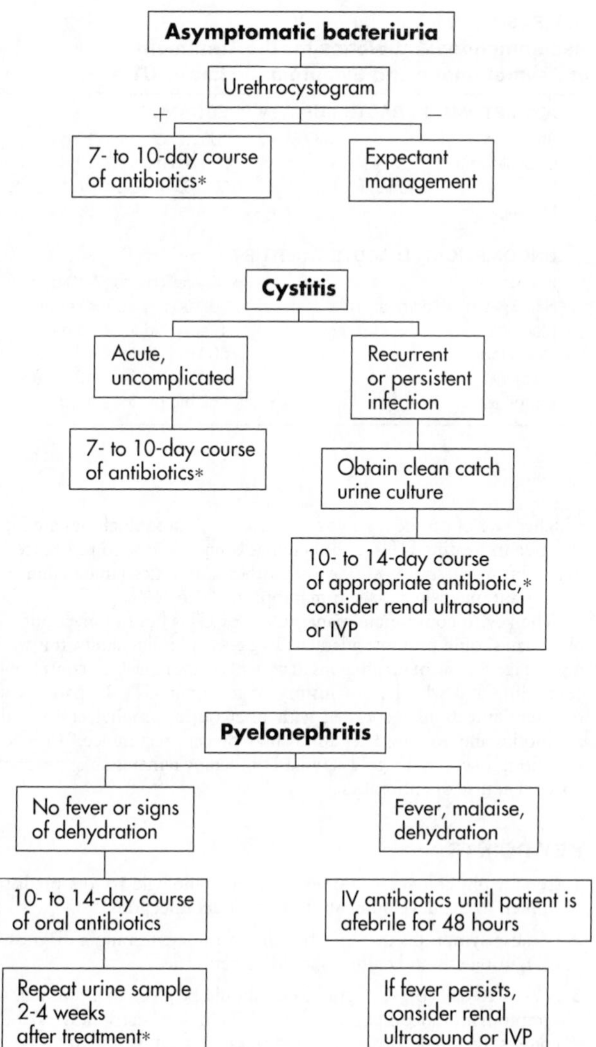

FIG. 63-1 Management and treatment of cystitis and pyelonephritis. *In pregnancy, repeat the urine sample 2 weeks after therapy and every 4 to 6 weeks until delivery.

TABLE 63-1
Recommended Antibiotics for the Treatment of Asymptomatic and Symptomatic Lower UTIs

ASYMPTOMATIC BACTERIURIA IN PREGNANCY	
Ampicillin	500 mg qid for 7-10 days
Cephalexin	500 mg qid for 7-10 days
Nitrofurantoin/Macrodantin	50-100 mg qid for 7-10 days
Macrobid	1 tablet bid for 7-10 days
UNCOMPLICATED ACUTE CYSTITIS	
Bactrim	DS orally bid for 7-10 days
Nitrofurantoin/Macrodantin	50-100 mg qid for 7-10 days
Macrobid	1 tablet bid for 7-10 days
Cephalexin	500 mg qid for 7-10 days
Ampicillin	500 mg qid for 7-10 days
Ciprofloxacin	250 mg bid for 7-10 days

a higher rate of candidal vulvovaginitis. The flouroquinalones are highly effective in treating UTIs, and there has been less in vitro resistance (less than 5%) to these drugs than with other antibiotics (amoxicillin 33%, nitrofurantoin 15% to 20%, trimethoprim 5% to 15%).

The key to appropriate management of UTIs lies in prevention. The physician should promote adequate hygiene and toilet habits. It is wise to discourage the use of diaphragms in patients who are seeking contraceptive counseling and who have a history of recurrent UTI. In patients with recurrent infections associated with intercourse, prophylactic low-dose antibiotics and voiding after coitus may prevent recurrence. With active infection, however, the gold standard of therapy remains an appropriately selected course of antibiotics.

KEY POINTS

1 Certain physiologic, anatomic, and microbiologic factors predispose women to the development of urinary tract infections.

2 Because symptoms may not be reliable in determining a diagnosis of UTI, urinalysis and culture should be performed.

3 A 7- to 10-day course of antibiotics should be given to all women with symptomatic uncomplicated lower UTI. The effectiveness of shorter courses or single doses of antibiotics in treating asymptomatic or symptomatic infections is debatable.

4 Upper UTI should be treated with an appropriately sensitive intravenous antibiotic until the patient is afebrile for 48 hours, followed by a 10- to 14-day regimen of oral antibiotics.

5 Recurrent or resistant infections can be evaluated by radiologic testing such as a renal ultrasound or pyelogram to rule out the presence of calculi or other source of obstruction.

SUGGESTED READINGS

Hooton TM et al: Randomized comparative trial and cost analysis of 3 day antimicrobial regimens for treatment of acute cystitis in women, *JAMA* 273:41-45, 1995.

Meade PB: Postoperative infections. In Thompson JD, Rock JA: *TeLinde's operative gynecology,* ed 7, Philadelphia, 1992, JB Lippincott.

Pappas PG: Laboratory in the diagnosis and management of urinary tract infections, *Med Clin North Am* 75:313-325, 1991.

Patton JP, Nash DB, Abrutyn E: Urinary tract infection: economic considerations, *Med Clin North Am* 75:495-513, 1991.

Stamm WE, Hooton TM: Management of urinary tract infections in adults, *N Engl J Med,* 329:1328-1334, 1993.

Wall LL, Norton PA, DeLancey JO, eds: *Practical urogynecology,* Baltimore, 1993, Williams and Wilkins.

64

Diarrhea—Chronic

James S. Ma and Thomas Y. Ma

The term *diarrhea* refers to a "loosening" of stools. Clinically, patients may complain of an increase in the frequency, volume, and/or fluidity of stools. The frequency and consistency of stools may vary greatly from individual to individual. For instance, normal frequency of bowel movements ranges from as few as three/week to three/day. For clinical purposes, diarrhea is defined as having stool volume >200 ml/24 hours or stool weight >200 g/24 hours. Most acute diarrheal syndromes resolve within 3 weeks and usually do not require therapy. When the diarrheal state persists for more than 3 to 4 weeks, it is considered a chronic diarrhea.

PHYSIOLOGY

On average, approximately 9 L of fluid pass through the gastrointestinal tract daily: 2 L from diet, 1 L from saliva, 2 L from gastric juice, 1 L from bile, 2 L from pancreatic juice, and 1 L from small bowel. On average, 7 to 8 L of fluid are absorbed by the small intestine, 1 to 1.5 L are absorbed by the colon, and <200 ml are lost in the stool. The maximum absorptive capacity of the small intestine and the colon is 12 L and 5 L, respectively. Diarrhea can result if (1) the maximal absorptive capacity of the colon (5 L) is exceeded (increased osmotic load or secretion), (2) the absorptive capacity of the small intestine/colon is pathologically decreased (e.g., mucosal injury in celiac disease), and/or (3) there is a decrease in the intestinal transit time (rapid transit), resulting in decreased luminal contact and absorption time.

The epithelial surface of the small intestine consists of two functionally and anatomically distinct regions, the villus and the crypt. Epithelial cells in the villi are functionally and structurally differentiated for absorption of nutrients and fluids. The crypt cells, on the other hand, lack the ability to absorb nutrients, but promote secretion of ions and fluid. In general, it may be assumed that the villus region is absorptive in nature, whereas the crypt is secretory. Thus diseases that result in destruction of the villus epithelium (e.g., inflammatory bowel disease, celiac disease) will decrease absorption of nutrients and fluid, and diseases that produce hypertrophy of the crypts (e.g., celiac disease) will increase fluid secretion.

CLASSIFICATION

The causes of chronic diarrhea can be divided into four major classes: (1) osmotic diarrhea, (2) secretory diarrhea, (3) mucosal injury or decreased absorptive capacity, and (4) disordered motility. In most chronic diarrheal states, more than one mechanism of action is present. For example, in celiac disease there is (1) extensive destruction of the villus (the absorptive component of the mucosa) resulting in a marked decrease in mucosal absorptive capacity, (2) hyperplasia of the crypts (the glandular component of the mucosa) leading to increased ion and fluid secretion, (3) destruction of brush border enzymes resulting in lactase deficiency and resultant osmotic diarrhea, and (4) increased luminal fluid load causing increased propulsive motor activity (decreased transit time).

Osmotic Diarrhea

Osmotic diarrhea is caused by the presence of poorly absorbable or nonabsorbable solutes in the intestinal lumen. The presence of these osmotically active solutes results in the accumulation of fluid in the intestinal lumen to achieve an isoosmotic state. The most common cause of osmotic diarrhea in clinical medicine is the malabsorption of lactose caused by deficiency of the brush border enzyme lactase. Brush border lactase hydrolyzes the disaccharide lactose into the monosaccharides glucose and galactose. Glucose and galactose are rapidly absorbed in the small intestine. Undigested lactose is poorly absorbed and remains in the lumen and may cause osmotic diarrhea. Lactase levels are high at birth, but progressively decrease with age. In most populations, lactase deficiency is present by age 50 or sooner. Typically, small amounts of malabsorbed carbohydrates do not cause diarrhea because colonic bacteria have the capability to metabolize carbohydrates into short-chain fatty acids that are absorbed in the colon. Diarrhea results when the colonic carbohydrate load exceeds the "threshold level" such that either the capability of the colonic bacteria to metabolize the carbohydrate load and/or the colonic absorptive capacity of short-chain fatty acids is exceeded.

Disaccharidase deficiency is caused by an inherited defect or an acquired loss of brush border disaccharidases. Lactase deficiency is the most common disaccharidase deficiency. Sucrase-isomaltase deficiency results in the intolerance of sweets (sucrose is present in high concentrations in many candies and medication syrups). Trehalase deficiency (trehalose present in mushrooms) is rare. The ingestion of excessive loads of poorly absorbed carbohydrates such as fructose, sorbitol, lactulose, mannitol, and cellulose (fiber) can also cause osmotic diarrhea. A transporter deficiency/defect (e.g., absence of specific disaccharide transporter), such as the glucose-galactose transporter deficiency, is often inherited and results in glucose malabsorption. Medications containing poorly absorbed anions (e.g., magnesium, sulfate, phosphate) are frequently found to be the cause of osmotic diarrhea and include laxatives and antacids.

The evaluation of osmotic diarrhea begins with a thorough history of ingestion of dairy (lactose-containing) products, sugar-free candies and/or dietary soft drinks (sorbitol), or laxatives. Symptoms may involve any or all of the following: abdominal bloating and cramping, abdominal pain, flatus, and diarrhea (usually within 4 hours of ingestion). Generally, symptoms subside with fasting. Elevation of the stool osmotic gap (>50) may be helpful in confirming the presence of an osmotic diarrhea. Stool osmotic gap may be calculated by subtracting twice the sum of the stool K^+ and Na^+ from the stool osmolality (obtained from stool analysis). The stool K^+ and Na^+ are multiplied by 2 to account for the stool anions. In carbohydrate-induced osmotic diarrhea, the stool pH is usually low (pH < 5.3) because of carbohydrate metabolism by colonic bacteria producing short-chain fatty acids (e.g., lactic acid).

Secretory Diarrhea

Secretory diarrhea is caused by an inappropriate intestinal secretion of ions (Cl^-, HCO_3^-, Na^+, K^+), namely the anions Cl^- and HCO_3^-, with the accompanying water. This is a component of most diarrheal syndromes. In some conditions (e.g., VIPoma, traveler's diarrhea), intestinal secretion of ions may be stimulated by hormones, neurotransmitters, or various exogenous sources, including bacterial toxins. In diseases such as celiac sprue, there is marked hypertrophy of the crypt epithelium resulting in an increase in ion and fluid secretion. Infectious causes (bacterial toxins) are commonly identified in travelers, areas of overcrowding, or under conditions of poor hygiene. Vibrio cholera toxin directly affects the enterocyte activating adenylate cyclase, causing increased production of cAMP. The stimulation of intracellular cAMP production results in secretion of chloride and bicarbonate and inhibition of NaCl uptake. *E. coli* heat stable enterotoxin increases production of cGMP, also resulting in anionic secretion. Medications including laxatives (phenolphthalein, bisacodyl, castor oil, senna, dioctyl sodium), cholinergic drugs, prostaglandins, diuretics, caffeine, and other methylxanthines can induce intestinal secretion. Bile acids stimulate colonic secretion of electrolytes and fluids. An increased colonic load of bile causes secretory diarrhea. Since the ileum is the only site of active bile acid absorption, surgical resection, bypass, or inflammatory disease of the ileum may result in secretory diarrhea. Primary bile acid malabsorption in the ileum may occur in some patients. Increased production or ingestion of bile acids (e.g., ingestion of ursodeoxycholic acid) above the absorptive capacity of the ileum may also cause diarrhea. Hydroxy fatty acids also cause colonic and electrolyte secretion. The following tumors can produce substances that act as secretagogues in the intestines: gastrinoma (gastrin), carcinoid syndrome (serotonin, histamine, catecholamines, kinins), and VIPoma (vasoactive intestinal peptide). In contrast to osmotic diarrhea, stool osmotic gap is normal in secretory diarrhea. Typically, diarrhea does not improve (or only minimally improves) with fasting. In general, secretory diarrhea tends to be larger in volume than osmotic diarrhea, and stool pH is usually >5.6.

Inflammatory Diarrhea

Inflammatory diarrhea may be caused by several mechanisms. Intestinal inflammation can produce extensive destruction of the absorptive villus epithelium and result in decreased absorptive capacity. Additionally, intestinal inflammation results in the production of a variety of inflammatory mediators that promote intestinal secretion and motility. Intestinal inflammation is characterized by the presence of blood, pus, mucus, and proteins in the intestinal lumen and stool.

Inflammatory bowel disease (ulcerative colitis, Crohn's disease) must always be a consideration. Invasive infections (*Entamoeba histolytica,* enteropathogenic *E. coli, Yersinia enterocolitica, Shigella, Salmonella, Campylobacter, Clostridium difficile*) may lead to inflammation. Other important causes include celiac sprue, tropical sprue, radiation colitis, microscopic (lymphocytic) colitis, and collagenous colitis. Often, patients may have systemic manifestations including fever and elevated WBC count and ESR. Typically, the stool is characterized by the presence of WBCs and RBCs indicating the presence of intestinal inflammation and mucosal injury. Depending on the site of involvement (small intestine versus colon), stool volume and frequency will vary. Frequently, components of both secretory and osmotic diarrhea may be present.

Altered Motility

Altered motility is a component of most diarrheal states. Increased intestinal fluid load or accumulation of luminal fluid stimulates intestinal contraction, thus further complicating the existing condition. Intestinal contraction may also be stimulated by various neural and inflammatory factors of the underlying disease process. The extent of the contribution of enhanced motility in diarrhea is variable depending on the disease process.

Irritable bowel syndrome (IBS, functional bowel disease, spastic colon) is a disorder defined by abdominal discomfort associated with an alteration in stool consistency characterized by diarrhea, constipation, or both in an alternating pattern. This functional syndrome has no identifiable organic pathology, and the etiology is not clear. However, an alteration in motility has been documented in many patients with this condition. Generally, patients may have a lower threshold to pain with balloon dilation in the rectum; a hyperstimulatory response in the colon to cholecystokinin, food, and stress; and an increase in slow wave motor activity in the colon. Altered bowel movements associated with the onset of pain, relief of pain with the passing of a bowel movement or flatus, or the sensation of incomplete evacuation are all symptoms suggestive of IBS. Hyperthyroidism, scleroderma, diabetes mellitus, postvagotomy, postgastrectomy, and medications are additional common causes.

DIAGNOSIS

The history is the key to an efficient evaluation and timely diagnosis. A good history alone often leads to the diagnosis. It not only directs the approach, but also the sequence in which tests are performed. For example, symptoms occurring during or following a trip to Mexico should alert the physician to the probability of an infectious etiology that may require a routine sigmoidoscopy and stool studies. The color of stool (brown, melena, bright red blood), the consistency (watery, soupy, greasy, mucous), and volume are all important factors. Large-volume stools, 4 to 5 episodes/day (3 to 4 L/day), may be consistent with small intestinal disease. On the other hand, small-volume, frequent (8 to 12/day) stools are more likely to involve the distal colon or rectum.

The presence (or absence) of pain, its nature, and its location may also reveal important clues. Intermittent, crampy, right upper quadrant/periumbilical pain reflects small intestinal or cecal origin. Pain located in either lower quadrant, hypogastrium, or sacrum may reflect distal colon or rectal pathology. Blood and/or pus (inflammatory or neoplastic); excessive flatus (carbohydrate malabsorption); frothy, oily (steatorrhea) changes with fasting; and a history of travel, diet, and medication are all important. In addition, a history of eating disorders, psychiatric history, family history, ill contacts, pets, sexual orientation, and possible causes of immunosuppression should be sought.

Certain characteristics have been strongly correlated with the presence with organic disease. These include daily, nonintermittent diarrhea, nocturnal diarrhea, onset at a specific point in time, evidence of malnutrition, dehydration, and weight loss.

During the physical examination, hydrational status must be evaluated. Any evidence of hypovolemia must be addressed, if necessary, with IV hydration. Some important findings include skin lesions (hyperpigmentation with Whipple's disease, dermatitis herpetiformis with sprue, pyoderma gangrenosa and erythema nodosum with IBD), glossitis (vitamin B_{12} deficiency), icterus (liver disease), exophthalmos, goiter, abdominal pain/mass, hepatosplenomegaly, ascites, evidence of anemia, perianal fistulas, rectal mass, edema, and lymphadenopathy.

Stool studies may include 24-hour volume/consistency to confirm the presence of diarrhea, Wright stain to assess the presence of WBCs, evaluation for the presence of blood, and, culture for ova and parasites × 3 and enteric pathogens. Other studies include stool osmotic gradient; alkalinization study ("laxative screen"), which may be useful in the evaluation of the surreptitious use of laxatives (1 drop of 1N NaOH added to 3 ml of urine or stool supernate will turn pink if phenolphthalein is present); a fecal fat analysis (qualitative [sudan stain] or quantitative [72-hour stool collection while patient is on 75 to 100 g of fat/24-hour diet]), which can be obtained for the determination of steatorrhea or malabsorption; and *Clostridium difficile* toxin, which may confirm the diagnosis of pseudomembranous colitis (if a history of antibiotic use is present in the previous 2 months). Blood tests may include CBC with differential to assess anemia (microcytic/macrocytic) and/or leukocytosis/leukopenia; chemistry panel to assess electrolytes, general nutritional state, and renal function; liver panel to assess hepatic and biliary status; and thyroid panel to assess hypothyroidism/hyperthyroidism. Other blood tests include betacarotene level for assessing nutritional status; folate, iron (Fe, ferritin, TIBC), and vitamin B_{12} studies for malabsorption syndromes (vitamin B_{12} absorbed in the terminal ileum, folate and iron in the proximal duodenum); gastrin, which is elevated in gastrinoma, a non–β-islet cell tumor of the pancreas (Zollinger-Ellison syndrome); vasoactive intestinal peptide (VIP), which is elevated in VIPoma (a.k.a. WDHA, pancreatic cholera, Verner-Morrison syndrome), another non-β-islet cell tumor of the pancreas; calcitonin, which may be elevated in medullary carcinoma of the thyroid; and amylase/lipase, which may be elevated in pancreatic cancer.

Urine tests are ordered as indicated. A laxative screen may be positive in surreptitious use. A drug screen may be performed if indicated. 5-hydroxyindoleacetic acid (5-HIAA) (a metabolite of serotonin) is elevated in a 24-hour urine sample in patients with carcinoid tumors. Metanephrine can be elevated in patients with pheochromocytoma.

Endoscopy with biopsy and culture may be helpful when indicated. Flexible sigmoidoscopy should be performed on the majority of patients with chronic diarrhea (without bowel preparation so as not to alter the current state of the mucosa). Esophagogastroduodenoscopy/enteroscopy should be considered if/when an upper gastrointestinal lesion is suspected. Colonoscopy should be considered if the sigmoidoscopy is unrevealing and a strong suspicion for a lower gastrointestinal lesion persists. When a lesion is believed to be located in the distal small intestine/proximal colon, colonoscopy is the procedure of choice. Radiologic examination also can frequently be of assistance. Plain abdominal films may reveal pancreatic calcifications suggestive of chronic pancreatitis. Other examinations should be considered as indicated (upper GI with small bowel follow through [UGI/SBFT], barium enema, ultrasound, CT scan).

Other specific examinations should be considered when necessary. The Schilling test can determine if/where a defect in the absorption of vitamin B_{12} exists. The D-xylose test determines small intestine mucosal integrity and may be helpful in distinguishing between a defect in digestion versus absorption. The H_2 breath test measures increased hydrogen in the exhaled breath after the consumption of a specific carbohydrate and, if positive, is suggestive of carbohydrate malabsorption or bacterial overgrowth. The secretin test may be helpful in determining pancreatic insufficiency.

In all patients having diarrhea for more than 3 to 4 weeks, a workup for chronic diarrhea should be initiated. A thorough history and physical examination is crucial in guiding the workup. In many cases, the diagnosis will be apparent after the history and physical examination. However, when the etiology of the diarrhea is unclear, a reasonable approach would be to examine stool for evidence of inflammation (WBCs and/or RBCs). Flexible sigmoidoscopy should also be performed to rule out an obvious colonic source. If stool WBCs and/or RBCs are present or if colitis is present, an inflammatory process is suggested. In the absence of these findings, the possibility of a secretory, osmotic, and/or motility disorder should be evaluated (Fig. 64-1).

THERAPY

The main goal in the therapy of chronic diarrhea is to efficiently identify and treat the specific underlying cause. For example, steroids and mesalamine are the mainstays in therapy for ulcerative colitis; a gluten-free diet is the treatment of choice for celiac sprue. Dietary and medication modifications should be made whenever appropriate. An empiric therapeutic trial may be appropriate initial treatment in some cases.

Generally, there are three major considerations: (1) hydrational status, (2) nutritional status, and (3) clinical symptoms. Regardless of the etiology of diarrhea, hydrational status of an individual must be addressed first. Fluids and electrolytes have to be replaced as needed. Oral replenishment is always preferred if feasible, if not, an intravenous route may be required. Hemodynamic stability must be maintained. Nutritional requirements and deficits should be assessed and managed aggressively. A dietitian may be able to diagnose specific deficiencies that may add to the diagnostic evaluation. Again, oral supplementation is preferred, but parenteral nutrition may be indicated, especially if the patient is unable to have oral intake, is severely malnourished, or needs aggressive preoperative or postoperative nutritional support. Despite treatment of the underlying cause of diarrhea, some patients remain symptomatic because of chronic organic or functional conditions. In these patients, attempts at symptomatic treatment to control the volume and frequency of stools is reasonable and desirable.

Nonspecific antidiarrheal agents are used for symptomatic therapy. Hydrophilic agents (psyllium, polycarbophil, methylcellulose) bind water. Although fewer, bulkier stools are passed, the total amount of stool is unchanged. In fact, diarrhea may worsen in some cases. Adsorbent agents (bismuth subsalicylate, kaolin/pectin) presumably adsorb intraluminal toxins and microbials and bismuth may have some intrinsic antimicrobial effect; salicylate may have a local antiinflammatory effect and/or local antisecretory effect. Opioids (diphenoxylate hydrochloride/atropine, loperamide, codeine) slow gastrointestinal transit time, decrease gastrointestinal secretions, and stimulate water and electrolyte absorption. Some caution must be exercised when using opioids, especially in the setting of an acute inflammatory colitis (infectious or IBD), because there is a risk of toxic megacolon and perforation. An addictive potential also exists.

Hydrophilic agents are not absorbed, are very safe, and should be considered as first-line therapy. They may cause constipation if taken in

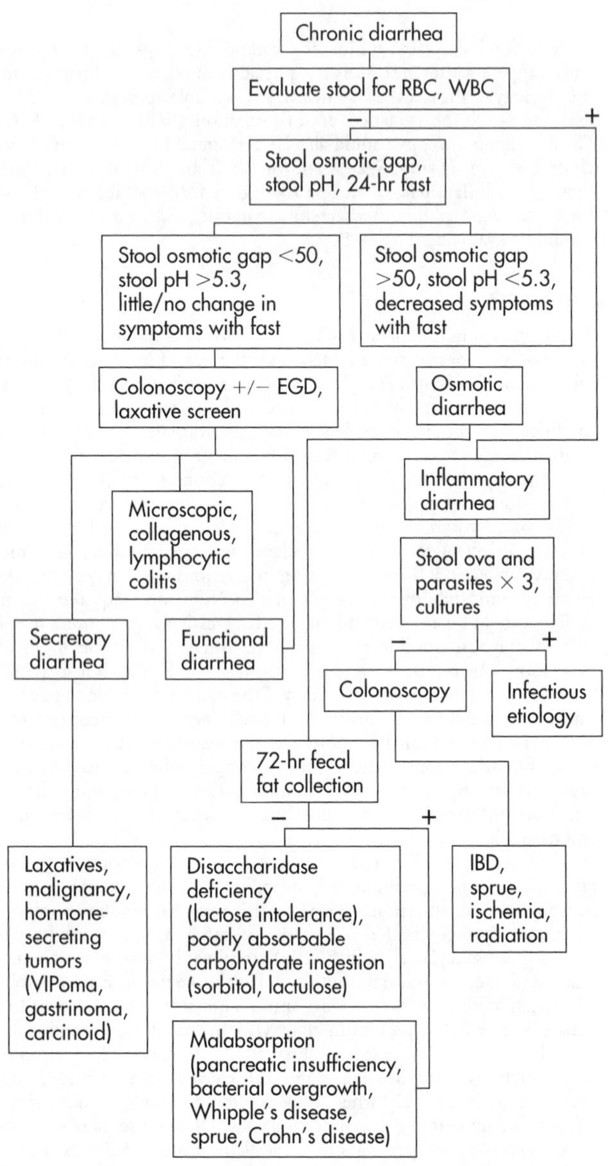

FIG. 64-1 Diagnostic workup of chronic diarrhea. *EGD,* esophagogastroduodenoscopy.

excess or impaction if a partial bowel obstruction is already present. Adsorbents are typically safe and should be considered first line therapy. Bismuth toxicity can be seen if large amounts of Pepto-Bismol are ingested. The opioids are very effective in controlling diarrhea but should be used only if first-line therapies are not effective. As mentioned, opioids must be used cautiously in the setting of an acute (infectious or noninfectious) colitis because toxin clearance may be hindered and toxic megacolon can result, especially in the setting of transmural inflammation.

Specific antidiarrheal agents are indicated according to the underlying disease process. Antibiotics are used in infectious diarrheas. Resins such as cholestyramine may be useful in diarrhea caused by excessive intraluminal bile (most commonly postsurgical) by binding bile salts. Antiinflammatory agents (sulfasalazine, mesalamine, corticosteroids) are used in the management of IBD. Anticholinergic/antispasmodic/antianxiety combination agents are available and may be helpful in irritable bowel syndrome (IBS) or other functional bowel syndromes.

KEY POINTS

1 Chronic diarrhea is defined as having stool volume >200 ml or stool weight >200 g/24 hours for more than 3 to 4 weeks duration.

2 Osmotic diarrhea is characterized by an elevated stool osmotic gap and a low stool pH.

3 Secretory diarrhea is caused by an increase in ionic and water secretion into the lumen and is characterized by a normal stool osmotic gap and a normal stool pH.

4 Inflammatory diarrhea is characterized by the presence of blood, pus, and/or fever.

5 A specific diagnosis can be made in up to 80% of cases with a thorough history and physical examination, focused laboratory tests, and sigmoidoscopy.

SUGGESTED READINGS

Ammon HV: Diarrhea and constipation. In Berk JE, ed: *Gastroenterology,* ed 5, Philadelphia, 1995, WB Saunders.

Fine KD, Krejs GJ, Fordtran JS: Diarrhea. In Sleisenger MH, Fordtran JS, eds: *Gastrointestinal disease: pathophysiology, diagnosis, management,* ed 5, Philadelphia, 1993, WB Saunders.

Powell DW: Approach to the patient with diarrhea. In Yamada T, ed: *Textbook of gastroenterology,* ed 2, Philadelphia, 1995, JB Lippincott.

Walfish JS: Diarrhea. In Sachar DB, Waye JD, Lewis BS: *Pocket guide to gastroenterology,* Baltimore, Md, 1991, Williams & Wilkins.

65

Domestic Violence and the Physician Response

JULIANNE STOODY TOOHEY AND CAROL A. MAJOR*

Four thousand women from all ages, races, ethnic backgrounds, occupations, religions, and socioeconomic groups are murdered each year in the United States by their current or former spouse or boyfriend. Approximately 4 million are injured seriously enough to necessitate medical or police intervention.

Experts in this field agree that domestic violence is about abuse of power and control. The batterer's low self-esteem instills a desperate need to control as many aspects of his life as possible, including his wife. He is usually a victim of abuse himself or has witnessed his mother's abuse at the hands of his father, and has learned to use jealousy, anger, and violence to achieve this control.

Domestic violence is a pattern of physical, sexual, and psychologic attacks by a member of a family against another member of the same family for the purpose of coercion without regard for the victim's rights. The U.S. Department of Justice estimates that 95% of domestic violence cases between spouses involves abusive behavior by men against women. Domestic violence occurs in both adult and adolescent, and heterosexual and homosexual intimate relationships.

Physical abuse may involve a push or a slap, and may escalate to repeated beatings with a closed fist, boot, or other weapon. For many women, physical abuse ends in death. Sexual abuse is often a component of domestic violence and includes rape, degrading acts, violent sex, or injury with objects during sex. It also includes intercourse when the victim is unconscious and may include sex without protection from pregnancy, HIV, and other STDs. Women often share that one of the most painful forms of abuse is psychologic. Continual threats of violence to either herself, her children, or others she loves may be coupled with threats of suicide by the abuser. Threats to report to immigration authorities or to kidnap the children leave the woman in constant terror. Attacks against property are common and directed against things that are precious to her. Psychologic abuse also includes continued, humiliating verbal attacks

* A grateful acknowledgment to Vivian Clecak and Shirley Gellatly of Human Options for their assistance in preparing this work.

about her sorrows or mistakes. Isolation from family or friends is an important method for further control and includes dictating how she may spend her time and with whom. Extreme jealousy colors the abuser's view of all of her encounters with others and reflects his fear of loss of control.

Economic control has obvious direct implications regarding the woman's options in her life and occurs even if the woman is working. It includes control over important decisions in the family, the checking account, use of the car, access to transportation, food, shelter–in short, the necessities of life. The coercive behavior in abusive relationships is not an isolated event but rather a repetitive, chronic pattern that has been called the *cycle of violence.* Phase I of the cycle involves a building of tensions in the home, with the perpetrator becoming increasingly irritable and angry. Typically, during this phase the woman and her children are desperately attempting to prevent his anger and subsequent outbursts. Eventually, however, no matter how hard they try, the battering occurs. Phase II is the actual battering incident. It may involve threats, a slap, a push, or may include severe beatings, rape, and even death. Phase III is often referred to as the *honeymoon period.* During this time, the abuser is apologetic, repentant, and even ashamed of his violent behavior. He reminds his wife that he loves her and promises never to hurt her again. He may blame increased stress at work or alcohol use for his lack of control. This phase gives the woman hope that her situation will change and therefore may be the most dangerous phase for her. It is important that women be reminded that no one deserves to be abused, that violence is never justified in a relationship, and that she is not responsible. Researchers are aware that the violence in Phase II escalates with time and that the honeymoon phase gets shorter and shorter. Eventually, the couple finds themselves alternating between the tension-building phase and the actual physical abuse.

CHARACTERISTICS OF THE BATTERED WOMAN

The battered woman is often very isolated and may have increased dependence on her spouse (e.g., she is pregnant, a teenager, lives in rural areas, does not drive, has a special handicap or disability, is an immigrant, or does not speak the language of the community). She has few friends and rarely attends social functions. If she does go to outings, she is usually accompanied by her spouse. While at work, she calls or frequently receives calls from her spouse or he may show up unexpectedly. He is usually with her during physician's appointments and is reluctant to leave her alone with a nurse or physician. She is unable to make decisions on her own and must always confer with her husband. The battered woman carries little or no money, credit cards, or checks. She often wears clothes that cover up injuries in various stages of healing (e.g., dark glasses, long sleeves, and long slacks). She misses work frequently because of injury and is also noncompliant with her physician's appointments. When a patients misses an appointment, remember to call and reschedule her appointment as soon as possible. The battered woman often has multiple somatic complaints or presents to the emergency room for insignificant symptoms such as a yeast infection or UTI.

THE PHYSICIAN AND DOMESTIC VIOLENCE

Domestic violence is the number one cause of injury to women in the United States. The numbers total more than motor vehicle accidents and muggings combined. All physicians will treat victims of abuse. However, it is estimated that only 1 in 25 battered women will be identified or diagnosed by her physician.

The woman herself erects several barriers to identification. Her shame, humiliation, protective feelings towards her partner, and also her real fear that revelation to others will further endanger her or her children are some of the factors that keep the battered woman from confiding in her physician, counselor, priest, or friend. In addition, it is important to recognize the multiple cultural barriers that may exist in an ethnically diverse population.

Physicians also erect barriers against proper diagnosis. Their lack of awareness as to the scope of this health care problem, their belief that domestic violence is really not a physician issue, time constraints, their feelings of discomfort and frustration in dealing with a complex medical-social issue, and their lack of knowledge on how to respond to the battered woman are all factors that prevent physicians from routinely screening and assessing their patients for abuse. The single most important reason why health care providers do not diagnose domestic violence is because they do not ask the question.

It is critical that physicians routinely assess all of their patients for domestic violence (Fig. 65-1). It is clear that following stereotypes regarding which woman is at risk prevents accurate diagnosis. In addition, routine assessment is a form of health education, acknowledges that domestic violence is a health care issue, and reminds the patient that they are not alone.

The physician should always assess the patient in private and provide literature and resource information where she may read it or pick it up in private (e.g., the woman's restroom). A common way for the physician to open up the topic is to say "Domestic violence is unfortunately a problem for many women. Are you or have you ever been in an abusive relationship? Are you safe at home?" If a suspicious injury or bruise is seen, the physician may say "In my experience, when a woman has a bruise like this, she has been hit by someone. Did this happen to you? Is someone hurting you?" The physician should always ask about sleeping and eating difficulties and other signs of depression. Also question her about sleep and pain medications and drug and alcohol use. These are red flags. Do not be judgmental and discriminatory to women who present under the influence of alcohol or drugs. These patients need you most of all.

Teach patients about the cycle of violence. Inform your patient that violence in abusive relationships escalates and that her life and the lives of her children are in danger. Always ask about child abuse. In over 50% of homes where there is spousal abuse the children are also injured. Assess your patient's immediate safety. Where is the family in the cycle of violence? Has the violence recently escalated in severity or frequency? Does he have a gun in the house? Has he threatened homicide or suicide? These are all serious risk factors for homicide. Help your patient formulate a safety plan. Does she have a safe place to go? As much as possible,

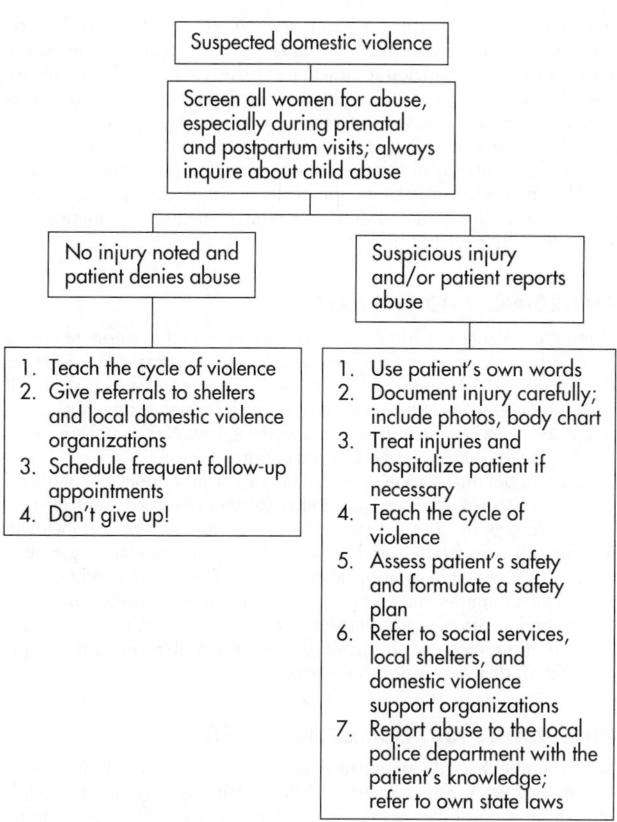

FIG. 65-1 Management of suspected domestic violence.

encourage entry into a woman's shelter. Professional counselors who are dedicated to helping women in this situation are available and can assist you in providing a safety plan. Does the patient need to be hospitalized and treated for injuries or does she require immediate psychiatric intervention? Also refer patients to social services workers who can assist you with appropriate referrals.

If your patient plans to return to her partner, suggest an emergency kit that includes an extra set of car keys, some cash, important documents (birth certificates, custody papers, immigration papers), important phone numbers, medications, diapers, etc. This kit should be kept at the home of a neighbor or friend where it can be easily obtained should she be required to flee. Encourage your patient to talk to someone about her fear. Battery depends on isolation, and a friend can be an important first step. Schedule the patient for frequent appointments. Be careful if you call her at home because this may endanger her. If your patient denies abuse but you are suspicious or if you think she is at high risk for violence teach her about the cycle of violence, provide her with information on helpful resources. Do not expect her to immediately trust in you or confide in you. Remember that this is a long-term, chronic problem and that your patient may not share your concerns. The most dangerous time for a woman is when she attempts to leave her abusive partner, and it may take her a long time to do so. Be nonjudgmental, informative, and supportive. Respect her decisions.

PHYSICIANS AND THE LAW

Domestic violence is a crime. Many states now have mandatory reporting laws for health care providers. For example, in California, AB 1652 states that any health care provider who knows or suspects an injury is the result of domestic violence must report this to the local police immediately by phone and by written report within 2 working days. Noncompliance with this law is punishable by fine and/or jail time.

Careful documentation is vitally important in all domestic violence cases. It is the physician's responsibility to complete the patient medical record. Always use the patient's own words to describe the incident. Measure all cuts, bruises, and burns and describe in detail any objects removed (i.e., splinters of wood, glass, or carpet fibers). Use a body chart to document all injuries and take photographs when possible. Document on the medical record the name of the police officer who took your report, the case report number, and the action that was taken. Remember to include the referrals that were given to the patient.

PREGNANCY AND DOMESTIC VIOLENCE

Several studies have documented an increased incidence of physical abuse during pregnancy. Some experts feel that pregnancy may represent a loss of control to the abuser even though the pregnancy itself is often a result of rape. Pregnant women who are abused tend to suffer more injuries to the breasts and abdomen and have an increased incidence of spontaneous abortions, stillbirth, and low-birth-weight infants.

It is estimated that one in six neonates will go home to a mother that has been abused during her pregnancy. Battering during pregnancy is more common than gestational diabetes or placenta previa. Pregnant women are more likely to seek medical attention after abuse than nonpregnant women. Obstetricians are therefore in a unique position to educate, assess, and treat victims of domestic violence.

KEY POINTS

1 Four thousand women from all ages, races, ethnic backgrounds, occupations, religions, and socioeconomic groups are murdered each year in the United States by a current or former partner.

2 Family violence may be physical, sexual, economic, and/or psychologic and is about abuse of power and control.

3 Abusive relationships are involved in a repetitive, chronic pattern of behavior called the *cycle of violence.*

4 In many states, physicians are required by law to report any injury that is the result of domestic violence.

5 Physical abuse may increase in incidence and severity during pregnancy.

6 Physicians play a vital role in providing a safe, nonjudgmental, and sensitive environment in which to assess, educate, and treat a victim of domestic violence.

SUGGESTED READINGS

Berrios DC, Grady D: Domestic violence: risk factors and outcomes, *West J Med* 155:133-135, 1991.

Campbell JC et al: Correlates of battering during pregnancy, *Res Nurs Health* 15:219-226, 1992.

Federal Bureau of Investigation: *Uniform crime reports for the United States,* Washington, DC, 1993, U.S. Dept of Justice.

Koss M: Testimony before the Senate Judiciary Committee, 1990.

McFarlane J et al: Assessing for abuse during pregnancy: severity and frequency of injuries and associated entry into prenatal care, *JAMA* 267:3176-3178, 1992.

National information centers

National Resource Center on Domestic Violence, Harrisburg, PA; (800) 537-2238

Health Resource Center on Domestic Violence, San Francisco, CA; (800) 313-1310

Resource Center on Family Violence: Child Protection and Custody, Reno, NV; (800) 52-PEACE

Battered Women's Justice Project; (800) 903-0111

National Coalition Against Domestic Violence, P.O. Box 18749, Denver, CO; (303) 839-1852

Domestic Abuse Awareness Project, New York, NY; (212) 353-1755

Centers for Disease Control and Prevention, Family and Intimate Violence Prevention Team, Atlanta, GA; (404) 639-3311

Gay and Lesbian Anti-Violence Project, New York, NY; (212) 807-0197

66

Gastritis—Chronic and Acute

Hooshang Meshkinpour

Gastritis is the most common disorder of the stomach. It is histologically characterized by an increased number of inflammatory cells in the gastric mucosa. Since histologic, endoscopic, and clinical findings poorly correlate, the classification of gastritis is difficult. A remarkable proportion of patients with gastritis are essentially asymptomatic. On the other hand, those who are symptomatic present either with upper gastrointestinal bleeding or they have vague, nonspecific upper abdominal complaints that are collectively identified as **non-ulcer dyspepsia.** There are three basic types of gastritis: acute, chronic, and specific.

Acute erosive gastritis is an inflammatory reaction that is often accompanied by superficial erosions and bleeding. The term *stress ulcers* generally refers to multiple erosions or ulcerations that develop in the clinical setting of severe physiologic stress in the form of trauma, thermal injury, sepsis, and multiorgan failure. In addition to physiologic stress, ingestion of drugs such as salicylates and NSAIDs and heavy alcohol consumption are the most common causes. Profound bleeding may occur in about 1% to 5% of these patients, with the exception of those patients with thermal injury where bleeding may occur in up to 30%. Diagnosis is primarily by endoscopy. Treatment includes correction of underlying conditions and discontinuing the predisposing factors. In this setting, the frequency of bacterial pneumonia complicating the prophylactic treatment with H_2-receptor antagonists has been estimated to be as high as 50%. It has been suggested that hypochlorhydria promotes bacterial growth in the stomach, which leads to aspiration pneumonia. A prophylactic regimen probably should be used in patients with a history of peptic ulcer disease or upper gastrointestinal bleeding and those with severe multisystem failure.

Acute nonerosive gastritis is usually caused by *Helicobacter pylori* infection, although salicylates and NSAIDs may also be considered. Because of the mild and transient nature of symptoms, these patients are rarely seen by a physician. Moreover, there is evidence that the majority of these patients are likely to progress to chronic gastritis. In fact, the term *chronic active gastritis* is applied to *H. pylori* infection, and implies that the process is almost always chronic with acute exacerbations. Diagnosis is primarily made by endoscopy.

Chronic gastritis is characterized by mononuclear infiltration of the gastric mucosa and is usually associated with colonization by *H. pylori*. In the early stage of the disease, when the underlying gastric glands are normal, it is called *chronic superficial gastritis*. This condition gradually advances into **chronic atrophic gastritis** when normal gastric glands are no longer present. **Type A,** or pernicious anemia-type of chronic gastritis, refers to severe atrophic changes involving the body and fundus of the stomach. This type of gastritis is usually associated with circulating antibodies to parietal cells and to an intrinsic factor and an increased risk of gastric cancer. The risk of cancer is five times higher in this group as compared with the general population. On the other hand, in **type B** gastritis histologic changes are confined to the antrum. It is this type of gastritis that is classically associated with *H. pylori* infection. Over 80% of this group are infected by this organism and carry a higher risk of peptic ulcer disease. Finally, **type C** or **AB gastritis** refers to situations where the entire gastric mucosa is involved.

Chronic gastritis is a common condition and its incidence increases with age. The condition is more prevalent in communities with a lower standard of living and poor hygiene. Chronic gastritis is a histologic diagnosis. The majority of these patients are essentially asymptomatic, and there are a lot of fluctuations among those who are symptomatic. In general, the symptoms are vague but are characteristically located in the upper abdominal region and occur after ingestion of a meal. Fullness, early satiety, abdominal discomfort, nausea, and rarely vomiting are the symptoms collectively known as *nonulcer dyspepsia*. Eradication of *H. pylori*, when it is associated with peptic ulcer disease, is justified. However, such a recommendation cannot easily be advanced to chronic gastritis. Treatment of *H. pylori* infection may not improve the clinical syndrome.

Specific types of gastritis are relatively uncommon. **Eosinophilic gastritis** is part of the spectrum of eosinophilic gastroenteritis and is characterized by eosinophilic leukocytes infiltrating the mucosa and submucosa. The etiology of the disease is unknown. Abdominal pain, nausea, and vomiting in association with an increase in eosinophils in the peripheral blood are seen, particularly in patients with a history of allergy. Steroid therapy is used with variable results. **Hypertrophic gastritis** or **Ménétrier's disease** is yet another rare condition. Hypertrophic gastric rugae, hypoproteinemia, edema, and anorexia are among cardinal features of this disease. Full-thickness biopsy obtained at laparotomy is usually required for diagnosis. Gastrectomy has been recommended as management of this condition. **Bile gastritis** or **alkaline-reflux gastritis** is caused by the reflux of duodenal contents, including bile acids and pancreatic enzymes. This type of gastritis usually develops in patients with a history of gastric surgery. Bile gastritis is suspected when there is persistent epigastric pain that is temporarily relieved after vomiting bile, anorexia and weight loss, or a history of gastric resection with a gastrojejunostomy anastomosis. Revision of the gastrojejunostomy to a Roux-en-Y anastomosis to divert the duodenal contents from the stomach is the treatment of choice for this condition. Binding agents such as cholestyramine have also been tried. **Granulomatous gastritis** is extremely rare and is usually found in patients with sarcoidosis, tuberculosis, Crohn's disease, or syphilis. Patients with portal hypertension, particularly those who have undergone sclerotherapy for variceal bleeding, often have characteristic changes in the gastric mucosa that are known as *portal hypertensive gastropathy*. These changes may be seen in about 30% of the patients with portal hypertension who present with an episode of upper gastrointestinal bleeding. Swelling and congestion of the mucosa, intramucosal hemorrhage, and erosions that are more prominent in the body and fundus are the endoscopic features of this type of gastritis. Treatment of this condition is directed at correction of the underlying portal hypertension and providing supportive measures.

KEY POINTS

1 Gastritis is the most common disease of the stomach.

2 The majority of patients with histologic or endoscopic diagnosis of gastritis are essentially asymptomatic. The minority who seek medical attention have either vague symptoms of non-ulcer dyspepsia or gastrointestinal bleeding.

3 Ingestion of aspirin and NSAIDs, heavy consumption of alcohol, *H. pylori* infection, and portal hypertension are among the common known causes of gastritis.

4 Management of symptomatic patients is aimed at removal of the contributing factors and correction of the underlying conditions. However, in the case of *H. pylori* infection, the results are controversial.

5 Special types of gastritis, except for portal hypertensive gastropathy, are rare, and their diagnosis and management usually require the skill of a specialist.

SUGGESTED READINGS

Graham DY, Go MF: *Helicobacter pylori:* current status, *Gastroenterol* 105:279-282, 1993.

Lingenfelser T, Krige JE: The stomach in cirrhosis, *J Clin Gastroenterol* 17:92-96, 1993.

Price AB: The Sydney system: histological division, *J Gastroenterol Hepatol* 6:209-222, 1991.

67

Headaches

Stanley van den Noort

There are three fundamental forms of headache–tension, migraine, and headache caused by neighborhood disease. The last form embraces aneurysms, meningitis, stroke, pituitary tumors, tumors of the posterior fossa and those near the tentorium, glaucoma, trigeminal neuralgia, other neuralgias, orbital and sinus pathology, mastoiditis, bone disease, metastases, and toothache.

DIAGNOSIS

Headache of substantial severity and of recent onset, particularly if associated with lethargy or confusion, should be promptly investigated. The warning leak of an aneurysm can cause a headache that simulates migraine but is either new to the patient or more severe than prior experiences.

One common neighborhood headache is spinal headache that occurs after epidural anesthesia. The brain normally floats in spinal fluid, and leakage of spinal fluid after arachnoid puncture produces an orthostatic headache of great severity caused by direct contact of the base of the brain with the skull. This usually responds over several days to recumbent posture, fluids, and the ingestion of caffeine and analgesics. An autologous blood patch is sometimes needed but should not be a routine treatment. Spinal headache rarely occurs spontaneously.

New onset headache in the elderly may be a harbinger of stroke and requires careful assessment. In the elderly, severe temporal or bitemporal headache with tenderness, malaise, and often arthralgia suggests temporal arteritis. The ESR is usually very high. Treatment with prednisone is urgent to prevent loss of vision.

Cranial herpes zoster, usually accompanied by severe pain, may precede vesicles for some days.

Trigeminal neuralgia in younger patients suggests multiple sclerosis. In older patients, it is probably caused by pulsation of tortuous vessels against the fifth nerve. It is best managed with carbamazepine or baclofen. A gamma knife treatment to the trigeminal ganglion is done in refractory cases. Atypical facial pain is a most difficult symptom to evaluate and treat. Some patients have Sjögren's syndrome with trigeminal neuropathy, sarcoid, or other causes, but many defy specific diagnosis.

Headache is also a hallmark of pseudotumor cerebri. This disorder is rare in men, is most often seen in morbidly obese young women, and may appear at any of the endocrine shifts in woman from menarche to pregnancy. It is also seen with long-term use of outdated tetracycline for treatment of acne, vitamin A intoxication, cerebral venous sinus thrombosis, and corticosteroid treatment or its withdrawal. Papilledema is usually evident, and sudden permanent loss of vision can occur. Mild cases respond to acetazolamide, diuretics, and weight loss. Protracted cases may benefit from lumboperitoneal shunts. Deteriorating vision dictates emergency optic nerve sheath decompression.

The (vascular) headache of eclampsia is obvious in its context. Postpartum headache (may be prepartum) of great severity, which may be accompanied by seizures and lethargy, suggests thrombophlebitis of cerebral veins with or without sinus thrombosis. Endovascular thrombolysis with thrombolytic agents may be life saving.

Aseptic meningitis caused by viral infections and/or Lyme disease often mimics vascular headache. Rarely, aseptic meningitis can be caused by ibuprofen and similar drugs.

Muscle tension headache is common. It may result from occupational straining at video terminals that are too high. Bruxism, or a pattern of teeth clenching when tense, can produce a dreadful headache that is usually worse in one temple. The temple and masseter are often tender. A history of changed bite from recent dental pathology is often present. Since the scalp is the "tendon" of the neck muscles and spasm produces pain at points where tendons insert into bone, one can have relatively constant frontal headache from neck pathology. Often the pain is like a headband and commonly is worse in back. Onset and offset of tension headache is usually slow, and headaches are often bilateral. Nausea and sensitivity to environmental stimuli such as light are uncommon. Whiplash is a common generator of tension headache. Cervical disc disease is almost ubiquitous, and rheumatoid involvement of the neck may cause intractable headache.

Migraine or vascular headache is the most common reason for seeking medical attention for headache. Keys to diagnosis are predilection for one side (migraine derives from hemigrania or hemicrania), rapid onset with or without warning, pulsation, nausea, and sensitivity to environmental stimuli (light, sound, smell). Auras include visual phenomenon of curved or angular moving light with areas of impaired sight, paresthesia, vertigo, aphasia, hemiparesis, diplopia, syncope, seizure, tachycardia, and even diarrhea. Gastrointestinal symptoms may overshadow the headache. Auras without subsequent headache are common. Headaches usually peak over a relatively brief period of time, last for hours, and then slowly abate. They most commonly occur on awakening, and the pain is severe. Vascular thrombosis and arterial dissection are uncommon but do occur and indicate the need to regard this as a substantial disease process. Some vascular headaches occur at the same time of day every day for weeks. Thunderclap headache is one of sudden onset that may occur with extreme exertion (e.g., coitus [5% or so of aneurysms bleed during intercourse]). Chronic daily headache is a problem of great morbidity that envelops aspects of migraine and tension headache and overuse of medication.

The pathogenesis of migraine seems to rest in irritation of the trigeminal vascular network, leading to release of agents promoting inflammation and fluid leakage from arteries and veins with associated irritation of the cerebral cortex and other structures.

In women, migraine is often aggravated by hormonal shifts. Onset with menarche and subsidence with menopause is common. Absence of migraine in pregnancy after the first two months is customary, but migraine may also first appear in pregnancy. Paramenstrual migraine is common. Migraine may also accompany ovulation. Birth control pills often make migraine worse. Traditional estrogenic birth control pills and smoking carry a substantial risk of stroke in migraine sufferers. Postmenopausal ERT, even in currently used doses, can initiate or aggravate migraine. Oophorectomy is rarely advised for intractable migraine.

DIFFERENTIAL DIAGNOSIS

The management of headache must begin with a diagnostic triage of neighborhood, tension, and vascular subtypes. Frontal sinusitis often produces pain in the middle of the day. Glaucoma pain may increase with pupillary dilation after sunset. The yield of pathology on routine screening of headaches with imaging procedures is very low. The strongest indication for imaging studies is new onset of very severe headache. A CT scan will show blood in more than 90% of subarachnoid hemorrhage. A lumbar puncture is in order when the new onset of very severe headache is accompanied by a negative CT scan. A majority of aneurysms that bleed are large enough to see on careful MRI. The treatment of neighborhood headache is generally directed at the neighborhood problem. Sinusitis of substantial severity is commonly seen in brain MRI on patients without complaints of local pain. Most so called *sinus headaches* are really facial migraines. However, acute bacterial sinusitis can surely cause a headache of great severity. Sudden headache, with or without hemorrhage and/or infarction, can be seen after the use of cocaine or amphetamines.

TREATMENT AND MANAGEMENT

The management of tension headache must address the likely source. Raising the chair of a work station, lowering a video terminal, physical therapy, and NSAIDs for neck pain are often helpful. (Ibuprofen and similar drugs can produce an allergic meningitis.) The temporomandibular joint can often be helped by bite splints for day and/or night use. Dental procedures to improve bite symmetry are often helpful. Direct intervention to the temporomandibular joint is rarely required. Chronic daily tension headache is often helped by small (5 to 10 mg) bedtime doses of amitriptyline.

Acetaminophen or aspirin at onset of headache is often better than much stronger analgesics given later. Analgesics with caffeine work better but contain the risk of caffeine withdrawal headache. Combinations of analgesics with caffeine, a barbiturate, and with or without codeine, should be used occasionally, but near daily use should be urgently discouraged.

Chlorzoxazone (Parafon Forte) is often helpful. Hydrocodone, oxycodone, and codeine are variably helpful. A small percentage of the population cannot metabolize these compounds to active opiate receptor agonists. Propoxyphene is useful in some people. The new tramadol (Ultram) appears to be safe and often effective (50 to 100 mg, every 6 hours as needed). Butorphanol nasal spray is an agent that often can prevent trips to the emergency room. Ketorolac, 30 mg orally or 60 mg intramuscularly, is often helpful.

In frequent migraine, the physician must evaluate environmental factors. Relaxation and long sleeps may trigger spells, as may certain smells (perfumes) and designs on clothing and wallpaper. Caffeine withdrawal is a common trigger. Most patients with migraines are well advised to abstain from alcohol. Sensitivity to nitrites in food; to amines in cheese, yogurt, nuts, wine, chocolate, and pickled foods; to aspartame, monosodium glutamate, beans, yeast, citrus, and highly individual food sensitivities are described.

Paramenstrual migraine is difficult to prevent. Estrogenic agents often increase migraine. Progesterone tends to help. Depo-Provera is sometimes quite useful. Some patients with migraines fare better on contraceptive pills, but most do not. High-dose ERT in the older patient has similar risks.

Imaging studies reveal that dissection of the internal carotid, vertebral, and intercranial arteries is more common than previously thought. It often occurs after neck trauma, but may be spontaneous. A background of migraine is commonly present. Early recognition of dissection and acute treatment with heparin may prevent cerebral embolism with disastrous consequences.

Functional hypoglycemia may also trigger migraines. Certain antihistamines, ephedrinelike agents, and diet pills may increase migraine. Low grades of variable hypertension may cause high grades of headache and may respond to simple measures to lower the blood pressure. Migraine may be a response to depression and responds to antidepressants. Lactose intolerance may also trigger migraine.

The prevention of migraine with drugs rests on five groups of agents.

1. Beta blockers, especially propanalol in long-acting preparations, and nadolol are helpful. More cardioselective beta blockers are less helpful. Avoid the use of beta blockers in asthmatics and in women who want to conceive. Mild depression and hair loss are sometimes side effects of beta blockers.
2. Verapamil and nicardipine are occasionally helpful, as are other agents used to lower blood pressure, including diuretics.
3. Two enteric-coated aspirin and/or NSAIDs can be helpful prophylactics, stomach permitting.
4. Antidepressants prevent migraine in people judged not to be depressed. Trazodone and desipramine are particularly useful.
5. Valproic acid (Depakote), with attention to blood levels is often helpful. Prolonged use of methylergonovine (0.2 mg orally tid) may be helpful.

Paroxysmal hemicrania and cluster headache may selectively, and sometimes dramatically, respond to indomethacin. A short course of prednisone may be helpful in some cycles. Lithium is often helpful in cluster headache. Oxygen inhalation often helps. Diazepam and its analogues should be avoided. Cluster headache is more common in men.

Pituitary tumors often produce headache. Prolactinomas with galactorrhea are often tied to severe vascular headaches. Slight elevations of prolactin are often caused by psychotropic medication. However, an episode of severe migraine with episodic galactorrhea and mild prolactin elevation is not rare. Dopamine agonists help the galactorrhea, but the headache is usually unaffected. Pituitary apoplexy (infarction) with adenomas, diabetes, and during the postpartum stage produces severe headaches and the potential for adrenal crisis.

The acute treatment of migraine after simple analgesics probably best begins with isometheptene (Midrin) with additives, two tablets, repeated if necessary once or twice in several hours. If this fails, the next trial should probably focus on the serotonin agonist sumatriptan (Imitrex), 25 to 50 mg by mouth or 6 mg intramuscularly. These preparations will greatly reduce the use of emergency rooms. For some people, Imitrex is not tolerated and is too expensive. Cafergot pills usually do not work, but in some patients they are quite sufficient. Cafergot suppositories are more reliable. It usually is best to precede Cafergot suppositories with oral trimethobenzamide (Tigan) or metoclopramide (Reglan). Usually a third of a suppository is enough. Ergotamine accumulates on continued use. Daily use is not prudent. Metoclopramide by mouth followed by dihydroergotamine (DHE), intramuscularly or intravenously, is often helpful. Intravenous metoclopramide or/and phenothiazines may help headaches. A brief hospital stay to stop analgesics, block withdrawal with clonidine, and administer periodic metoclopramide/DHE, intramuscularly or intravenously, is a useful technique. Even simple, acute migraine can provoke severe vomiting with dehydration and require a hospital stay for observation, fluid replacement, and analgesics.

KEY POINTS

1 There are three fundamental forms of headache–tension, migraine, and headache caused by neighborhood disease.

2 Headache of substantial severity and of recent onset, particularly if associated with lethargy or confusion, should be promptly investigated.

3 The strongest indication for imaging studies is new onset of very severe headache. A CT scan will show blood in more than 90% of subarachnoid hemorrhage. A lumbar puncture is in order when the new onset of very severe headache is accompanied by a negative CT scan.

4 The prevention of migraine with drugs rests on five groups of agents: (1) beta blockers, (2) verapamil and nicardipine, (3) enteric-coated aspirin, (4) antidepressants, and (5) valproic acid.

5 The acute treatment of migraine after simple analgesics probably best begins with isometheptene (Midrin) with additives, two tablets, repeated if necessary once or twice in several hours. If this fails, the next trial should probably focus on the serotonin agonist sumatriptan (Imitrex). If Imitrex is not tolerated, Cafergot suppositories are more reliable.

SUGGESTED READINGS

Anderson KE, Vigre E: (beta)-Adrenoceptor blockers and calcium antagonists in the prophylaxis and treatment of migraine, *Drugs* 39:355-373, 1990.

Bank J: A comparative study of amitriptyline and fluvoxamine in migraine prophylaxis, *Headache* 34(8):476-478, 1994.

Buzzi MG, Moskowitz MA: The antimigraine drug sumatriptan (GR43175) selectively blocks neurogenic plasma extravasation from blood vessels in dura mater, *Br J Pharmacol* 99:202-206, 1990.

Mochan E: Analgesics in the treatment of headaches. In: Gallagher RM, ed: *Drug therapy for headache,* New York, 1990, Marcel Dekker.

Morewood GH: A rational approach to the cause, prevention and treatment of postdural puncture headache [see comments], *Can Med Assoc J* 149(8):1087-1093, 1993.

Ratinahirana H, Darbois Y, Bousser MG: Migraine and pregnancy: a prospective study in 703 women after delivery, *Neurology* 40:437, 1990.

Silberstein SD, Merriam G: Estrogen, progesterone, and headache, *Neurology* 41:786-793, 1991.

Tek DS et al: A prospective, double-blind study of metoclopramide hydrochloride for the control of migraine in the emergency department, *Ann Emerg Med* 19:1083-1087, 1990.

68

Hypertension

Nancy E. Gin

Uncontrolled hypertension is a major risk factor in the development of myocardial infarctions, heart failure, strokes, and renal failure. Because many of those who have hypertension are asymptomatic, the disease may progress for years before the patient receives medical attention. Despite such a paucity of symptoms, nearly 2 million people/year are newly diagnosed with hypertension; the prevalence is higher among African Americans than Caucasians. Because of the enormous potential psychologic and socioeconomic impact the diagnosis of hypertension carries, however, the label must be applied carefully.

PATHOGENESIS

Although there is no clear delineation between normal and high blood pressure, hypertension has been defined as a diastolic pressure >90 mm Hg. A systolic pressure >140 mm Hg is also considered hypertensive.

Approximately 95% of all hypertensive patients will have no identifiable cause. These patients are considered to have "essential" hypertension. Renal parenchymal disease constitutes the largest proportion of secondary causes of hypertension. Other causes of secondary hypertension include renal vascular disease, primary hypoaldosteronism, Cushing's syndrome or hypercortisolemia, pheochromocytoma, hyperparathyroidism, hyperthyroidism, coarctation of the aorta, obesity, and sleep apnea.

Prescription, over-the-counter, and illicit drugs, including cyclosporine, erythropoietin, NSAIDs, tricyclic antidepressants, phenylpropanolamine, pseudoephedrine, cocaine, and estrogen-containing oral contraceptives may cause hypertension. The effects of oral contraceptives on blood pressure are especially pronounced in women who are over age 35, obese, or consume large quantities of alcohol. ERT in postmenopausal women, however, does not induce hypertension. Alcohol use greater than 2 oz of ethanol per day, smoking, and high lead content have all been implicated in causing hypertension.

PATHOPHYSIOLOGY

Cardiovascular effects are the most common complications of hypertension. Multiple studies have shown a clear relationship between hypertension and the development of vascular events such as stroke and coronary heart disease. Concentric left ventricular hypertrophy develops in response to the increased work load caused by an elevated systemic pressure. The hypertrophic myocardium may also lead to accelerated coronary arterial disease and increased myocardial oxygen demand, leading to myocardial ischemia and infarction, sudden death, and arrhythmias. Eventually, the left ventricle cannot hypertrophy any further, and dilation begins. Dilation of the left ventricle heralds the clinical onset of CHF.

The same accelerated atherogenesis observed in the coronary arteries of hypertensive patients may occur in the cerebral circulation as well, leading to cerebral infarction. Microaneurysms in hypertensive patients also increase the risk of cerebral hemorrhage. The risk of a vascular event increases substantially in patients who have multiple risk factors (i.e., diabetes mellitus, hyperlipidemia, left ventricular hypertrophy on ECG, cigarette smoking).

Likewise, changes in the renal circulation, both afferent and efferent, from nephrosclerosis may ultimately lead to end-stage renal disease. Hypertensive African-Americans have a greater prevalence of end-stage renal disease. Hypertension is also a major etiologic factor in the development of peripheral vascular disease, including aortic aneurysms and dissection.

Another complication of long-standing hypertension is retinopathy, which may result in decreased visual acuity or even blindness. Retinopathy may progress from arteriolar narrowing to arteriovenous nicking to hemorrhages and exudates, and finally, to papilledema. The hypertensive changes visible in the arterial circulation of the retina often reflect similar changes in the systemic circulation.

DIAGNOSIS

The history of a patient with hypertension should focus on risk factors for vascular disease as well as signs and symptoms of end-organ complications of hypertension. Typically, the patient with uncomplicated hypertension is completely asymptomatic. Inquiries should be made regarding medications, diabetes mellitus, hyperlipidemia, cigarette smoking, alcohol use, illicit drug use, and any family history of vascular disease diagnosed at a young age.

Symptoms of angina pectoris as well as CHF (i.e., orthopnea, paroxysmal nocturnal dyspnea, pedal edema) should be elicited along with any history of documented stroke, transient cerebral ischemia, or myocardial infarction. Headaches of any type may occur, as well as epistaxis and changes in vision. Pain caused by a dissecting aortic aneurysm may occasionally be elicited in the history.

Symptoms referable to secondary causes of hypertension should be reviewed with the patient. For example, episodic flushing, palpitations, headaches, and dizziness would be characteristic of a pheochromocytoma, whereas easy bruising and hirsutism might suggest Cushing's syndrome.

The physical examination in a patient with uncomplicated essential hypertension is often unremarkable except for the blood pressure. The pressure should be taken in a nonthreatening environment once the patient has had a chance to relax. Generally, it is prudent for the physician to recheck any borderline or higher blood pressure reading. In a minority of patients with markedly elevated pressures (systolic ≥210 mm Hg and/or diastolic ≥120 mm Hg), the diagnosis of hypertension may be made and treatment initiated during the same office visit. The majority of patients, however, will exhibit pressures that require substantiation over time. A diagnosis of hypertension in this group should be made only after a minimum of three readings at least a week apart.

The remainder of the physical examination should focus on evidence of any end-organ damage, including fundoscopic exam, and auscultation for carotid, renal, and femoral bruits. Renal bruits are best auscultated in the flanks or just lateral and cranial to the umbilicus. The femoral pulses should be compared to radial pulses and if diminished or delayed, lower extremity blood pressure should be measured.

The cardiopulmonary examination should focus on evidence of CHF and pulmonary edema, left ventricular hypertrophy (i.e., a lift), and third and fourth heart sounds. The abdomen should be examined for palpable polycystic kidneys or an aortic aneurysm. The patient should also be evaluated for any signs of a previous stroke.

Laboratory evaluation should include a CBC, BUN, serum creatinine, serum potassium, fasting glucose, serum calcium, total cholesterol and subtypes, triglyceride, urinalysis, and an ECG. An echocardiogram should be obtained in patients with evidence of end-organ damage caused by hypertension, but not in the uncomplicated patient.

Patients whose diastolic pressures are intermittently at or above 90 mm Hg are considered to have borderline hypertension. These people should be advised of their status and rechecked in 6 to 12 months. Because some in this group may experience "white coat" hypertension, the use of ambulatory blood pressure monitoring may be useful in diagnosing hypertension. Other patients who might require ambulatory monitoring are those in whom the physician suspects nocturnal pressure changes or episodic hypertension, and those whose pressure seems resistant to pharmacologic intervention. In general, the diagnosis of hypertension is made without such monitoring.

TREATMENT

Treatment varies depending on the degree of hypertension (Fig. 68-1). For patients with mild hypertension (i.e., diastolic pressure between 90 and 95 mm Hg) without additional vascular risk factors, conservative treatment with weight reduction, decreased alcohol intake (less than one ounce of alcohol or the equivalent of 24 oz of beer/day), regular aerobic exercise, and reduced sodium intake (less than 6 g of NaCl/day) may be sufficient. A weight reduction of 10 lbs, for instance, may result in a substantial decrease in pressure. Sodium restriction, on the other hand, does not necessarily result in a commensurate decrease in pressure in all patients. However, since sodium restriction has virtually no complications in most patients, a trial should be attempted in all patients with hypertension. Additionally, smoking cessation and reduction in dietary fat and cholesterol, though unrelated to hypertension, are additional risk factors in the development of cardiovascular disease that should be modified in the hypertensive patient.

Angiotensin-Converting Enzyme (ACE) Inhibitors

Generally well-tolerated, ACE inhibitors include benazepril, captopril, enalapril, fosinopril, lisinopril, quinapril, and ramipril. The antihypertensive of choice in patients with a codiagnosis of diabetes mellitus, ACE inhibitors exert a renal protective effect. In particular, the rate of progression of microalbuminuria to frank nephrotic syndrome is markedly reduced with prolonged use of ACE inhibitors. The beneficial effect is not as clearly delineated in patients who have already demonstrated macroproteinuria (>500 mg/day).

This class of agents is also effective for the uncomplicated general population of patients with hypertension and for those with a concurrent diagnosis of CHF. However, ACE inhibitors tend to be less effective among the elderly and African-Americans. Except for captopril, most ACE inhibitors may be given once daily in low to moderate doses and twice daily with higher doses.

Common side effects of ACE inhibitors include hyperkalemia and a dry cough. More serious side effects include angioedema, leukopenia, and the precipitation of renal insufficiency or failure in patients with preexisting bilateral renal artery stenosis. Renal function and potassium level should be checked within 1 week of starting an ACE inhibitor and rechecked after each dosage adjustment.

Systolic	Diastolic	Stage	Intervention	Follow-up
<130	<85	Normal	Recheck in 2 years	
130-139	85-89	High Normal	Recheck in 1 year, consider lifestyle modification counseling	
140-159	90-99	Stage I	Confirmation within 2 months, lifestyle modification, counseling	
160-179	100-109	Stage II	Recheck within 1 month, lifestyle modification, counseling	Systolic <140 Diastolic <85 → Continue lifestyle modification
180-209	110-119	Stage III	Recheck within 1 week, lifestyle modification, counseling	Blood pressure still elevated → Begin pharmacologic therapy (monotherapy) ↓
>210	>120	Stage IV	Refer to source of care immediately, begin pharmacologic treatment	→ Recheck blood pressure in 3-7 days; if still elevated, add second agent

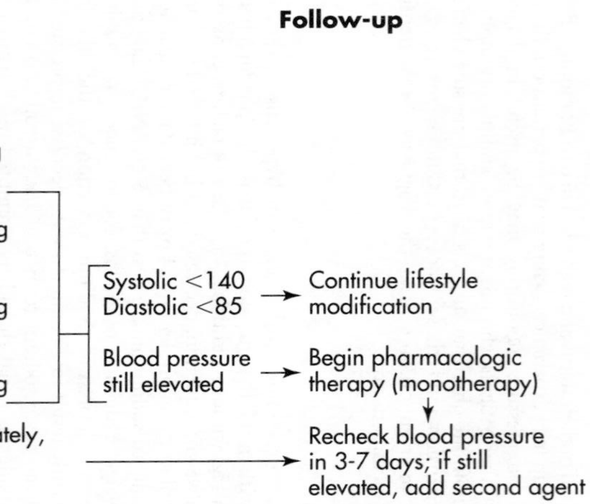

FIG. 68-1 Treatment of hypertension. (Modified from Joint National Committee on Detection, Evaluation, and Treatment of High Blood Pressure: The fifth report of the Joint National Committee on Detection, Evaluation, and Treatment of High Blood Pressure (JNC V), *Arch Intern Med* 153:154-183, 1993.)

Calcium Channel Antagonists

Also generally well-tolerated, the calcium channel blockers include amlodipine, diltiazem, felodipine, isradipine, nicardipine, nifedipine, and verapamil. Except for diltiazem and verapamil, all the others are dihydropyridines, which exert a greater vasodilatory effect than nondihydropyridines. The calcium channel blockers tend to be effective for uncomplicated hypertension in the general population. Dosing with the short-acting calcium channel blockers is 3 to 4 times/day, whereas the longer-acting preparations may be administered daily.

The side effects associated with vasodilation include peripheral edema, flushing, palpitations, and headaches. The nondihydropyridines may depress atrioventricular conduction and sinus node automaticity, resulting in bradycardia. Verapamil also tends to constipate. All calcium channel blockers exert a negative inotropic effect, and may cause or exacerbate CHF in predisposed patients. A few studies indicate amlodipine and felodipine may have less of a negative inotropic effect.

Some reports have found an increased risk of mortality in patients with preexisting coronary artery disease taking calcium channel blockers, in particular the dihydropyridines. The reports show that moderate to high doses of short-acting agents such as nifedipine increased the risk of myocardial infarction and all-cause mortality. Literature is lacking for the longer-acting preparations, including the sustained-release form of nifedipine.

Diuretics

Thiazide diuretics constitute a relatively inexpensive class of antihypertensive agents, which includes hydrochlorothiazide, chlorthalidone, metolazone, and indapamide. Hydrochlorothiazide is the most commonly used preparation. Thiazide diuretics seem to be particularly effective in the elderly and African-American populations. The metabolic complications of these agents, however, have decreased their routine use in the general hypertensive population.

The primary metabolic complication of thiazide diuretics is hypokalemia. Since most of the antihypertensive effect of thiazides is seen at lower doses than previously believed, hypokalemia may often be offset by eating a diet high in potassium. Hyperuricemia, hypercholesterolemia, hyperglycemia, and hypercalcemia may all occur with thiazide diuretics. Thus gout, hyperlipidemia, diabetes mellitus, and hyperaldosteronism are relative contraindications.

Several products are available combining hydrochlorothiazide with potassium-sparing agents, such as amiloride, triamterene, and spironolactone, to counterbalance the potassium loss from hydrochlorothiazide. However, these preparations are generally much more expensive, and hyperkalemia may be a consequence.

Potassium levels should be checked regularly on all patients taking diuretics in any form, especially within 1 to 2 weeks after the initiation of therapy, after any change in the dose, and at regular intervals on a stable dose. Glucose, lipids, uric acid, and calcium may be checked less often, but should also be evaluated after initiation of diuretics and dosage changes.

Loop diuretics, which include furosemide, torsemide, and bumetanide, should not be considered first-line antihypertensive agents for the general population. The short half-life of loop diuretics restricts their antihypertensive use primarily to patients with renal dysfunction.

Beta-Adrenergic Receptor Antagonists

The beta-blockers belong to a diverse group of agents including acebutolol, atenolol, betaxolol, carteolol, metoprolol, nadolol, pindolol, propranolol, and timolol. Labetalol is the only mixed alpha- and beta-blocker. All decrease heart rate and cardiac output by reducing cardiac sympathetic activity. Therefore patients with increased sympathetic activity, such as angina pectoris, a history of myocardial infarction, migraine headaches, and anxiety disorders producing palpitations, often respond well to this class of antihypertensive. Beta-blockers also work well in conjunction with agents such as hydralazine and the alpha-adrenergic blockers by decreasing the reflex tachycardia resulting from these vasodilators.

Complications of beta-blockers include bronchospasm and CHF caused by the negative inotropic effects, and are therefore contraindicated in patients with symptomatic bronchospasm or CHF. Beta-blockers with relative specificity to the cardiac $\beta_1$receptors have less effect on the $\beta_2$receptors in the bronchi and vasculature, but the cardioselectivity disappears at higher doses. Elevation in triglyceride levels; depression of high-density lipoproteins; atrioventricular conduction defects; CNS effects, such as confusion or depression, especially in the elderly; lethargy; and impotence are additional side effects of this class of agents. The lipid solubility of each beta-blocker determines the extent of movement across the blood-brain barrier, with more lipid-soluble preparations such as propranolol crossing more easily and causing CNS side effects.

Beta-blockers are relatively contraindicated in patients with insulin-using diabetes because the sympatholytic action of the drugs may mask the early signs and symptoms of hypoglycemia. Finally, beta-blockers should not be considered as a first-line antihypertensive in a poorly-compliant patient, because sudden cessation of the medication may result in rebound hypertension. In general, glucose and lipids should be checked after initiation of beta-blockers, after any dosage adjustment, and at least annually on patients on a stable regimen.

Second-Line Therapy

Once a patient has failed a combination of first-line therapies, other classes should be considered, including the vasodilators (e.g., hydralazine, minoxidil), the central acting $\alpha_2$agonists (e.g., clonidine, guanabenz, guanfacine, methyldopa), agents with postganglionic adrenergic effects (e.g., guanethidine, reserpine), and peripheral alpha-adrenergic receptor antagonists (e.g., doxazosin, prazosin, terazosin). Poorly compliant patients should not be prescribed clonidine or any of the other $\alpha_2$agonists, because rebound hypertension may occur. Prazosin and terazosin may be used effectively in men who also have benign prostatic hypertrophy to improve urinary flow rate.

Approximately 5% of all patients with hypertension will have a recognizable underlying cause. Patients in whom secondary hypertension should be suspected and who should be referred to an internist include those with onset of hypertension before the age of 20 or after 50; dramatic worsening of pressure in a compliant, previously well-controlled patient; presence of abdominal bruits; and renal insufficiency or a family history of renal disease.

Additional "red flags" include a poor response to normally effective therapy; pressure greater than 180/110; labile pressures associated with flushing, diaphoresis, tachycardia, and tremor; unexplained hypokalemia; fundoscopic changes; and evidence of left ventricular hypertrophy. Patients who have failed first-line therapy, including those who have worsening of renal function with the use of ACE inhibitors, should also be referred to a general internist.

KEY POINTS

1. Diastolic blood pressures greater than 90 mm Hg and systolic pressures greater than 140 are considered hypertensive.
2. The history, physical, and laboratory examinations should be directed toward determining the presence of end-organ damage as well as evaluating for cardiovascular risk factors and secondary causes of hypertension.
3. Pharmacologic treatment of hypertension should be individualized for each patient based on possible etiologies of the hypertension as well as compatibility with potential side effects of the medications.
4. The primary classes of treatment are ACE inhibitors, calcium channel blockers, diuretics, and beta-blockers.

SUGGESTED READINGS

Furberg CD et al: Nifedipine: Dose-related increase in mortality in patients with coronary heart disease, *Circulation* 92:1326-1331, 1995.

Hollenberg NK, Raij L: Angiotensin converting enzyme inhibition and renal protection: an assessment of implications for therapy, *Arch Intern Med* 153:2426-2435, 1993.

Joint National Committee on Detection, Evaluation, and Treatment of High Blood Pressure: The fifth report of the Joint National Committee on Detection, Evaluation, and Treatment of High Blood Pressure (JNC V), *Arch Intern Med* 153:154-183, 1993.

Kaplan NM: Systemic hypertension: mechanisms and diagnosis. In Braunwald E, ed: *Heart disease,* ed 4, Philadelphia, 1992, WB Saunders.

Law MR, Frost CD, Wald NJ: By how much does dietary salt reduction lower blood pressure? III: Analysis of data from trials of salt reduction, *BMJ* 302:819-824, 1991.

MacMahon S et al: Blood pressure, stroke, and coronary heart disease. I. Prolonged differences in blood pressure: prospective observational studies corrected for the regression dilution bias, *Lancet* 335:765-774, 1990.

National High Blood Pressure Education Program Working Group: National High Blood Pressure Education Program Working Group report on primary prevention of hypertension, *Arch Intern Med* 153:186-208, 1993.

Psaty BM et al: The risk of myocardial infarction associated with antihypertensive drug therapies, *JAMA* 274:620-625, 1995.
Witteman JC et al: Relation of moderate alcohol consumption and risk of systemic hypertension in women, *Am J Cardiol* 65:633-637, 1990.

69

Influenza

THOMAS C. CESARIO

Influenza is a disease caused by an orthomyxovirus of the same name, the *influenza virus.* This agent is a unique virus that has a genome composed of single-stranded RNA. The RNA is associated with a nucleoprotein, the nature of which determines the type of the virus (i.e., influenza A, B, or C). The nucleoprotein and RNA form a helical structure called the *nucleocapsid,* which in turn is surrounded by the matrix or membrane protein. Protruding from the membrane are two specific glycoproteins. The first is termed the *hemagglutinin (HA),* which functions to attach the virus to the receptor site on the cell surface. The second is the neuraminidase (NA), which may function to release the virus from the cell surface. Both hemagglutinin and neuraminidase may vary in biochemical composition, and alterations in these glycoproteins constitute the basis for the major antigenic variations in the virus. These two components of the virus are of further importance because immunity to the hemagglutinin and neuraminidase offers protection to the host from illness caused by the virus. Two types of antigenic variation are known. The first is antigenic drift. This is the year-to-year variation in the composition of either the HA or NA and likely is the result of mutation affecting the RNA. Antigenic shift, however, is the major change in predominant circulating influenza type. This is likely the result of either reintroduction into a very susceptible population of an influenza strain long gone from human society or reassortment (i.e., new mixing of two strains of the virus, one or both of which could be a strain or strains found in the animal world).

Major variations in the nature of the circulating virus have occurred several times in this century. Thus we know influenza A strains have carried three different types of hemagglutinin (called H_1, H_2, and H_3) and two types of neuraminidase (called N_1 and N_2). Introduction of a strain of the A virus with a totally different HA, or HA and NA, than the strain circulating in the previous year has generally led to a new epidemic or pandemic with the virus. Epidemics caused by the influenza B are less common and by influenza C are rare.

The introduction of a new virus strain has generally occurred at 10-year intervals, although it has now been some years since a true influenza pandemic has occurred. Influenza epidemics in the northern hemisphere generally occur in the winter months of December to April. Typically, such epidemics initially are detected because of increased illnesses among children, followed by additional illnesses in adults, and finally increased hospitalizations in patients with either respiratory illnesses or deterioration of chronic conditions initiated by the virus. The epidemics usually run their course in approximately 6 weeks.

DIAGNOSIS

Influenza is spread by the respiratory route. Typically susceptible patients are best defined by the absence or inadequacy of antibody titers to the hemagglutinin, although local IgA antibodies and nonspecific defense mechanisms are likely important in preventing disease. The virus itself attaches to the respiratory epithelium and begins the cycle of viral replication. Live virus can be detected in respiratory secretions within a short time (24 to 48 hrs) after infection. Subsequently, fever begins to occur. The body's own response to the presence of the influenza virus includes the production of interferon, which follows the ability to culture the virus, and the elaboration of specific antibodies, including local IgA antibodies, systemic hemagglutination-inhibiting antibodies, antineuraminidase antibodies, and neutralizing antibodies. The role of cell-mediated immunity has not yet been entirely defined.

The incubation period of influenza is 1 to 3 days. A range of signs and symptoms may follow the onset of illness, but the most typical ones include fever, malaise, cough, and severe myalgias. Presumably, the systemic symptoms are the result of the body's own response to the virus, as detectable viremia is uncommon. Other symptoms occurring with some frequency include headache and mild coryza. The clinical illness usually runs its course in 3 to 5 days and may be followed by prolonged fatigue.

The most important features of the clinical illness are the complications. Often these center on the respiratory tract and include tracheobronchitis and croup, the latter in children. The most severe respiratory complication is pneumonia, of which there are two types. The first type is fortunately the less common, is caused by the virus itself, and is called *primary influenzal pneumonia.* This is the more severe of the two types and though it occurs in otherwise healthy young adults, it is likely most common in individuals with underlying cardiovascular disease (especially mitral stenosis) and pregnancy. Primary influenzal pneumonia is characterized by the rapid onset of tachypnea and cyanosis often followed by respiratory failure, extensive pulmonary changes compatible with adult respiratory distress syndrome, severe hypoxemia, and death.

Secondary pneumonia is attributable to the presence of pathogenic bacteria that are able to invade the host because of the severe destructive effects of the influenza virus on the respiratory epithelium. The bacteria in question includes *Streptococcus pneumoniae, Haemophilus influenza,* and *Staphylococcus aureus.* Bacterial pneumonia as a complication of influenza follows a different pattern than that of primary influenzal pneumonia. Typically, the patient appears to improve transiently, then suffers a relapse of the fever. The infiltrates tend to be alveolar in nature, and the sputum contains leukocytes and bacteria. Antibiotic treatment generally ameliorates the condition.

Other important complications of influenza include exacerbations of chronic obstructive pulmonary disease, myositis, myocarditis, pericarditis, and Reye's syndrome, although the latter may be more attributable to the use of aspirin in children rather than caused by the effects of the influenza virus.

The usual diagnosis of influenza is presumptively based on clinical criteria (Fig. 69-1). Thus a patient with a moderate respiratory infection characterized by cough, intense myalgias, and fever that occurs in the appropriate season and often in light of a flurry of similar cases should always raise the spectre of influenza.

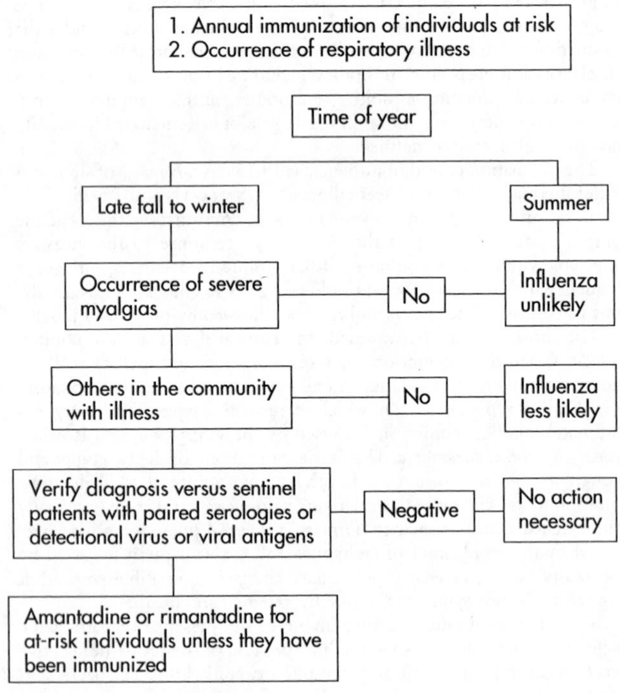

FIG. 69-1 Diagnosis of influenza.

A specific diagnosis can be established by culture of the agent from throat washings, although this may not be readily available for most cases, or by rapid identification of the agent in respiratory secretions using other means such as immunofluorescence of exfoliated pharyngeal cells (throat scraping) or ELISA identification of viral antigens in throat washings. Serologic tests have also been a traditional means of establishing the diagnosis. These generally rely, however, on a fourfold rise in antibody titers to establish the diagnosis and thus require the passage of 10 to 14 days to generally observe such a change. Hemagglutination-inhibiting antibodies have been used most commonly for this purpose.

TREATMENT

The usual treatment of influenza is symptomatic (i.e., fluids, rest, and acetaminophen). Specific therapy is available for influenza A, but not for influenza B or C. Two oral agents are amantadine and rimantadine. The former is a synthetic amine that inhibits replication of the virus in tissue culture and experimental animal systems. The drug appears to work by inhibiting viral uncoating. It is reasonably absorbed from the gastrointestinal tract and is excreted largely by the kidney. The drug is effective in reducing the duration of both fever and symptoms if taken promptly. On the other hand, a few troublesome side effects can be seen, including insomnia, agitation, and disorientation. These effects are most likely seen in the elderly, a group that may benefit from such a therapeutic intervention. The dose in patients with normal renal function is 100 mg twice a day; in the elderly, the dose is reduced to 100 mg once a day. Rimantadine is a related agent that differs from amantadine in that it is excreted by the liver and may be less associated with toxic symptoms. The dose is similar.

PREVENTION

Because influenza can be a devastating infection, particularly in the compromised, and because therapy is not optimal, prevention remains the best strategy. It is generally accepted that immunization can be 60% to 90% effective. Those most likely to be seriously affected by influenza are those most in need of the vaccine. Thus patients over the age of 65 and those with serious underlying disease, especially chronic cardiac or pulmonary disease, should be immunized annually. In addition, individuals in high-risk situations (i.e., health care personnel) should consider receiving the vaccine. There are several forms of the vaccine currently available, including the whole inactivated vaccine generally recommended for adults and split virus vaccines or subunit vaccines that may be better for children.

The only adverse effects reported with any frequency with current vaccines include local pain in 20% to 25% of vaccines and systemic symptoms that occur in 5% of these individuals. Guillain-Barré syndrome, associated with the swine flu, does not appear to be an increased risk for other influenza vaccines. Split virus and subunit vaccines are less immunogenic and also less reactogenic.

Each year vaccine is prepared from the strains most frequently found in the preceding 12 months. Current vaccines will contain H_1 N_1 and H_3 N_2 strains of influenza A and a current strain of influenza B. The vaccine must be administered annually in the late fall when it becomes available.

For those individuals unable to receive the vaccine for fear of an adverse reaction or for those at high risk, particularly when there has been significant antigenic drift or even antigenic shift, amantadine or rimantadine are effective prophylaxis if taken in the doses mentioned above for the duration of the epidemic. In some individuals who inadvertently failed to receive the vaccine, amantadine or rimantadine may be given simultaneously with the vaccine and for 2 weeks thereafter.

KEY POINTS

1 Immunity to the influenza virus is associated with antibodies to hemagglutinin and neuraminidase.

2 The important clinical feature of influenza is intense myalgias.

3 The diagnosis of influenza is made by detection of virus or viral antigens in respiratory secretions or by a fourfold rise in antibody titers.

4 Treatment is largely supportive, but amantadine and rimantadine reduce the duration of fever and other symptoms.

5 Annual immunization for certain high-risk groups is important.

SUGGESTED READINGS

Couch R: Advances in influenza virus vaccine research, *Ann N Y Acad Sci* 685:803-812, 1993.

LaForce F, Nichol K, Cox N: Influenza: virology, epidemiology, disease and prevention, *Am J Prev Med* 10 Suppl:31-44, 1994.

Laufer D, Stan S: Resistance to antivirals, *Pediatr Clin North Am* 42:583-599, 1995.

Peschke T et al: Role of macrophage cytokines in influenza A virus infections, *Immunobiology* 189:340-355, 1993.

Wiselka M: Influenza: diagnosis, management and prophylaxis, *BMJ* 308:1341-1345, 1994.

70

Laryngitis and Pharyngitis

David B. Keschner and William B. Armstrong

PHARYNGITIS

Pharyngitis is an inflammation of the pharyngeal mucosa and submucosal tissues. The name does not imply an etiology, and the condition may result from multiple infectious and noninfectious causes (Box 70-1). Acute viral or bacterial infections produce the majority of cases of pharyngitis. Noninfectious etiologies, however, may produce significant morbidity, and their clinical features must be recognized by the primary care physician, who is often the first physician to encounter, evaluate, and treat this condition.

Diagnosis

Viral infections produce the majority of cases of pharyngitis. These are most often caused by respiratory viruses including rhinovirus, coronavirus, influenza, and parainfluenza viruses. Group A β-hemolytic Streptococcus (GABHS) is the most common bacterial cause of pharyngitis and is the etiology of up to 30% of cases of pharyngitis treated by physicians. Differentiating between GABHS and viral pharyngitis is difficult on clinical grounds alone, but diagnosis is aided by clinical studies, such as culturing for GABHS, and rapid diagnostic tests that use latex particle agglutination or enzyme-linked immunoassays. Viral pharyngitis is usually associated with rhinitis, cough, conjunctivitis, and systemic symptoms. Fever, tonsillar exudate, cervical adenopathy, and pharyngeal injection may be present, but are more often seen with GABHS pharyngitis. GABHS is associated with a higher incidence of temperature over 101° F, tender cervical adenopathy, tonsillar exudate, and absence of cough. Onset is rapid, and a preceding rhinitis is unusual. Unfortunately, the accuracy of clinical diagnosis alone to distinguish GABHS from viral pharyngitis is only 50% to 75% by experienced physicians. Throat cultures for GABHS and rapid reagent streptococcal tests have been utilized to improve diagnostic accuracy. Throat cultures are sensitive and specific when properly obtained from the tonsillar and posterior pharyngeal surfaces, but have a 24- to 48-hour delay for growth. Rapid streptococcal tests have over 90% sensitivity and are useful when positive, but their specificity (i.e., ability to exclude streptococcal infection) is only 50% to 75%. Use of symptoms scores to aid in clinical decision making has also been advocated by some authors. Symptoms to be scored include the presence of tonsillar exudate, tender cervical adenopathy, temperature over 101° F,

BOX 70-1

Causes of Pharyngitis

INFECTIOUS

Bacterial

Group A β-hemolytic streptococcus
Staphylococcus aureus
Bordetella pertussis
Haemophilus influenzae
Neisseria gonorrhoeae
Actinomyses sp.
Chlamydia trachomatis
Haemophilus influenzae type B
Streptococcus influenzae
Non-Group A Streptococcus
Corynebacterium diphtheriae
Mycobacterium sp.
Treponema pallidum (syphilis)
Klebsiella rhinoscleromatis
Peptostreptococcus
Coxiella burnetii (Q fever)
Streptococcus pneumoniae

Viral

Parainfluenza
Rhinovirus
Epstein-Barr virus
Herpes simplex virus
Influenza
Respiratory syncytial virus
Cytomegalovirus

Fungal

Candida albicans
Cryptococcus neoformans
Blastomyces dermatitdites
Rhinosporidium seeberi
Histoplasma capsulatum
Paracoccidioides brasiliensis

NONINFECTIOUS

Neoplastic

Leukemia
Squamous cell carcinoma
Lymphoma
Other carcinomas

Traumatic

Penetrating trauma
Thermal injury
Environmental pollutants (e.g., smog)
Caustic agents (Iye)
Cigarette/marijuana smoke

Medical/Systemic

Allergy
Sinusitis
Crohn's disease
Stevens-Johnson syndrome
Bullous pemphigoid
Other dermatologic diseases

and absence of cough. When two or more of these signs or symptoms are present, presumptive treatment for GABHS is recommended. Scoring systems have sensitivities and specificities around 80%.

The rationale for aggressive diagnosis and treatment of GABHS is predicated on the prevention of suppurative and nonsuppurative complications. Suppurative complications include peritonsillar abscess, deep neck abscess, and scarlet fever. Peritonsillar abscess is the most common suppurative complication of pharyngitis. It is characterized by unilateral severe throat pain, bulging of the soft palate, deviation of the uvula, and often trismus (restriction of mouth opening). Scarlet fever is an uncommon complication that appears to be associated with certain toxigenic strains of GABHS. Scarlet fever produces a fine macular rash that appears on the second day of illness, starts on the neck and chest and spreads to the entire body, with sparing of the perioral area, palms, and soles. The rash is punctate and blanches under pressure. Often there is a "strawberry tongue" present, which is considered to be pathognomonic.

Rheumatic fever and poststreptococcal glomerulonephritis are examples of nonsuppurative complications of GABHS pharyngitis. Acute rheumatic fever usually presents as a symmetric polyarthritis beginning about 2 weeks after the onset of pharyngitis. Later, carditis, chorea, erythema marginatum (blanching, painless erythematous rash on trunk and proximal extremities), and fever may develop. After recovery from the acute episode, patients are subject to relapse with subsequent streptococcal infections. Poststreptococcal acute glomerulonephritis is an acute inflammatory disorder that produces hematuria, proteinuria, peripheral edema, and hypertension. The disorder is usually self-limited, and the incidence is not decreased by treatment of GABHS infections with antibiotic therapy.

Although streptococcal infections are the most common causes of pharyngitis, several other bacterial species contribute significantly to the development of acute bacterial pharyngitis. Non-Group A streptococci, *S. aureus,* oral anaerobes, *Mycoplasma pneumoniae, H. influenzae,* N. gonorrhoeae, T. pallidum (syphillis), and *Corynebacterium* diphtheriae also produce pharyngitis. *H. influenzae* type B is a common cause of epiglottitis in the pediatric population and also occurs in the adult population. Although it may progress to airway compromise in both age groups, this complication is more common in children because of the anatomy of the pediatric hypopharynx.

N. gonorrhoeae and *T. pallidum* are uncommon causes of pharyngitis, but should also be considered in sexually active patients. Gonococcal pharyngitis can be diagnosed by plating throat swabs on appropriate culture media, and syphilis can be diagnosed with darkfield examination of swabs from the pharynx or more commonly through serologic testing.

Pharyngitis is but one of the many manifestations of infection with *C. trachomatis.* Some studies have reported that approximately 20% of the pharyngitides may be the result of chlamydial infection. Although this figure may overestimate the incidence of chlamydial pharyngitis, it is nonetheless an important and relevant etiologic agent. Treatment includes supportive care and the administration of appropriate enteral or parenteral antibiotic.

C. diphtheriae, the causative agent of diphtheria, is now an extremely rare cause of pharyngitis in the United States as a result of widespread immunization. It is characterized by the presence of a gray pseudomembrane in the pharynx that bleeds when removed. This may be mimicked by or confused with Vincent's angina, caused by anaerobic fusospirochetal infection, and occasionally infectious mononucleosis. If diphtheria is contemplated, cultures and serum are obtained, diphtheria antitoxin is given, and antimicrobial therapy is administered. Antitoxin administration is critical to prevent cardiac and neurologic complications.

Epstein-Barr virus is an important cause of pharyngitis. Infectious mononucleosis primarily affects adolescents and young adults. The disease is characterized by acute tonsillopharyngitis, fatigue, coryza, and often a tonsillar exudate. Petechia at the junction of the soft and hard palate may be noted. Anterior and posterior lymphadenopathy are often present. Splenomegaly is present in approximately half the cases and hepatomegaly in approximately 10%. The monospot test (a rapid slide test) and serum heterophile antibody tests are used to diagnose infectious mononucleosis. Patients with the clinical picture resembling infectious mononucleosis but with negative antibody tests may be infected with cytomegalovirus (CMV).

Primary and secondary infections with HSV I and II may present with pharyngitis. Presence of a vesicular eruption with fever, pain, and malaise, or a history of previous similar infections points toward this diagnosis. Minor or major aphthous stomatitis will appear as punched-out ulcers in the pharynx. In addition, the Group A coxsackie virus may produce a clinical syndrome in which ulcerations or papules may appear in the oral mucosa, soft palate, or tonsillar fossae (herpangina). HSV infections, on the other hand, may cause ulcerations of the tonsils or vesicular eruptions in the pharyngeal mucosa.

Candida albicans is the most common fungal agent causing pharyngitis. White areas or patches may be present on the tongue, floor of the mouth, buccal mucosa, palate, and tonsillar pillars. When scraped, there is an erythematous base. A history of recent antibiotic use or conditions impairing systemic immunity may be present. Rarely, other fungal agents may produce pharyngitis, although these are usually extensions of a more deep-seated infection. Other causative fungal agents include *Aspergillus, Cryptococcus, Rhinosporidium,* and *Histoplasma* organisms. As the incidence of immunoincompetence caused by viral infection (e.g., HIV) or advanced medical treatment modalities (e.g., chemotherapy, corticosteroid regimens) rises, the fungal pharyngitides become increasingly important to the primary care physician. Although once immediately discarded as an etiologic agent because of its rarity, fungal disease can no longer be so quickly dismissed, in the pharynx or elsewhere.

Noninfectious causes of pharyngitis can be divided into neoplastic and nonneoplastic causes. Leukemia and lymphoma can present with pharyngitis, but often this is overshadowed by other systemic manifestations. Squamous cell carcinoma may present as a painful area in the throat, sometimes with associated odynophagia, dysphagia, and weight loss. Squamous cell carcinoma in the oral cavity or pharynx is linked to cigarette and alcohol use, and over 90% of cases occur in patients over 40 years. In this population, pharyngitis failing to resolve within 2 weeks should be referred for otolaryngologic evaluation. Early tumors are characterized by velvety red areas or leukoplakic patches that may be nontender. Early diagnosis is imperative because oropharyngeal carcinomas are potentially curable in the early stages.

Irritants and trauma, including thermal burns from hot liquid, topical aspirin placement for a toothache, cigarette or marijuana smoke, and environmental pollutants, may all produce symptoms of pharyngitis. Several systemic disorders including Crohn's disease and certain dermatologic conditions (such as bullous pemphigoid and Stevens-Johnson syndrome) may manifest primarily or secondarily as pharyngitis.

Treatment

Management of viral pharyngitis is symptomatic, with use of analgesics and hydration constituting the mainstays of treatment. Topical anesthetic sprays or lozenges are also helpful. Management of presumed GABHS consists of a 10-day course of oral penicillins, or a single intramuscular dose of penicillin G benzathine. Penicillin-allergic patients may be treated with erythromycin or cephalosporins. The decision to prescribe antibiotics for possible GABHS depends on the diagnostic modalities used. If available, rapid streptococcal tests may be used to determine eligibility for treatment. If the rapid test is positive, treatment is instituted for 10 days. If the test is negative, a culture should be obtained and treatment empirically initiated. If the culture is negative (usually available after 3 days), treatment may be discontinued. Finally, if symptom scoring for pharyngitis is used for management of pharyngitis, patients with at least two of the symptomatic criteria described earlier may be treated empirically with antibiotics. Patients with scarlet fever are treated empirically, as are patients with a previous history of rheumatic fever.

Treatment of other causes of pharyngitis depends on the etiology. For mononucleosis, treatment is supportive. Ampicillin should be avoided to prevent allergic reactions and Stevens-Johnson syndrome, a severe form of erythema multiforme. Treatment of candidal pharyngitis includes use of topical nystatin or other antifungal agents and, when possible, elimination of underlying cause for immunosuppression. If a neoplastic process is suspected, immediate referral for biopsy is indicated.

LARYNGITIS AND HOARSENESS

Hoarseness is the most common and specific symptom of laryngeal disease. As with pharyngitis, laryngitis is a nonspecific term that denotes inflammation of the laryngeal mucosa and submucosa. Acute hoarseness is generally a self-limited problem caused by viral laryngitis or voice abuse. An accurate history can often point to the correct diagnosis. Important historic factors include patient's age; duration of hoarseness; associated smoking or alcohol consumption; presence of shortness of breath; voice use patterns; presence of pain, dysphagia, or odynophagia; preceding URI; presence of a neck mass; history of neck surgery, intubation, or a lung tumor; and exposure to toxic or allergic compounds.

Diagnosis

It is useful to divide hoarseness into acute and chronic varieties because their etiologies and management differ markedly. Acute hoarseness lasting under 2 weeks is most often the result of a viral infection or voice abuse. The voice is rough, and there is often a history of cigarette smoking that exacerbates the vocal fold edema. Environmental allergens and inhalation of toxic fumes can produce mild laryngeal edema, resulting in voice change.

Three serious causes of acute hoarseness that are important for the physician to recognize are anaphylactic reactions, angioedema, and adult epiglottitis. Allergic reactions to foods (e.g., shellfish) or medications (e.g., penicillin) can produce rapid onset of shortness of breath and hoarseness from laryngeal edema. This usually occurs in conjunction with systemic shock and is easily recognized. Treatment with epinephrine and protection of the airway are key points in management of this emergency. Hereditary angioedema is an inherited disorder caused by the lack of (85%) or malfunction of (15%) C1-esterase inhibitor. This defect in the complement cascade results in sporadic episodes of mucosal and cutaneous edema. The syndrome is characterized by repeated attacks of rapid onset of diffuse edema that is indurated and tender. Swelling often involves the face and lips and may extend to the hypopharynx and larynx, resulting in rapid onset of airway compromise. Airway management is of primary concern in these patients, and many patients will require emergent endotracheal intubation. The swelling and induration from hereditary angioedema respond poorly to epinephrine and corticosteroids. Adult epiglottitis is usually polymicrobial in nature. This disorder is associated with sore throat, odynopagia, dysphagia, muffled voice, and respiratory difficulty, and may occasionally progress to airway obstruction.

Chronic hoarseness (over 2 weeks) has a much more extensive differential diagnosis. In general, hoarseness lasting over 2 weeks requires visualization of the larynx to determine etiology. Examination of the larynx will provide a diagnosis in the majority of cases.

Chronic laryngitis often results from repeated or chronic voice abuse. Often, cigarette smoking is a contributing factor. Chronic irritation of the mucosa and submucosa of the vocal cords produces swelling and inflammation. The voice is rough, with symptoms worsening as the day progresses. Pain and systemic symptoms indicative of infection are absent.

Gastroesophageal reflux disease (GERD) is also a very common and underrecognized cause of chronic hoarseness, accounting for up to 15% of cases of chronic laryngitis. Patients present with varying degrees of hoarseness and intermittent sore throats. The voice is typically worse in the morning, improving as the day progresses. Typically, patients do not complain of heartburn or regurgitation, but may note a bitter taste in the mouth on awakening or during the night. Patients may note a foreign body sensation in the throat ("globus pharyngeus") or exhibit chronic throat clearing. Laryngeal examination reveals erythema or pale edema in the posterior larynx adjacent to the esophageal inlet.

Tumors of the larynx often produce hoarseness as the only early symptom. Often these may be simple benign nodules or cysts, but squamous cell carcinoma occurs with increasing frequency with cigarette use and increasing age. When diagnosed early, it is highly curable. This is a major reason why early laryngeal evaluation of hoarseness is so important.

Vocal cord paralysis is an uncommon cause of hoarseness in the primary care setting. Most commonly, the paralysis is iatrogenic, a result of cardiothoracic or thyroid surgery. Paralysis is almost always unilateral. Clinically, the voice is breathy. The differential diagnosis is extensive. Nerve disruption from trauma, neoplasm, infection, or inflammatory disorders anywhere in the course of the proximal vagus nerve and recurrent laryngeal nerve from the brainstem through the larynx will result in paralysis.

Hoarseness may also result from external trauma to the vocal cords and surrounding structures. Toxic inhalants, including cigarette smoke, can cause edema and inflammation in the hypopharynx. Endotracheal intubation may produce erosions and granulomas along the posterior portions of the vocal cords, producing acute and chronic hoarseness.

A number of other localized and systemic diseases may cause laryngitis (Box 70-2), although they are difficult to identify, diagnose, and treat in the primary care setting. The responsibility of the primary care physician is to identify those etiologies that may be life threatening, including malig-

BOX 70-2

Causes of Laryngitis

ACUTE

Infectious

Haemophilus influenzae
β-hemolytic streptococcus
Streptococcus pneumoniae
Bordetella pertussis
Parainfluenza, types 1-4
Staphylococcus
Corynebacteria diphtheriae
Paramyxovirus (measles)

Noninfectious

Environmental allergens
Inhalational irritants
Anaphylaxis
Vocal abuse
Angioedema

CHRONIC

Infectious

Mycobacterium sp.
Klebsiella rhinoscleromatis
Blastomyces
Candida albicans
Coccidioides immitis
Treponema pallidum
Mycobacterium leprae
Histoplasma capsulatum
Actinomyces bovis

NonInfectious

Benign masses
Vocal abuse
GERD
Wegener's granulomatosis
Malignant neoplasms
Inhalational irritants
Vocal cord paralysis
Sarcoidosis

nancy, and to refer patients with such voice derangements for definitive evaluation and management.

Treatment

Management of hoarseness depends on the etiology. Treatment of viral laryngitis is supportive. Viral laryngitis is self-limited and resolves with voice rest (soft voice but no whispering), increased fluid intake, and humidified mist. Cessation of smoking and avoidance of caffeine are important treatment measures. Mucolytic agents (guaifenesin, iodinated glycerol) thin secretions and are very helpful. Antibiotics are not indicated for treatment of acute viral laryngitis, but may be helpful when a bacterial superinfection is suspected. Bacterial laryngitis generally causes a sore throat, odynophagia, dysphagia, and muffled voice. Adult epiglottitis, resulting from bacterial infection of the glottic and supraglottic larynx, is managed aggressively with parenteral antibiotics to cover oral aerobes (including *S. aureus* and *H. influenzae*) and anaerobes, serial airway examinations, and hydration. If airway encroachment ensues, a tracheostomy must be performed.

Treatment of reflux laryngitis addresses the underlying disorder of GERD. Elevating the head of the bed, eating smaller meals, and avoiding late-night meals are all easily instituted measures. Pharmacotherapy, including H_2-blockers and proton-pump inhibitors, is also effective as an adjunctive method of treatment. Patients failing conservative medical management will require gastroenterologic workup and consideration for possible surgical intervention.

Finally, it is worthwhile to note that hoarseness does not imply laryngitis. Indeed, although laryngitis may cause hoarseness, it is but one of a wide spectrum of disorders, ranging from singer's nodules to vocal cord paralysis to laryngeal carcinoma, that are capable of producing hoarseness. Almost invariably, hoarseness that is insidious in onset or that does not subside quickly mandates formal evaluation of the larynx.

KEY POINTS

1. Group A β-hemolytic streptococcus and respiratory viruses account for the majority of cases of pharyngitis.
2. GABHS is more likely to be present when there is a temperature over 101° F, tender anterior cervical adenopathy, pharyngeal exudate, and absence of a previous rhinorrhea, cough, or myalgias.
3. Treatment of GABHS is aimed at prevention of suppurative and nonsuppurative complications of infection.
4. Throat cultures are the gold standard for diagnosis of streptococcal infections. Rapid diagnostic tests are sensitive, but not specific. Use of symptom scores increases the sensitivity and specificity of diagnosis to approximately 80%.
5. Penicillin is the agent of choice for treatment of GABHS. A dose of 1.2 million units penicillin G benzathine intramuscularly, or a 10-day

course of oral penicillin is administered. Erythromycin or cephalosporins may be used in penicillin-allergic patients.

6 Definite indications for treatment of GABHS are history of rheumatic fever, scarlet fever, or a positive throat culture.

7 Hoarseness lasting over 2 weeks requires visual evaluation of the larynx; the majority of chronic causes of hoarseness can be diagnosed by visualization of the larynx.

8 Laryngitis causes hoarseness, but not all hoarseness is caused by laryngitis. Acute hoarseness usually results from viral laryngitis or voice abuse. Chronic hoarseness is usually from noninfectious etiology.

9 Treatment of voice abuse includes cessation of cigarette smoking, cool mist, and voice rest. It is important to remind patients to avoid whispering, which causes more irritation to the vocal cords than merely speaking in a soft voice.

SUGGESTED READINGS

Bonilla JA, Bluestone CD: Pharyngitis: when is aggressive treatment warranted? *Postgrad Med* 97:61-69, 1995.

Denny FW: Current management of streptococcal pharyngitis: a review of pathophysiology, diagnosis, and management, *J Emerg Mgt* 36:619-620, 1992.

Farizo KM et al: Fatal respiratory disease due to *Corynebacterium diphtheriae:* case report and review of guidelines for management, investigation, and control, *Clin Infect Dis* 16:59-68, 1993.

Goldstein MN: Office evaluation of the sore throat, *Otolaryngol Clin North Am* 25(4):837-842, 1992.

Guzman L: Rheumatic fever. In: HR Schumacher Jr, ed: *Primer of the rheumatic diseases,* ed 10, 1993, Arthritis Foundation, pp 168-171.

Kiselica D: Group A β-hemolytic streptococcal pharyngitis: current clinical concepts, *Am Fam Physician* 49:1147-1154, 1994.

Kline JA et al: Streptococcal pharyngitis: a review of pathophysiology, diagnosis and management, *J Emerg Med* 12:665-680, 1994.

Paisley JW et al: Infections: viral and rickettsial. In WE Hathaway et al, eds: *Current pediatric diagnosis and treatment,* ed 10, 1991, Appleton & Lange, pp 815-843.

Wenig BM, Kornblut AD: Pharyngitis. In Byron Bailey, ed: *Head and neck surgery–otolaryngology,* volume 1, 1993, JB Lippincott, pp 551-567.

71

Nutrition

DIANA YAO AND THOMAS Y. MA

Nutrition is defined as the sum of the processes involved in taking in the food and liquid requirements that are essential for normal physiologic function. Malnutrition results from a deficit of these required elements and is associated with an increase in morbidity and mortality. A relationship exists between nutritional status and disease, indicating the importance of adequate nutrition. Recommended Dietary Allowances (RDAs) represent the amount of nutrient intake for healthy individuals that is required to prevent the development of nutritional deficiency states. Ideally, dietary recommendations should meet the RDAs and the following guidelines: (1) eat a variety of foods, (2) decrease fat consumption to <30% of total calories, (3) decrease cholesterol intake, (4) increase fiber intake to 20 to 30 g/day, (5) decrease sodium intake, (6) drink alcohol only in moderation, and (7) maintain ideal body weight. A multidisciplinary team approach to nutritional management should include physicians, dietitians, pharmacists, nurses, and the patients themselves.

NUTRIENT REQUIREMENTS

Nutrients are made up of macronutrients and micronutrients. Macronutrients consist of carbohydrates, fats, and proteins. Micronutrients consist of vitamins and minerals. Essential nutrients are those whose removal from dietary sources results in a deficiency state.

Carbohydrates constitute 50% of a typical U.S. diet and are essential nutrients that provide 4 kcal/g of energy. A minimum daily carbohydrate intake of 400 kcal is recommended. Carbohydrates require digestion by digestive enzymes (including amylase and brush border enzymes such as lactase) and are absorbed as monosaccharides. These substrates may be utilized directly by cells as an energy source or stored as glycogen or fat. Glycogen is only a small storage form of carbohydrates and at the body's maximal capacity can only provide energy requirements for 12 to 24 hours or approximately 900 kcal of energy.

Fats provide 9 kcal/g of energy. In an average U.S. diet, 90% of fat is in the form of triglycerides, and fat provides 35% of the total calories. The essential fatty acids are linoleic acid and linolenic acid. The caloric value of fat is eight times that of carbohydrates, and fat is the major storage form of calories.

Proteins constitute 15% of a typical U.S. diet. Although proteins provide 4 kcal/g of energy, this value is not included in the calculation of energy needs. The major function of ingested proteins is to provide amino acids for endogenous protein synthesis. No storage form of proteins exist in the body.

The vitamins are a group of 13 essential micronutrients, the majority of which are available in an average U.S. diet. Vitamins B and C are water soluble, and vitamins A, D, E, and K are fat soluble. Vitamin deficiency states result from reduced dietary intake, decreased storage forms, decreased absorption, reduced endogenous synthesis, increased loss, or increased utilization. The minerals include the major minerals sodium, potassium, calcium, magnesium, and phosphorous. The trace elements with a known role in nutrition include iron, zinc, copper, manganese, iodide, fluoride, selenium, chromium, and molybdenum.

Energy Requirements

Activity factors account for the amount of energy required for different levels of activity. At rest, the activity factor is 1.0. For light activity, moderate activity, and heavy activity, the activity factors are 1.5 to 2.5, 5.0, and 7.0, respectively. The following general values may also be used to estimate the energy expenditure of activity: 400 to 800 kcal/day for sedentary activity, 800 to 1200 kcal/day for light work, 1200 to 1800 kcal/day for moderate work, and 1800 to 4500 kcal/day for heavy exercise. In hospitalized, bedridden patients, this value is low.

Stress is an additional factor that must be considered with specific clinical situations. For example, in the setting of starvation, the stress factor is 0.8. to 1.0. For elective surgery and a major operation, the stress factors are 1.0 to 1.1 and 1.1 to 1.2, respectively. For mild infections, moderate infections, and severe infections, the values are 1.0 to 1.2, 1.2 to 1.4, and 1.4 to 1.6, respectively. Total energy requirements during illness may be estimated as follows: none to mild stress: 25 kcal/kg/day (elective surgery), mild to moderate stress: 25 to 35 kcal/kg/day (severe infection), and severe stress: 45 kcal/kg/day (severe burns or hepatic failure).

Any combination of carbohydrates and fats can provide the total daily energy requirements, with the provision that 400 to 700 kcal/day must be provided by glucose. The source of glucose may be from ingested carbohydrates or gluconeogenesis from protein catabolism. Glucose is essential because it is required by the glucose-dependent organs, including the brain, bone marrow, renal medulla, and peripheral nerves.

Protein Requirements

The usual daily protein requirement for healthy individuals is 0.8 g/kg, and this amount provides the protein necessary to maintain a positive nitrogen balance. Daily protein requirements increase during growth periods, pregnancy, lactation, and illness. Illness increases protein losses as a result of excess catabolism and losses in body fluids from organs with large surface areas such as the bowel, lungs, or skin. If an insufficient number of calories are provided by carbohydrates and fats, body proteins are catabolized to meet the body's energy needs, resulting in a negative nitrogen balance. Protein requirements may be estimated as follows: normal–0.6 to 0.8 gm/kg ideal body weight (IBW)/day, mild metabolic stress–1.0 to 1.1 gm/kg IBW/day, moderate metabolic stress–1.2 to 1.4 gm/kg IBW/day, severe metabolic stress–1.5 to 2.5 gm/kg IBW/day, and pregnancy–an additional 10 g above calculated needs.

ASSESSMENT OF MACRONUTRIENT DEFICIENCY

The purpose of a complete nutritional assessment is to evaluate nutritional deficiencies, to determine the impact of diet on diseases, and to predict systemic dysfunction (Fig. 71-1). The assessment is valuable in guiding the nutritional needs of individual patients depending on their disease states. Unfortunately, no single test is able to predict an individual's nutritional status. Components of the clinical assessment include (1) a complete history and physical, (2) a complete nutritional history, (3) weight measurement, and (4) anthropometry.

A complete history and physical are essential in the nutritional assessment. A history obtained from the patient or patient's family members is a simple tool for identifying malnutrition or risk factors for its development. The history should emphasize the presence or absence of weight loss, anorexia, edema, nausea, vomiting, diarrhea, abdominal pain, or chronic illness. Other conditions that may result in decreased food intake should be identified, such as dysphagia, immobility, depression, impaired smell or taste, or dental problems. Other important aspects of the history include the presence of polypharmacy or heavy alcohol or drug usage. A social history is also essential to identify factors that may contribute to the development of malnutrition, including employment status and income, social isolation, or size of patient's family.

A thorough physical examination must be conducted, with specific attention to the findings of decreased mobility, loss of subcutaneous fat, muscle wasting, edema, jaundice, changes in hair color and texture, cheilosis, or glossitis. Height and weight should be recorded. A nutritional history must be obtained in a complete evaluation. Diet diaries may expose unusual food intake and dietary habits. Daily calorie counts can be very helpful in identifying the presence of inadequate dietary intake.

Weight loss may be an important indicator of malnutrition and should be assessed in the context of weight loss over time. Severe weight loss may be characterized as >5% weight loss over 1 month, >7.5% loss over 3 months, or >10% loss over 6 months. If the weight loss is >40%, survival is unusual. An alternative evaluation of weight is to determine what percentage of IBW is present in a given patient. IBW for males is 106 lbs for the first 5 ft of height and 6 lbs for each additional inch. IBW for females is 100 lbs for first 5 ft of height and then 5 lbs for each additional inch. Mild malnutrition is present at 80% to 90% of IBW, moderate at 70% to 79% of IBW, and severe at <70% of IBW. Weight loss may be underestimated in the presence of edema or ascites, so a careful history is essential.

Anthropometry uses specific body measurements to assess body fat and protein stores. The triceps skinfold thickness (TSF) is measured with calipers and assesses subcutaneous fat, which represents approximately

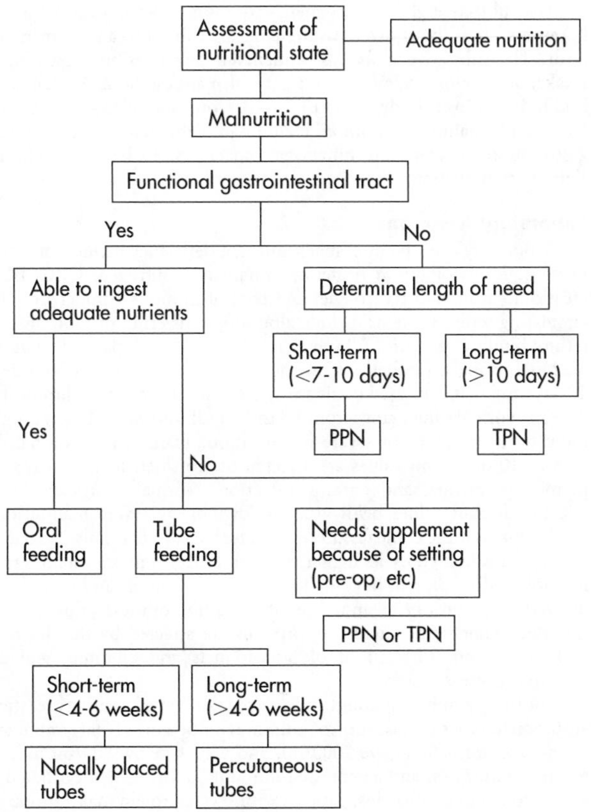

FIG. 71-1 Management of nutrition. *PPN,* peripheral parenteral nutrition; *TPN,* total parenteral nutrition.

50% of body fat. The midarm circumference (MAC) is measured with a tape measure and is used in the calculation of the midarm muscle circumference (MAMC).

$$\text{MAMC(cm)} = \text{MAC(cm)} - (0.314 \times \text{TSF in mm})$$

A significant loss of protein stores is present if MAC is less than the fifth percentile and MAMC is less than the tenth percentile. The MAC and MAMC assess skeletal muscle, which represents approximately 60% of the total body protein stores.

The subjective global assessment score is a better nutritional marker because each of the above measurements are subject to a wide margin of error. The subjective global assessment encompasses an evaluation of intake, absorption, digestion, and clinical manifestations of changes in bodily function or body composition. A score is applied to six separate features of a patient's condition, including weight change, dietary intake, gastrointestinal symptoms, functional capacity, stress level, and physical signs of malnutrition.

Laboratory Assessment

The laboratory assessment of macronutrient deficiency includes measurement of levels of serum proteins, urinary urea nitrogen, CBC, BUN, creatinine, iron, and β-carotene, and tests of immune competence. The circulating serum proteins include albumin, transferrin, prealbumin, and retinol-binding protein. Albumin is obtained as a part of standard chemistry panels. Limitations on the use of albumin are its half-life of 20 days and that decreased levels are often seen with sepsis or chronic liver disease. Normal values range from 3.5 to 4.5 g/dl, and values below 2.1 g/dl indicate the presence of severe malnutrition. Transferrin has a half-life of 8 to 10 days, and values are affected by iron deficiency, pregnancy, pernicious anemia, and chronic infection. Normal values are above 200 mg/dl, and values below 100 mg/dl indicate severe malnutrition. Prealbumin is more clinically useful because its half-life is only 2 to 3 days, but its use is limited by its higher cost and longer time to obtain results. Retinol-binding protein has a half-life of 10 to 12 hours and may also be utilized. Care must be taken in the interpretation of these values because the measurements of circulating proteins are affected by the degree of hydration, administration of blood products and albumin, and any underlying disease states.

The total lymphocyte count and delayed skin hypersensitivity reactions are useful tests in the evaluation of immune competence. Total lymphocyte counts are normally above 2000/ml, and values below 800/ml indicate severe malnutrition and a depressed immune status. As demonstrated by anergy to common proteins, patients with severe protein malnutrition are not able to mount an appropriate immune response to foreign antigens.

NUTRITIONAL SUPPORT

The nutritional needs of individuals can be assessed by the above parameters. The average, well-nourished individual is capable of tolerating up to 7 days of starvation if given supplemental fluid and glucose. After 1 to 2 weeks of decreased intake (earlier if already malnourished), nutritional support should be instituted. Up to 40% of hospitalized patients may be malnourished and should have early and aggressive nutritional support. These patients often have increased protein mobilization caused by a "hypermetabolic" state secondary to their illness. If the ultimate goal of nutritional support is weight gain, an additional 500 to 1000 kcal/day should be given to a malnourished patient; this will generally result in a weight gain of 1 to 2 lbs/week.

Enteral Alimentation

Enteral alimentation is the preferred method for nutritional support whenever possible. The enteral route is more physiologic and less costly than parenteral nutrition. Intraluminal nutrients have a trophic effect on the intestinal epithelium that helps to maintain mucousal integrity and epithelial barrier function. Enteral nutrition also provides nutrients that are not available through the parenteral route, including the gut-specific fuels of glutamine and short chain fatty acids. Glutamine is essential for normal intestinal structure and function. Short chain fatty acids are the products of bacterial fermentation of undigested carbohydrates (e.g., cellulose). In some patients, the absence of or low levels of short chain fatty acids has been associated with the development of colitis.

Oral feeding is the preferred method of nutritional support in patients who are able to eat. Typical types of hospital diets include clear liquids, full liquids, low fiber, high fiber, low fat, low sodium, and regular. Clear-liquid diets should not be used long-term because they do not provide adequate caloric, mineral, or vitamin requirements. Full-liquid diets can provide all the needed nutrients if given appropriately. Commercial formulas are palatable and may be used either as supplements or to supply all the necessary nutrients. Protein supplements containing modified amino acids are also available and are useful in the setting of hepatic or renal disease. Medium chain triglyceride (MCT) oil is useful in the setting of fat malabsorption and pancreatic insufficiency because it does not require pancreatic enzymes or bile salts for digestion or absorption. The maximally tolerated dose of MCT oil is 3 to 4 tablespoons/day and supplies 400 kcal/day. MCT oil does not provide the essential fatty acid linoleic acid.

Enteral tube feeding is indicated for patients with functioning bowels who are unable to ingest an adequate amount of nutrients to meet their nutritional needs (Fig. 71-1). Tube feeding may also be instituted in settings when patients are expected to become malnourished given their particular disease states (e.g., development of swallowing disorders or enlarging esophageal tumors). Tube feeding may also be used for the goal of small intestinal adaptation after surgical resection of bowel or as part of the management strategy for active inflammatory bowel disease. The only absolute contraindication to tube feeding is mechanical bowel obstruction.

Feeding tubes may be placed nasally or percutaneously. Of the transnasal tubes, the smaller caliber, more pliable tubes, such as the Keofeed or Dobbhoff tubes, should be used over standard nasogastric tubes. Transnasal tubes are usually placed in the stomach, but may be advanced into the duodenum or jejunum endoscopically or with the help of intravenous metoclopramide. The transnasal tubes should be used only for short-term (less than 4 to 6 weeks) supplementation.

Complications of nasally placed feeding tubes include epistaxis, sinusitis, local irritation, gastrointestinal bleeding or perforation, tube obstruction, reflux esophagitis or ulceration, tracheoesophageal fistula, and pulmonary aspiration.

Percutaneous feeding tubes should be considered when a longer period of feeding is necessary. Gastrostomy or jejunostomy tubes may be placed with the assistance of endoscopy or radiologic guidance, or during surgery. Jejunal access is appropriate in patients with a history of recurrent aspiration, reflux esophagitis, or an obstructive lesion involving the duodenum. Ideally, the tube should be placed beyond the third portion of the duodenum or past the ligament of Treitz.

Elemental diets may be used if the patient has limited digestive capability, because these formulas do not require intraluminal digestion. Elemental diets contain little fat and they should be combined with MCT oil. Specialty diets exist, including renal formulations rich in essential amino acids and restricted electrolytes and hepatic formulations that are rich in branched chain amino acids. Pulmonary formulations have a higher fat content and result in a lower ratio of carbon dioxide production to oxygen consumption compared with formulas containing higher carbohydrate contents.

Chronic enteral alimentation can result in a number of complications such as electrolyte abnormalities or vitamin and mineral deficiencies caused by the fixed nutrient content of the formulas. Volume overload may also occur from chronic excess sodium load. Diarrhea may be caused by individual product characteristics (e.g., fiber or lactose content), the rate of delivery, and concomitant medications (e.g., antibiotics). The diarrhea frequently resolves with a change in the strength or rate of infusion or a change in the type of formula. Other complications include tracheobronchial aspiration, which may be decreased by elevating the head of the patient's bed and avoiding large bolus feedings. A surgical jejunostomy or percutaneous endoscopic jejunostomy tube should be considered if aspiration persists. Tube obstruction may be caused by improper care of the tube (such as poor flushing), use of thick formulas, or medications. The obstruction may be relieved with infusion of 30 to 60 ml of diet carbonated soda, full strength cranberry juice, or one teaspoon of papain (Adolph's meat tenderizer) in 30 ml of water. Probing the tube blindly with a stylet in an attempt to open the obstruction should be avoided because it may perforate the tube. High gastric residuals can occur because of gastric outlet obstruction, partial small bowel obstruction, motility disorders, or an ileus. Residuals may be decreased by enhancing gastric emptying, which can be done by decreasing the fat content in the formula (fat slows gastric emptying), avoiding the use of narcotics and anticholinergics, using small caliber intestinal feeding tubes, and adding promotility drugs (e.g., metoclopramide or cisapride). Reflux esophagitis can also occur and may be treated with H_2 blockers (cimetidine or ranitidine), promotility drugs, or proton pump inhibitors (omeprazole). Trace mineral deficiencies may be seen after long-term enteral feeding and are usually caused by selenium and zinc deficiency. A hyperosmolarity syndrome may also occur; it often presents with lethargy, dehydration, obtundation, and fever and can be treated by an increase in free water intake.

Parenteral Nutrition

Parenteral nutrition is indicated when more than 5 to 7 days of bowel rest is anticipated, patients cannot meet nutritional needs enterally, or bowel dysfunction precludes enteral feeding (e.g., bowel obstruction, short gut syndrome, enterocutaneous fistulas, inflammatory bowel disease, radiation or chemotherapy-induced enteritis) (Fig. 71-1). Parenteral nutrition may also be instituted when complications of pancreatitis occur or a patient develops hepatic failure with encephalopathy. Its use should also be considered in the perioperative period and used preoperatively in patients with >15% weight loss or a low albumin state.

Parenteral nutrition should not be utilized when the bowel is functional or if the expected length of usage is less than 7 days. If the patient's prognosis does not warrant aggressive intervention (e.g., advanced malignancies with no available treatment options), parenteral nutrition does not improve prognosis. Parenteral nutrition should also be avoided in patients who do not want aggressive therapy.

Parenteral nutrition may be administered peripherally (peripheral parenteral nutrition [PPN]) or centrally (total parenteral nutrition [TPN]). PPN does not provide adequate nutrition to meet daily nutritional requirements and should only be used for short-term support (no longer than 10 to 14 days) in patients who are expected to resume enteral diets. This form of nutrition relies heavily on lipids as the major calorie source at 1 to 2 kcal/ml and provides only limited nutritional support. PPN should not be used in patients with severe malnutrition, severe metabolic stress, large nutrient needs, or in the setting of fluid restriction. When PPN is used, peripheral catheters must be changed every 72 hours, and the solutions must have an osmolarity less than 900 to 1000 mOsm to avoid phlebitis.

Total peripheral nutrition is provided through a central vein. Energy requirements are provided by carbohydrates in the form of dextrose and fats in lipid emulsions. Proteins are supplied by amino acids. The caloric value and osmolarity of the TPN solutions are adjusted depending on the concentration and amount of each component. Before ordering TPN, the individual patient's fluid, calorie, and protein requirements must be determined.

Standard TPN solutions utilize dextrose (3.4 kcal/g), which provides 40% to 65% of the total calories delivered. Dextrose solutions above 10% must be infused via a central line. Lipid emulsions are derived from soybean or safflower oils and provide the essential fatty acids. Approximately 4% of TPN calories must be in the form of linoleic acid and 0.5% as linolenic acid to avoid essential fatty acid deficiency. A 20% lipid emulsion provides 2 kcal/ml; a 10% solution provides 1.1 kcal/ml. The use of the lipid emulsions is advantageous because they concentrate calories into a smaller volume and decrease carbon dioxide production. Occasionally, patients may have a severe, immediate reaction to the lipids that may include dyspnea, nausea, vomiting, headaches, or flushing. Delayed complications may include hepatomegaly, jaundice, splenomegaly, thrombocytopenia, leukopenia, or elevated liver function tests. Contraindications to the use of lipid emulsions include prior adverse reaction to lipids, egg allergy, or pancreatitis secondary to hypertriglyceridemia. Standard amino acid solutions contain both the essential and nonessential amino acids, and their caloric value is not calculated into the daily energy needs.

TPN solution is usually formulated based on whether a glucose or a glucose-lipid system is to be utilized (both contain the required proteins mixed in the dextrose solution). In a glucose system, dextrose is used as the primary source of calories and only enough lipids are infused separately to prevent essential fatty acid deficiency (in general, 500 ml of 10% lipid emulsion is given 2 to 3 times/week). The glucose-lipid system is better tolerated by patients who are under moderate stress or who are glucose intolerant because 50% of calories are provided by dextrose and 50% by lipids. In this system, the dextrose and amino acids are mixed together and the patient receives a separate, daily lipid infusion. If a patient is lipid intolerant and has elevated serum triglycerides, lipids cannot be used for a daily energy source, and this system must not be used. Under these conditions, only enough lipids should be infused to prevent essential fatty acid deficiency. Alternatively, the TPN solution may be given as a 3-in-1 admixture that combines the carbohydrates, fats, and proteins into one single daily bag.

Electrolytes and micronutrients should be added to the TPN solution, and standard recommendations exist for their addition. In addition, vitamin K (5 to 10 mg) should be given once a week, either subcutaneously or added to the TPN solution, as long as the patient has no history of thrombotic events and is not on anticoagulants such as coumadin or heparin. For patients on long-term TPN, iodine (50 to 75 μg), selenium (40 to 120 μg), molybdenum (20 μg), and iron (1 to 3 mg) should also be added to the solution.

Monitoring of Total Parenteral Nutrition

A baseline chemistry panel, CBC, and lipid profile should be obtained on the first day of parenteral feeding at least weekly thereafter. Glucose levels are checked four times a day to detect hyperglycemia or hypoglycemia. Prothrombin time, albumin levels, and liver function tests should be initially obtained and periodically monitored. Nitrogen balance levels should be obtained weekly. The patient should be weighed daily, and fluid intake and output should be strictly monitored.

Central line placement for TPN can result in mechanical complications such as pneumothorax, injury of the great vessels, brachial plexus injury, thoracic duct injury, or air embolism. Metabolic complications are also possible. Hyperglycemia may occur and be severe enough to cause hyperosmolarity with subsequent coma and death. Hypoglycemia can occur if TPN is abruptly stopped for any reason. Electrolyte abnormalities are common. Essential fatty acid deficiency may occur if fat-free TPN is given for 3 to 4 weeks. Vitamin and mineral deficiencies may also occur. Elevated liver function tests occur in 30% to 60% of patients, with a twofold to threefold elevation in 1 to 2 weeks. Hepatic steatosis is the most common finding; it is usually benign and may be treated with a decrease in the total daily calories and a mixture of fat and dextrose. Gallbladder disease with development of biliary sludge or stones occurs in 30% of cases. Catheter-related sepsis can also occur, and central vein thrombosis occurs in about 5% of cases.

KEY POINTS

1. A relationship exists between nutritional status and disease, indicating the importance of adequate nutrition.
2. Total energy requirements are increased proportionally to the severity of illness.
3. The laboratory assessment of nutritional status includes measurement of serum protein, tests of urinary urea nitrogen, CBC, BUN, creatinine, iron, and β-carotene levels and tests of immune competence.
4. Enteral alimentation is the preferred method of nutritional support whenever possible.
5. Parenteral nutrition is indicated when more than 5 to 7 days of bowel rest is anticipated, patients cannot meet nutritional needs enterally, or bowel dysfunction precludes enteral feeding.

SUGGESTED READINGS

American Gastroenterological Association technical review on tube feeding for enteral nutrition, *Gastroenterology* 108:1282, 1995.

Cerda JJ: Diet and gastrointestinal disease, *Med Clin North Am* 77:881, 1993.

Fleming CR, Jeejeebhoy KN: Advances in clinical nutrition, *Gastroenterology* 106: 1365, 1994.

Sax HC, Souba WW: Enteral and parenteral feedings, *Med Clin North Am* 77:863, 1993.

Smith LC, Mullen JL: Nutritional assessment and indications for nutritional support, *Surg Clin North Am* 71:449, 1991.

Williams SR: *Basic nutrition and diet therapy,* ed 9, St. Louis, 1992, Mosby.

72

Peptic Ulcer Disease

Hooshang Meshkinpour

Peptic ulcer disease is a chronic inflammatory condition that affects as many as 10% of the U. S. population at some point in their lives. It remains one of the most prevalent and costly gastrointestinal diseases. The spectrum of the disease is broad and includes microscopic mucosal injury, erythema, erosion, and ulceration. An erosion is a sloughed patch superficial to the muscularis mucosa, whereas an ulcer extends through the muscularis mucosa. Peptic ulcers usually occur in those regions of the gastrointestinal tract that are exposed to the action of acid and pepsin, including the gastric mucosa, duodenal bulb, distal esophagus, and Meckel's diverticulum (where metaplastic gastric mucosa are often found).

EPIDEMIOLOGY

The annual incidence of peptic ulcer disease in the United States is about 1.8% or 500,000 new cases each year. In addition, there are approximately 4 million ulcer recurrences reported annually. In 1985 about 400,000 patients were hospitalized because of peptic ulcer disease and its complications; 130,000 of them underwent surgical interventions and 9000 of those eventually died. The total direct and indirect cost of peptic ulcer disease was estimated at around $7 billion. Although the number of hospital admissions for uncomplicated duodenal ulcer is declining, admissions for bleeding gastric ulcer are on the rise. This is probably a result of increased use of NSAIDs. The incidence of duodenal ulcer is about three times higher in men than in women. In the past, gastric ulcer affected men and women equally. However, higher NSAID use by women has increased the incidence of gastric ulcer and has changed this ratio during the past two decades.

PATHOPHYSIOLOGY

Peptic ulcer disease is caused when gastroduodenal mucosal integrity is disrupted. Mucosal integrity is maintained because of the existing balance between aggressive or damaging factors and protective or defensive factors. Therefore peptic ulcer disease results from either an increase in damaging factors, a decrease in protective factors, or a combination of both. Acid and pepsin are the most important aggressive factors in the pathogenesis of peptic ulcer disease. *H. pylori* infection and NSAID ingestion are responsible for decreased defense; the proportions of patients with duodenal and gastric ulcers associated with *H. pylori* infection or NSAID use are shown in Table 72-1.

Hydrochloric acid plays a prime role in the pathogenesis of peptic ulcer disease. A pH of between 1 and 2 maximizes the activity of pepsin. Moreover, aspirin, other NSAIDs, and bile, in contrast to alcohol, are more damaging in the presence of acid.

Normally the gastroduodenal mucosa has mechanisms to protect itself against the injurious effects of acid and pepsin. Those mechanisms that are collectively called *cytoprotection* include (1) prostaglandins that stimulate mucous and bicarbonate secretion from surface epithelial cells, (2) cellular tight junction, (3) mucosal blood flow and the alkaline tide that it creates, (4) an unstirred water layer that protects the surface epithelium, and (5) proliferation of new cells and the subsequent migration to replace the old cells.

H. pylori is almost always associated with histologic gastritis. Some patients may even have a normal-appearing mucosa by endoscopy and be

TABLE 72-1
Proportion of Patients Associated with *H. Pylori* Infection and NSAID Use

	H. pylori	NSAIDs	Both	Neither
Duodenal Ulcer	82%	5%	10%	3%
Gastric Ulcer	46%	22%	21%	11%

asymptomatic. The *H. pylori* bacterium is a curved, gram-negative rod that adheres to the gastric mucosa, grows in the mucous layer, and produces a highly active urease. Urease-negative mutants of the bacteria are unable to colonize in the stomach. Its natural habitat outside the human stomach is unclear, but person-to-person transmission is suspected. Patients infected with *H. pylori* usually have a high serum gastrin level. This phenomenon has been attributed to destruction of somatostatin-producing D cells that normally exercise a negative feedback on gastrin-producing G cells. *H. pylori* has been widely accepted as a cause of gastritis, which results in damage to the mucosal defense mechanism and predisposes to ulcer formation.

The prevalence of duodenal and gastric ulcers in arthritic patients on NSAIDs is 10 to 50 times higher, respectively. Further, chronic NSAID users are approximately three times more likely to develop a serious adverse event than nonusers. It has been hypothesized that NSAIDs, through the inhibition of prostaglandins, exert their damaging effect. In support of this, it has been found that misoprostol, a synthetic prostaglandin E_2, is effective in the prevention of gastric ulceration in chronic NSAID users. There is no scientific evidence to suggest that peptic ulcer disease is caused by psychologic stress, ingestion of spicy food, or drinking alcohol.

DIAGNOSIS

Clinical Presentation

Although a distinct minority of patients with peptic ulcer disease are asymptomatic, abdominal pain is the most common symptom. Pain in its typical presentation is located in the epigastrium and usually is relieved by ingestion of a meal (hunger pain) or antacids. It is difficult, if not impossible, to distinguish the pain of duodenal ulcer from that of gastric ulcer. Probably the most characteristic feature of pain in peptic ulcer disease, if present, is its periodic feature. Often, patients with peptic ulcer disease complain of more vague symptoms of dyspepsia, such as ill-defined abdominal distress, nausea, bloating, early satiety, and a sense of fullness. In about 10% of patients, an episode of upper gastrointestinal bleeding may be the first manifestation of the disease. When the ulcer is located in the distal antrum or in the prepyloric region, the patient may present with persistent vomiting and weight loss. The correlation between the severity of symptoms and the presence of an ulcer is poor. Ulcer healing is not synonymous with symptom relief and conversely, relief of symptoms does not necessarily mean that the ulcer has healed. Physical examination in patients with uncomplicated peptic ulcer disease is usually normal. In practice, a significant proportion of patients labeled as having peptic ulcer disease are in actuality suffering from gastroesophageal reflux disorders (GERD).

Diagnostic Studies

Most patients, regardless of whether they present with typical abdominal pain or atypical dyspeptic symptoms, do not require a diagnostic study (Fig. 72-1). An empiric treatment course of 2 to 6 weeks, aimed at the control of acid secretion is all most patients need. Those who do not respond to such treatment may then undergo either an upper gastrointestinal series or endoscopy.

A conventional contrast study detects about 70% of ulcer craters. The yield of this diagnostic method can be further improved when the double-contrast technique is used. This study is most valuable in the differentiation of benign and malignant gastric ulcers. For benign gastric ulcers, the ulcer crater is located beyond the barium-filled gastric lumen in a profile view. A thin, lucent line with parallel, straight margins is seen at the base of the crater. The ulcer crater is found within a radiolucent zone (ulcer collar). Above and below the crater is a smooth, concave impression (ulcer mound). Smooth, slender mucosal folds radiate to the edge of the ulcer crater. The shape, number, and location of the ulcers have little practical value. However, ulcers larger than 2 cm in diameter are more likely to be malignant.

Multiple gastric ulcers and postbulbar duodenal ulcers associated with diarrhea are suggestive of a gastrinoma. Up to 4% of radiologically diagnosed benign gastric ulcers are malignant. The chance of malignancy is even higher when the radiologist is unable to make such a differentiation.

Fiberoptic or video endoscopy detects ulcers with a sensitivity of almost 95%. Endoscopic features of a benign gastric ulcer include a smooth and homogeneous base; sharp, regular margins; and uniform merging of mucosal folds. Six to eight biopsy specimens are taken from the margin, from all quadrants of the ulcer, and any nodularities. Brush cytology is performed at the time of endoscopy. All radiologically defined benign ulcers must be evaluated endoscopically after 4 to 6 weeks of treatment. Larger ulcers may require a longer treatment period for complete healing. Delayed healing is usually seen in smokers, those who use aspirin and NSAIDs, patients with a large ulcer, those with a gastrinoma or malignant ulcer, or when the diagnosis of peptic ulcer disease is incorrect. Coexisting *H. pylori* infection can be established at the time of endoscopy or by other tests that do not require endoscopy. (The currently available tests for detection of *H. pylori* are listed in Table 72-2.)

The hormone gastrin is secreted by the antral G-cells that are normally under the inhibitory feedback of hydrochloric acid. Therefore any condition that suppresses acid secretion can increase the serum gastrin level. An increased fasting serum gastrin level of more than 500 pg/ml is diagnostic of a gastrinoma. In the case of refractory peptic ulcer disease, repeated gastrin determinations are indicated. In addition to gastrinoma, other

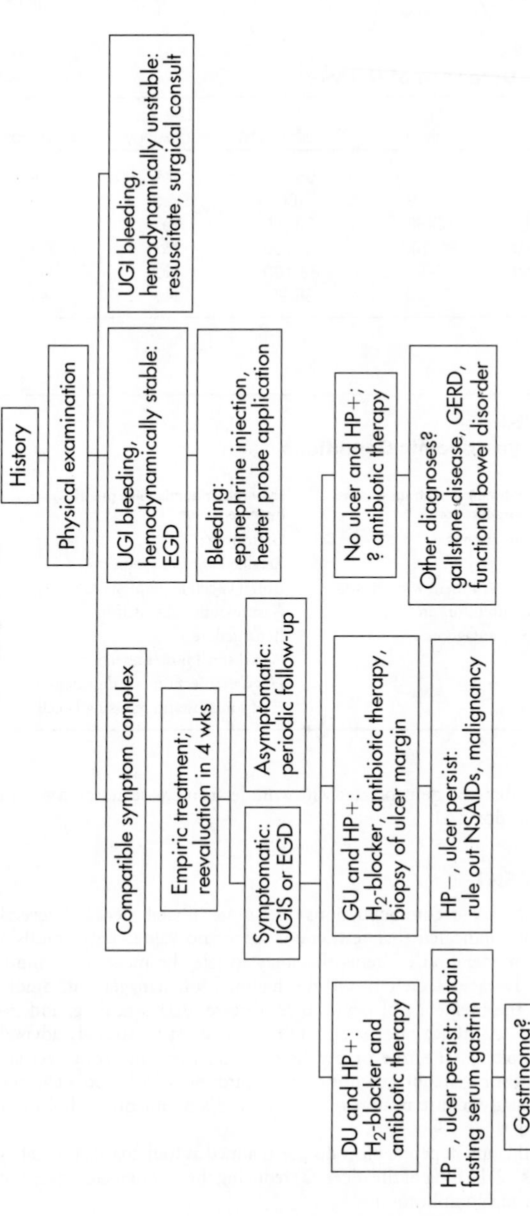

FIG. 72-1 Diagnosis of peptic ulcer disease. *EGD,* esophagogastroduodenoscopy; *UGI,* upper gastrointestinal; *UGIS,* upper gastrointestinal series; *DU,* duodenal ulcer; *HP,* Helicobacter pylori; *GU,* gastric ulcer.

TABLE 72-2
Tests for Detection of *H. Pylori*

Test	Sensitivity (%)	Specificity (%)	Need for encoscopy	Relative cost
Histology	93-99	95-99	Yes	+++
Culture	77-92	100	Yes	+++
Urease test	89-98	93-98	Yes	+
C breath test	90-100	98-100	No	++
C breath test	90-97	89-100	No	++
Serology	88-99	86-95	No	+

BOX 72-1
Hypergastrinemic Conditions

Hypergastrinemia without gastric acid hypersecretion

Pernicious anemia
Gastric atrophy
Prolonged treatment with proton pump inhibitors and H_2-receptor antagnoists

Hypergastrinemia with gastric acid hypersecretion

Gastrinoma
Retained antrum syndrome
Antral G-cell hyperplasia
Gastric outlet obstruction
Renal failure
Partial small bowel resection
H. pylori infection and destruction of somatostatin-releasing D cells

conditions that may be associated with a moderate increase in serum gastrin are listed in Box 72-1.

TREATMENT

Current dietary recommendations are quite liberal because several studies have indicated that restrictions are of no value. Three meals a day, with moderation of items that may irritate the mucosa or stimulate excessive acid secretion, are the hallmark of management. Smoking raises the incidence of peptic ulcer disease, delays healing, and increases the recurrence rate. Therefore patients must be strongly advised against smoking. The role of psychologic stress is quite controversial. Patients must be encouraged not to use aspirin or NSAIDs on a chronic basis. Similarly, consumption of an excessive amount of alcohol must be avoided.

Drug therapy in peptic ulcer disease is aimed at four goals: (1) relief of symptoms, (2) healing of the ulcer, (3) reducing the rate of recurrence, and (4) preventing complications.

TABLE 72-3
Medical Management of Acute Peptic Ulcer Disease

Action	Drug	Dose
Antacids	Maalox or Mylanta	30 ml, 1 and 3 hr after meals and at bedtime
H_2-receptor antagonists	Cimetidine (Tagamet)	300 mg 4 times daily or 400 mg twice daily
	Ranitidine (Zantac)	150 mg twice daily or 300 mg at bedtime
	Famotidine (Pepcid)	400 mg daily
	Nizatidine (Axid)	300 mg daily
Proton pump inhibitor	Omeprazole* (Prilosec)	20 mg daily
Mucosal protective agents	Sucralfate (Carafate)	1 g before meals and at bedtime

*Treatment with omeprazole for a period longer than 3 months is not recommended. This precaution is based on animal studies where carcinoid tumors have been reported after prolonged use of larger doses of this drug.

Antacids, H_2-receptor antagonist, proton pump inhibitor, and sucralfate are the cornerstones of treatment of peptic ulcer disease. These agents relieve symptoms, and numerous studies show they are superior to placebo in promoting the healing process. Table 72-3 lists the acid-reducing agents commonly used in the management of acute peptic ulcer disease.

Maintenance therapy using acid-reducing agents and sucralfate, eradication of *H. pylori* infection, and abstinence from aspirin and other NSAIDs are measures utilized to reduce the rate of ulcer recurrence. In chronic NSAID users, the recurrence of duodenal lesions (but not gastric lesions) can be reduced by low H_2-receptor antagonist maintenance therapy. Misoprostol is effective for the prevention of chronic NSAID-induced gastric ulcers.

Patients with gastric or duodenal ulcers who are infected with *H. pylori* should be treated with antimicrobials regardless of whether they are suffering from the initial presentation of the disease or from a recurrence. The presence of aspirin or NSAIDs as contributing factors should not alter the antimicrobial regimen. In asymptomatic *H. pylori*-infected patients without ulcers, the data is not sufficient to support prophylactic therapy to prevent future ulcer development.

Table 72-4 lists regimens for *H. pylori* infection.

Intractibility is considered when peptic ulcer disease does not yield to usual medical management. With introduction of the modern therapy during the past two decades, the incidence of intractable ulcers has drastically declined. However, in those circumstances, poor patient compliance, smoking, chronic use of aspirin and NSAIDs, untreated *H. pylori* infection, a gastrinoma, and a malignant gastric ulcer must be considered. Finally, a distinct minority of patients exist who require a larger dose of antisecretory agents for a longer period of time.

TABLE 72-4
Treatment Regimens for *H. pylori* Infection

Therapy	Drug 1	Drug 2	Drug 3	Notes*	Success
Triple	Tetracycline 500 mg qid	Metronidazole 250 mg tid	Bismuth subsalicylate† 2 tablets qid	With meals for 14 days plus an antisecretory drug	>90%
Triple	Tetracycline 500 mg qid	Clarithromycin 500 mg tid	Bismuth subsalicylate 2 tablets qid	With meals for 14 days plus an antisecretory drug	>90%
Triple	Amoxicillin 500 mg qid	Clarithromycin 500 mg tid	Bismuth subsalicylate 2 tablets qid	With meals for 14 days plus an antisecretory drug	>90%
Triple	Amoxicillin 500 mg qid	Metronidazole 250 mg tid	Bismuth subsalicylate 2 tablets qid	With meals for 14 days plus an antisecretory drug for 7-14 days	>80%
Double	Clarithromycin 250 mg bid	Metronidazole 500 mg bid	Omeprazole 20 mg bid		>90%
Double	Amoxicillin 750 mg tid	Clarithromycin 500 mg tid		With meals for 14 days plus an antisecretory drug	>90%
Double	Amoxicillin 750 mg tid	Metronidazole 500 mg tid		With meals for 14 days plus an antisecretory drug	>85%
Double	Clarithromycin 500 mg tid	Omeprazole 40 mg every morning		With meals for 14 days	65%-75%
Double	Amoxicillin 750 mg tid	Omeprazole 40 mg tid		With meals for 14 days	>90%
Double	Amoxicillin 1 g tid	Omeprazole 20 mg bid		With meals for 14 days	35%-60%

*Generally, antisecretory drugs should be continued for 6 weeks to ensure ulcer healing.
†Bismuth subsalicylate is the only bismuth compound available in the United States; bismuth subcitrate can be substituted.

DIAGNOSIS AND MANAGEMENT OF COMPLICATED PEPTIC ULCER DISEASE

Peptic ulcer disease is responsible for almost 50% of all gastrointestinal bleeding, which carries an overall mortality rate of 10% to 14%. This rate is higher in patients older than 60 who have concomitant medical problems. Clinically, bleeding presents either as vomiting bright red blood (hematemesis); coffee ground emesis; passing a black, tarry bowel movement (melena); or occult bleeding associated with anemia. Over 80% of episodes of upper gastrointestinal bleeding usually stop on their own.

Clinical Features

The patient who presents with gastrointestinal bleeding is usually managed in an intensive care unit by the primary care physician in consultation with a gastroenterologist and a surgeon. The gastrointestinal bleeding is systematically approached through four stages. First, the patient's age, concomitant medical and surgical problems, and magnitude of blood loss are assessed. In the second stage, efforts are directed toward hemodynamic resuscitation of the patient, utilizing fluid replacement and transfusions of packed RBCs and other blood products. In the third step, empiric treatment is instituted based on the data collected. Finally, in the fourth stage, specific diagnostic and therapeutic approaches are undertaken. The first three stages of this approach can be safely handled by a primary care physician and only the fourth stage requires the help of a specialist. Despite the lack of proof that raising the gastric pH above 3.5 stops bleeding from peptic ulcer disease sooner, most physicians give parenteral H_2-blockers, either in bolus form or by a drip infusion.

Early endoscopy is the procedure of choice for use in diagnosing upper gastrointestinal bleeding and must be considered as soon as the patient is hemodynamically stable. Over 50% of the cases of upper gastrointestinal bleeding are the result of peptic ulcer disease. Endoscopy, in addition to locating the site of bleeding, reveals endoscopic features of the bleeding ulcer that have prognostic significance (Table 72-5).

Oozing is usually indicative of bleeding from granulation tissue at the base of the ulcer. When melena precedes hematemesis or coffee ground emesis, it is more likely that a duodenal ulcer is the source. Injection therapy, utilizing a 1:10,000 epinephrine solution, is inexpensive and

TABLE 72-5
Endoscopic Features of a Bleeding Peptic Ulcer

Endoscopic feature of the ulcer	Relative risk of rebleeding
Clean ulcer base	5%
Flat pigmented spots	10%
Presence of an adherent clot	22%
Visible blood vessel	43%
Active bleeding in the form of oozing or spurting	55%

effective in 76.5% of cases. Bicap and heater probe, treatments that are aimed at cooking the base of the ulcer, are equally effective. Endoscopic homeostasis reduces the need for emergency surgery by two thirds and hospital mortality by one third. The timing for surgical intervention depends on (1) the number of transfusions and the rapidity with which they must be given, (2) rebleeding on the same hospital admission, and (3) bleeding from a visible vessel in patients with evidence of vascular disease.

The incidence of gastric outlet obstruction is about 5% and increases with duration of the peptic ulcer disease. It usually complicates the ulcers that are located in the prepyloric region of the antrum, pyloric channel, or duodenal bulb. Symptoms of obstruction include early satiety, fullness, and epigastric pain that usually does not respond to acid-reducing agents or food but is characteristically relieved by vomiting. The presence of a large amount of fluid and air in the obstructed stomach causes the characteristic splashing sound when the patient's abdomen is shaken. When a gastric outlet obstruction is suspected, nasogastric aspiration through a large bore tube is instituted for 72 hours while the patient receives intravenous fluid replacement and H_2-blockers. At the end of this period, a radiologic contrast study or endoscopy is performed to assess the cause and severity of obstruction. It is at this point that nasogastric aspiration is discontinued and an oral feeding of liquid is allowed. In most cases, where obstruction is caused by edema and inflammation around the ulcer, recovery is complete. However, in patients whose obstruction is caused by scarring, an endoscopic dilation or surgical intervention is indicated.

An ulcer crater may perforate through the wall into the abdominal cavity, penetrate into adjacent solid organs such as the pancreas or liver, or form a fistula with a hollow organ such as the gallbladder or common bile duct. The incidence of perforation, thanks to modern treatment of peptic ulcer disease, is on the decline. Characteristically, ulcer craters located in the anterior wall of the duodenal bulb may perforate, whereas ulcers of the posterior aspect of the bulb and, rarely, the lesser curvature of stomach penetrate. Sudden onset, persistent, severe abdominal pain is the hallmark symptom of perforation. This is usually accompanied by a striking tenderness of the abdomen and the absence of bowel sounds. Loss of fluids into the peritoneal cavity is often associated with a shocklike syndrome. Hemoconcentration, leukocytosis, and a mild hyperamylasemia may be present. Under certain circumstances, such as in the elderly and infants and those who are on steroid therapy, these clinical findings may not be so striking; this condition is known as *"silent perforation."* Diagnosis is usually confirmed on abdominal x-rays by the presence of an air collection in the peritoneal cavity and under the diaphragm when the patient is in an upright position. The absence of free air does not exclude perforation. If a perforated peptic ulcer is suspected, the next step is to perform a radiologic study to delineate the site of perforation, using a water-soluble contrast medium. Diagnosis of a perforation usually prompts surgical intervention. To prepare the patient, intravenous fluid replacement, gastrointestinal decompression, and broad-spectrum antibiotic therapy are instituted. Rarely will a perforation seal spontaneously.

KEY POINTS

1 Peptic ulcer disease is mainly related to *H. pylori* infection or chronic use of aspirin and NSAIDs.

2 Hypergastrinomas are often associated with multiple ulcers that are usually located in odd locations and are frequently intractable to usual medical management.

3 To reduce the recurrence rate of peptic ulcer disease, aspirin and NSAIDs must be discontinued and *H. pylori* infection should be vigorously treated; in the absence of these two factors, a low-dose maintenance therapy should be instituted.

4 Peptic ulcer disease is the single most common cause of upper gastrointestinal bleeding, with an overall mortality rate of about 10%.

SUGGESTED READINGS

Brown KE, Peura DA: Diagnosis of *Helicobacter pylori* infection, *Gastroenterol Clin North Am* 22:105-115, 1993.

Collins PW: Misoprostol: discovery, development, and clinical applications, *Med Res Rev* 10(2):149-172, 1990.

Gabriel SE, Jaakkimaineu L, Bombardier C: Risk for serious gastrointestinal complications related to use of nonsteroidal anti-inflammatory drugs: a meta-analysis, *Ann Intern Med* 115:787-796, 1991.

Graham DY: Treatment of peptic ulcers caused by *Helicobacter pylori, N Engl J Med* 328:349-350, 1993.

Lane L, Peterson WL: Bleeding peptic ulcer, *N Engl J Med* 331:717-727, 1994.

Peterson WL: *Helicobacter pylori and* peptic ulcer disease, *N Engl J Med* 324:1043-1048, 1991.

73

Pneumonia: Viral and Bacterial

THOMAS C. CESARIO AND DOUGLAS A. CESARIO

Pneumonia is one of the most common serious infections encountered in the treatment of infectious diseases. It has been estimated that 2 to 4 million cases of community-acquired pneumonia occur each year in the United States. The overall attack rate is 10 to 12 cases/1000 individuals/year but increases in the incidence occur at the extremes of age, with young children and the elderly being 5 to 25 times more prone to this disease.

Pneumonia is the sixth leading cause of death in the United States and the leading cause of death caused by infectious diseases.

PATHOPHYSIOLOGY

Community-acquired pneumonia is differentiated from nosocomial pneumonia because the etiologies and approach to therapy are considerably different. Thus in hospitalized patients who acquire the infection during their period of confinement, the nature of the causative organisms is such that they are considerably more resistant to antibiotics. In the hospital setting, gram-negative organisms predominate, whereas in the community setting these organisms are far less prevalent. In fact, even in those cases of community-acquired pneumonia where gram-negative organisms are present, the nature of the organism may differ depending on the population under discussion. Thus patients coming from skilled nursing facilities or debilitated patients with serious underlying diseases may acquire pneumonia with organisms more closely resembling those acquired in the hospital setting. Patients with AIDS are also prone to distinct types of pneumonia that are not often seen in less compromised individuals. Thus in predicting the nature of the infecting organism it becomes important to understand the underlying nature of the patients themselves.

Streptococcus pneumoniae accounts for 5% to 18% of community-acquired pneumonia. *H. influenzae* accounts for about 10% of the cases, and *S. aureus* and enteric gram-negative rods account for 3% to 10% of the cases. *Legionella* appears to be responsible for 1% to 15% of cases of community-acquired pneumonia. Other less common organisms to consider include *Moraxella, Streptococcus pyogenes,* and anaerobic bacteria. The role of the latter has never been clearly defined in patients not known to aspirate.

Among the nonbacterial agents known to cause community-acquired pneumonia are *Mycoplasma pneumoniae* and *Chlamydia pneumoniae.* These two agents account for 10% to 20% of the pneumonias occurring in this setting. Finally, the true viruses such as influenza and adenovirus appear to be responsible for about 5% to 15% of the known cases. *Mycobacterium tuberculosis* and fungal agents such as *Coccidioides immitis* and *Histoplasma capsulatum* also likely account for a small number of cases. The fungi, of course, will vary in the frequency with which they cause disease, depending on the geographic area under consideration. Of further importance is the fact that agents such as *Haemophilus* and *Legionella* usually prey on individuals with some underlying predisposition such as chronic lung disease, hypogammaglobulinemia, or alcoholism. Up to 50% of the cases of community-acquired pneumonia never have their specific etiologies determined.

DIAGNOSIS

Chest x-ray examination should be done in patients who appear ill and have respiratory symptoms, in patients with moderately severe respiratory symptoms and underlying problems, and in patients with physical findings suggestive of pulmonary infection and systemic signs pointing to an infectious problem (Fig. 73-1). Of major importance is establishing an etiologic diagnosis with as much confidence as possible. Recovery of a microbiologic agent from an uncontaminated specimen obtained from blood or pleural fluid is extremely valuable, and care should be taken to collect such specimens if possible. Isolation of an organism from a transthoracic lung aspiration or protected bronchoscopic brushing is also very valuable.

Sputum collection with appropriate gram stain and culture may be useful. One of the most important aspects of sputum collection is the care taken to obtain a specimen from the lung itself and not merely from oral secretions. Furthermore, direct observation and assessment of the quality of the sample by review of its color, character, and microscopic appearance contribute to determining the value of the specimen. Cultures can only be of assistance when it is clear the specimen reflects the flora of the infected area. Gram stain may not be diagnostic in half or more of the cases, especially with those individuals who cannot produce a quality specimen. In addition to culture, serologies may be of value in pneumonias caused by

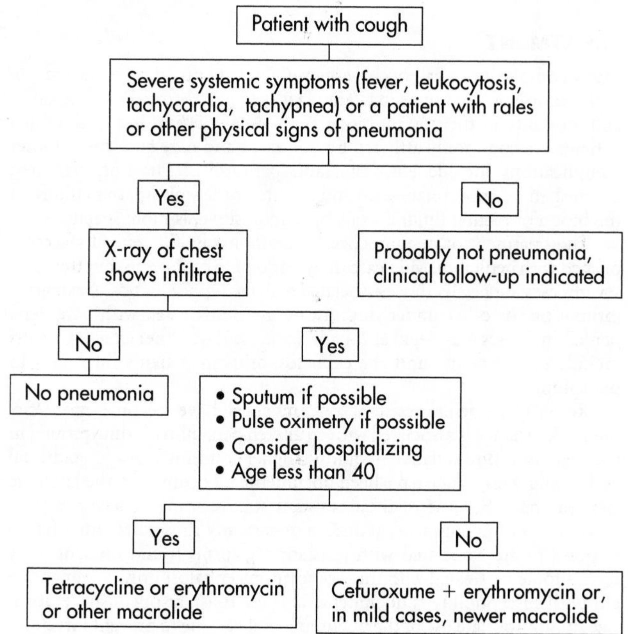

FIG. 73-1 Management of pneumonia.

agents such as mycoplasma, chlamydia, the true viruses, *Legionella pneumophila,* Coxiella, or the fungi. Urinary antigen detection is of value with Legionella.

At least 84 different capsular types of *Streptococcus pneumoniae* can cause pneumonia, although certain types are more frequently responsible for severe lower respiratory tract infection. The organism is a frequent inhabitant of the upper respiratory tract but has the ability to multiply rapidly in the lower tract. Most cases (75%) of pneumococcal pneumonia are preceded by coryza. The onset of the pneumonia itself is usually abrupt and associated with a shaking chill. This is followed by fever and a cough that produces blood-tinged sputum (rusty sputum). Pleuritic chest pain is very common, and malaise and general prostration are frequent. The physical findings typically include tachycardia, tachypnea, and the signs of either bronchopneumonia or frank pulmonary consolidation. Abdominal findings such as distension may be present.

Leukocytosis is most typical, but leukopenia may occur often in overwhelming cases. Radiographically, bronchopneumonia is more common in children and lobar pneumonia is more common in adults. The extent of the pneumonia will depend on any delay on the part of the patient in seeking medical attention.

TREATMENT

Many complications can occur, especially in patients who are treated late in the course of the disease. Bacteremia is seen in 25% to 30% of the cases, and mortality in the postantibiotic era is usually 5% or less. Debilitated patients are commonly afflicted by this agent and may fare worse. Other complications include empyema and pericarditis. Diagnosis is often established by appropriate stain and culture of the sputum, but culture of the blood or pleural fluid, if available and positive, is more specific.

The treatment of pneumococcal pneumonia is still generally accomplished with penicillin. Mild cases may respond to oral agents, but the more severe cases, especially those associated with tachypnea, hypoxia, extensive infiltration, or other underlying disease are best treated with parenteral penicillin. Doses may begin at 2.4 million units/day. Other effective agents include erythromycin and the cephalosporins in patients intolerant to penicillin.

Recently penicillin-resistant pneumococci have become more frequent. Resistance is associated with an altered penicillin binding protein in the organism. Both relative (requiring higher concentrations to eradicate) and absolute resistance have been documented. Fortunately, the latter are less common. Because of these resistant strains, some believe the most severe cases of pneumococcal disease or certainly those that either fail to respond or are associated with resistant organisms found on sensitivity tests, should be treated with third generation cephalosporins or vancomycin until susceptibility is documented. These resistant organisms emphasize the appropriate use of the pneumococcal vaccine to prevent infection.

Haemophilus influenzae is another important bacterial cause of pneumonia. The organism is another frequent inhabitant of the upper airways. In the past, capsular type B was believed to be the most likely type to cause pneumonia, but recently even unencapsulated types have been reported to cause lower respiratory infections. The organism itself will most commonly cause infection in the very young or the elderly. It will also prey on the compromised, especially those with chronic lung disease or agammoglobulinemia. The clinical picture resembles that of pneumonia associated with *S. pneumoniae,* although some believe there is a greater frequency of associated infection outside the lung, such as epiglotittis, otitis, or meningitis. This is more likely true in children. Diagnosis is again established from sputum, blood, or pleural fluid cultures.

Because almost half of the strains now produce beta lactamase, currently recommended antibiotics include second generation cephalosporins such as cefuroxime, ampicillin, or amoxicillin in combination with an inhibitor of beta lactamase such as sulbactam or quinolones. More recently newer macrolides such as clarithromycin or azithromycin have been found to be effective, especially for milder cases. The case fatality rate for pneumonia associated with *H. influenzae* is believed to be higher than that associated with *S. pneumoniae,* perhaps because of comorbidity caused by other disease processes.

In recent years other bacterial agents have also been found to be occasional causes of pneumonia. These include *Moraxella catarrhalis,* which produces disease under the circumstances likely associated with conditions such as chronic pulmonary disease. It responds to the same type of antibiotics used to treat *H. influenzae.*

The other common type of pneumonia associated with a bacterial agent is that attributed to *Legionella pneumophila.* This organism appears to have an affinity for water, particularly areas in air conditioning systems where water can accumulate and allow the organism to grow and disseminate. Legionella can become sporadic or epidemic in certain nosocomial situations. Typically patients with pneumonia caused by Legionella are predisposed by cigarette smoking, chronic lung disease, advanced age, immunosuppression, and possibly excessive alcohol intake. The organism exists intracellularly, and in contrast to the other forms of pneumonia discussed up to this point, cell-mediated immunity may be the body's most important defense against Legionella.

Clinically, Legionella infection may exist as a brief febrile illness called *Pontiac fever* or as the more typical pneumonia called *legionnaires' disease.* After a brief incubation period (2 to 10 days), the patient experiences the onset of cough and chest pain. Extrapulmonary manifestations are common, as they may be in any severe pneumonic process, and include diarrhea, nausea, vomiting, abdominal pain, headache, and encephalopathy.

Physical findings progress from a few rales to typical signs of consolidation. Laboratory confirmation can be made by culture of the sputum on charcoal yeast extract agar by direct fluorescent antibody stain of sputum smears although the method is not especially sensitive. The diagnosis can also be made by measurement of serum antibody levels or detection of Legionella-specific antigen in urine or by use of a DNA probe.

Treatment is best accomplished with erythromycin 2 to 4 gs/day for at least 14 days. Rifampin has some activity against the agent, as do the quinolones. Overall, the mortality from appropriately treated legionnaires' disease is under 10%.

In addition to the bacterial agents, other types of organisms may produce community-acquired pneumonia. Among these is *Mycoplasma pneumoniae.* The organism is resistant to antibiotics active on the cell wall. The organism requires yeast extract and supplementary serum for growth, but can be grown on artificial media. *M. pneumoniae* can be endemic, but distinct epidemic periods may be recognized and distinct outbreaks have been reported. Infection rates have been highest in school-age children and young adults, and mycoplasma are known to spread extensively within the family unit. Although lesser forms of respiratory illness can be seen with mycoplasma, 5% to 10% of the infections appear to result in pneumonia. Most important to the spread of the agent is the fact it may be detectable in respiratory secretions for many weeks. Although immunity to the organism exists, recurrent mycoplasma infections can occur.

The incubation period for *M. pneumoniae* infections is 15 to 25 days. The disease begins with the gradual onset of constitutional symptoms, fever, and headache. Only about 10% of *M. pneumoniae* infections actually result in pneumonia. The rest are either asymptomatic or present as pharyngitis or tracheobronchitis. The pneumonia itself is usually mild. After the period of constitutional symptoms, cough occurs and initially it is dry. Coryza, sore throat, hoarseness, and substernal pain may occur. Auscultatory findings are usually mild but include wheezes, rhonchi, and rales. Arthralgias and rash occur.

Roentgenographic findings include a subsegmental bronchopneumonia. The peripheral WBC count is usually normal. Gram stain should reveal polymorphonuclear cells and mononuclear cells with no bacteria or only bacteria from contamination. The best known antibody used to diagnose mycoplasma infections is the cold agglutinin. This IgM antibody to the I antigen of red blood cells usually becomes evident at the end of the first week of illness. It is seen in about half the cases, although the sicker the patient, the more likely the antibody is to be detected. Specific mycoplasma antibody may be detected by ELISA, and it is possible to culture the organism. The clinical course of the pneumonia generally is completed in 1 to 2 weeks, although 6 weeks may be required to resolve the roentgenographic findings.

Complications of *M. pneumoniae* include erythema multiforme, erythema nodosum, sinusitis, bullous myringitis, intravascular hemolysis, meningoencephalitis, and both myocarditis and pericarditis. The treatment of *M. pneumoniae* is best undertaken with tetracyclines, erythromycin, and newer macrolides. It is likely that quinolones will be effective as well. Therapy should be given for 1 week and shortens the clinical course. No vaccine is currently available.

Another recently identified cause of nonbacterial pneumonia likely seen in the community is that caused by *Chlamydia pneumoniae* (also known as *chlamydia TWAR*). This organism does not appear to have a bird or animal reservoir as does, for example, *Chlamydia psittaci.* In adults, approximately 25% to 50% of individuals have antibodies to this organism.

Its pathogenesis has not been well defined, but it is known that it can cause a variety of mild respiratory infections.

Pneumonia is perhaps the best described of the clinical illnesses associated with *C. pneumoniae.* This agent is known to cause 6% of pneumonias in one study of community-acquired pneumonias. A higher proportion has been noted in college students. The illness has many similarities to mycoplasma, except the cold agglutinin test can be expected to be negative. Fever, cough, and sore throat are all common features of pneumonic infections associated with *C. pneumoniae.* Infiltrates are typically modest, and rales are typically present. The best treatment for *C. pneumoniae* is considered to be tetracycline for 10 to 14 days.

A number of true viruses are also associated with pneumonia. In children under the age of 1, respiratory syncytial virus (RSV) is probably the most common cause of pneumonia. Parainfluenza virus is also common as a cause of pneumonia in children. In older children and young adults, adenoviruses are an occasional cause of pneumonic infection. Typically these resemble illnesses caused by mycoplasma, with the exception that the cold agglutinin test is typically negative and the course of disease is mild. No treatment or prophylaxis is generally available.

During the influenza season and during epidemic periods, the influenza virus may produce pneumonia. This is usually severe and is best known to occur in patients with mitral stenosis, although pregnancy is a reported risk factor. This is commonly a progressive illness, with bilateral infiltrates and severe hypoxia. Death is common, and no proved effective therapy is known, although amantadine and rimantadine are worthy of trial.

Finally, many milder cases of pneumonia in otherwise healthy individuals can be treated at home. Indications for hospitalization include serious underlying disease, hypoxia or tachypnea (respiratory rate >25 in adults), hypotension, systemic toxicity, patient's social circumstances do not allow careful follow-up, and extensive pulmonary infiltration.

KEY POINTS

1 Pneumonia is one of the most common serious infections encountered in the treatment of infectious diseases.

2 Among the nonbacterial agents known to cause community-acquired pneumonia are *Mycoplasma pneumoniae* and *Chlamydia pneumoniae* (TWAR).

3 At least 84 different capsular types of *Streptococcus pneumoniae* can cause pneumonia.

4 Penicillin-resistant pneumococci have become more frequent.

74

Thyroid Disorders

Jorge H. Mestman*

Hyperthyroidism

Hyperthyroidism is one of the most common endocrinologic problems encountered in women. In the majority of cases, the etiology is Graves' disease, with a predominance in women of 8:1 as compared with men. In many cases, women may present with mild or nonspecific complaints (i.e., shortness of breath, proximal muscle weakness, abnormal menses). With the advent of more sensitive and simple tests of thyroid function (sensitive TSH), diagnosis is now made earlier in the course of the disease.

Hyperthyroidism or thyrotoxicosis is defined as the constellation of symptoms and physical and biochemical findings as a consequence of chronic tissue exposure to excessive amounts of thyroid hormones.

PATHOPHYSIOLOGY

Common causes of hyperthyroidism are Graves' disease (the etiology in over 90% of women), toxic adenoma, multinodular goiter (occurring mostly in older individuals), and iatrogenic hyperthyroidism. Less common causes are subacute painful thyroiditis, subacute painless thyroiditis, and iodine-induced thyroiditis. Rare causes include TSH-producing pituitary tumor, struma ovari, and choriocarcinoma. In addition, molar pregnancy, transient hyperthyroidism of hyperemesis gravidarum, and postpartum hyperthyroidism consisting of recurrent Graves' disease or, transient postpartum thyroiditis are pregnancy-related causes.

CLINICAL PRESENTATION

A complete history, physical examination, and proper use and interpretation of thyroid tests will allow the physician to confirm the diagnosis of thyrotoxicosis and establish the etiology in the majority of cases. A family history of thyroid disease is not uncommon. The classic symptoms may be interpreted by the patient in different ways, emphasizing the importance of a careful medical history (Box 74-1). The patient's inability

*The author gratefully acknowledges the expert secretarial assistance of Elsa C. Ahumada.

BOX 74-1
Common Symptoms of Hyperthyroidism

Nervousness, irritability, tremor
Increased perspiration
Emotional instability
Hypersensitivity to heat
Hyperactivity
Sleep disturbances
Palpitations
Fatigue, decreased exercise tolerance
Exertional dyspnea
Weight loss
Proximal muscle weakness
Hyperdefecation
Eye complaints
- Photophobia
- Eye irritation
- Diplopia
- Change in visual acuity

Menstrual dysfunction
- Oligohypomenorrhea
- Anovulation
- Amenorrhea

to perform routine exercises because of excessive fatigue or palpitations along with shortness of breath may be perceived by the patient to be a heart problem.

A history of radiologic procedures using iodine contrast materials performed in the few weeks before the onset of symptoms may be a clue to the etiology of hyperthyroidism (iodine-induced hyperthyroidism). In patients on thyroid therapy, the type of preparation and its daily dose should be carefully checked to allow better interpretation of thyroid function tests (iatrogenic thyrotoxicosis). The development of hyperthyroidism within 1 year after pregnancy or miscarriage (postpartum thyroid dysfunction), a painful neck with low-grade fever and malaise (subacute painful thyroiditis), and mild hyperthyroid symptoms in the absence of goiter (painless thyroiditis) are other causes that should be considered.

The presence of eye signs and a diffusely enlarged thyroid gland are typical findings in Graves' disease. However, classic eye signs (stare, eyelid retraction, and exophthalmus) are only present in 50% of women with Graves' disease. In about 3% of patients and in up to 20% of older women, the thyroid gland is not enlarged. In the majority of women with Graves' disease, the size of the goiter is two to three times normal, nontender to palpation, and consistency varies from soft to firm. A bruit is frequently heard over the gland. A very tender thyroid gland on palpation usually rules out painful subacute thyroiditis. A goiter with several nodules favors a diagnosis of toxic multinodular goiter because the presence of a single nodule favors toxic nodular goiter (Plummer's disease). Other common signs of hyperthyroidism are tachycardia; warm, moist, smooth skin; tremor; proximal muscle weakness; hyperreflexia; and systolic murmur.

After the initial clinical evaluation, the physician will be able to select the proper thyroid tests. The common practice of ordering a battery of routine tests for all clinical situations should be discouraged.

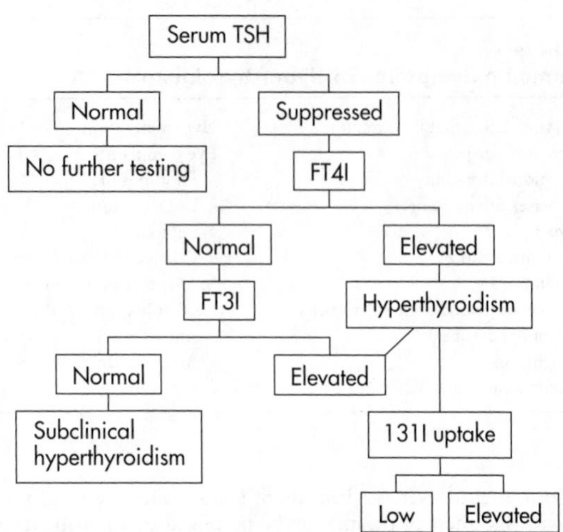

FIG. 74-1 Diagnosis of hyperthyroidism. *FT4I,* Free thyroxine index or its equivalent free thyroxine; *FT3I,* free triiodothyronine index or its equivalent free triiodothyronine.

DIAGNOSIS

Regardless of the etiology of hyperthyroidism, serum TSH is suppressed in almost every patient (the exception is the rare case of pituitary hyperthyroidism) (Fig. 74-1). Indeed, serum TSH (sensitive assay or second or third generation test) is the most useful test for screening thyroid disease in the outpatient setting; it discriminates euthyroid from hyperthyroid individuals. A determination of serum free thyroxine (FT4) or its estimate, free thyroxine index (FT4I) is included at the time of the initial evaluation. If the serum TSH is suppressed and the FT4 or FT4I is elevated, the diagnosis of hyperthyroidism is confirmed.

If Graves' disease is suspected by the presence of a diffuse goiter and ophthalmologic signs and confirmed by an elevation in FT4 or FT4I and suppressed serum TSH, no other tests are required, and the different therapeutic modalities should be discussed with the patient.

Further tests are indicated when mild symptoms of thyrotoxicosis and small or no palpable thyroid gland are present. In this situation, a 6- or 24-hour radioactive iodine uptake test (RAIU) is very useful. A suppressed test is consistent with subacute painless or painful thyroiditis, iatrogenic hyperthyroidism, or iodine-induced thyrotoxicosis (Box 74-2). An elevated RAIU is consistent with Graves' disease. Further tests also are needed with nodular goiter (multinodular or single adenoma). A radioactive scan, iodine-123 (123I) or 99mTc pertechnetate (99mTc), will localize the

BOX 74-2
Radioactive Iodine Thyroid Uptake in Hyperthyroidism by Etiology

Elevated	Low
Graves' disease	Subacute painful thyroiditis
Toxic nodule	Subacute painless thyroiditis
Multinodular goiter	Iatrogenic hyperthyroidism*
Postpartum Graves' disease	Postpartum thyroiditis
Choriocarcinoma	Iodine-induced hyperthyroidism
TSH dependent	Struma ovarii

*Caused by excessive thyroid administration.

presence of an autonomous (hot) nodule. In the presence of a suppressed serum TSH and normal FT4 or FT4I, a determination of serum free triiodothyronine (FT3) or the equivalent calculated free triiodothyronine index (FT3I) is indicated; an elevated FT3 or FT3I confirms the diagnosis of hyperthyroidism, the so called *T3-toxicosis.*

Consultation with an endocrinologist is needed in the following situations:

1. Hyperthyroid symptoms in the presence of elevated situations: FT4 and/or FT3 and normal TSH values
2. Hyperthyroidism caused by Graves' disease and the presence of a single nodule in a diffuse goiter
3. Normal serum TSH and elevated FT4 in a euthyroid patient
4. Suppressed serum TSH and normal FT4 and FT3 (subclinical hyperthyroidism)
5. Abnormal thyroid tests in critically ill or psychiatric patients (euthyroid sick syndrome)

TREATMENT

The management of hyperthyroidism depends on the patient's age, etiology of the disease, severity of symptoms, and physician preference and experience in a given treatment. It is essential for the physician to discuss with the patient the different therapeutic alternatives, potential side effects, and the need in many cases for long-term thyroid replacement therapy after ablation. Women of childbearing age are anxious to learn about the potential complications of the disease and/or treatment in future pregnancies.

A short course of beta-adrenergic blocker agents is effective in controlling the symptoms of hyperthyroidism; propranolol 20 to 40 mg every 6 hours is recommended.

Three treatments are acceptable for patients with hyperthyroidism caused by Graves' disease. Ablation with radioactive iodine is the treatment of choice for most patients. Well tolerated, it is an outpatient procedure. The main side effect is permanent hypothyroidism in the majority of patients. Contraindicated in pregnancy and breastfeeding women, its use is controversial in patients younger than 20. It is mandatory to perform a pregnancy test in women of childbearing age before treatment is administered. Second, antithyroid drug therapy entails treatment with methimazole or propylthiouracil (PTU) for 12 to 24 months and may result in remission of hyperthyroidism in 20% to 40% of patients. Patients with short duration of symptoms, small goiters, and minimum exophthalmopathy are most likely to go into remission on completion of treatment. Methimazole 10 to 40 mg or PTU 100 to 400 mg/day in divided doses are the usual starting doses. Thereafter patients should be monitored regularly and the dose adjusted according to patient's symptoms and results of laboratory tests. Patients should be instructed about potential side effects (skin rash, pruritus, arthralgia) that affect about 5% of patients. The most serious complication is agranulocytosis (presenting with sore throat, fever, oral mucosa ulcerations), which occurs in less than 0.2% of patients treated and requires prompt recognition and treatment. Finally, surgery is rarely recommended, but it is indicated for patients with very large goiters, patients younger than 20, patients with Graves' disease and a coincidental thyroid nodule, for those refusing ablation with radioiodine, and in selective cases in the second trimester of pregnancy. It should be performed by surgeons experienced in neck surgery and after proper medical preparation.

Hyperthyroidism caused by nodular goiter is treated by surgery or radioactive iodine. Symptoms of thyrotoxicosis respond well to beta-adrenergic blocker agents; antithyroid drugs are ineffective. In the painful form of thyroiditis, aspirin or acetaminophen given every 4 to 6 hours may be effective in some patients; in others, prednisone 40 to 60 mg/day may be required.

Most patients receiving ablation therapy (surgery or radioactive iodine) will become hypothyroid and in need of long-term thyroid replacement therapy. The goal of replacement therapy is to keep the serum TSH and the FT4 or FT4I within normal limits; patients should be followed at regular intervals (yearly in most cases). Hyperthyroidism may recur in some patients, even many years after the original treatment.

KEY POINTS

1. The most common etiology of hyperthyroidism in women is Graves' disease; not all patients present with the classic symptoms.
2. Laboratory tests confirm the diagnosis of hyperthyroidism.
3. A radioactive iodine thyroid uptake test is indicated when etiology is in doubt.
4. Treatment does not begin until the diagnosis is confirmed. Beta-adrenergic drugs may be used to control symptoms.

SUGGESTED READINGS

Franklyn JA: The management of hyperthyroidism, *N Engl J Med* 330:1731-1738, 1994.

Franklyn JA et al: Comparison of second and third generation methods for measurements of serum thyrotropin in patients with overt hyperthyroidism, patients recovering from thyroxine therapy, and those with nonthyroidal illness, *J Clin Endocrinol Metab* 78:1368-1371, 1994.

Goodwin TM, Montoro M, Mestman JH: Transient hyperthyroidism and hyperemesis gravidarum: clinical aspects, *Am J Obstet Gynecol* 167:648-652, 1992.

Loughney MH, Burman KD: Unusual forms of thyrotoxicosis, *Adv Endocrinol Metab* 5:349, 1994.

Klein I, Becker DV, Levey GS: Treatment of hyperthyroid disease, *Ann Intern Med* 121:281-288, 1994.

Mestman JH, Goodwin TM, Montoro M: Thyroid disorders of pregnancy, *Endocrinol Metab Clin North Am* 24:41-71, 1995.

Ross DS: Subclinical thyrotoxicosis, *Adv Endocrinol Metab* 2:89-105, 1991.

Singer PA et al: Treatment guidelines for patients with hyperthyroidism and hypothyroidism, *JAMA* 273:808-812, 1995.

Smith SA: Concise review for primary-care physicians: commonly asked questions about thyroid function, *Mayo Clin Proc* 70:573-577, 1995.

Hypothyroidism

Hypothyroidism is common in adults, affecting women five to eight times more than men. The incidence increases with age, particularly over the age of 50. The onset is insidious in the majority of cases, and the symptoms may be nonspecific, requiring a high level of suspicion on the nonspecific part of the physician.

A constellation of symptoms and signs is seen in hypothyroidism as a result of decreased action of thyroid hormones at the peripheral tissues. The term *myxedema* is used in cases of advanced disease in the presence of nonpitting edema, the result of accumulation of a mucopolysaccharide substance in subcutaneous tissues.

CLASSIFICATION OF HYPOTHYROIDISM

Over 95% of hypothyroid patients suffer from primary hypothyroidism resulting from a failure of the thyroid gland to secrete the normal amount of thyroid hormones; the most common causes are chronic thyroiditis, with or without the presence of a goiter, and surgical ablation for the treatment of hyperthyroidism or thyroid cancer. Other causes include ^{131}I therapy for hyperthyroidism, congenital origin, external x-ray treatment to the neck, drugs such as lithium carbonate and amidiorone, and infiltrative disease such as amyloidosis. Congenital hypothyroidism is diagnosed in 1 in 4000 births in countries where screening programs are routinely performed.

Secondary hypothyroidism is caused by failure of the pituitary gland to secrete TSH or failure of the secretion of TSH releasing hormone (TSHRH) by the hypothalamus. Other causes include neoplasms, pituitary surgery or radiation, Sheehan's syndrome, and idiopathic hypopituitarism. Hypothalamic causes also include therapeutic irradiation and infiltrative disease (sarcoidosis). Peripheral resistance to the action of thyroid hormones is a rare but intriguing cause of hypothyroidism.

The prevalence of primary hypothyroidism increases with age, and is estimated to be 10% at age 50 and almost 15% by age 60 if subclinical hypothyroidism is included. Therefore it has been suggested that women over age 50 should have serum TSH levels checked.

CLINICAL PRESENTATION

In the vast majority of women, hypothyroidism develops over many months or years. With the most liberal use of routine thyroid tests, the diagnosis is made before myxedema is manifested. Early in the course of the disease, symptoms are nonspecific and it may be difficult to recognize the disease.

Menstrual abnormalities are not uncommon, particularly menometrorrhagia. Hypothyroidism may present with amenorrhea and galactorrhea; because the serum prolactin may be elevated in primary hypothyroidism, serum TSH tests should be ordered for every woman with the galactorrhea-amenorrhea syndrome. (The most classic symptoms of hypothyroidism are shown in Box 74-3.)

The physical findings of bradycardia; dry, cold, and sallow skin; periorbital edema; delayed relaxation of the deep tendon reflexes; and brittle, thin hair are not always evident. Goiter may be absent in 40% of women with chronic thyroiditis.

SUBCLINICAL HYPOTHYROIDISM

Subclinical hypothyroidism is characterized by an asymptomatic state associated with an increase in serum TSH in the presence of normal or low normal FT4 or FT4I. Although most patients are asymptomatic, subtle abnormalities may be detected, such as an increase in serum cholesterol or impaired cardiovascular performance. The etiology is the same as primary

BOX 74-3
Most Common Symptoms of Hypothyroidism

Weakness, fatigue
Tiredness
Muscle cramps
Cold intolerance
Deepness of the voice
Dry, coarse skin
Modest weight gain
Periorbital edema
Menorrhagia
Amenorrhea with galactorrhea
Constipation
Decreased memory
Stiffness of the hands on awakening

hypothyroidism. A great proportion of patients eventually will develop overt hypothyroidism. Goiter is present in 30% to 60% of women with subclinical hypothyroidism. It is prudent to treat patients with subclinical hypothyroidism with thyroid therapy, particularly those women with positive thyroid antibodies because they will progress into frank hypothyroidism.

For screening purposes, serum TSH is the best test. In those women in whom the physician is entertaining the diagnosis of hypothyroidism, a serum TSH with the determination of FT4 or FT4I are the tests of choice. Antimicrosomal thyroid antibody (anti-TPO antibodies) are markers for autoimmune disease, and are helpful in establishing the etiology of hypothyroidism (Figs. 74-2 and 74-3).

In the presence of low FT4 or FT4I, a serum TSH test must be performed before thyroid therapy is started. In the case of normal serum TSH and low FT4 or FT4I, the diagnosis of secondary hypothyroidism is very likely, and further tests should be carried out to assess for other pituitary hormonal deficiencies. Isolated TSH deficiency as a cause of hypothyroidism is extremely rare and should be confirmed by additional endocrine tests.

Other laboratory abnormalities are not uncommon in hypothyroid patients and may include elevated levels of serum cholesterol and triglycerides, creatine phosphokinase (CPK), and transaminases.

When the laboratory tests are confusing or not diagnostic, consultation with an endocrinologist is indicated. Examples of such situations include the following:

1. Normal serum TSH in the presence of low FT4I
2. Abnormal thyroid tests in patients taking nonthyroid medications

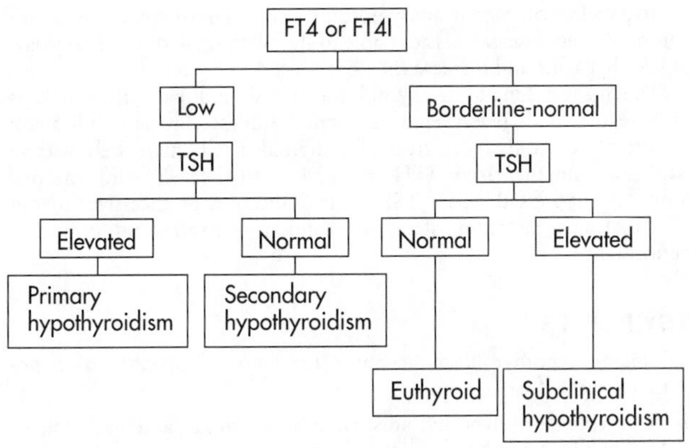

FIG. 74-2 Interpretation of thryoid tests.

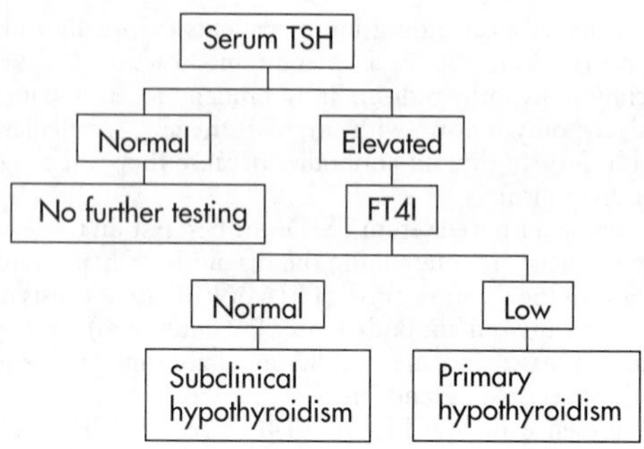

FIG. 74-3 Diagnosis of hypothyroidism.

3. Hospitalized patients with low serum FT4 or FT4I values
4. Elevated serum TSH levels in patients taking adequate doses of thyroid hormones

TREATMENT

The drug of choice in the treatment of hypothryoidism is levothyroxine. Most patient will require between 75 and 125 μg/day (1.7 μg/g body weight/day). In older individuals the total replacement dose is somewhat lower. It is advisable to start with 75 μg daily and repeat the thyroid tests in 6 to 8 weeks. Once serum TSH levels are normalized, tests are performed every 6 to 12 months.

In patients with significant symptoms, or in older patients or those with coronary artery disease, it is advisable to start with small doses, 25 μg/day, of levothyroxine and increase the dose every 4 to 8 weeks.

Patients on long-term thyroid therapy should have thyroid tests on a regular basis (every 6 to 12 months, unless clinically indicated); with few exceptions (postsurgery for thyroid carcinoma), the objective is to maintain the serum TSH and FT4 or FT4I levels within normal limits. A suppressed serum TSH is an indication of excessive thyroid hormone, a risk factor for osteoporosis, and may also affect cardiovascular performance.

KEY POINTS

1 Primary hypothyroidism accounts for 95% of all cases of hypothyroidism.

2 The incidence of hypothyroidism increases with age, and reaches up to 15% of all women over age 50.

3 The initial symptoms of hypothyroidism may be nonspecific.

4 Subclinical hypothyroidism is characterized by an elevated serum TSH value in the presence of normal FT4 and FT4I levels.

SUGGESTED READINGS

Cooper DS: Subclinical hypothyroidism, *Adv Endocrinol Metab* 2: 77-88, 1991.

Duncan WE et al: Influence of clinical characteristics and parameters associated with thyroid hormone therapy on the bone density of women treated with thyroid hormone, *Thyroid* 4:183-190, 1994.

LaFranchi S: Congenital hypothyroidism: a newborn screening success story? *The Endocrinologist* 4:477-486, 1994.

LiVolsi VA: The pathology of autoimmune thyroid disease: a review, *Thyroid* 4:333-339, 1994.

Roti E et al: The use and misuse of thyroid hormone, *Endo Rev* 14:401, 1993.

Singer PA: Thyroiditis: acute, subacute, and chronic, *Med Clin North Am* 75:61-77, 1991.

Toft AD: Thyroxine therapy, *N Engl J Med* 331:174-180, 1994.

75

Varicose Veins

MITCHEL P. GOLDMAN AND JOHN J. BERGAN

Varicose veins occur with increasing frequency as one ages. In addition to their objectionable cosmetic appearance, varicose and even smaller telangiectatic veins are symptomatic in at least 50% of female patients. Women commonly report a heaviness and fullness in the legs with various types of neuropathic pain over clinically apparent veins. Symptoms are usually more pronounced after standing or sitting for prolonged periods of time. Varicose veins may also lead to significant superficial thrombophlebitis, external bleeding, and chronic venous insufficiency. Therefore these unsightly vessels warrant evaluation and treatment.

The incidence in women approaches 30% by age 30 and 80% by age 80. Women are affected at least five times as often as men. Although many patients fail to correlate symptoms with the vein and claim only cosmetic embarrassment, most will acknowledge symptoms of pain, ache, and heaviness in the affected legs in the last half of the menstrual cycle and especially during the first day of a menstrual period and after prolonged standing. In addition to symptoms and cosmetic appearances, varicose veins may cause conditions as serious as chronic venous insufficiency, deep vein thrombosis, and pulmonary embolism or as minor as spontaneous bruising.

PATHOPHYSIOLOGY

The etiology of varicose veins is multifactorial and the pathophysiology not widely appreciated. A familial causation has been demonstrated in numerous studies and in clinical experience. The incidence increases with increasing numbers of family members affected. This factor cannot be modified. High levels of progesterone during pregnancy and the last half of the menstrual cycle inhibit smooth muscle contraction and are associated with development of varicose veins, telangiectasia, and their symptoms. Standing for prolonged periods of time in occupations such as teaching, nursing, sales, factory work, and as airline flight attendants both increases symptoms and accentuates the development of varicose veins. Some studies link increased body weight to an increased incidence of varicose veins. Straining when having a bowel movement and eating foods low in fiber are thought by a few researchers to be associated with varicose veins. Both estrogen and progesterone found in hormone replacement therapy/birth control pills have been found to increase the distensibility of vessel walls. Wearing of tight abdominal garments (garter belts, girdles, control-top pantyhose, or even tight pants) may impede venous return from the leg and raise distal venous pressure. Impedance of venous flow may also occur from crossing the legs when sitting. In addition, a sedentary lifestyle results in a relative stagnation of blood flow in the legs. Calf and foot muscle movement is required to propel blood to the heart. Wearing of high-heeled shoes forces walking with gluteal instead of calf muscles and results in a relative stagnation of blood flow in the legs.

DIAGNOSIS

Although clinical diagnosis is straightforward, recognizing potential medical problems (chronic venous insufficiency and thrombophlebitis) may be difficult. Numerous grading systems exist to help describe the extent of varicose vein disease. A simplified classification is provided in Box 75-1. Diagnostic tests are not required in many patients. Certainly, any suspicion of venous thrombosis (superficial or deep) must be evaluated with duplex ultrasound. Before planning surgical treatment, duplex and/or Doppler ultrasound is recommended. Other functional tests may be useful to determine the extent of venous disease. These include duplex ultrasound of superficial veins, which determines their extent and extent of reflux. Competence of venous valves and luminal thrombosis are easily ascertained. Doppler ultrasound may also be helpful in determining competence of deep valves and in localizing points of maximal reflux of blood flow. Photoplethysmography (PPG) measures cutaneous blood volume and gives an indirect measure of venous flow during calf muscle pumping. Normally, cutaneus blood volume should decrease with calf muscle movement and return to baseline after more than 25 seconds after muscular activity. A more rapid return to baseline cutaneous blood volume indicates improper function of venous valves. Air or impedance plethysmography directly measures total leg volume as suggested by the PPG.

BOX 75-1
Classification of Varicose Vein Disease

1. Truncal varicose veins
   Greater and lessor saphenous vein
2. Accessory varicose veins
   Veins (usually greater than 4 mm in diameter) connected to truncal varicose veins
3. Perforating veins
   Veins that connect the deep veins to superficial veins, "perforating" the fascial sheath
4. Reticular veins
   Veins (usually 2-4 mm in diameter) coursing in a superficial plane and connecting superficial veins and telangiectasia to perforating and accessory veins
5. Venulectases
   Veins connecting reticular veins to telangiectasia, usually 1 mm in diameter
6. Telangiectasia
   Veins less than 1 mm in diameter that are superficial in location; they represent the beginning or end of clinically visible veins

DIFFERENTIAL DIAGNOSIS

The differential diagnosis of varicose veins is limited. Subcutaneous tumors (lipoma, epidermal inclusion cysts) and muscle herniation may mimic the appearance of a bulging varicose vein. Doppler or duplex ultrasound (or even puncture with a needle) will establish the correct diagnosis.

TREATMENT

Prevention consists of minimizing superficial venous pressure and stimulating deep venous flow. Treatment consists of removing abnormal veins to reestablish centripetal venous flow (Fig. 75-1).

Sclerotherapy involves the introduction of a caustic solution into the vessel lumen to cause its destruction and resorption. Normalization of venous flow will follow. This improved circulation limits symptoms. Modern surgical techniques use selective procedures for various types of venous pathology. When reflux occurs at the junction of the saphenous vein and femoral or popliteal veins, surgical ligation and stripping is curative. Tributary and accessory veins can be selectively avulsed through stab incisions 2 to 3 mm in length or smaller. Results of modern surgical techniques are cosmetic and curative. These procedures can be performed under local anesthesia in an ambulatory setting. Various rutinosides have been found to augment venous flow by stimulating venous wall smooth muscle. These agents are not approved by the FDA,

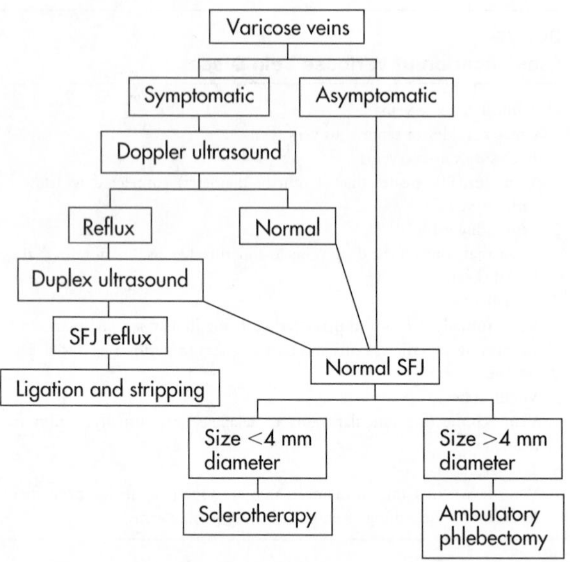

FIG. 75-1 Diagnosis and treatment for varicose veins. *SFJ,* saphenofemoral junction

but are in widespread use throughout the world. They can be found in health food stores and are labeled "rutin."

KEY POINTS

1. Varicose veins may be symptomatic and may cause potentially serious medical problems.
2. Safe and effective treatment for varicose and telangiectatic leg veins is available.

SUGGESTED READINGS

Bergan JJ, Goldman MP, eds: *Varicose and telangiectatic leg veins: diagnosis and treatment,* St. Louis, 1993, Quality Medical Publishing Inc.

Feid CF: Deep vein thrombosis: the risk of sclerotherapy in hypercoagulable states, *Semin Dermatol* 12:135, 1993.

Goldman MP, Bergan JJ, eds: *Ambulatory treatment of varicose and telangiectatic leg veins: an illustrative guide,* St. Louis, 1996, Mosby.

Goldman MP: *Sclerotherapy treatment of varicose and telangiectatic leg veins,* ed 2, St. Louis, 1995, Mosby.

Ricci S, Geogiev M, Goldman MP, eds: *Ambulatory phlebectomy: treatment of varicose veins,* St. Louis, 1995, Mosby.

Tibbs DJ: *Varicose veins and related disorders,* Oxford, 1992, Butterworth-Heineman Ltd.

Weiss RA, Weiss MA, Goldman MP: Physicians' negative perception of sclerotherapy for venous disorders: a review of a 7-year experience with modern sclerotherapy, *South Med J* 85:1101, 1992.

Weiss RA, Weiss M: Resolution of pain associated with varicose and telangiectatic leg veins after compression sclerotherapy, *J Dermatol Surg Oncol* 16:333, 1990.

Index

A

Abdomen, fetal, ultrasonographic evaluation of, 263, 265, 279-281
Abdominal hysterectomy, total, for treatment of endometriosis, 54
Abdominal pregnancy, 51
Abdominal radiotherapy for ovarian cancer, 129
Abdominal wall block, anterior, local infiltration and, for cesarean section, 473
Ablation
  for adenomyosis, 205
  for coagulation defects, 205
  for condyloma, 89
  for hyperthyroidism, 637-638
ABO incompatibility, 413; *see also* Alloimmunization
Abruption, placental; *see* Placental abruption
Abscess
  breast, 23
  liver, amebic, 346
  peritonsillar, pharyngitis and, 601
  tuboovarian, 145; *see also* Pelvic inflammatory disease
Abstinence, periodic, for contraception, 39-40
Abuse
  childhood, 156
  physical, 572-577
  psychologic, 572-573; *see also* Domestic violence
  sexual; *see* Domestic violence; Sexual abuse
  substance; *see* Substance abuse
Accelerations in fetal heart rate, 467
Accessory varicose veins, 645
Acebutolol for hypertension, 592
Acetaminophen
  for headache, 583-584
  for influenza, 597
  for osteoarthritis, 528
Acetazolamide for pseudotumor cerebri, 582
Acid-aspiration syndrome, 349
Acidosis, fetal, heart rate abnormalities indicating, 469
Acquired immunodeficiency syndrome, 499-505
  congenital infection with, 372
  diagnosis of, 499, 501
  opportunistic infections with, prophylaxis for, 502-503
  treatment of, 500, 501-504
Acquired sexual dysfunction, 179
Actinomycin-D
  for choriocarcinoma, 61-62
  for ovarian germ cell tumors, 132
Active gastritis, chronic, 578
Activity log for chronic pelvic pain, 162
Acupressure for menopausal symptoms, 113
Acyclovir
  for herpes simplex virus infection, 84
  for herpes simplex virus prophylaxis, 503
  for varicella pneumonia during pregnancy, 299
Addison's disease during pregnancy, 319
Adductor tendonitis causing chronic pelvic pain, 160-161
Adenocarcinoma
  cervical, therapy for, 30
  of endometrium, estrogen replacement therapy and, 94
  vaginal, 223

Adenoma(s)
adrenal, virilizing, hirsutism with, 69
lactational, 22
liver cell, 347
of nipple, 22
prolactin-producing, during pregnancy, 317-318
Adenomyosis
dysmenorrhea caused by, 42
hysterectomy for, 203
symptoms and treatment of, 205
Adhesions, pelvic, causing infertility, therapy for, 80
Adolescent
palpable breast lesions in, 22
psychosocial development of, 483
uterine bleeding in, causes of, 201
Adolescent pregnancy
nutrition for, 483-484
prenatal care for, 483
repeat, 484
risks of, 483
Adrenal adenomas, virilizing, hirsutism with, 69
Adrenal hyperandrogenemia, therapy for, 72
Adrenal hyperplasia
anovulatory bleeding caused by, 202
hirsutism caused by, 64
Adrenal insufficiency during pregnancy, 319
Adrenal rest tumors, hirsutism with, 67
Adrenocorticotropic hormone for gout, 531
Adriamycin
for invasive breast cancer, 18
for metastatic breast disease, 19
Adult epiglottitis causing hoarseness, 604
Adult immunizations, 373
guidelines for, 374
Advanced extrapelvic disease, therapy for, 32
Advanced pelvic disease, therapy for, 31-32
Affective disorder, seasonal, 99
Aging, bone loss with; *see* Osteoporosis
Agoraphobia, panic disorders with or without, 522-523
AIDS, 499-505; *see also* Acquired immunodeficiency syndrome
Albuterol for asthma, 446
during pregnancy, 297
Alcohol
abuse of; *see* Substance abuse
breastfeeding and maternal use of, 481
gastritis caused by, 578
hypertension caused by, 587
mood disorders caused by, 98-99
use of, during pregnancy, 487; *see also* Substance abuse
Aldomet; *see* Methyldopa
Alendronate for osteoporosis, 120, 121
Alimentation, enteral, 613-614
Alkaline-reflux gastritis, 579
Alkalosis, respiratory, maternal, changes in, during pregnancy, 294
Allergic reactions causing hoarseness, 604
Alloimmune thrombocytopenia, neonatal, 328
Alloimmunization, 413-419
Allopurinol for gout, 531
Alpha-1-antitrypsin deficiency, 255-256
α-blockers for pheochromocytoma, 319
Alprazolam
for generalized anxiety disorder, 524
for premenstrual syndrome, 176
Amantadine
for influenza, 597
for mood disorders, 103
Ambulatory phlebectomy for varicose veins, 645-646
Amebic liver abscess, 346
Amenorrhea, 3-10
Aminoglycoside for acute pyelonephritis, 360
Aminophylline for asthma, 446
during pregnancy, 298
Aminopterin, teratogenic effects of, 247
Aminosalicylic acid for inflammatory bowel disease, 350
Amitriptyline
for chronic pelvic pain, 161
for mood disorders, 103
for tension headache, 583
Amlodipine for hypertension, 591
Amniocentesis
for alloimmunization, 415, 417

Amniocentesis–cont'd
to screen for birth defects, 243
Amniotic fluid, 272-273
Amniotic fluid embolism, 446-447
Amniotic fluid index, 273, 286
Amniotic fluid volume
to diagnose intrauterine growth restriction, 427
scoring for, 267
Amoxicillin
for chlamydial infection, 90
for *H. pylori* infection, 624
for mastitis, 480
for pneumonia, 631
during pregnancy, 299
for urinary tract infections, 562
Amoxicillin-clavulanate for pneumonia during pregnancy, 299
Amphetamines
abuse of, during pregnancy, 488; *see also* Substance abuse
in urine specimens, 485
Ampicillin
for group B β-hemolytic streptococcal infection, 373
for mastitis, 235, 480
for papillomavirus infections, 137
for pneumonia, 631
for systemic sclerosis, 552
for urinary tract infections, 562
Amylophagia during pregnancy, 239
Anabolic steroids
hirsutism caused by, 64
for osteoporosis, 120
Analgesia, inhalation, for vaginal delivery, 473
Analgesics for pharyngitis, 603
Anaphylactic reactions causing hoarseness, 604
Androgen insensitivity syndrome
amenorrhea caused by, 7
treatment of, 9
Androgen-producing ovarian tumors
evaluation to rule out, 68
hirsutism with, 67
therapy for, 72
Androgen-producing tumors, hirsutism caused by, 64
Androgenic evaluation in evaluation of amenorrhea, 4
Androgenic hormones, teratogenic effects of, 248
Androgenic progestins to treat hirsutism, 71
Anemia
iron deficiency, during pregnancy 320-322
megaloblastic, during pregnancy, 322-323
during pregnancy, evaluation of, 321
sickle cell, 324-326
Anencephaly, 253
ultrasonography to detect, 275
Anesthesia
for cesarean delivery, 473-474
epidural, 471-472
for pregnant woman with cardiac problems, 305
for labor, 471-472
obstetric, 470-474
spinal, 471-472
for vaginal delivery, 472-473
Aneurysm, headache with, 581
Angioedema causing hoarseness, 604
Angiography, pulmonary
radiation exposure to fetus from, 421
to diagnose thromboembolism, 422
Angiotensin-converting enzyme inhibitors
for hypertension, 589
teratogenic effects of, 248
Angleman's syndrome, 256
Ankylosing spondylitis, 532-533
Annual examination, 506-518
Anorexia nervosa, amenorrhea caused by, 6
Anovulation
amenorrhea caused by, 4
hyperandrogenic chronic, hirsutism caused by, 64
hypoestrogenic
amenorrhea caused by, 6
treatment of, 9
infertility caused by, therapy for, 80
treatment of, 8
Anovulatory bleeding, 200
in adolescent, treatment of, 201
in reproductive age women, 201-202
Antacids for peptic ulcer disease, 623
Antenatal testing, 282-287
Anterior abdominal wall block, local infiltration and, for cesarean section, 473
Anthropometry, 610-611

Antiarrhythmic agents to prevent myocardial infarction complicating pregnancy, 306
Antibiotics
for advanced pelvic disease, 32
for asymptomatic bacteriuria in pregnancy, 562
for cholecystitis, 546
for diarrhea, 571
for endometritis, 204
for impetigo herpetiformis, 383
for infectious or septic arthritis, 534
for laryngitis, 606
for male factor infertility, 80
for pelvic inflammatory disease, 144
for pharyngitis, 603
for pneumonia during pregnancy, 299
for premature PROM, 395
for systemic sclerosis, 552
teratogenic effects of, 247-248
for tuboovarian abscess, 145
for urinary tract infections, 560, 562
Antibodies, antisperm, determination of presence of, 79
Anticoagulant(s)
bleeding caused by, symptoms and treatment of, 205
lupus, 334, 336; *see also* Lupus anticoagulant/antiphospholipid antibody syndrome
Anticoagulation for thromboembolism, 422-424
Anticonvulsants for chronic pelvic pain, 161
Antidepressants
for migraine headache, 584
mood disorders caused by, 99
for mood disorders, 101-103
tricyclic; *see* Tricyclic antidepressants
Antiepileptics, teratogenic effects of, 248-249
Antifungal medications
for candidiasis, 87
for papillomavirus infections, 137
Antigenic drift in influenza virus, 594
Antihistamines
for herpes gestationis, 380
for intrahepatic cholestasis of pregnancy, 343
Antihypertensives
mood disorders caused by, 99
Antihypertensives–cont'd
for preeclampsia, 343-344
Antiinflammatory drugs for asthma during pregnancy, 297
Antimalarials
fetal effects of, 340
for systemic lupus erythematosus, 550
Antineoplastic drugs, teratogenic effects of, 247
Antioxidants, need for, during menopause, 111-112
Antiphospholipid syndrome, 549-550
Antiprostaglandins
for adenomyosis, 205
excessive bleeding caused by, symptoms and treatment of, 205
Antipruritics for prurigo gestationis, 382
Antiretroviral therapy for HIV, 503-504
Antisperm antibodies, determination of presence of, 79
Anxiety, performance, causing orgasmic disorder, 182
Anxiety disorder, generalized, 523-524
Anxiety reaction, 519-526
management of, 520
Aortic stenosis complicating pregnancy, 307-308
Apgar score, 490
Apical prolapse, 169
Apoplexy, pituitary, headache with, 585
Appendicitis, 350
Arias-Stella reaction, 45
Arrhythmias, fetal cardiac, ultrasonography to detect, 278-279
Arteriovenous fistulas, uterine, bleeding caused by, symptoms and treatment of, 205
Arteritis, 555, 581
Artery, renal, stenosis of, pregnancy and, 362
Arthritis
enteropathic, 533
gouty, 530
infectious or septic, 533-534
nonbacterial, 534-535
psoriatic, 533
and related musculoskeletal disorders, 527-536
rheumatoid, 338-339, 528-530

Arthrotomy for septic arthritis, 534
ASCUS; *see* Atypical squamous cells of uncertain significance
Aseptic meningitis, headache with, 582
Asherman's syndrome
  amenorrhea caused by, 7
  curettage causing, 449
Aspiration
  fine-needle, to diagnose breast cancer, 13
  meconium, 494-495
  pneumonia during pregnancy caused by, 298
  thin-needle, to diagnose breast cancer, 13
  tracheobronchial, complicating enteral alimentation, 614
Aspirin
  for headache, 583-584
  for lupus anticoagulant/antiphospholipid antibody syndrome, 337-338
  for migraine headache, 584
  for osteoarthritis, 528
  for rheumatoid arthritis, 339, 529
Assisted reproductive procedures, 80-82
Asthenospermia, 76
Asthma, 444-446
  during pregnancy, 295-298
Asymptomatic bacteriuria, 359
  in pregnancy, antibiotics for, 562
Atenolol
  for chronic hypertension during pregnancy, 356
  for hypertension, 592
Atony, uterine, treatment of, 448-449
Atresia, duodenal, ultrasonography to detect, 279, 280
Atrial septal defects complicating pregnancy, 308
Atrophic gastritis, chronic, 579
Atrophy, Leber's hereditary optic, 253
Atropine
  for asthma during pregnancy, 297
  breastfeeding and maternal use of, 480
  for diarrhea, 569
Atypical squamous cells of uncertain significance, 135
Auscultation, intermittent, for fetal heart rate monitoring, 466-467
Autoimmune disease during pregnancy, 332-341
  considerations for drug therapy for, 340-341
Autoimmune disorder evaluation in evaluation of amenorrhea, 4
Autosomal dominant chromosomal abnormalities, 252
Autosomal recessive chromosomal abnormalities, 252, 253
Axid; *see* Nizatidiine
Axillary dissection for invasive breast cancer, 17-18
Azathioprine
  fetal effects of, 340-341
  for herpes gestationis, 380
  for pregnant woman on long-term dialysis, 365
  for rheumatoid arthritis, 530
  for systemic lupus erythematosus, 336, 550
Azithromycin
  for chancroid, 83
  for chlamydial infection, 89
  for pneumonia, 631
AZT; *see* Zidovudine

B

Backache, 536-543
Baclofen for trigeminal neuralgia, 581
Bacterial endocarditis during pregnancy, prophylaxis against, 305
Bacterial laryngitis, treatment of, 606
Bacterial pharyngitis, 601
Bacterial pneumonia, 627-633
Bacterial vaginosis, 86-87
Bacteriuria
  asymptomatic, 359, 558
    in pregnancy, antibiotics for, 562
  testing for, indications for, 517
Bactrim for urinary tract infections, 562
Banana sign in spina bifida, 276, 277
Barbiturate abuse during pregnancy, 488; *see also* Substance abuse
Barrier methods of contraception, 36-37
Basal body temperature in evaluation of ovulation, 78
Battered woman, characteristics of, 573
Beck Depression Inventory, 101

Behavioral therapy
for generalized anxiety disorder, 524
for obsessive-compulsive disorder, 521
Benazepril for hypertension, 589
Benign breast disease, 21-25
Bentyl; *see* Dicyclomine
Benzathine penicillin
for rheumatic heart disease complicating pregnancy, 307
for syphilis, 85
Benzodiazepine
for generalized anxiety disorder, 524
for intrahepatic cholestasis of pregnancy, 343
for panic disorders with or without agoraphobia, 523
Bereavement, differentiation of, from depressive disorder, 100-101
Beta-adrenergic receptor antagonists for hypertension, 592
β-agonists for asthma, 445, 446
during pregnancy, 297
Beta-blockers
for hypertension, 592
for hyperthyroidism, 637
for Marfan syndrome complicating pregnancy, 309
for maternal tachycardia, 307
for migraine headache, 584
to prevent myocardial infarction complicating pregnancy, 306
for social phobia, 525
β-HCG levels
to diagnose ectopic pregnancy, 47
to diagnose hydatidiform mole, 56
β-hemolytic streptococcus, group B, congenital infection with, 372-373
Betamethasone for preeclampsia/eclampsia, 433
Beta-sympathomimetics for preterm labor, protocol for, 391, 392-393
β-thalassemia, treatment of, 256
Betaxolol for hypertension, 592
Bethanechol for voiding dysfunction, 197
Bile gastritis, 579
Biliary colic, 544
Billings method for contraception, 40
Bimanual examination, procedure for, 515-516
Biochemical testing to diagnose osteoporosis, 118
Biophysical profile
for antenatal testing, 283-284
fetal assessment by, 266, 267, 268
Biopsy
cone, for abnormal Pap smear, 135, 136
core-needle, to diagnose breast cancer, 13, 14
to diagnose cervical cancer, 26
endometrial
to diagnose pelvic inflammatory disease, 141
in evaluation of ovulation, 79
excisional, to diagnose breast cancer, 13, 14
placental, 244
stereotactic, to diagnose breast cancer, 14
surgical, needle localization, to diagnose breast cancer, 14
Biparietal diameter of fetal head, ultrasonographic evaluation of, 261, 262
Bipolar disorders, 97-98; *see also* Mood disorders
Birth, premature, 384-397; *see also* Premature birth
Birth control, breastfeeding and, 481
Birth defects, maternal serum analyte screening for, 241-243
Birth weight, low or very low, 384
Bismuth subsalicylate
for diarrhea, 569
for *H. pylori* infection, 624
Bisphosphonates for osteoporosis, 120, 121
Black cohash for menopausal symptoms, 113
Bladder diary, 186, 189
to diagnose urge incontinence, 194
Bladder training for urge incontinence, 194
Bleeding
anovulatory; *see* Anovulatory bleeding
breakthrough, with oral contraception, 35
from choriocarcinoma, 61
contraceptive-related, 203
midcycle, symptoms and treatment of, 204

Bleeding–cont'd
ovulatory
causes, symptoms, and treatment of, 204-206
in reproductive age women, 202-203
peptic ulcer, endoscopic features of, 625
perimenopausal, symptoms and treatment of, 206
postmenopausal, 206
third trimester, 403-413
uterine; *see* Uterine bleeding
Bleomycin
for ovarian germ cell tumors, 132
for sex cord–stromal tumors, 133
Block
anterior abdominal wall, local infiltration and, for cesarean section, 473
epidural, for vaginal delivery, 472
pudendal, for vaginal delivery, 472
"saddle," for vaginal delivery, 473
spinal, for vaginal delivery, 473
Blood pressure
of hypertensive patient, 588-589
maternal, changes in, during pregnancy, 293, 294
Blood volume, maternal, changes in, during pregnancy, 293, 294
Bloody nipple discharge, 22, 25
"Bloody show," 410
Body movements, gross, fetal, scoring for, 267
Body weight, maintaining appropriate, during menopause, 112
Bone loss; *see also* Osteoporosis
Bone mineral density, assessment of, to diagnose osteoporosis, 115, 117
Bouchard's nodes, 527
Bowel
fetal, ultrasonography to evaluate, 279
functional or follicular disease of, 566-567
inflammatory disease of, 349-350
irritable, 348
treatment of, 571
Bowstring test, 538
Brachytherapy implants for advanced pelvic disease, 31-32
Bradycardia, fetal, 467
ultrasonography to detect, 278-279
Braxton-Hicks contractions, 390
BRCA-1 and risk of breast cancer, 11
BRCA-2 and risk of breast cancer, 11
Breakthrough bleeding with oral contraception, 35
Breast
abscess of, 23
of adolescent, palpable lesions in, 22
cancer of, 10-20; *see also* Malignant breast disease
benign breast disease versus, 21
estrogen replacement therapy and, 94-95
disease of
benign, 21-25; *see also* Benign breast disease
malignant, 10-20; *see also* Malignant breast disease
examination of, 511
fibrocystic changes in, 23
inflammation of, 23-24
Paget's disease of, 15
Breast milk, pumping and storing, 481
Breast-ovarian cancer syndrome, hereditary, 126
Breastfeeding
AIDS as contraindication for, 504
birth control and, 481
common difficulties with, 478-480
getting started with, 477-478
medications safe for use during, 480-481
nutritional requirements for, 239
practical information about, 475, 477
prenatal education about, 475
weaning from, 481
Breathing movements, fetal, scoring for, 267
Breech presentation, 451-454
delivery of fetus in, 451, 453-454
risks of, 451
Bromhexine for Sjögren's syndrome, 553
Bromides, breastfeeding and maternal use of, 480
Bromocriptine
for hyperprolactinemia and pituitary tumors, 8
to induce ovulation, 81
for male factor infertility, 80
for premenstrual syndrome, 176
for prolactin-producing adenomas during pregnancy, 318

Bronchodilators for asthma during pregnancy, 297
Bronchogenic carcinoma, hyperprolactinemia caused by, 6
Brow presentation, 455-457
Bruxism, headache with, 582
Bulky cervical disease, therapy for, 31
Bumetanide for hypertension, 592
Bupivacaine for spinal anesthesia for labor, 471
Bupropion
  for mood disorders, 102-103
  for panic disorders with or without agoraphobia, 523
  in pregnancy, 106
Burch culposuspension for stress incontinence, 192
Buspar; *see* Buspirone
Buspirone
  for generalized anxiety disorder, 524
  for mood disorders, 103
  for premenstrual syndrome, 173, 176
Busulfan, teratogenic effects of, 247
Butorphanol
  for headache, 584
  for labor, 471
Bypass, gastrointestinal, pregnancy and, 349

C

Cafergot for migraine headache, 585
Caffeine for headache, 583
Caffeine withdrawal headache, 583, 584
CAGE questionnaires for substance abuse, 485
Calamine lotion for prurigo gestationis, 382
Calcitonin for osteoporosis, 120, 122
Calcitriol for osteoporosis, 123
Calcium
  for hypoparathyroidism, 317
  need for, during menopause, 110-111
  osteoporosis and, 119, 120
Calcium 125 levels in diagnosis of ovarian cancer, 128, 131
Calcium channel antagonists for hypertension, 591
Calcium channel blockers
  to prevent myocardial infarction complicating pregnancy, 306
Calcium channel blockers–cont'd
  for systemic sclerosis, 552
Calcium pyrophosphate disease, 531-532
Calcium supplements, 111
  for premenstrual syndrome, 176
  to prevent osteoporosis, 119, 120
Calculi, renal tract, 360
Cancer; *see also* Carcinoma
  breast, 10-20; *see also* Malignant breast disease
    benign breast disease versus, 21
    estrogen replacement therapy and, 94-95
  cervical, 26-33; *see also* Cervical cancer
    causing third trimester bleeding, 410
    metastatic, therapy for, 32
  oral contraceptives and, 35
  ovarian, 124-133; *see also* Ovarian cancer
  uterine, 209-216
  vaginal, 222-224; *see also* Vaginal cancer
  vulvar, 216-222; *see also* Vulvar cancer
Candida albicans infection, 87
Candidal pharyngitis, 602
Candidiasis, vulvovaginal, 87
Captopril
  for hypertension, 589
  teratogenic effects of, 248
Carafate; *see* Sucralfate
Carbamazepine
  for mood disorders, 103-105
  side effects of, 104-105
  teratogenic effects of, 249
  for trigeminal neuralgia, 581
  use in pregnancy of, 106
Carbohydrates, 608
Carboplatin for ovarian cancer, 129
Carcinoma in situ
  of breast, ductal or lobular, 11
    noninvasive, treatment of, 15, 17
  of cervix complicating pregnancy, 287-288
Carcinoma; *see also* Cancer
  bronchogenic, hyperprolactinemia caused by, 6
  cervical
    complicating pregnancy, 287-292
    symptoms and treatment of, 204

Carcinoma–cont'd
endometrial, of uterus, 209-214; *see also* Endometrial carcinomas of uterus
hepatocellular, primary, 347
renal cell, hyperprolactinemia caused by, 6
Carcinosarcoma, uterine, 215
Cardiac activity, fetal, ultrasonographic visualization of, 260
Cardiac arrhythmias, fetal, ultrasonography to detect, 278-279
Cardiac catheterization to diagnose heart disease in pregnancy, 305
Cardiac changes in pregnancy, 227-228
Cardiac diseases during pregnancy, 302-309
Cardiac output
maternal, changes in, during pregnancy, 293
with mitral stenosis, 306
Cardiopulmonary examination of hypertensive patient, 588
Cardiovascular disease after menopause, 93-94
Cardiovascular risk factors, counseling about, 516
Carrier screening tests, 256
Carteolol for hypertension, 592
Catheterization, cardiac, to diagnose heart disease in pregnancy, 305
CBC as carrier screening test, 256
CC; *see* Clomiphene citrate
CD4 lymphocyte count to diagnose AIDS, 501
Cefixime for gonorrhea, 88
Cefotaxime
for gonorrhea, 88
for pelvic inflammatory disease, 144
Cefotetan
for gonorrhea, 88
for pelvic inflammatory disease, 144
Cefoxitin
for gonorrhea, 88
for pelvic inflammatory disease, 144
Cefpodoxime proxetil for gonorrhea, 88
Ceftizoxime
for gonorrhea, 88
for pelvic inflammatory disease, 144
Ceftriaxone
for chancroid, 83
for gonorrhea, 88
for pelvic inflammatory disease, 144
Cefuroxime for pneumonia, 631
Cefuroxime axetil for gonorrhea, 88
Celestone before preterm birth to reduce severity of respiratory distress syndrome, 389-390
Celiac sprue, 565
therapy for, 569
Central cystocele, 167
Central nervous system
anomalies of, ultrasonography to measure, 273-276
lesions of, hyperprolactinemia caused by, 6
Cepalosporins for pneumonia, 630, 631
Cephalexin
for mastitis, 235
for urinary tract infections, 562
Cephalic index, ultrasonographic evaluation of, 261
Cephalic version, external, 453-454
Cephalosporin(s)
for acute pyelonephritis, 360
for gonorrhea, 88
for pharyngitis, 603
for pneumonia during pregnancy, 299
for urinary tract infections, 560, 562
Cerclage, cervical; *see* Cervical cerclage
Cerebral infarction, hypertension and, 587
Cerebral malformations, ultrasonography to detect, 273
Cerebral ventricle diameters of fetus, posterior, ultrasonographic evaluation of, 261
Cervical cancer, 26-33; *see also* Cervical carcinoma
third trimester bleeding caused by, 410
Cervical cap for contraception, 36
Cervical carcinoma; *see also* Cervical cancer
complicating pregnancy, 287-292

Cervical carcinoma–cont'd
symptoms and treatment of, 204
Cervical cerclage
for abnormal cervical competence, 399-400, 401-403
McDonald, placement of, 401-403
perioperative care of, 402
Cervical competence, abnormal, 397-403
diagnosis of, 397-398
management of, 399-403
risk factors for, 398
Cervical conization for microinvasive cervical cancer, 30
Cervical disc disease, headache with, 582
Cervical factors in infertility evaluation, 77
Cervical fibroid causing third trimester bleeding, 410
Cervical infections, 87-90
Cervical leiomyoma causing third trimester bleeding, 410
Cervical mucus, lack of, therapy for, 80
Cervical pain, 535
Cervical polyps causing third trimester bleeding, 410
Cervical pregnancy, 51
Cervical stenosis, 42-43
Cervicitis
symptoms and treatment of, 204
third trimester bleeding caused by, 410
Cervix; *see also* Cervical cancer; Cervical carcinoma
adenocarcinoma of, therapy for, 30
dysplastic lesions of, high-grade, 135, 136
high-grade squamous epithelial lesions of, 135, 136
incompetent; *see* Cervical competence, abnormal
low-grade squamous intraepithelial lesions of, 135-137
Cesarean delivery
amenorrhea caused by, 7
anesthesia for, 473-474
for breech fetus, 451, 453
for transverse lie fetus, 454
Chancre of syphilis, 84
Chancroid, vulvar, 83
Charcot-Marie-Tooth disease, 253
Chasteberry for menopausal symptoms, 113
Chemotherapy
for advanced pelvic disease, 32
for androgen-producing ovarian neoplasms, 72
for choriocarcinoma, 61-62
for condyloma, 89
for hydatidiform mole, 59
for invasive breast cancer, 17-19
for metastatic breast disease, 18, 19
for ovarian cancer, 128-131
for ovarian germ cell tumors, 132
for sex cord–stromal tumors, 132-133
for Sjögren's syndrome, 553
for vulvar cancer, 220, 221
Chest expansion in diagnosis of cause of backache, 537-538
Chest x-ray, radiation exposure to fetus from, 421
Chickenpox, congenital infection with, 369-370
Childhood, uterine bleeding in, causes of, 200-201
Childhood abuse, 156
Chlamydia, 88-90
pelvic inflammatory disease and, 142, 143
Chlamydia cultures, 515
Chlamydia pneumoniae causing pneumonia, 632-633
Chlamydia trachomatis
causing cervical chlamydia, 88
causing lymphogranuloma venereum, 85
Chlamydial pharyngitis, 601
Chloasma, 375-376
Chloramphenicol, breastfeeding and maternal use of, 480
Chloroquine, fetal effects of, 340
Chlorthalidone for hypertension, 591
Chlorzoxazone for headache, 584
"Chocolate cysts," 152
Cholangiopancreatography, endoscopic retrograde, 350
Cholecystectomy for cholecystitis, 546, 547
Cholecystitis, 543-547
Cholestasis of pregnancy, 376-377, 378
intrahepatic, 341, 343
Cholesterol, menopause and, 111
Cholestyramine
for bile gastritis, 579
for diarrhea, 571

Cholestyramine–cont'd
for intrahepatic cholestasis of pregnancy, 343
Chondrocalcinosis, 532
Chorioadenoma destruens, 59-60
Choriocarcinoma, 55-56, 60-62
Chorionic gonadotropin, human; *see* Human chorionic gonadotropin
Chorionic villus sampling to screen for birth defects, 243-244
Chromosomal abnormalities, 251-252
Churg-Strauss syndrome, 555-556
Cigarettes, breastfeeding and maternal use of, 481
Cimetidine
breastfeeding and maternal use of, 480
for peptic ulcer disease, 623
for reflux esophagitis, 614
Ciprofloxacin
for gonorrhea, 88
for urinary tract infections, 562
Cisplatin
for advanced pelvic disease, 32
for endometrial stromal sarcoma of uterus, 215
for ovarian cancer, 129
for ovarian germ cell tumors, 132
for sex cord–stromal tumors, 133
for uterine carcinosarcoma, 215
Cisterna magna, fetal, ultrasonographic evaluation of, 262, 263
Clarithromycin
for *H. pylori* infection, 624
for pneumonia, 631
Clear-liquid diet, 613
Cleft lip, 253
treatment of, 256
Cleft palate, 253
treatment of, 256
Climara for hormone replacement therapy, 96
Clindamycin
for bacterial vaginosis, 86-87
for pelvic inflammatory disease, 144
Clitoral index, diagnosis of causes of hirsutism using, 70
Clomid; *see* Clomiphene citrate
Clomiphene citrate
for anovulation, 8, 80
to induce ovulation, 81
Clomiphene citrate–cont'd
multiple ovulation induced by, as risk factor for ectopic pregnancy, 45
twinning caused by, 459
Clomipramine
for obsessive-compulsive disorder, 521
for premenstrual syndrome, 176
Clonazepam for generalized anxiety disorder, 524
Clonidine
for hypertension, 592
for opiate withdrawal, 488
for posttraumatic stress disorder, 524
Clotting time, whole-blood, to screen for coagulopathy, 405
Club foot, 253
Cluster headache, 584
Coagulation defects
menorrhagia caused by, 201
pregnancy and, 326-331
symptoms and treatment of, 205
Coagulation, intravascular, disseminated, 328-331
Coagulopathy, whole-blood clotting time to screen for, 405
Cocaine
abuse of, during pregnancy, 488; *see also* Substance abuse
hypertension caused by, 587
placental abruption and, 405
in urine specimens, 485, 488
withdrawal from, 488
Codeine
for chronic pelvic pain, 162
for diarrhea, 569, 571
for headache, 584
Coelomic metaplasia, theory of, to explain endometriosis, 53
Colchicine for gout, 531
Colic, biliary, 544
Colitis, ulcerative, 349-350, 566
therapy for, 569
Colonoscopy
to diagnose cause of diarrhea, 568
indications for, 517
Colpectomy for vaginal vault prolapse, 169
Colpocleisis for vaginal vault prolapse, 169
Colporrhaphy for cystocele, 167
Colposacral suspension for vaginal vault prolapse, 169

Colposcopic examination for abnormal Pap smear, 135, 136
Colpotomy for tubal occlusion, 185
Combined factor sexual dysfunction, 179
Commercial formulas for enteral alimentation, 613
Community-acquired pneumonia, 628; *see also* Pneumonia
Competence, cervical, abnormal, 397-403
Complete breech, 451, 452
Complicated peptic ulcer disease, diagnosis and management of, 625-626
Compound presentation, 457-458
Compulsions, 519, 521
Computed tomography to evaluate chronic pelvic pain, 162
Condoms for contraception, 37
Condyloma, 90
  treatment options for, 89
Condyloma acuminata, 134-139
Condylox; *see* Podofilox
Cone biopsy for abnormal Pap smear, 135, 136
Congenital anomalies
  of müllerian duct, amenorrhea caused by, 6-7
  prenatal diagnosis of, 240-244
Congenital heart disease, ultrasonography to detect, 276
Congenital infections, 366-373
Congestion, pelvic, dysmenorrhea caused by, 42
Congestive heart failure in pregnant woman, 306-307
Conization, cervical, for microinvasive cervical cancer, 30
Connective tissue diseases, 548-557
  mixed, 551
Constipation during pregnancy, management of, 238
Continuous-wave Doppler ultrasound, 266
Contraception, 34-41
  sterilization for, 184-185
Contraceptives, oral; *see* Oral contraceptives
Contraction stress test, 284-285
Contractions
  Braxton-Hicks, 390
  impaired, detrusor hyperactivity with, 193; *see also* Urge incontinence
Contractions–cont'd
  of preterm labor, 390
Contrast study to diagnose peptic ulcer disease, 620
Copper IUD for contraception, 38-39
Cord insertion, velamentous, 410
Cordocentesis
  for alloimmunization, 415
  for antenatal testing, 285-286; *see also* Percutaneous umbilical blood sampling
Core-needle biopsy to diagnose breast cancer, 13, 14
Coronary heart disease, hypertension and, 587
Corpus luteum, 3
Corpus luteum cyst, hemorrhagic, 149, 150, 151
Corticosteroids
  for asthma, 445, 446
    during pregnancy, 297
  before preterm birth to reduce severity of respiratory distress syndrome, 389-390
  for diarrhea, 569, 571
  fetal effects of, 340
  for gout, 531
  for HELLP syndrome, 344
  for herpes gestationis, 380
  for hyperandrogenism, 8
  for idiopathic inflammatory myopathies, 553
  for impetigo herpetiformis, 383
  for inflammatory bowel disease, 350
  for male factor infertility, 80
  mood disorders caused by, 99
  for osteoarthritis, 528
  for premature PROM, 395
  for PUPPP syndrome, 381
  for rheumatoid arthritis, 530
  for sarcoidosis in pregnancy, 300
  for spondyloarthropathies, 533
  for systemic lupus erythematosus, 335, 550
  for vasculitides, 556-557
Cosmetic therapy for hirsutism, 73
Coumadin
  breastfeeding and maternal use of, 481
  intrauterine growth restriction caused by, 426
  teratogenic effects of, 246-247
Coumarin derivatives for thromboembolism during pregnancy, 423, 424

Counseling, genetic, common indications for, 241
Couvelaire uterus, 405
Crack cocaine abuse during pregnancy, 488; *see also* Substance abuse
Cranial arteritis, 555
Craniopharyngioma, hyperprolactinemia caused by, 6
Creatine kinase levels, serum, measurement of, as carrier screening test, 256
CREST syndrome, 339, 551
Cri du chat syndrome, 256
Critical periods in exposure to teratogens, 245
Crixivan; *see* Indinavir
Crohn's disease, 349-350, 566
Cromolyn sodium for asthma during pregnancy, 297
Crown-rump length, ultrasonographic visualization of, 260
Cryoglobulinemia, 556
Cryoprecipitate for disseminated intravascular coagulation, 331
Cryotherapy
  for condyloma, 89
  for high-grade cervical dysplasia, 135
Culdoplasty for enterocele, 169-170
Cultures
  chlamydia, 515
  gonorrhea, 515
Curettage
  suction, evacuation by, to treat hydatidiform mole, 56
  for uterine inversion, 449
Cushing's disease causing anovulatory bleeding, 202
Cushing's syndrome, 69
  in pregnancy, 318-319
Cutaneous scleroderma, limited, 339
Cyclophosphamide
  for endometrial stromal sarcoma of uterus, 215
  fetal effects of, 340-341
  for invasive breast cancer, 18
  for metastatic breast disease, 19
  for ovarian germ cell tumors, 132
  for rheumatoid arthritis, 530
  for sex cord–stromal tumors, 133
  for systemic lupus erythematosus, 550
  teratogenic effects of, 247
Cyclophosphamide–cont'd
  for vasculitides, 556-557
Cyclosporine
  hirsutism caused by, 69
  hypertension caused by, 587
  for rheumatoid arthritis, 530
Cyclosporine A, fetal effects of, 340-341
Cyclothymic disorders, 97; *see also* Mood disorders
Cyproheptadine for mood disorders, 103
Cyproterone acetate for hirsutism, 71, 73
Cystectomy for recurrent cervical cancer, 32-33
Cystic fibrosis, ethnic groups at risk for, 255
Cystic teratoma, 151, 152
Cystitis, 359
  diagnosis of, 559
  and pyelonephritis, 558-563; *see also* Urinary tract infections
  treatment of, 560, 562
Cystocele, 165, 167
Cystometrogram to diagnose urge incontinence, 194
Cystospaz; *see* Hyoscyamine
Cystourethrocele, 165, 167
Cysts
  "chocolate," 152
  corpus luteum, hemorrhagic, 149, 150, 151
  dermoid, 152
  follicular, of ovary, 149, 154
  functional, of ovary, 154
    symptoms and treatment of, 204
  hepatic, 346-347
  ovarian
    dysmenorrhea caused by, 42
    treatment of, 43, 154
  paraovarian, 153
    therapy for, 155
  theca-lutein, 151-152
    hydatidiform mole associated with, 56
    management of, 57
Cytology, atypical, and papillomavirus infections, 138
Cytomegalovirus
  congenital, 367-368
  prophylaxis for, 502-503
Cytoprotection, 618
Cytoreduction for ovarian cancer, 129

D

D4T; *see* Stavudine
Danazol
  for endometriosis, 204
  for premenstrual syndrome, 176
  teratogenic effects of, 248
  for treatment of endometriosis, 54
Dandy-Walker malformation, ultrasonography to detect, 273
Danocrine, hirsutism caused by, 69
Dapsone
  for herpes gestationis, 380
  for prophylaxis in HIV-infected woman, 502
DDC; *see* Zalcitabine
DDI; *see* Didanosine
Death, leading causes of, among women, 507
Decelerations in fetal heart rate, 467
  prolonged, 467
Decompressive laminectomy for backache, 542
Deep venous thrombosis, 419; *see also* Thromboembolic disease
Degenerative joint disease, 527-528
Dehydroepiandrosterone
  diagnosis of causes of hirsutism using, 70
  measurement of, in evaluation of amenorrhea, 4
Delivery
  for eclamptic patient, management of, 435
  for multiple gestation, 465
  of postterm/postdate infant, 441
  for preeclampsia/eclampsia, 434
  preterm, spontaneous versus indicated, 387-388
  vaginal, anesthesia for, 472-473
  in woman with gestational diabetes mellitus, 313
Delivery room resuscitation for depressed neonate, 490-491
Dementia, differentiation of, from mood disorder, 101
Demerol; *see* Meperidine
Depakote; *see* Divalproex sodium; Valproic acid
Depo-Provera
  bleeding related to, 203
    symptoms and treatment of, 205
  breastfeeding and maternal use of, 481
  for contraception, 37-38
  for migraine headache, 584
  teratogenic effects of, 248
Depression
  and hypoactive sexual desire disorder, 180
  neonatal, 489-490
  postpartum, 235
Depressive disorders
  major, 97, 98; *see also* Mood disorders
  not otherwise specified, 97; *see also* Mood disorders
Depressive episodes
  diagnosis of, 99-100
  postpartum, 98
Dermatitis, papular, of pregnancy, 382
Dermatologic disorders, common, 375-384
Dermatomyositis, 552-553
Dermatoses, pruritic, of pregnancy, 378
Dermoid cyst, 152
Desipramine
  for migraine headache, 584
  for mood disorders, 103
Desonorgesteryl to treat hirsutism, 71
Detrusor hyperactivity with impaired contractions, 193; *see also* Urge incontinence
Detrusor hyperreflexia, 193; *see also* Urge incontinence
Detrusor instability, 193; *see also* Urge incontinence
Dexamethasone
  for adrenal hyperandrogenemia, 72
  for anovulation, 80
  for HELLP syndrome, 344
  for hyperandrogenism, 8
Dexamethasone suppression test
  to diagnose Cushing's syndrome, 69
  to diagnose virilizing adrenal adenomas, 69
Diabetes insipidus during pregnancy, 318
Diabetes mellitus
  gestational, 310-315; *see also* Gestational diabetes mellitus
  pregestational, management of, 312
Diabetic ketoacidosis, 442-444
Diabetic nephropathy, pregnancy and, 362
Diagnosis, prenatal, 241-244
  and teratology, 240-251
Diagnostic laparoscopy to diagnose ectopic pregnancy, 47-48

Diagnostic procedures in annual examination, 516-517
Diagnostic studies for peptic ulcer disease, 620-622
Dialysis, long-term, pregnancy in women on, 364-365
Diaphragms for contraception, 36
DIAPPERS mnemonic of causes of urinary incontinence, 189
Diarrhea, 563
 chronic, 563-571
 hydrational status in, 569
 inflammatory, 566
 osmotic, 564-565
 secretory, 565-566
 traveler's, 565
Diazepam for generalized anxiety disorder, 524
Dicloxacillin for mastitis, 235, 480
Dicyclomine for urge incontinence, 195
Didanosine for HIV therapy, 503, 504
Diet(s)
 balanced, during menopause, 110-112
 elemental, 614
 hospital, 613
 prenatal, 237
Diethylstilbestrol
 in utero exposure to, as risk factor for ectopic pregnancy, 45
 teratogenic effects of, 246
Diffuse scleroderma, 339
Diffuse sclerosis, 550; *see also* Systemic sclerosis
Diflucan for thrush mastitis, 480
DiGeorge syndrome, 256
Digoxin to prevent myocardial infarction complicating pregnancy, 306
Dihydroergotamine for migraine headache, 585
Dilantin; *see* Phenytion
Diltiazem for hypertension, 591
Diphenhydramine for PUPPP syndrome, 381
Diphenoxylate hydrochloride for diarrhea, 569
Diphtheria, pharyngitis and, 601-602
Direct fluorescent antibody staining to diagnose chlamydia, 88
Disaccharidase deficiency causing osmotic diarrhea, 565
Disc
 cervical, disease of, headache with, 582
Disc–cont'd
 herniated, 537, 538
Discectomy for backache, 542
Discharge, nipple, 24-25
 bloody, 22
Disomy, uniparental, 253
Displacement cystocele, 167
Dissection, axillary, for invasive breast cancer, 17-18
Disseminated intravascular coagulation, 328-331
Distention cystocele, 167
Ditropan; *see* Oxybutynin chloride
Diuretics
 for hypertension, 591-592
 for pseudotumor cerebri, 582
 thiazide, for osteoporosis, 123
Divalproex sodium
 for mood disorders, 103-105
 side effects of, 104
 use in pregnancy of, 106
Dizygotic pregnancy, 459-461
DNA analysis to screen for genetic diseases, 256
DNA linkage analysis to screen for genetic diseases, 256
Dobbhoff tube, 613
Domestic violence, 572-577
Dong quai for menopausal symptoms, 113
Donor sperm insemination for male factor infertility, 79
Dopamine
 low levels of, hyperprolactinemia caused by, 6
 for neonatal depression, 494
Doppler ultrasound, 266-271
 to diagnose thromboembolism, 421
 to diagnose varicose veins, 644
Doppler velocimetry for antenatal testing, 285
Down syndrome, 251-252
 prenatal diagnosis of, 243
Doxazosin for hypertension, 592
Doxorubicin
 for endometrial stromal sarcoma of uterus, 215
 for sex cord–stromal tumors, 133
 for uterine leiomyosarcoma, 215
Doxycycline
 for chlamydial infection, 89
 for lymphogranuloma venereum, 86
 for pelvic inflammatory disease, 144

Doxycycline–cont'd
for syphilis, 85
teratogenic effects of, 247-248
Drainage for tuboovarian abscess, 145
Drug-induced lupus, 550
Dual energy x-ray absorptiometry (DEXA) to diagnose osteoporosis, 117
Ductal carcinoma in situ of breast, 11
noninvasive, treatment of, 15, 17
Ducts, plugged, with breastfeeding, diagnosis and treatment of, 478
Duodenal atresia, ultrasonography to detect, 279, 280
Duodenal ulcer; *see* Peptic ulcer disease
D-xylose test to diagnose cause of diarrhea, 568
Dysgerminomas, ovarian, 131, 132
Dysmature placenta, 438
Dysmenorrhea, 41-44
Dyspepsia, non-ulcer, 578, 579
Dysplastic lesions of cervix, high-grade, diagnosis and treatment of, 135, 136
Dyspnea of pregnancy, 295
Dyssexualis history, 156-157, 158
Dysthymic disorder, 97, 98; *see also* Mood disorders
diagnosis of, 100

E

Early decelerations in fetal heart rate, 467
Echinococcal disease, 346
Echocardiography to diagnose heart disease in pregnancy, 305
Eclampsia, 430-436; *see also* Preeclampsia
headache with, 582
incidence of, 355
Ectopic pregnancy, 44-52
future reproductive outcome after, 50
nontubal, 51
pelvic inflammatory disease causing, 146
persistent, 50
risk factors associated with, 45
sites of, 45
Ectopic prolactin production, hyperprolactinemia caused by, 6
Effexor; *see* Venlafaxine
Efudex; *see* 5-Fluorouracil
Ehlers-Danlos syndrome, 253
Eisenmenger syndrome complicating pregnancy, 308
Elavil; *see* Amitriptyline
Electrical stimulation of pelvic floor muscles for stress incontinence, 192
Electrocardiography to diagnose heart disease in pregnancy, 305
Electroconvulsive therapy for mood disorders, 105
Electromyography to diagnose idiopathic inflammatory myopathies, 552
Electrophoresis, hemoglobin, 256
Electrotherapy for condyloma, 89
Elemental diets, 614
ELISA to diagnose HIV, 499
Embolism
amniotic fluid, 446-447
pulmonary, 419; *see also* Thromboembolic disease
Embolization for uterine inversion, 449
Embryonic period, teratogen exposure during, 245
Embryopathy, retinoic acid, 247
Emergencies, medical, in obstetrics, 442-450
Emergency contraception, 40
Emulsions, lipid, for parenteral nutrition, 615-616
Enalapril
for hypertension, 589
teratogenic effects of, 248
Encephalocele, ultrasonography to detect, 276
Encephalomyopathy, mitochondrial, 253
End-organ defects
as cause of amenorrhea, 6-7
treatment of, 9
End-stage renal disease, hypertension and, 587
Endocarditis, bacterial, during pregnancy, prophylaxis against, 305
Endocrine abnormalities during pregnancy, 315-320
Endocrine changes in pregnancy, 230-231
Endometrial ablation
for adenomyosis, 205

Endometrial ablation–cont'd
for coagulation defects, 205
Endometrial biopsy
to diagnose pelvic inflammatory disease, 141
in evaluation of ovulation, 79
Endometrial carcinomas of uterus, 209-214
Endometrial sampling, for postmenopausal bleeding, 206
Endometrial stromal sarcoma, uterine, 215
Endometrioma, 151, 152
of ovary, 53
therapy for, 154
Endometriosis, 52-55
causing chronic pelvic pain, 160
diagnosis of, 53
differential diagnosis of, 53
dysmenorrhea caused by, 42
pathophysiology of, 52-53
symptoms and treatment of, 204
treatment of, 43, 53-54
Endometritis; *see also* Pelvic inflammatory disease
postpartum, 234
symptoms and treatment of, 204
Endometrium, adenocarcinoma of, estrogen replacement therapy and, 94
Endoscopic retrograde cholangiopancreatography, 350
Endoscopy
for bleeding peptic ulcer, 625
to diagnose cause of diarrhea, 568
to diagnose peptic ulcer disease, 620
Endotracheal intubation
causing hoarseness, 605
elective, indications for, 494
for neonatal depression, 493
Energy requirements, 609
Engorgement, treatment of, 478
Enoxacin for gonorrhea, 88
Enteral alimentation, 613-614
Enteral tube feeding, 613
Enterocele, 169-170
Enteropathic arthritis, 533
Enthesopathy, 532
Environmental agents, teratogenic effects of, 250
Enzyme blockers for ovarian hyperandrogenism, 71
Enzyme defects, hirsutism caused by, 64, 67
Enzyme immunoassay to diagnose chlamydia, 88
Eosinophilic fasciitis, 551
Eosinophilic gastritis, 579
Ephedrine for stress incontinence, 191
Epidural anesthesia
for cesarean section, 473
for labor, 472
for pregnant woman with cardiac problems, 305
Epidural block for vaginal delivery, 472
Epiglottitis causing hoarseness, 604
Epilepsy, myoclonus, 253
Epinephrine
for asthma, 446
during pregnancy, 297
for hoarseness, 604
for neonatal depression, 493
Episiotomy, care of, 234
infections at site of, 234-235
Epithelial ovarian cancer, 125-131
Epivir; *see* Lamivudine
Epstein-Barr virus, pharyngitis and, 602
Ergotamine
for migraine headache, 585
for uterine atony, 448
Erosion, peptic ulcer, 617-618
Erosive gastritis, acute, 578
Eruptions, polymorphic, of pregnancy; *see* Pruritic urticarial papules and plaques of pregnancy
Erythema infectiosum, 370
Erythroblastosis, 413, 414; *see also* Alloimmunization
Erythromycin
for chancroid, 83
for chlamydial infection, 89, 90
for lymphogranuloma venereum, 86
for mastitis, 480
for pharyngitis, 603
for pneumonia, 630, 631-632
during pregnancy, 299
Erythropoietin, hypertension caused by, 587
Esophagitis, reflux, 614
Esophagogastroduodenoscopy/enteroscopy to diagnose cause of diarrhea, 568
Essential fatty acids, 608
Essential hypertension, 587

Essential nutrients, 608
Estimated date of confinement (EDC), calculation of, 232-233
Estrace
  for hormone replacement therapy, 96
  to prevent osteoporosis, 93
Estraderm
  for hormone replacement therapy, 96
  to prevent osteoporosis, 93
Estradiol
  for hormone replacement therapy, 96
  measurement of, in evaluation of amenorrhea, 4
  in menstrual cycle, 3
  for premenstrual syndrome, 176
Estrogen
  for anovulatory bleeding, 202
    in adolescent, 201
  for contraceptive-related bleeding, 203
  endogenous, production of, evaluation of, in evaluation of amenorrhea, 4
  for hormone replacement therapy, 96
  hyperprolactinemia caused by, 6
  for irregular bleeding with Depo-Provera or Norplant, 205
  for midcycle bleeding, 204
  for perimenopausal bleeding, 206
  for stress incontinence, 191
  for urge incontinence, 195
Estrogen replacement therapy, 93-94
  complications of, 94-95
  for hypoestrogenic anovulation/amenorrhea, 9
  to prevent osteoporosis, 119-120
  to prevent vaginal prolapse, 170
Ethanol, teratogenic effects of, 246
Ethnic groups at risk for genetic diseases, 255
Etidronate for osteoporosis, 120, 121
Etoposide
  for ovarian germ cell tumors, 132
  for sex cord–stromal tumors, 133
Etretinate, teratogenic effects of, 247
Evacuation
  by suction curettage to treat hydatidiform mole, 56
  to treat partial mole, 59
Examination
  annual, 506-518; *see also* Annual examination
  bimanual, procedure for, 515-516
  breast, 511
  neurologic, in diagnosis of cause of backache, 538
  physical, annual, 511-516; *see also* Annual examination
Excisional biopsy to diagnose breast cancer, 13, 14
Exenteration, pelvic, for recurrent cervical cancer, 32-33
Exercise
  Kegel; *see* Kegel exercises
  pelvic floor muscle
    for mixed urinary incontinence, 195
    for stress incontinence, 191-192
    for urge incontinence, 195
  for premenstrual syndrome, 176
  to prevent osteoporosis, 119
  strenuous, amenorrhea caused by, 6
  weight maintenance and, 112
External cephalic version, 453-454
External genitalia, examination of, 511
Extrapelvic disease, advanced, therapy for, 32
Extrauterine life, adaptation of infant to, 490
Extremities, fetal, ultrasonographic evaluation of, 263

F

Face presentation, 455-457
Facial migraines, 583
Factor IX levels, measurement of, as carrier screening test, 256
Factor VIII levels, measurement of, as carrier screening test, 256
Fallopian tube
  ectopic pregnancy in, 44-45
  pregnancy in; *see* Ectopic pregnancy
  reconstructive surgery of, as risk factor for ectopic pregnancy, 45
  rupture of, from ectopic pregnancy, 45, 46
Famciclovir for herpes simplex virus prophylaxis, 503

Familial hypercholesterolemia, ethnic groups at risk for, 255
Familial ovarian cancer syndromes, 126
Family pedigree, genetic diseases and, 254
Famotidine for peptic ulcer disease, 623
Fasciitis, eosinophilic, 551
Fasting glucose test, indications for, 517
Fat, 608
Fatty acids, essential, 608
Fatty liver of pregnancy, acute, 345, 364
Feeding, enteral tube, 613
Feeding tubes, 613-614
Felodipine for hypertension, 591
Female factor infertility, therapeutic considerations for, 80
Female orgasmic disorder, 182
Female sexual arousal disorder, 181
Female sterilization, 184-185
Feminization, testicular
  amenorrhea caused by, 7
  treatment of, 9
Femoral neck fractures, 93
Femur, fetal, length of
  ratio of, to abdominal circumference to diagnose intrauterine growth restriction, 427
  ultrasonographic evaluation of, 263, 264
Fentanyl for spinal anesthesia for labor, 471
Fertilization, in vitro
  for infertility, 81-82
  for male factor infertility, 80
Fetal alcohol effect, 246
Fetal alcohol syndrome, 246, 487
Fetal carbamazepine syndrome, 249
Fetal distress, 467
Fetal hydantoin syndrome, 249
Fetal karyotype to diagnose intrauterine growth restriction, 428
Fetal lie, 450-451
Fetal tachycardia, paroxysmal, 467
Fetal tone, scoring for, 267
Fetal valproate syndrome, 249
Fetal warfarin syndrome, 246
Fetal-maternal hemorrhage causing alloimmunization, 413
Fetoscopic and ultrasonographic fetal sampling to screen for birth defects, 244
Fetus
  abdomen of, ultrasonographic evaluation of, 279-281
  acidosis of, heart rate abnormalities indicating, 469
  anatomic evaluation of, using ultrasound, 261
  breathing movements of, scoring for, 267
  breech, 451-454
  cardiac activity of, ultrasonographic visualization of, 260
  cardiac arrhythmias of, ultrasonography to detect, 278-279
  of chronic hypertensive mother, antenatal evaluation of, 356
  congenital infections of, 366-373
  evaluation of
    with fetal heart rate monitoring, 467-469
    in preeclampsia/eclampsia, 433
  extremities of, ultrasonographic evaluation of, 263
  fetoscopic and ultrasonographic sampling of, to screen for birth defects, 244
  fibronectin from, in cervicovaginal secretions, assay for
    to diagnose preterm labor, 390
    to diagnose preterm PROM, 394
  gross body movements of, scoring for, 267
  head, ultrasonographic evaluation of, 261-263
  heart of, ultrasonographic evaluation of, 276, 278-279
  heart block of, 467
  heart rate of
    abnormalities in, 467
      treatment of, 469
    monitoring of, 466-470
    scoring for, 267
    variability of, 467
  malpresentation of, 450-458
  metastatic lesions to, complicating pregnancy, 292
  monitoring of, during labor in postterm/postdate pregnancy, 441
  movement of, counting, 283
  position of, 451
  presentation of, 451
Fever, Pontiac, 631

Fiber, need for, during menopause, 111
Fiberoptic endoscopy to diagnose peptic ulcer disease, 620
Fibrinogen for placental abruption, 406-407
Fibrinolytics for thromboembolism during pregnancy, 423
Fibroadenoma, 14-15
  breast, 22
Fibrocystic changes in breast, 23
Fibrocystic mastopathy, 14-15
Fibroid(s)
  cervical, causing third trimester bleeding, 410
  ovulatory bleeding caused by, 203
  submucous, causing infertility, therapy for, 80
Fibroma, ovarian, 132
Fibromyalgia causing arthritis, 535
Fibronectin, fetal, in cervicovaginal secretions, assay for
  to diagnose preterm labor, 390
  to diagnose preterm PROM, 394
"Fifth" disease, 370
FIGO; *see* International Federation of Obstetrics and Gynecology
Finasteride for hirsutism, 73
Fine-needle aspiration to diagnose breast cancer, 13
First trimester, ultrasound examination in, 259-260
FISH; *see* Fluorescence in situ hybridization
Fistulas, arteriovenous, uterine, bleeding caused by, symptoms and treatment of, 205
Fitz-Hugh–Curtis syndrome, 142-143
Florinef for adrenal insufficiency, 319
Fluconazole for candidiasis, 87
Fluorescence in situ hybridization to diagnose genetic diseases, 254, 256
Fluorescent treponemal antibody-absorbed (FTA-ABS) test to diagnose syphilis, 84
Fluoride for osteoporosis, 120, 121-122
Fluoroquinolones
  teratogenic effects of, 248
  for urinary tract infections, 562
5-Fluorouracil
  for advanced pelvic disease, 32
  for choriocarcinoma, 61-62
  for condyloma, 89
5-Fluorouracil–cont'd
  for invasive breast cancer, 18
  for metastatic breast disease, 19
  for papillomavirus infections, 138
Fluoxetine
  for mood disorders, 102-103
  for obsessive-compulsive disorder, 521
  orgasmic disorder caused by, 182
  for premenstrual syndrome, 173, 176
  use in pregnancy of, 106
Fluvoxamine
  for obsessive-compulsive disorder, 521
  for panic disorders with or without agoraphobia, 523
Focal nodular hyperplasia of liver, 347
Focal vulvitis causing chronic pelvic pain, 161
Folate supplements during pregnancy, 238
Folic acid deficiency, 322-323
Folic acid supplementation for multiple gestations, 464
Follicle-stimulating hormone
  measurement of, in evaluation of amenorrhea, 4
  in menstrual cycle, 3
Follicular cysts of ovary, 149
  therapy for, 154
Follicular therapy for hirsutism, 72-73
Foot
  club, 253
  fetal, ultrasonographic evaluation of, 263
Foot drop, 537
Footling breech, 451, 452
Foreign bodies causing uterine bleeding in childhood and adolescence, 200
45,X, 251
45,X gonadal dysgenesis, ovarian failure caused by, 9
46,XX syndrome, amenorrhea caused by, 7
Foscarnet for herpes simplex virus prophylaxis, 503
Fosinopril for hypertension, 589
Fossa, posterior, fetal, ultrasonographic evaluation of, 262, 263
Four-chamber view to evaluate fetal heart, 263, 264, 276, 278

Fractures
femoral neck, 93
sacral, osteoporotic, causing chronic pelvic pain, 161
Fragile X syndrome, 253
Frank breech, 451, 452
Free thyroxine index
to diagnose hyperthyroidism, 636
to diagnose hypothyroidism, 641
5-FU; *see* 5-Fluorouracil
Full-liquid diet, 613
Functional bowel disease, 566-567
Functional cysts, symptoms and treatment of, 204
Functional ovarian cyst, 149, 150
therapy for, 154
Fungal infections, prophylaxis for, 503
Furosemide for hypertension, 592

G

Galactorrhea, 24
Galactosemia, treatment of, 256
Gallbladder disease, 350
Gallstone disease; *see* Cholecystitis
Gamete intrafallopian transfer
for infertility, 81-82
for male factor infertility, 80
Ganciclovir for prophylaxis for cytomegalovirus
Gastric outlet obstruction from peptic ulcer disease, 626
Gastric ulcer; *see* Peptic ulcer disease
Gastrin, serum, level of, to diagnose peptic ulcer disease, 620, 622
Gastrinoma, 620
conditions associated with, 622
Gastritis
alkaline-reflux, 579
atrophic, chronic, 579
bile, 579
chronic, 579
chronic active, 578
chronic and acute, 578-580
eosinophilic, 579
erosive, acute, 578
granulomatous, 579-580
hypertrophic, 579
nonerosive, acute, 578
superficial, chronic, 579
type A, 579
type AB, 579
type B, 579
Gastritis–cont'd
type C, 579
Gastroesophageal reflux disease, 348
causing hoarseness, 604
Gastrointestinal bypass, pregnancy and, 349
Gastrointestinal changes in pregnancy, 229-230
Gastrointestinal disease in pregnancy, 347-351
evaluation of, 342
Gastrojejunostomy for bile gastritis, 579
Gastropathy, portal hypertensive, 580
Gastroschisis
screening for, 242
ultrasonography to detect, 279, 280
Gastrostomy tube, 614
Gaucher's disease, ethnic groups at risk for, 255
Gene transfer therapy, 256
General anesthesia for cesarean delivery, 473-474
Generalized anxiety disorder, 523-524
Generalized type sexual dysfunction, 179
Genetic amniocentesis, 243
Genetic counseling, common indications for, 241
Genetic diseases
diagnosis of, 254-256
ethnic groups at risk for, 255
family pedigree in diagnosis of, 254
karyotype in diagnosis of, 254, 256
laboratory assessment in diagnosis of, 254, 256
nonclassic patterns in, 253
physical examination in diagnosis of, 254
treatment of, 256
types of, 251-253
Genetics, 251-257
Genital tract, lower, infections of, 83-90
Genital trauma, treatment of, 449
Genital warts, 90, 134; *see also* Papillomavirus infections
Genitalia, external, examination of, 511
Genitofemoral nerve disorders causing chronic pelvic pain, 159
Gentamicin
for acute pyelonephritis, 360
for pelvic inflammatory disease, 144

Geophagia during pregnancy, 239
Germ cell tumors
  causing uterine bleeding in childhood and adolescence, 200
  of ovary, 131-132
Gestational age, estimation of, using ultrasonography, 261
Gestational diabetes mellitus, 310-315
Gestational sac, ultrasonographic visualization of, 259
Gestational thrombocytopenia, 327
Gestational trophoblastic disease, 55-63
  hyperthyroidism caused by, 316
  morphologic diagnosis of, 56-62
Gestational trophoblastic neoplasia
  management of, 57, 59
  recurrent, 62-63
Gestations, multiple, 459-466
Giant cell arteritis, 555
Ginseng for menopausal symptoms, 113
Gittes urethropexy for stress incontinence, 192
Globulin
  immune, intravenous
    for immune thrombocytopenic purpura, 328
    for neonatal alloimmune thrombocytopenia, 328
  Rh immune, for alloimmunization, 416-418
  steroid hormone binding, 64
Glomerulonephritis
  chronic, pregnancy and, 362
  poststreptococcal, pharyngitis and, 601
Glucocorticoid replacement therapy for adrenal hyperandrogenemia, 72
Glucocorticoids
  for immune thrombocytopenic purpura, 327
  for rheumatoid arthritis, 529-530
Glucola test for multiple gestation, 464
Glucose for diabetic ketoacidosis, 443, 444
Glucose-galactose transporter deficiency causing osmotic diarrhea, 565
Glycerol, iodinated, for laryngitis, 606
Glycogen, 608
GOG; *see* Gynecologic Oncology Group
Goiter, 635, 640, 641
  toxic nodular, causing hyperthyroidism, 316
Gold salts for rheumatoid arthritis, 530
Gonadal dysgenesis, amenorrhea caused by, 7
Gonadectomy, 9
Gonadotropin(s)
  chorionic; *see* Human chorionic gonadotropin
  deficiency of, amenorrhea caused by, 6
  for hypoestrogenic anovulation, 9
  for male factor infertility, 80
Gonadotropin-releasing hormone
  for hypoestrogenic anovulation, 9
  to induce ovulation, 81
  in menstrual cycle, 3
Gonadotropin-releasing hormone agonists
  for coagulation defects, 205
  for endometriosis, 204
  for leiomyoma, 204
  for ovarian hyperandrogenism, 71
  for ovulatory bleeding in reproductive age women, 203
  for premenstrual syndrome, 176
  for treatment of endometriosis, 54
Gonadotropin-resistant ovary syndrome, amenorrhea caused by, 7, 8
Gonococcal pharyngitis, 601
Gonorrhea, 87
  pelvic inflammatory disease and, 142, 143
  treatment of, 88
Gonorrhea cultures, 515
Gottron's papules, 552
Gout, 530-531
Gouty arthritis, 530
Gouty nephropathy, 530
Granulomatosis, Wegener's, 555, 556
  pregnancy and, 362
Granulomatous gastritis, 579-580
Granulomatous lesions, hyperprolactinemia caused by, 6
Granulosa cell tumors, 132
  causing uterine bleeding in childhood and adolescence, 200
Graves' disease, 635
  causing hyperthyroidism, 316

Gross body movements, fetal, scoring for, 267
Group A β-hemolytic streptococcus, pharyngitis and, 599-601
Group B β-hemolytic streptococcus, congenital infection with, 372-373
Growth, intrauterine, restriction of, 426-430
Guaifenesin for laryngitis, 606
Guanabenz for hypertension, 592
Guanethidine for hypertension, 592
Guanfacine for hypertension, 592
Gynandroblastoma, 132
Gynecologic Oncology Group on staging of gynecologic cancer, 27

H

H_2 breath test to diagnose cause of diarrhea, 568
H_2 receptor antagonists for peptic ulcer disease, 623
Haemophilus ducreyi infection of vulva, 83
Haemophilus influenzae causing pneumonia, 630-631
Hair changes during pregnancy, 376
HAIR-AN syndrome, 66
  therapy for, 71
Hallucinogen abuse during pregnancy, 488; *see also* Substance abuse
Haloperidol, hyperprolactinemia caused by, 6
Hands, fetal, ultrasonographic evaluation of, 263
Hashimoto's thyroiditis, Turner's syndrome with, 9
Head, fetal
  circumference of, ultrasonographic evaluation of, 261
  ultrasonographic evaluation of, 261-263
Headache(s), 581-586
  caffeine withdrawal, 583, 584
  cluster, 584
  migraine, 582, 583
  sinus, 582
  spinal, 581
  tension, 582
  vascular, 582
Health promotion screening and review, 516
Heart, fetal, ultrasonographic evaluation of, 263, 276, 278-279
Heart block, fetal, 467
Heart disease
  congenital, ultrasonography to detect, 276
  rheumatic, complicating pregnancy, 307
Heart rate, fetal
  monitoring of, 466-470
  scoring for, 267
  variability in, 67
Heartburn during pregnancy, management of, 238-239
Heberden's nodes, 527
Helicobacter pylori, tests for detection of, 622
Helicobacter pylori infection
  peptic ulcer disease caused by, 618-619
  treatment regimens for, 624
HELLP syndrome, 344
  DIC caused by, 330
Hemagglutinin in influenza virus, 594
Hemangiomas, hepatic, 346
Hematemesis, 625
Hematologic changes in pregnancy, 227
Hematologic complications during pregnancy, 320-331
Hematoma
  liver, 344-345
  pyramidal muscle, causing chronic pelvic pain, 160
Hemicrania, paroxysmal, 584
Hemodynamic monitoring to diagnose heart disease in pregnancy, 305
Hemoglobin A_1, 323
Hemoglobin A_2, 323
Hemoglobin AS, 324
Hemoglobin electrophoresis, 256
Hemoglobin F, 323
Hemoglobin S, 324-326
Hemoglobin SS, 324
Hemoglobin testing, indications for, 517
Hemoglobinopathies during pregnancy, 323-326
Hemophilia A, treatment of, 256
Hemorrhage
  fetal-maternal, causing alloimmunization, 413

Hemorrhage–cont'd
postpartum, 447-449
after delivery of multiple gestations, 465
uterovaginal, severe, management of, 206, 207
Hemorrhagic corpus luteum cyst, 149, 150, 151
Heparin
breastfeeding and maternal use of, 481
for thromboembolism during pregnancy, 422-423, 424
Hepatic disease in pregnancy, 341-347
Hepatitis, viral
acute, during pregnancy, 345-346
chronic, pregnancy and, 346
Hepatitis A during pregnancy, 345-346
Hepatitis A vaccine, guidelines for adult immunization with, 374
Hepatitis B
congenital infection with, 370-371
during pregnancy, 345
Hepatitis B immunoglobulin, 345
Hepatitis B infection causing arthritis, 534
Hepatitis B vaccine, guidelines for adult immunization with, 374
Hepatitis C, 346
Hepatitis immune globulin, 371
Hepatocellular carcinoma, primary, 347
Hepatoiminodiacetic acid scan for cholecystitis, 546
Herbs for menopausal symptoms, 113
Herniated disc, 537, 538
Herpes gestationis, 378, 379-380
neonatal, 380
Herpes gestationis factor, 379
Herpes simplex virus infections
congenital, 368-369
pharyngitis and, 602
prophylaxis for, 503
of vulva, 83-84
Herpes virus, vulvar cancer and, 217
Herpes zoster, 369-370
headache with, 581
Hexosaminidase A activity, 256
HGSIL; *see* Cervix, high-grade squamous intraepithelial lesions of
Hilus cell tumors
hirsutism with, 67
therapy for, 72
Hip joints in diagnosis of cause of backache, 538
Hirsutism, 64-74
in pregnancy, 376
History
patient, 511
sexual, 516
HIV testing, 499
indications for, 499, 517
HIV-infected patient, management of, 500
Hivid; *see* Zalcitabine
HLA-B27 antigen study to diagnose cause of backache, 538-539
HMG; *see* Human menopausal gonadotropin
Hoarseness, 604
laryngitis and, 603-606
Homans' sign to diagnose thromboembolism, 420
Homeopathy for menopausal symptoms, 113
Hormonal preparations causing mood disorders, 98-99
Hormonal therapy for metastatic breast disease, 19
Hormone(s)
androgenic, teratogenic effects of, 248
follicle-stimulating
measurement of, in evaluation of amenorrhea, 4
in menstrual cycle, 3
gonadotropin releasing; *see* Gonadotropin-releasing hormone
luteinizing
measurement of, in evaluation of amenorrhea, 4
in menstrual cycle, 3
thyroid-releasing, hyperprolactinemia caused by, 6
thyroid-stimulating; *see* Thyroid-stimulating hormone
Hormone replacement therapy, 93-95
Hormone therapy for invasive breast cancer, 18-19
Hormone-producing tumors causing uterine bleeding in childhood and adolescence, 200
Horsetail for menopausal symptoms, 113

Hospital diets, 613
Hot flashes, 93
Human chorionic gonadotropin, high levels of, hydatidiform mole associated with, 56
Human immunodeficiency virus infection, 499; *see also* Acquired immunodeficiency syndrome
  congenital, 372
  during pregnancy, special considerations with, 504
Human menopausal gonadotropin
  for anovulation, 8, 80
  to induce ovulation, 81
  multiple ovulation induced by, as risk factor for ectopic pregnancy, 45
Human papillomavirus, 134; *see also* Papillomavirus infections
Humerus, fetal, length of, ultrasonographic evaluation of, 263
Huntington's disease, 253
Hydantoin, teratogenic effects of, 249
Hydatid of Morgagni, 153
  therapy for, 155
Hydatidiform mole, 56-59
Hydralazine
  for chronic hypertension during pregnancy, 355, 356
  for hypertension, 592
  for preeclampsia/eclampsia, 344, 432
Hydrocephalus, ultrasonography to detect, 273, 274
Hydrochlorothiazide for hypertension, 591
Hydrocodone for headache, 584
Hydrocortisone for asthma, 446
Hydronephrosis, 360
Hydrophilic agents for diarrhea, 569
Hydrops fetalis, 414
Hydroureter, 360
Hydroxychloroquine, fetal effects of, 340
11β-Hydroxylase deficiency, hirsutism caused by, 64, 67
21-Hydroxylase deficiency, hirsutism caused by, 64, 67, 69
3β-Hydroxysteroid dehydrogenase, hirsutism caused by, 64, 67
Hydroxyurea for advanced pelvic disease, 32
Hydroxyzine
  during labor, 471
  for PUPPP syndrome, 381
Hymen, imperforate
  amenorrhea caused by, 7
  treatment of, 9
Hymenal syndrome causing chronic pelvic pain, 159
Hyoscyamine for urge incontinence, 195
Hyperactivity, detrusor, with impaired contractions, 193; *see also* Urge incontinence
Hyperandrogenemia, ovarian, therapy for, 69, 71-72
Hyperandrogenic chronic anovulation, hirsutism caused by, 64
Hyperandrogenism, treatment of, 8
Hypercholesterolemia, familial, ethnic groups at risk for, 255
Hypercoagulability of pregnancy, 227
Hyperemesis, hydatidiform mole associated with, 56
Hyperemesis gravidarum, 347-348
Hypergastrinemic conditions, 622
Hyperlordosis, 539
Hyperosmolarity syndrome, 614
Hyperparathyroidism during pregnancy, 317
Hyperpigmentation during pregnancy, 375-376
Hyperplasia
  adrenal, causing anovulatory bleeding, 202
  nodular, focal, of liver, 347
Hyperprolactinemia
  amenorrhea caused by, 4, 6
Hyperreflexia, detrusor, 193; *see also* Urge incontinence
Hypersensitivity vasculitis, 556
Hypertension, 586-594
  chronic, during pregnancy, 351-358
    antepartum fetal evaluation in mother with, 356
    diagnosis of, 352-353
    labor and delivery considerations for, 356
    pathophysiology and blood pressure regulation for, 352
    postpartum considerations for 356-357
    therapy and management of, 353-355, 356
  pulmonary, complicating pregnancy, 308
  renal disease and, 363
  secondary, 587, 588

Hypertensive gastropathy, portal, 580
Hyperthecosis, hirsutism caused by, 64
Hyperthyroidism, 634-639
  in pregnancy, 316
Hypertrophic gastritis, 579
Hypoactive sexual desire disorder, 179-181
Hypoestrogenic anovulation/amenorrhea, 6
Hypoglycemics, oral, for ovarian hyperandrogenism, 71
Hypogonadism as cause of amenorrhea, 6
Hypomanic episode, diagnosis of, 100
Hypoparathyroidism during pregnancy, 317
Hypoplastic left heart syndrome, ultrasonography to detect, 278
Hypothalamus
  dysfunction of, amenorrhea caused by, 6
  evaluation of, in evaluation of amenorrhea, 4
  tumor of, amenorrhea caused by, 6
Hypothyroidism, 639-643
  anovulatory bleeding caused by, 202
  congenital, treatment of, 256
  hyperprolactinemia caused by, 6
  in pregnancy, 316-317
Hysterectomy
  for adenomyosis, 205
  for benign pelvic masses, 155
  for bulky cervical disease, 31
  for chorioadenoma destruens, 60
  for early stage invasive cervical cancer, 30-31
  for endometrial carcinomas of uterus, 211
  for endometriosis, 54
  for hydatidiform mole, 57
  for invasive cervical carcinoma complicating pregnancy, 290
  for leiomyoma, 204
  for microinvasive cervical cancer, 30
  for ovulatory bleeding in reproductive age women, 203
  for recurrent cervical cancer, 32-33
  for uterine arteriovenous fistulas, 205
Hysterectomy–cont'd
  for uterine inversion, 449
  for uterine prolapse, 169
  for vaginal cancer, 223
Hysterosalpingography to evaluate tubal patency, 77
Hysteroscopy
  to evaluate tubal patency, 78
  for intrauterine synechiae or submucous fibroids, 80
  for leiomyoma, 204
Hysterotomy to treat partial mole, 59

I

Iatrogenic thyrotoxicosis, 635
Ibuprofen
  for mastitis, 480
  for systemic lupus erythematosus, 550
"Ice" abuse during pregnancy, 488; *see also* Substance abuse
Idiopathic hirsutism, 69
Idiopathic inflammatory myopathies, 552-553
Idiopathic postpartum renal failure, 364
Ifosfamide, 215
Ilioinguinal and iliohypogastric nerve disturbances causing chronic pelvic pain, 159
Imaging studies in diagnosis of cause of backache, 539-540
Imipramine
  for mixed urinary incontinence, 195
  for mood disorders, 103
  for panic disorders with or without agoraphobia, 523
  for posttraumatic stress disorder, 524
  for urge incontinence, 195
Imitrex; *see* Sumatriptan
Immune globulin, intravenous, 328
Immune thrombocytopenic purpura, 327-328
Immunizations
  adult, 373
  perinatal, 366-375
Immunodeficiency virus, human; *see* Human immunodeficiency virus
Immunoglobulin
  for hepatitis A, 346
  hepatitis B, 345

Immunoglobulin A nephropathy, pregnancy and, 362
Immunosuppressants, fetal effects of, 340-341
Immunotherapy for condyloma, 89
Impedance plethysmography to diagnose thromboembolism, 421
Imperforate hymen
amenorrhea caused by, 7
treatment of, 9
Impetigo herpetiformis, 378, 383
Implants, brachytherapy, for advanced pelvic disease, 31-32
In vitro fertilization
for infertility, 81-82
for male factor infertility, 80
Inclusion body myositis, 552
Incompatibiity, ABO, 413; *see also* Alloimmunization
Incompetent cervix; *see* Cervical competence, abnormal
Incomplete breech, 451, 452
Incontinence
overflow, 196
stress, 189-192; *see also* Stress incontinence
urge, 192-195; *see also* Urge incontinence
urinary, 186-189; *see also* Urinary incontinence
mixed, 195
Indapamide for hypertension, 591
Indicated preterm delivery, 387-388
Indinavir for HIV therapy, 503
Indomethacin
for cluster headache, 584
for preterm labor, protocol for, 391, 393
for rheumatoid arthritis, 529
Infant
adaptation of, to extrauterine life, 490
low-birth-weight, 384
very-low-birth-weight, 384
morbidity in, 386
Infarction
cerebral, hypertension and, 587
myocardial, complicating pregnancy, 306
Infection(s)
cervical, 87-90
congenital, 366-373
episiotomy, 234-235
fungal, prophylaxis for, 503
Infection(s)–cont'd
herpes simplex virus; *see* Herpes simplex virus infections
HIV, 499; *see also* Acquired immunodeficiency syndrome
management of, 500
in pregnancy, special considerations with, 504
lower genital tract, 83-98
opportunistic, with AIDS, prophylaxis for, 502-503
papillomavirus; *see* Papillomavirus infections
perinatal, 366-375
urinary tract, 558-563; *see also* Urinary tract infections
during pregnancy, 358-360
vaginal, 86-87
of vulva, ulcerative, 83-86
wound, after cesarean delivery, 234
yeast, wet mount to diagnose, 515
Infectious arthritis, 533-534
Infectious mononucleosis, pharyngitis and, 602
Infertile couple
factors affecting, 75; *see also* Infertility
history and examination of, 76
Infertility, 74-82
pelvic inflammatory disease causing, 146
Inflammation of breast, 23-24
Inflammatory bowel disease, 349-350, 566
Inflammatory diarrhea, 566
Inflammatory disease, pelvic; *see* Pelvic inflammatory disease
Inflammatory myopathies, idiopathic, 552-553
Influenza, 594-598
Influenza vaccine, guidelines for adult immunization with, 374
Influenza virus, 594
causing pneumonia, 633
Influenzal pneumonia, primary, 595
Inhalation analgesia for vaginal delivery, 473
Injection, intracytoplasmic sperm, for male factor infertility, 80
Insemination
donor sperm, for male factor infertility, 79
intrauterine
for infertility, 79-81

Insertion, velamentous, 410
Inspection to find cause of backache, 537
Instability, pelvic joint, causing chronic pelvic pain, 160
Insulin for diabetic ketoacidosis, 443-444
Insulin levels, diagnosis of causes of hirsutism using, 70
Interferon
  for condyloma, 89
  for papillomavirus infections, 138
Intermittent auscultation for fetal heart rate monitoring, 466-467
International Continence Society Committee on Standardization of Terminology classification of vaginal prolapse, 164, 165
International Federation of Obstetrics and Gynecology definitions for staging of gynecologic cancer, 26, 27
International Reference Standard test for ectopic pregnancy, 47
Interorbital diameter of fetus, ultrasonographic evaluation of, 263
Intracytoplasmic sperm injection
  for infertility, 81-82
  for male factor infertility, 80
Intraductal tumors of breast, 11
Intraepithelial lesions, squamous
  high-grade, of cervix, diagnosis and treatment of, 135, 136
  low-grade, of cervix, diagnosis and treatment of, 135-137
Intrafallopian transfer
  gamete
    for infertility, 81-82
    for male factor infertility, 80
  zygote, for infertility, 81-82
Intrahepatic cholestasis of pregnancy, 341, 343
Intraperitoneal ^{32}P for ovarian cancer, 129
Intrathecal narcotics for labor, 471-472
Intrauterine device for contraception, 38-39
  as risk factor for ectopic pregnancy, 45
Intrauterine growth restriction, 426-430
Intrauterine insemination
  for infertility, 79-81
Intrauterine synechiae causing infertility, therapy for, 80
Intrauterine transfusion for alloimmunization, 415
Intravascular coagulation, disseminated, 328-331
Intrinsic urethral sphincter deficiency, 190
  surgery for, 192
Intubation, endotracheal
  elective, indications for, 494
  hoarseness caused by, 605
  for neonatal depression, 493
Invasive carcinoma of breast, treatment of, 17-19
Invasive cervical cancer, early stage, therapy for, 30-31
Invasive cervical carcinoma complicating pregnancy, 290, 291
Invasive malignant breast disease, 11
Invasive mole, 59-60; *see also* Chorioadenoma destruens
Inversion, uterine, treatment of, 449
Inverted nipple, 476
Invirase; *see* Saquinavir
Iodides, breastfeeding and maternal use of, 480
Iodine, radioactive
  for hyperthyroidism, 637-638
  teratogenic effects of, 249
Iodine-induced hyperthyroidism, 635
Iron deficiency anemia during pregnancy, 320-322
Iron supplementation
  for multiple gestations, 464
  during pregnancy, 237-238
Irritable bowel syndrome, 348, 566-567
  treatment of, 571
Isoetharine for asthma, 446
Isoflavonoids for menopausal symptoms, 113
Isometheptene for migraine headache, 585
Isoniazid
  for prophylaxis in HIV-infected woman, 502
  for tuberculosis during prgnancy, 302
Isotretinoin
  intrauterine growth restriction caused by, 426
  teratogenic effects of, 247
Isradipine for hypertension, 591

J

Jarisch-Herexheimer reaction in syphilis, 85
Jaundice during pregnancy, 345
Jejunoileal bypass, pregnancy and, 349
Jejunostomy tube, 614
Joint(s)
  degenerative disease of, 527-528
  pelvic, instability of, causing chronic pelvic pain, 160
  sacroiliac and hip, in diagnosis of cause of backache, 538

K

Kallmann's syndrome, amenorrhea caused by, 6
Kanamycin, teratogenic effects of, 248
Kaolin/pectin for diarrhea, 569
Karyotype/karyotyping
  to diagnose genetic diseases, 254, 256
  to diagnose intrauterine growth restriction, 428
  in evaluation of amenorrhea, 4
  for multiple gestation, 464
Kearns-Sayre syndrome, 253
Kegel exercises
  instructions in performing, 516
  for mixed urinary incontinence, 195
  to prevent vaginal prolapse, 170
  for stress incontinence, 191-192
  for urge incontinence, 195
Keofeed, 613
Ketoacidosis, diabetic, 442-444
Ketoconazole for candidiasis, 87
Ketorolac for headache, 584
Kidney
  alterations in, during normal pregnancy, 358
  chronic disease of, pregnancy in women with, 361-363
  complications of, during pregnancy, 358-366
  decreased function of, during pregnancy, 361, 363
  pelvic, pregnancy and, 362
  solitary, pregnancy and, 362
Kidney failure
  acute, obstetric, 363-364
  postpartum, idiopathic, 364
Kidney stones, 360
Krukenberg tumor of ovary, 133, 154
Kyphosis, 539

L

Labetalol
  for chronic hypertension during pregnancy, 354, 355, 356
  for preeclampsia/eclampsia, 344, 432
Labia majora and minora, cancer on, 217; *see also* Vulvar cancer
Labor
  anesthesia for, 471-472
  for eclamptic patient, management of, 435
  in postterm/postdate pregnancy, monitoring during, 441
  preterm
    diagnosis of, 390-391
      guidelines for, 396
  trial of, for frank breech, 454
  of woman with chronic hypertension, 356
Laboratory assessment
  to diagnose cause of backache, 538-539
  to diagnose urinary tract infections, 559-560
  for hypertension, 588
  of macronutrient deficiency, 612
Lactase deficiency causing osmotic diarrhea, 565
Lactational adenoma, 22
Lactobacillus acidophilus, 86
Lady's slipper for menopausal symptoms, 113
Lamaze training for pain of labor, 471
Laminectomy, decompressive, for backache, 542
Lamivudine for HIV therapy, 503
Laparoscopic examination to diagnose pelvic inflammatory disease, 141
Laparoscopic tubal occlusion, 184
Laparoscopy
  to diagnose ectopic pregnancy, 47-48
  for ectopic pregnancy, 48, 50
  to evaluate chronic pelvic pain, 161, 162
  to evaluate tubal patency, 77-78
Laparotomy for early stage invasive cervical cancer, 30-31
Laryngitis, 599-607

Larynx, tumors of, causing hoarseness, 604
Laser ablation for condyloma, 89
Laser vaporization for high-grade cervical dysplasia, 135
Late decelerations in fetal heart rate, 467
Latent syphilis, 84-85
Lateral cystocele, 167
Law regarding domestic violence, physician and, 576
L-deamino-8-d-arginine for diabetes insipidus during pregnancy, 318
Leber's hereditary optic atrophy, 253
LEEP; *see* Loop electrical excision procedure
LeFort procedure for vaginal vault prolapse, 169
Leg pain, treatment of, 540
Leg raise, straight, in diagnosis of cause of backache, 538
Legionella pneumophila causing pneumonia, 631-632
Legionnaires' disease, 631-632
Leiomyoma
  cervical, causing third trimester bleeding, 410
  dysmenorrhea caused by, 42
  ovulatory bleeding caused by, 203
  symptoms and treatment of, 204
  therapy for, 154
  uterine, 153
Leiomyosarcoma, uterine, 215
Lemon sign in spina bifida, 276, 277
Levothyroxine for hypothyroidism, 642
Levsinex; *see* Hyoscyamine
Lichen sclerosis et atrophicus causing uterine bleeding in childhood and adolescence, 200
Lidocaine for pudendal block, 472
Lie
  fetal, 450-451
  oblique, 454
  transverse, 454-455
Lifelong sexual dysfunction, 179
Lip, cleft, 253
  treatment of, 256
Lipid emulsions for parenteral nutrition, 615-616
Lipid profile, indications for, 517
Lipoma, breast, 22
Lisinopril
  for hypertension, 589
  teratogenic effects of, 248
Lithium
  breastfeeding and maternal use of, 480
  for cluster headache, 584-585
  for mood disorders, 103-105
  side effects of, 104
  teratogenic effects of, 248
  use of, in pregnancy, 106
Liver
  abscess of, 346-347
  disease of, in pregnancy, 341-347
    evaluation of, 342
  fatty, acute, of pregnancy, 345, 364
  hematoma of, 344-345
  tumors of, 346-347
Liver cell adenoma, 347
Lobular carcinoma in situ of breast, 11
  noninvasive, treatment of, 17
Local infiltration
  with anterior abdominal wall block for cesarean section, 473
  for vaginal delivery, 472
Lomefloxacin for gonorrhea, 88
Long-term dialysis, pregnancy in women on, 364-365
Loop diuretics for hypertension, 592
Loop electrical excision procedure
  for abnormal Pap smear, 135
  for papillomavirus infections, 138
Loperamide for diarrhea, 569, 571
Lorazepam for generalized anxiety disorder, 524
Lotrimin for thrush mastitis, 480
Low back pain; *see* Backache
Low birth weight, 384
Lower genital tract infections, 83-90
LSD abuse during pregnancy, 488; *see also* Substance abuse
Lumbar spasm, 537
Lumbar spine, x-rays of, to diagnose cause of backache, 539
Lumpectomy
  for invasive breast cancer, 17-18
  for noninvasive breast cancer, 17
Lung scans, radiation exposure to fetus from, 421
Lungs, fetal, ultrasonographic evaluation of, 263
Lupus anticoagulant, 334, 336
Lupus anticoagulant/antiphospholipid antibody syndrome, 336-338
  diagnosis of, 337
  treatment of, 337-338

Morbidity, leading causes of, among women, 507
Morgagni, hydatid of, 153
  therapy for, 155
Morning sickness, management of, 238
Morphine
  for chronic pelvic pain, 162
  during labor, 471
  for spinal anesthesia for labor, 471
Mortality
  leading causes of, among women, 507
  neonatal, factors affecting, 385
Mortality risk, maternal, associated with pregnancy, 303-304
Mosaicism, 253
  chorionic villus sampling and, 244
Motherwort for menopausal symptoms, 113
Motility, altered, causing diarrhea, 566-567
Motion, range of, examining for, 537
Movement, fetal, counting, 283
Mucus, cervical, lack of, therapy for, 80
Müllerian agenesis, treatment of, 9
Müllerian duct, congenital malformation of, amenorrhea caused by, 6-7
Müllerian fusion anomalies
  amenorrhea caused by, 7
  treatment of, 9
Multifactorial genetic diseases, 253
Multiple gestations, 459-466
Multiple ovulation, drug-induced, as risk factor for ectopic pregnancy, 45
Murphy's sign, 546
Muscle, pyramidal, hematoma of, causing chronic pelvic pain, 160
Muscle tension headache, 582
Musculoskeletal disorders
  arthritis and related, 527-536
  regional, common, 535
Mycelex for thrush mastitis, 480
Mycobacterium avium complex disease, 501
  prophylaxis for, 502
Mycoplasma pneumoniae causing pneumonia, 632
Mycostatin for thrush, 480
Myelography to diagnose cause of backache, 539
Mylanta for peptic ulcer disease, 623
Myocardial infarction complicating pregnancy, 306
Myoclonus epilepsy, 253
Myoma(s)
  therapy for, 155
  uterine, 153
    treatment of, 43
Myomectomy
  amenorrhea caused by, 7
  for myoma, 155
  for ovulatory bleeding in reproductive age women, 203
Myopathies, idiopathic inflammatory, 552-553
Myositis, inclusion body, 552
Myxedema, 639; *see also* Hypothyroidism

N

Nadolol
  for hypertension, 592
  for migraine headache, 584
Nafazodone, use in pregnancy of, 106
Nafcillin for mastitis, 480
Nalbuphine during labor, 471
Naprosyn; *see* Naproxen sodium
Naproxen sodium for premenstrual syndrome, 176
Narcotic addiction, 487; *see also* Substance abuse
Narcotic analgesics causing mood disorders, 98-99
Narcotics, intrathecal, for labor, 471-472
Nardil; *see* Phenelzine
Nasally placed feeding tubes, 613
Nausea during pregnancy, 347
  management of, 238
Neck pain, 535
Necrotizing vasculitis, systemic, 555
Needle localization surgical biopsy to diagnose breast cancer, 14
Needle urethropexy for stress incontinence, 192
Nefazodone for mood disorders, 102-103
Neisseria gonorrhea causing gonorrhea, 87
Neonatal alloimmune thrombocytopenia, 328
Neonatal depression, 489-496
Neonatal herpes gestationis, 380

Lupus erythematosus, systemic, 332-336, 548-550; *see also* Systemic lupus erythematosus
pregnancy and, 362
Luteal phase deficiency, 78
Luteinizing hormone
measurement of, in evaluation of amenorrhea, 4
in menstrual cycle, 3
Luteoma of pregnancy
hirsutism with, 67
therapy for, 72
Lyme disease causing arthritis, 534-535
Lymph node sampling
for early stage invasive cervical cancer, 30-31
for endometrial carcinomas of uterus, 211
Lymphadenectomy
for early stage invasive cervical cancer, 30-31
for invasive cervical carcinoma complicating pregnancy, 290
for vaginal cancer, 223-224
for vulvar cancer, 218, 220
for vulvar melanoma, 222
Lymphatic dissemination, theory of, to explain endometriosis, 53
Lymphogranuloma venereum, 85-86
Lynch syndrome II, 126
Lysergic acid diethylamide abuse during pregnancy, 488; *see also* Substance abuse
Lysis of pelvic adhesions, 80

M

Maalox for peptic ulcer disease, 623
Macroadenoma
amenorrhea caused by, 6
treatment of, 8
Macrobid for urinary tract infections, 562
Macrodantin for urinary tract infections, 560, 562
Macronutrient deficiency, assessment of, 610-612
Macronutrients, 608
Magnesium sulfate
breastfeeding and maternal use of, 480-481
osmotic diarrhea caused by, 565
for placenta previa, 410
Magnesium sulfate–cont'd
for placental abruption, 40
for preeclampsia/eclampsia 432, 433, 434
for preterm labor, protocol f 391, 392
Magnesium supplements for pr strual syndrome, 176
Magnetic resonance imaging
to diagnose cause of backache 540
to evaluate chronic pelvic pain 162
Male
evaluation of, for infertility, 76
sterilization of, 185
Male factor infertility, therapeutic considerations for, 79-80
Malignant breast disease, 10-20
Malnutrition, 608
weight loss and, 610
Malpresentation, 450-458
Mammogram/mammography
to diagnose breast cancer, 11-14
fibrocystic changes shown in, 23
indications for, 517
Manic episode, diagnosis of, 100
MAO inhibitors for mood disorders, 103
Marfan syndrome complicating pregnancy, 308-309
Marginal placenta previa, 407
Marginal sinus separation, 412
Marijuana abuse during pregnancy, 488; *see also* Substance abuse
Marshall-Marchetti-Krantz culposuspension for stress incontinence, 192
Mass on mammogram, 14
Massage, uterine, for uterine atony, 448
Mastalgia, 23
Mastectomy
for invasive breast cancer, 17-18
for noninvasive breast cancer, 17
Mastitis, 23-24
from breastfeeding, diagnosis and treatment of, 480
postpartum, 235
Mastodynia, 23
Mastopathy, fibrocystic, 14-15
Maternal mortality risk associated with pregnancy, 303-304
Maternal serum analyte screening for birth defects, 241-243

Neonatal mortality, factors affecting, 385
Neonatal tetany, 317
Neoplasia, gestational trophoblastic, recurrent, 62-63; *see also* Gestational trophoblastic disease
Neoplasms
  breast, common benign, 22-23
  ovarian, androgen-producing, therapy for, 72
Neosalpingostomy for tubal occlusion and pelvic adhesions, 80
Neovagina, creation of, for end organ/outflow defects, 9
Nephrectomy, pregnancy after, 362
Nephritis, systemic lupus erythematosus causing, differentiation of, from preeclampsia, 335
Nephrolithiasis, 530
Nephropathy
  diabetic, pregnancy and, 362
  gouty, 530
  IgA, pregnancy and, 362
  reflux, pregnancy and, 362
Nerve(s)
  genitofemoral, disorders of, causing chronic pelvic pain, 159
  ilioinguinal and iliohypogastric, disturbances of, causing chronic pelvic pain, 159
Nerve root impingement, 537
Nettles for menopausal symptoms, 113
Neural tube defects
  ethnic groups at risk for, 255
  folic acid to prevent, 232, 233
  screening for, 242
Neuralgia, trigeminal, 581
Neuraminidase in influenza virus, 594
Neurectomy, presacral, for dysmenorrhea, 43
Neurologic examination in diagnosis of cause of backache, 538
Neurosyphilis, diagnosis of, 85
New York Heart Association classification of risks of pregnancy in women with cardiac lesions, 303, 304
Newborn
  congenital infections of, 366-373
  resuscitation of, 489-496
Nicardipine
  for hypertension, 591
  for migraine headache, 584
Nifedipine
  for chronic hypertension during pregnancy, 354, 355, 356
  for hypertension, 591
  for preeclampsia/eclampsia, 432
  for preterm labor, protocol for, 391, 392
Nipple(s)
  adenoma of, 22
  bloody discharge from, 22
  breastfeeding and, 476
  discharge from, 24-25
  sore, from breastfeeding, diagnosis and treatment of, 478
Nitrates to prevent myocardial infarction complicating pregnancy, 306
Nitrazine test for preterm PROM, 394
Nitrofurantoin for urinary tract infections, 560, 562
Nizatidine for peptic ulcer disease, 623
Nodes
  Bouchard's, 527
  Heberden's, 527
Nodular goiter, toxic, causing hyperthyroidism, 316
Nodular hyperplasia, focal, of liver, 347
Nodules, rheumatoid, 529
Nomifensine, hyperprolactinemia caused by, 6
Nonbacterial arthritis, 534-535
Nonerosive gastritis, acute, 578
Noninvasive ductal carcinoma in situ of breast, treatment of, 15, 17
Noninvasive lobular carcinoma in situ of breast, treatment of, 17
Noninvasive malignant breast disease, 11
Nonprimary herpes simplex virus infection, 83-84
Nonpuerperal mastitis, 23
Nonsteroidal antiinflammatory drugs
  for backache, 540
  for chronic pelvic pain, 161
  for dysmenorrhea, 42, 43
  gastritis caused by, 578
  for gout, 531
  hypertension caused by, 587

Nonsteroidal antiinflammatory drugs–cont'd
  for migraine headache, 584
  for osteoarthritis, 528
  peptic ulcer disease caused by, 618-619
  for rheumatoid arthritis, 529
  for spondyloarthropathies, 533
  for systemic lupus erythematosus, 550
Nonstress testing, 283, 286
Nontubal ectopic pregnancy, 51
Nonulcer dyspepsia, 578, 579
Norethindrone
  for anovulatory bleeding, 202
  for hormone replacement therapy, 96
Norfloxacin for gonorrhea, 88
Norgestimate to treat hirsutism, 71
Norplant
  bleeding caused by, 203
    symptoms and treatment of, 205
  breastfeeding and maternal use of, 481
  for contraception, 37-38
Norpramine; *see* Desipramine
Nortriptyline
  for mood disorders, 103
  for premenstrual syndrome, 176
Norvir; *see* Ritonavir
Nosocomial pneumonia, 628; *see also* Pneumonia
Nubain; *see* Nalbuphine
Nuclear medicine studies to diagnose cause of backache, 539
Nucleocapsid, 594
Nutrient requirements, 608-610
Nutrients, essential, 608
Nutrition, 608-617
  breastfeeding and, 239
  and menopause, 110-114
  parenteral, 615-616
  and pregnancy, 236-240
  for pregnant adolescent, 483-484
  for substance-abusing pregnant woman, 487
Nutritional assessment, 610-612
Nutritional supplements
  during pregnancy, 237-238
  for premenstrual syndrome, 174, 176
Nutritional support, 612-617
Nystatin
  for pharyngitis, 603
  for thrush mastitis, 480

O

Oblique lie, 454
Obsessions, 519, 521
Obsessive-compulsive disorder, 519, 521
Obstetric anesthesia, 470-474
Obstetric ultrasound; *see* Ultrasound
Obstetrics, 225-496
  medical emergencies in, 442-450
Occipitofrontal diameter of fetal head, ultrasonographic evaluation of, 261, 262
Occlusion, tubal, 184-185
  causing infertility, therapy for, 80
Ocular diameter of fetus, ultrasonographic evaluation of, 263
Ofloxacin
  for chlamydial infection, 89
  for gonorrhea, 88
  for pelvic inflammatory disease, 144
Ogen for hormone replacement therapy, 96
17OH P_4, diagnosis of causes of hirsutism using, 70
Oligohydramnios, 272-273
Oligomenorrhea, 199-200
Oligospermia, 76
Omeprazole
  for *H. pylori* infection, 624
  for peptic ulcer disease, 623
  for reflux esophagitis, 614
Omphalocele
  screening for, 242
  ultrasonography to detect, 279, 280-281
Oophorectomy
  for androgen-producing ovarian neoplasms, 72
  for ovarian hyperandrogenism, 71-72
  for premenstrual syndrome, 176-177
Opiates
  addiction to, 487; *see also* Substance abuse
  hyperprolactinemia caused by, 6
  in urine specimens, 485
Opioids
  addiction to, 487; *see also* Substance abuse
  for diarrhea, 569, 571
  for labor, 471-472
Opioid-type drugs for chronic pelvic pain, 161-162

Opportunistic infections with AIDS, prophylaxis for, 502-503
Optic atrophy, Leber's hereditary, 253
Optivite for premenstrual syndrome, 176
Oral contraceptives, 34-36
for anovulatory bleeding, 202
in adolescent, 201
benefits of use of, 35-36
for bleeding caused by spironolactone, 205
bleeding related to, 203
cancer and, 35
for coagulation defects, 205
compliance when using, 34-35
contraindications to use of, 34
for dysmenorrhea, 42-43
erratic use of, bleeding caused by, symptoms and treatment of, 205
for hirsutism, 73
for hyperandrogenism, 8
hyperprolactinemia caused by, 6
hypertension caused by, 587
for ovulatory bleeding in reproductive age women, 203
for premenstrual syndrome, 176
side effects to use of, 35
to treat amenorrhea, 8
to treat endometriosis, 54
to treat hirsutism, 71
Oral feeding, 613
Oral hypoglycemics for ovarian hyperandrogenism, 71
Orbital diameter, outer, of fetus, ultrasonographic evaluation of, 263
Orgasmic disorders, 182
Osmotic diarrhea, 564-565
Osteitis pubis causing chronic pelvic pain, 160
Osteoarthritis, 527-528
Osteoporosis, 93, 115-124
calcium and, 110-111
Osteoporotic sacral fractures causing chronic pelvic pain, 161
Outer orbital diameter of fetus, ultrasonographic evaluation of, 263
Outflow defects
as cause of amenorrhea, 6-7
Ovarian cancer, 124-133
epithelial, 125-131; *see also* Epithelial ovarian cancer
Ovarian cancer–cont'd
metastatic, 133
modified WHO classification of, 125
recurrent or persistent, 131
Ovarian cancer syndromes, familial, 126
Ovarian cysts
dysmenorrhea caused by, 42
follicular, 149, 154
functional, 149, 150, 154
treatment of, 43
Ovarian drilling to induce ovulation, 81
Ovarian failure
amenorrhea caused by, 6, 7-9
Ovarian hyperandrogenemia, therapy for, 69, 71-72
Ovarian pregnancy, 51
Ovarian wedge resection for ovarian hyperandrogenism, 71
Ovary; *see also* Ovarian cancer; Ovarian cysts
androgen-producing tumors of
evaluation to rule out, 68
hirsutism with, 67
therapy for, 72
endometriomas of, 53
injury to, amenorrhea caused by, 7
polycystic disease of; *see* Polycystic ovarian disease
stromal tumors of, 132-133
ultrasound of, diagnosis of causes of hirsutism using, 70
Overflow incontinence, 196
Ovulation
induction of, methods for, 81
multiple, drug-induced, as risk factor for ectopic pregnancy, 45
Ovulation suppression for premenstrual syndrome, 176
Ovulatory bleeding
causes, symptoms, and treatment of, 204-206
in reproductive age women, 202-203
Ovulatory cycle, key events in, 3
Ovulatory factors in infertility evaluation, 78-79
Oxandrolone, hirsutism caused by, 69
Oxybutynin chloride for urge incontinence, 195
Oxycodone
for chronic pelvic pain, 162
for headache, 584

Oxygen
for amniotic fluid embolism, 447
for asthma, 445
for neonatal depression, 493, 494
for pulmonary edema, 422
Oxygen consumption, maternal, changes in, during pregnancy, 294-295
Oxytocin
for contraction stress test, 285
for uterine atony, 448

P

Paget's disease of breast, 15
Pain
back; *see* Backache
cervical, 535
leg, treatment of, 540
neck, 535
pelvic; *see* Pelvic pain
Pain generators, 536
Painful thyroiditis, subacute, 635
Painless thyroiditis, 635
Palate, cleft, 253
treatment of, 256
Pamelor; *see* Nortriptyline
Pancreatitis, 350-351
Panic attacks, 522-523
Panic disorders with or without agoraphobia, 522-523
Pap smears
abnormal
management of, 135-137, 288, 289
papillomavirus infections and, 134-139
for HIV-infected women, 502
procedure for, 515
Papillomavirus infections
and abnormal Pap smear, 134-139
typing of, 137, 138
Papular dermatitis of pregnancy, 382
Papules, Gottron's, 552
Parafon Forte; *see* Chlorzoxazone
Paraguard IUD for contraception, 38
Parainfluenza virus causing pneumonia, 633
Paralysis, vocal cord, causing hoarseness, 604-605
Paramenstrual migraine, 584
Paramethadione, teratogenic effects of, 249
Paraortic lymph node sampling for early stage invasive cervical cancer, 30-31
Paraovarian cysts, 153
therapy for, 155
Paravaginal repair for cystocele, 167
Parenteral nutrition, 615-617
Parnate; *see* Tranylcypromine
Paroxetine
for mood disorders, 102-103
for obsessive-compulsive disorder, 521
orgasmic disorder caused by, 182
for panic disorders with or without agoraphobia, 523
use in pregnancy of, 106
Paroxysmal fetal tachycardia, 467
Paroxysmal hemicrania, 584
Partial mole, 59
Partial previa, 407
Parvovirus B19
arthritis caused by, 534
congenital infection with, 370
Patient history, 511
Patient/physician relationship, 507
Paxil; *see also* Paroxetine
PCP abuse during pregnancy, 488; *see also* Substance abuse
Peak expiratory flow rate, measuring, to diagnose asthma, 296
Peau d'orange, 15
Pederson hypothesis from diabetes, 310
Pelvic adhesions causing infertility, therapy for, 80
Pelvic congestion, dysmenorrhea caused by, 42
Pelvic disease, advanced, therapy for, 31-32
Pelvic examination, 511, 515-516
Pelvic exenteration for recurrent cervical cancer, 32-33
Pelvic floor muscle exercises
for mixed urinary incontinence, 195
for stress incontinence, 191-192
for urge incontinence, 195
Pelvic floor support, 163-171
Pelvic inflammatory disease, 140-147
chlamydia and, 142, 143
diagnosis of, 141-142
dysmenorrhea caused by, 42
epidemiology of, 140-141
gonorrhea and, 142, 143
hospitalization for, indications for, 143
inpatient treatment of, 144
microbiology of, 142-143

Pelvic inflammatory disease–cont'd
outpatient treatment of, 144
as risk factor for ectopic pregnancy, 45
sequelae of, 145-146
Pelvic joint instability causing chronic pelvic pain, 160
Pelvic kidney, pregnancy and, 362
Pelvic lymphadenectomy for early stage invasive cervical cancer, 30-31
Pelvic masses, benign, 147-155
Pelvic pain
chronic, 156-163
differential diagnosis of, 53
pelvic inflammatory disease causing, 146
Pelvic surgery as risk factor for ectopic pregnancy, 45
Pelvis, fetal, ultrasonographic evaluation of, 265
Pemphigoid gestationis, 379
Penicillamine
for rheumatoid arthritis, 530
for systemic sclerosis, 552
teratogenic effects of, 249
Penicillin
for acute pyelonephritis, 360
for labor to reduce neonatal group B streptococcal sepsis, 389
for mastitis, 23, 480
for pharyngitis, 603
for pneumonia, 630
during pregnancy, 299
for rheumatic heart disease complicating pregnancy, 307
for syphilis, 85, 369
Penicillin G for syphilis, 85
Penicillin G benzathine for pharyngitis, 603
Pentazocine for chronic pelvic pain, 162
Pepcid; *see* Famotidine
Peptic ulcer disease, 349, 617-627
bleeding with, endoscopic features of, 625
clinical presentation of, 619-620
complicated, diagnosis and management of, 625-626
diagnostic studies for, 620-622
H. pylori infection and NSAID use associated with, 619
intractable 623
perforation of ulcer in, 626
Percutaneous feeding tubes, 614
Percutaneous umbilical blood sampling
for antenatal testing, 285-286
to screen for birth defects, 244
Pereyra urethropexy for stress incontinence, 192
Perforating veins, 645
Perforation of peptic ulcer, 626
Performance anxiety causing orgasmic disorder, 182
Perfusion lung scan, radiation exposure to fetus from, 421
Pergonal causing twinning, 459
Periarteritis nodosa, pregnancy and, 362
Perimenopausal bleeding, symptoms and treatment of, 206
Perinatal infections and immunizations, 366-375
Periodic abstinence for contraception, 39-40
Peripheral parenteral nutrition, 615
Peritonitis; *see also* Pelvic inflammatory disease
Peritonsillar abscess, pharyngitis and, 601
Pessary, vaginal; *see* Vaginal pessary
Pharyngitis, 599-603
Phencyclidine abuse during pregnancy, 488; *see also* Substance abuse
Phenelzine
for mood disorders, 103
for posttraumatic stress disorder, 524
for social phobia, 525
Phenergan; *see* Promethazine
Phenobarbital for intrahepatic cholestasis of pregnancy, 343
Phenothiazines, hyperprolactinemia caused by, 6
Phenylketonuria
ethnic groups at risk for, 255
treatment of, 256
Phenylpropanolamine
hypertension caused by, 587
for stress incontinence, 191
Phenytoin, hirsutism caused by, 69
Pheochromocytoma during pregnancy, 319
Phlebectomy, ambulatory, for varicose veins, 645-646
Phobias, 525-526
Phosphate
for hyperparathyroidism, 317

Phosphate–cont'd
osmotic diarrhea caused by, 565
Photoplethysmography to diagnose varicose veins, 644
Phototherapy for mood disorders, 106
Phyllode tumors of breast, 22
Physical abuse, 572-577
Physical examination, annual, 511-516; *see also* Annual examination
Physician, domestic violence and, 574-576
Physician/patient relationship, 507
Phytoestrogens for menopausal symptoms, 113
Pi typing, 256
Pica during pregnancy, management of, 239
PID; *see* Pelvic inflammatory disease
Pindolol for hypertension, 592
Piperacillin for acute pyelonephritis, 360
Pituitary apoplexy, headache with, 585
Pituitary evaluation in evaluation of amenorrhea, 4
Pituitary insufficiency during pregnancy, 318
Pituitary tumor(s)
amenorrhea caused by, 4, 6
hyperprolactinemia caused by, 6
headache with, 585
Placenta
biopsy of, 244
dysmature, 438
grade of, to diagnose intrauterine growth restriction, 427
metastatic lesions to, complicating pregnancy, 292
monochorionic, 461
in monozygotic and dizygotic pregnancies, 460, 461
retained, treatment of, 449
ultrasonographic evaluation of, 266
Placenta accreta, 407, 409
Placenta increta, 407
Placenta percreta, 407
Placenta previa, 407-410
diagnosis of, 409
incidence of, 409
pathophysiology and natural history of, 407, 409
Placental abruption, 405-407
Placental site trophoblastic tumor, 60
Plant hormones for menopausal symptoms, 113
Plasma replacement for disseminated intravascular coagulation, 330-331
Plasmanate for neonatal depression, 494
Platelet count, low, during pregnancy, management of, 329
Plethysmography
to diagnose varicose veins, 644
impedance, to diagnose thromboembolism, 421
Plugged ducts with breastfeeding, diagnosis and treatment of, 478
Plummer's disease, 635
PMS; *see* Premenstrual syndrome
Pneumococcal pneumonia, treatment of, 630
Pneumococcal vaccine, guidelines for adult immunization with, 374
Pneumocystis carinii pneumonia, 501
Pneumonia
influenzal, 595
pneumococcal, treatment of, 630
during pregnancy, 298-299
viral and bacterial, 627-633
Podofilox
for condyloma, 89
for papillomavirus infections, 137-138
Podophyllin compounds for papillomavirus infections, 137
Podophyllin resin for condyloma, 89
Polyarteritis nodosa, 555-556
Polybrominated biphenyls, teratogenic effects of, 250
Polycarbophil for diarrhea, 569
Polychlorinated biphenyls, teratogenic effects of, 250
Polycystic disease, pregnancy and, 362
Polycystic ovarian disease
anovulatory bleeding caused by, 202
hirsutism caused by, 64-66
Polyhydramnios, 272, 273
ultrasonography to detect, 275
Polymenorrhea, 199
Polymorphic eruptions of pregnancy; *see* Pruritic urticarial papules and plaques of pregnancy

Polymyositis, 552-553
Polypectomy for uterine polyps, 204
Polyps
cervical, causing third trimester bleeding, 410
uterine
symptoms and treatment of, 204
treatment of, 43
Ponstel; *see* Mefenamic acid
Pontiac fever, 631
Porphyria, ethnic groups at risk for, 255
Portal hypertensive gastropathy, 580
Position
fetal, 451
mentum anterior, 455, 456
mentum posterior, 455, 456
mentum transverse, 455, 456
Positive end-expiratory pressure
for amniotic fluid embolism, 447
for pulmonary edema, 422
Postcoital test in infertility evaluation, 77
Postmenopausal bleeding, 206
Postmenopausal nipple discharge, 25
Postpartum care, 234-235
Postpartum depression, 235
Postpartum depressive episodes, 98
Postpartum headache, 582
Postpartum hemorrhage, 447-449
after delivery of multiple gestations, 465
Postpartum renal failure, idiopathic, 364
Postpartum thyroid dysfunction, 317, 635
Poststreptococcal glomerulonephritis, pharyngitis and, 601
Postterm/postdate pregnancy, 437-442
Posttraumatic stress disorder, 524
Potassium chloride for treatment of ectopic pregnancy, 48
Potassium iodide
teratogenic effects of, 250
for thyroid storm, 444
PPD test, indications for, 517
Prader-Willi syndrome, 256
Prazosin for hypertension, 592
Precocious puberty, causes of, 200
Preconceptional care, 232
Prednisone
for adrenal hyperandrogenemia, 72
for adrenal insufficiency, 319
Prednisone–cont'd
for asthma during pregnancy, 297, 298
for cluster headache, 584
for gout, 531
for headache caused by temporal arteritis, 581
for herpes gestationis, 380
for hyperandrogenism, 8
for hyperthyroidism, 638
for immune thrombocytopenic purpura, 327
for lupus anticoagulant/antiphospholipid antibody syndrome, 337-338
for pregnant woman on long-term dialysis, 365
for rheumatoid arthritis, 339
for systemic lupus erythematosus, 336
for vasculitides, 556-557
Preeclampsia, 343-344, 363-364, 430-436; *see also* Eclampsia
DIC caused by, 330
renal disease and, 363
severe, 432
remote from term (<30 weeks), 434, 436
systemic lupus erythematosus nephritis differentiated from, 335
treatment and management of, 432-436
Pregestational diabetic pregnancy, management of, 312
Pregnancy
abdominal, 51; *see also* *Ectopic pregnancy*
acute fatty liver of, 345, 364
acute renal failure during, 363-364
Addison's disease during, 319
adolescent, 482-484
adrenal insufficiency during, 319
anatomic and physiologic changes in, 227-231
anemia during, 320-323
evaluation of, 321
appendicitis during, 350
asthma during, 295-298, 444-446
asymptomatic bacteriuria in, antibiotics for, 562
autoimmune disease during, 332-341
considerations for drug therapy for, 340-341

Pregnancy–cont'd
back pain in, 542
cardiac changes in, 227-228
cardiac diseases during, 302-309
cardiac and pulmonary diseases complicating, 293-309
central hemodynamic changes during, 293
cervical, 51; *see also* *Ectopic pregnancy*
cervical carcinoma complicating, 287-292
cholestasis of, 376-377, 378
chronic hypertension during, 351-358
chronic renal disease and, 361-363
coagulation disorders and, 326-331
complications of, bleeding caused by, symptoms and treatment of, 205
dermatologic conditions associated with, 375-384
diabetes during, 310-315; *see also* Gestational diabetes mellitus
diabetes insipidus during, 318
diabetic ketoacidosis in, 442-444
dizygotic, 459-461
domestic violence and, 576
dyspnea of, 295
ectopic; *see* Ectopic pregnancy
endocrine abnormalities during, 315-320
endocrine changes in, 230-231
exclusion of, as cause of amenorrhea, 4
gallbladder disease in, 350
gastroesophageal reflux during, 348
gastrointestinal bypass and, 349
gastrointestinal changes in, 229-230
gastrointestinal disease in, 347-351
evaluation of, 342
hair changes during, 376
hematologic changes in, 227
hematologic complications during, 320-331
hemoglobinopathies during, 323-326
hepatic disease in, 341-347
evaluation of, 342
hepatitis during, 345-346
HIV infection and, 504
hypercoagulability of, 227
hyperparathyroidism during, 317

Pregnancy–cont'd
hyperpigmentation during, 375-376
hyperthyroidism during, 316
hypoparathyroidism during, 317
hypothyroidism during, 316-317
intrahepatic cholestasis of, 341, 343
jaundice during, 345
liver tumors during, 346-347
low platelet count during, management of, 329
luteoma of
hirsutism with, 67
therapy for 72
maternal mortality risk associated with, 303-304
medical diseases in, 287-366
molar; *see* Hydatidiform mole
monozygotic, 459-461
mood disorders and, 106
nausea and vomiting during, 347
nutrition and, 236-240
ovarian, 51; *see also* *Ectopic pregnancy*
pancreatitis during, 350-351
pheochromocytoma during, 319
pituitary insufficiency during, 318
pneumonia during, 298-299
polymorphic eruptions of; *see* Pruritic urticarial papules and plaques of pregnancy
postterm/postdate, 437-442; *see also* Postterm/postdate pregnancy
prolactin-producing adenomas during, 317-318
pruritus during, 376-378
renal alterations during, 229, 358
renal complications of, 358-366
respiratory changes in, 228-229
rheumatoid arthritis in, 338-339
sarcoidosis during, 299-300
scleroderma during, 339-340
Sjögren's syndrome in, 340
skin changes during normal, 375-376
substance abuse in, 485-489
supplements taken during, 237-238
thrombocytopenia during, 326-327, 329
thyroid storm in, 444
tuberculosis during, 300-302
urinary tract infections during, 358-360

Pregnancy–cont'd
weight gain during, recommendations for, 236-237
in women on long-term dialysis, 364-365
Premarin
for hormone replacement therapy, 96
to prevent osteoporosis, 93
Premature birth, 384-397
Premature ovarian failure, amenorrhea caused by, 7-8
Premature rupture of membranes, preterm, 391, 394-395
Premenstrual syndrome, 172-177
Prenatal care, 232-234
for pregnant adolescent, 483
Prenatal diagnosis, 241-244
and teratology, 240-251
Prenatal diet, 237
Prenatal testing, indications for, 241
Presacral neurectomy for dysmenorrhea, 43
Presentation
breech, 451-454
compound, 457-458
face and brow, 455-457, 458
fetal, 451
Preterm delivery, spontaneous versus indicated, 387-388
Preterm labor, 390-393
guidelines for, 396
Preterm premature rupture of membranes, 391, 394-395
Prilosec; *see* Omeprazole
Primary amenorrhea, 3
Primary care, 497-647
Primary dysmenorrhea, 41
Primary herpes simplex virus infection, 83
Primary hypothyroidism, 639, 640
Primary infertility, 74
Primary influenzal pneumonia, 595
Primary ovarian failure, treatment of, 9
Primary pain generators, 536
Primary Sjögren's syndrome, 553
Primary syphilis, 84
Pro-Banthine; *see* Propantheline
Probenecid for pelvic inflammatory disease, 144
Progestasert IUD for contraception, 38
Progesterone
for hormone replacement therapy, 96
Progesterone–cont'd
in menstrual cycle, 3
for migraine headache, 584
for premenstrual syndrome, 176
serum, levels of, in evaluation of ovulation, 78
Progestin(s)
androgenic, to treat hirsutism, 71
for anovulatory bleeding, 202
for endometrial stromal sarcoma of uterus, 215
for hormone replacement therapy, 96
long-acting, for contraception, 37-38
for ovulatory bleeding in reproductive age women, 203
for perimenopausal bleeding, 206
Progestin challenge in evaluation of amenorrhea, 4
Prolactin
ectopic production of, hyperprolactinemia caused by, 6
galactorrhea associated with elevated levels of, 24-25
serum, measurement of, in evaluation of amenorrhea, 4
Prolactinomas
headache with, 585
treatment of, 8
Prolactin-producing adenomas during pregnancy, 317-318
Prolactin-secreting tumors, treatment of, 8
Prolapse
examination for, 515
urethral, causing uterine bleeding in childhood and adolescence, 200
uterine, 168-169
vaginal, 163-171; *see also* Vaginal prolapse
vaginal vault/apical, 169
PROM; *see* Premature rupture of membranes
Promethazine during labor, 471
Propantheline for urge incontinence, 195
Prophylactic cerclage for abnormal cervical competence, 399-400
Propoxyphene for headache, 584
Propranolol
for chronic hypertension during pregnancy, 356

Propranolol–cont'd
for hypertension, 592
for hyperthyroidism, 637
for migraine headache, 584
for posttraumatic stress disorder, 524
for thyroid storm, 444
Propylthiouracil
for hyperthyroidism, 316, 638
for thyroid storm, 444
Prostaglandin synthetase inhibition for dysmenorrhea, 42-43
Prostaglandins
for ectopic pregnancy, 48
for uterine atony, 449
Protease inhibitors for HIV therapy, 503
Protein requirements, 609-610
Protein supplements for enteral alimentation, 613
Proteins, 609
Prozac; *see* Fluxoxetine
Prurigo gestationis, 378, 382
Pruritic dermatoses of pregnancy, 378
Pruritic urticarial papules and plaques of pregnancy (PUPPP syndrome), 378, 380-382
Pruritus, during pregnancy, 376-378
Pseudoephedrine
hypertension caused by, 587
for stress incontinence, 191
Pseudogout, 532
Pseudotumor cerebri, headache with, 582
Psoriatic arthritis, 533
Psychologic abuse, 572-573; *see also* Domestic violence
Psychologic sexual dysfunction, 179
Psychosexual dysfunction
classification of, according to phase of sexual response cycle, 179-183
Psychotherapy for mood disorders, 105
Psyllium for diarrhea, 569
Puberty, precocious, causes of, 200
Pudendal blocks for vaginal delivery, 472
Puerperal mastitis, 23
Pulmonary angiography
to diagnose thromboembolism, 422
radiation exposure to fetus from, 421
Pulmonary capillary wedge pressure in pregnant woman, 306
Pulmonary diseases complicating pregnancy, 293-309
Pulmonary embolism, 419; *see also* Thromboembolic disease
Pulmonary hypertension complicating pregnancy, 308
Pulsed Doppler ultrasound, 266, 269, 270
Pumping and storing breast milk, 481
Pumps, breast, 481
PUPPP syndrome; *see* Pruritic urticarial papules and plaques of pregnancy
Purpura, thrombocytopenic, immune, 327-328
Pyelonephritis
acute, 359-360, 558
cystitis and, 558-563; *see also* Urinary tract infections
diagnosis of, 559
pregnancy and, 362, 364
treatment of, 560
Pyogenic liver abscess, 346
Pyramidal muscle hematoma causing chronic pelvic pain, 160
Pyridoxine for prophylaxis in HIV-infected woman, 502
Pyrimethamine for toxoplasmosis, 371

Q

Quinapril for hypertension, 589
Quinolones for pneumonia, 631, 632

R

Radiation
for cervical carcinoma, 204
for endometrial carcinomas of uterus, 214
Radiation therapy
abdominal, for ovarian cancer, 129
for advanced extrapelvic disease, 32
for advanced pelvic disease, 31-32
for bulky cervical disease, 31
for early stage invasive cervical cancer, 30-31
for invasive breast cancer, 17-18
for noninvasive breast cancer, 17
for recurrent cervical cancer, 32-33
for Sjögren's syndrome, 553
for vaginal cancer, 223

Radiation therapy–cont'd
for vulvar cancer, 218, 220-221
for vulvar melanoma, 222
Radioactive iodine
for hyperthyroidism, 637-638
teratogenic effects of, 249
Radioactive iodine uptake test to diagnose hyperthyroidism, 636, 637
Radioactive scan to diagnose hyperthyroidism, 636-637
Radioactive therapeutic agents, breastfeeding and maternal use of, 480
Radiologic evaluation in evaluation of amenorrhea, 4
Radiologic studies to diagnose osteoporosis, 117-118
Raise, straight leg, in diagnosis of cause of backache, 538
Ramipril for hypertension, 589
Range of motion, examining for, 537
Ranitidine
for peptic ulcer disease, 623
for reflux esophagitis, 614
Rapid plasma reagin (RPR) test to diagnose syphilis, 84-85
Raynaud's phenomenon, 551
treatment of, 552
Raz urethropexy for stress incontinence, 192
Recommended Dietary Allowances, 608
Reconstruction following treatment for invasive breast cancer, 18
Reconstructive surgery of fallopian tubes as risk factor for ectopic pregnancy, 45
Rectocele, 167-168
Rectosigmoid resection for recurrent cervical cancer, 32-33
Recurrent cervical cancer, therapy for, 32-33
Recurrent gestational trophoblastic neoplasia, 62-63
Reflux, gastroesophageal, 348
causing hoarseness, 604
Reflux esophagitis, 614
Reflux laryngitis, treatment of, 606
Reflux nephropathy, pregnancy and, 362
Reglan; *see* Metoclopramide
Reiter's syndrome, 533
Renal artery stenosis, pregnancy and, 362
Renal cell carcinoma, hyperprolactinemia caused by, 6
Renal changes in pregnancy, 229
Renal complications of pregnancy, 358-366
Renal disease
chronic, pregnancy in women with, 361-363
hypertension and, 587
Renal failure
acute, obstetric, 363-364
postpartum, idiopathic, 364
symptoms and treatment of, 205
Renal tract calculi, 360
Repeat adolescent pregnancy, 484
Reproductive age women, uterine bleeding in, 201-206
Reproductive procedures, assisted, 80-82
Resection, rectosigmoid, for recurrent cervical cancer, 32-33
Reserpine
hyperprolactinemia caused by, 6
for hypertension, 592
Resistance, vascular, systemic, maternal, changes in, during pregnancy, 293
Respiratory alkalosis, maternal, changes in, during pregnancy, 294
Respiratory changes in pregnancy, 228-229
Respiratory diseases complicating pregnancy, 294-309
Respiratory syncytial virus causing pneumonia, 633
Resuscitation of newborn, 489-496
Retained placenta, treatment of, 449
Retardation, intrauterine growth, 426; *see also* Intrauterine growth restriction
Reticular veins, 645
Retin-A; *see* Tretinoin
Retinitis pigmentosa, 253
Retinoic acid embryopathy, 247
Retinopathy, hypertension and, 587
Retracted nipple, 476
Retrograde cholangiopancreatography, endoscopic, 350
Retrograde menstruation, theory of, to explain endometriosis, 52-53
Retrovir; *see* Zidovudine

Reverse transcriptase inhibitors for HIV therapy, 503
Rh alloimmunization, frequency of, 414
Rh immune globulin for alloimmunization, 416-418
Rheumatic fever, pharyngitis and, 601
Rheumatic heart disease complicating pregnancy, 307
Rheumatoid arthritis, 338-339, 528-530
"Rhythm" for contraception, 39-40
Rifampin
  for pneumonia, 632
  for tuberculosis during prgnancy, 302
Rimantadine for influenza, 597
Ritodrine for preterm labor, protocol for, 391, 392
Ritonavir for HIV therapy, 503
Rokitansky-Küster-Hauser syndrome
  amenorrhea caused by, 7
  treatment of, 9
Rokitansky's protuberance, 152
Rubella, congenital, 368
Rubella infection causing arthritis, 534
Rubella titer, 517
Rupture, uterine, causing third trimester bleeding, 412
Rutinosides to augment venous flow, 645-646

S

Sacral fractures, osteoporotic, causing chronic pelvic pain, 161
Sacroiliac joints in diagnosis of cause of backache, 538
Sacrospinous suspension for vaginal vault prolapse, 169
"Saddle block" for vaginal delivery, 473
Salicylates
  for chronic pelvic pain, 161
  for diarrhea, 569
  gastritis caused by, 578
Saline for neonatal depression, 494
Salpingectomy for treatment of ectopic pregnancy, 50
Salpingitis, treatment of, 143-144; *see also* Pelvic inflammatory disease
Salpingoophorectomy for endometrial carcinomas of uterus, 211
Salpingostomy for treatment of ectopic pregnancy, 50
Sampling
  chorionic villus, to screen for birth defects, 243-244
  endometrial, for postmenopausal bleeding, 206
  fetal, fetoscopic and ultrasonographic, to screen for birth defects, 244
  paraortic lymph node, for early stage invasive cervical cancer, 30-31
  percutaneous umbilical blood; *see* Percutaneous umbilical blood sampling
Saquinavir for HIV therapy, 503
Sarcoidosis
  hyperprolactinemia caused by, 6
  during pregnancy, 299-300
Sarcoma(s)
  stromal, endometrial, uterine, 215
  uterine, 214-215
    bleeding from, 206
  vaginal, 223
Sarcoma botyroides causing uterine bleeding in childhood and adolescence, 200
Savage syndrome, amenorrhea caused by, 7, 8
Scarlet fever, pharyngitis and, 601
Schilling test to diagnose cause of diarrhea, 568
School of fish pattern in chancroid, 83
Sciatica, treatment of, 540
Scleroderma, 339-340, 550; *see also* Systemic sclerosis
  pregnancy and, 362
Scleromalacia perforans, 529
Sclerosis
  diffuse, 550; *see also* Systemic sclerosis
  systemic, 339-340, 550-552; *see also* Systemic sclerosis
Sclerotherapy for varicose veins, 645-646
Screening programs, successful, criteria for, 506
Screening tests
  carrier, 256
  indications for, 517
Seasonal affective disorder, 99
Second International Standard test for ectopic pregnancy, 47

Second trimester, ultrasound examination in, 260-266
Secondary amenorrhea, 3
Secondary dysmenorrhea, 41
Secondary hypertension, 587
Secondary hypothyroidism, 639-640
Secondary infertility, 74
Secondary influenzal pneumonia, 595-596
Secondary osteoporosis, differential diagnosis of, 118
Secondary syphilis, 84
Secretory diarrhea, 565-566
Sedative-hypnotics causing mood disorders, 98-99
Selective serotonin reuptake inhibitor
 for generalized anxiety disorder, 524
 for obsessive-compulsive disorder, 521
 for panic disorders with or without agoraphobia, 523
Self-catheterization for voiding dysfunction, 197
Self-help strategies for premenstrual syndrome, 174, 176
Semen, analysis of, 76
 in evaluation of infertility, 76
Sensate focus for sexual desire disorders, 181
Separation, marginal sinus, 412
Sepsis, uterine, pregnancy and, 364
Septic arthritis, 533-534
Septum, transverse, of vagina
 amenorrhea caused by, 7
 treatment of, 9
Serology for alloimmunization, 415
Serous nipple discharge, 25
Sertoli-Leydig cell tumors, 132
 hirsutism with, 67
 therapy for, 72
 uterine bleeding in childhood and adolescence caused by, 200
Sertraline
 for mood disorders, 102-103
 for obsessive-compulsive disorder, 521
 orgasmic disorder caused by, 182
 for panic disorders with or without agoraphobia, 523
 use in pregnancy of, 106
Serum analyte screening, maternal, for birth defects, 241-243
Serzone; *see* Nefazodone
Sex cord–stromal tumors, 132-133
Sexual abuse, 572; *see also* Domestic violence
 causing uterine bleeding in childhood and adolescence, 200
Sexual desire disorders, 179-181
Sexual dysfunction, 178-183
Sexual history, 516
 to evaluate sexual dysfunction, 178
Sexual response cycle, phases of, 179
 psychosexual dysfunctions according to, 179-183
Sexually transmitted diseases
 barrier contraceptives and, 36-37
 discussion of prevention of, 516
 testing for, indications for, 517
Sheehan's syndrome, 318
 amenorrhea caused by, 6
Shingles, 369-370
Shprintzen's syndrome, 256
Sickle cell anemia, 324-326
Sickle cell disease, 324-326
 ethnic groups at risk for, 255
Sigmoidoscopy to diagnose cause of diarrhea, 568
Silent pelvic inflammatory disease, 142
"Silent perforation" of ulcer, 626
Simple phobia, 525-526
Sims-Huhner test in infertility evaluation, 77
Single-gene disorders
 by pattern of inheritance, 252
 treatment of, 256
Sinus headaches, 582
Sinusoidal pattern in fetal heart rate, 469
Situational type sexual dysfunction, 179
Sjögren's syndrome, 340, 553, 554
Skin changes during normal pregnancy, 375-376
Skinfold thickness, triceps, 610-611
Sleep, normalizing, in bipolar patients, 108
Smear, Pap; *see* Pap smear
Smith-Magenis syndrome, 256
Social phobia, 525
Sodium bicarbonate
 for diabetic ketoacidosis, 444
 for neonatal depression, 494
Sodium restriction for hypertension, 589
Solitary kidney, pregnancy and, 362
Somatic cell disorders, 253

Sonography, transvaginal; *see* Ultrasound
Sore nipples from breastfeeding, diagnosis and treatment of, 478
Spasm, lumbar, 537
Spastic colon, 566-567
Specific phobia, 525-526
Specimen collection to diagnose pneumonia, 629-630
Spectinomycin for gonorrhea, 88
Sperm injection, intracytoplasmic; *see* Intracytoplasmic sperm injection
Spermicides for contraception, 36
Spina bifida, 253
  ultrasonography to detect, 275-276
Spinal anesthesia
  for cesarean section, 473
  for labor, 471-472
Spinal block for vaginal delivery, 473
Spinal decompression for backache, 542
Spinal headache, 581
Spironolactone
  bleeding caused by, symptoms and treatment of, 205
  for hirsutism, 73
  for premenstrual syndrome, 176
Splenectomy for immune thrombocytopenic purpura, 328
Spondylitis, ankylosing, 532-533
Spondyloarthropathies, 532-533
Spondylolisthesis, 539
Spontaneous preterm delivery, 387-388
Sprue, celiac, 565, 569
Sputum collection to diagnose pneumonia, 629-630
Squamous cells, atypical, of uncertain significance, 135
Squamous intraepithelial lesions
  high-grade, of cervix, diagnosis and treatment of, 135, 136
  low-grade, of cervix, diagnosis and treatment of, 135-137
Squamous metaplasia, 24
Stadol; *see* Butorphanol
Stamey urethropexy for stress incontinence, 192
Standing stress test to diagnose stress incontinence, 190-191
Status asthmaticus during pregnancy, 295
Stavudine for HIV therapy, 503, 504
Stenosis
  aortic, complicating pregnancy, 307-308
  cervical, 42, 43
  mitral, complicating pregnancy, 306-307
  renal artery, pregnancy and, 362
Stereotactic biopsy to diagnose breast cancer, 14
Sterilization, 184-185
  female, 184-185
  male, 185
  tubal, as risk factor for ectopic pregnancy, 45
Steroid hormone binding globulin, 64
Steroids; *see* Anabolic steroids; Corticosteroids
Stimulants causing mood disorders, 99
Stimulation, vibroacoustic, for nonstress testing, 283
Stomach, fetal, ultrasonography to evaluate, 279
Stomach ulcer; *see* Peptic ulcer disease
Stones, kidney, 360
Stool studies to diagnose cause of diarrhea, 569-570
Straight leg raise in diagnosis of cause of backache, 538
Streptococcus
  group A β-hemolytic, pharyngitis and, 599-601
  group B β-hemolytic, congenital infection with, 372-373
Streptococcus pneumoniae causing pneumonia, 628-630, 631
Streptokinase for thromboembolism during pregnancy, 423
Streptomycin, teratogenic effects of, 248
Stress
  amenorrhea caused by, 6
  energy requirements and, 609
Stress disorder
  acute, 524-525
  posttraumatic, 524
Stress incontinence, 189-192
Stress test
  contraction, 284-285
  standing, to diagnose stress incontinence, 190-191
Stress ulcers, 578
Striae distensae, 376

Stroke
headache with, 581
hypertension and, 587
Stroke volume, maternal, changes in, during pregnancy, 293
Stromal sarcoma, endometrial, uterine, 215
Stromal tumors, sex cord–, 132-133
Struma ovarii, 152
Subacute painful thyroiditis, 635
Subclinical hypothyroidism, 640-642
Subcutaneous pump for thromboembolism during pregnancy, 423-424
Sublimaze; *see* Fentanyl
Submucous fibroids causing infertility, therapy for, 80
Substance abuse, in pregnancy, 485-489
Sucralfate for peptic ulcer disease, 623
Sucrase-isomaltase deficiency causing osmotic diarrhea, 565
Suction curettage, evacuation by, to treat hydatidiform mole, 56
Sufentanil for spinal anesthesia for labor, 471
Suicide, mood disorders and, 99
Sulbactam for pneumonia, 631
Sulfadiazine for toxoplasmosis, 371
Sulfasalazine
for diarrhea, 571
fetal effects of, 341
for inflammatory bowel disease, 349-350
for rheumatoid arthritis, 530
Sulfisoxazole for lymphogranuloma venereum, 86
Sulfonamides, breastfeeding and maternal use of, 480
Sumatriptan for migraine headache, 585
Superficial gastritis, chronic, 579
Supplements
nutritional, during pregnancy, 237-238
protein, for enteral alimentation, 613
Surgery
of fallopian tubes, reconstructive, as risk factor for ectopic pregnancy, 45
to induce ovulation, 81
pelvic, as risk factor for ectopic pregnancy, 45
Surgery–cont'd
urinary tract, previous, pregnancy and, 362
Surgical biopsy, needle localization, to diagnose breast cancer, 14
Swan-Ganz catheter to diagnose heart disease in pregnancy, 305
Sympathetic pelvic syndrome causing chronic pelvic pain, 160
Syndesmophyte, 532
Synechiae, intrauterine, causing infertility, therapy for, 80
Synthroid; *see* Thyroxine
Syphilis, 84-85
congenital, 369
Systemic lupus erythematosus, 332-336, 548-550
pregnancy and, 362
Systemic necrotizing vasculitis, 555
Systemic sclerosis, 339-340, 550-552
Systemic vascular resistance, maternal, changes in, during pregnancy, 293

T

TACE questionnaires for substance abuse, 485
Tachycardia
fetal, 467
ultrasonography to detect, 278
paroxysmal fetal, 467
Takayasu's arteritis, 555
Tamoxifen
bleeding caused by, symptoms and treatment of, 205
for invasive breast cancer, 19
for metastatic breast disease, 18
for premenstrual syndrome, 176
Taxol
for metastatic breast disease, 19
for ovarian cancer, 129
Tay-Sachs disease, ethnic groups at risk for, 255
3TC; *see* Lamivudine
TCU-308A for contraception, 38
Tegison; *see* Etretinate
Tegretal; *see* Carbamazepine
Telangiectasia, 645
Teletherapy for advanced pelvic disease, 31-32
Telogen effluvium, 376
Temporal arteritis, 555
headache with, 581

"Tender points," 535
Tendonitis, adductor, causing chronic pelvic pain, 160-161
TENS; *see* Transcutaneous electrical nerve stimulation
Tension headache, 582, 583
Teratogenic drugs, 245
Teratogens, 244-245
Teratology, 244-250
  prenatal diagnosis and, 240-251
Teratoma
  cystic, 151, 152
  therapy for, 154
Terazosin for hypertension, 592
Terbutaline
  for asthma, 445, 446
    during pregnancy, 297
  for preterm labor, protocol for, 391, 392-393
Tertiary syphilis, 84
Test(s)/testing
  antenatal, 282-287
  bacteriuria, indications for, 517
  bowstring, 538
  carrier screening, 256
  contraction stress, 284-285
    interpretation of, 284
  to detect *H. pylori*, 622
  D-xylose, to diagnose cause of diarrhea, 568
  fasting glucose, indications for, 517
  hemoglobin, indications for, 517
  H_2, to diagnose cause of diarrhea, 568
  HIV, indications for, 499, 517
  Nitrazine, for preterm PROM, 394
  nonstress, 283, 286
  postcoital, in infertility evaluation, 77
  PPD, indications for, 517
  prenatal, indications for, 241
  Schilling, to diagnose cause of diarrhea, 568
  screening, indications for, 517
  Sims-Huhner, in infertility evaluation, 77
  standing stress, to diagnose stress incontinence, 190-191
  STD, indications for, 517
  thyroid, interpretation of, 641
  urine, to diagnose cause of diarrhea, 568
Testicular feminization
  amenorrhea caused by, 7
Testicular feminization–cont'd
  treatment of, 9
Testosterone
  diagnosis of causes of hirsutism using, 70
  exogenous, teratogenic effects of, 248
  serum, measurement of, in evaluation of amenorrhea, 4
Tetanus-diphtheria vaccine, guidelines for adult immunization with, 374
Tetany, neonatal, 317
Tetracycline
  breastfeeding and maternal use of, 480
  for *H. pylori* infection, 624
  for pneumonia, 632, 633
  for syphilis, 85
  for systemic sclerosis, 552
  teratogenic effects of, 247-248
Thalassemia, ethnic groups at risk for, 255
Thalidomide, teratogenic effects of, 247
Theca-lutein cysts, 151-152
  hydatidiform mole associated with, 56
  management of, 57
Theophylline for asthma, 446
  during pregnancy, 297, 298
Thiazide diuretics
  for hypertension, 591
  for osteoporosis, 120, 123
Thick meconium, 494-495
Thin meconium, 494-495
Thin-needle aspiration to diagnose breast cancer, 13
Third trimester, ultrasound examination in, 260-266
Third trimester bleeding, 403-413
Thorax, fetal, ultrasonographic evaluation of, 263
Thrombectomy for thromboembolism during pregnancy, 423
Thrombocytopenia
  alloimmune, neonatal, 328
  during pregnancy, 326-327, 329
  symptoms and treatment of, 205
Thrombocytopenic purpura, immune, 327-328
Thromboembolic disease, 419-425
Thromboembolism
  acute, during pregnancy, 424

Thromboembolism–cont'd
antepartum prophylaxis for, 424-425
Thrombophlebitis, headache with, 582
Thrombosis, venous, deep, 419; *see also* Thromboembolic disease
Thrush mastitis from breastfeeding, diagnosis and treatment of, 480
Thunderclap headache, 582
Thyroid
disorders of, 634-643
postpartum dysfunction of, 317, 635
Thyroid medications
for male factor infertility, 80
teratogenic effects of, 249-250
Thyroid storm, 444
Thyroid tests, interpretation of, 641
Thyroid-binding globulin to assess endocrine abnormalities during pregnancy, 316
Thyroid-releasing hormone, hyperprolactinemia caused by, 6
Thyroid-stimulating hormone, level of
to diagnose hyperthyroidism, 636
to diagnose hypothyroidism, 640-641
in evaluation of amenorrhea, 4
Thyroid-stimulating hormone test, indications for, 517
Thyroiditis
Hashimoto's, Turner's syndrome with, 9
painful, subacute, 635
painless, 635
Thyrotoxicosis; *see* Hyperthyroidism
Thyrotoxicosis factitia causing hyperthyroidism, 316
Thyroxine
for hypothyroidism, 317
serum free
to diagnose hyperthyroidism, 636
to diagnose hypothyroidism, 641
Tigan; *see* Trimethobenzamide
Timolol for hypertension, 592
Tissue, connective, diseases of, 548-557
TNM staging of breast cancer, 15, 16
Tobramycin for acute pyelonephritis, 360
Tocolysis
contraindications to, 391
for placenta previa, 410
for placental abruption, 407
for premature PROM, 395
protocols for, 392-393
Tofranil; *see* Imipramine
Tolmetin for rheumatoid arthritis, 529
Tone, fetal, scoring for, 267
Tophi, 530
Torsemide for hypertension, 592
Torsion of pelvic masses, 155
Total abdominal hysterectomy for treatment of endometriosis, 54
Total parenteral nutrition, 615-616
monitoring of, 616-617
Total previa, 407
Total V/Q scan, radiation exposure to fetus from, 421
Toxemia, hydatidiform mole associated with, 56
Toxic nodular goiter causing hyperthyroidism, 316
Toxoplasma, prophylaxis for, 502
Toxoplasmosis, congenital, 371-372
Tracheobronchial aspiration complicating enteral alimentation, 614
Tramadol for headache, 584
Transcerebellar diameter of fetal head, ultrasonographic evaluation of, 262, 263
Transcutaneous electrical nerve stimulation for dysmenorrhea, 43
Transfusion, intrauterine, for alloimmunization, 415
Transnasal tube feeding, 613
Transporter deficiency/defect causing osmotic diarrhea, 565
Transvaginal sonography; *see* Ultrasound
Transvaginal ultrasonography to diagnose ectopic pregnancy, 47
Transverse lie, 454-455
Transverse septum of vagina
amenorrhea caused by, 7
treatment of, 9
Tranylcypromine for mood disorders, 103

Trauma
causing uterine bleeding in childhood and adolescence, 200
genital, treatment of, 449
vocal cord, causing hoarseness, 605
Traveler's diarrhea, 565
Trazodone
for migraine headache, 584
for panic disorders with or without agoraphobia, 523
Trehalase deficiency causing osmotic diarrhea, 565
Treponema pallidum causing syphilis, 84
Tretinoin, teratogenic effects of, 247
Triceps skinfold thickness, 610-611
Trichloroacetic acid
for condyloma, 89
for papillomavirus infections, 138
Trichomonas, wet mount to diagnose, 515
Trichomonas vaginalis infection, 86
Trichomoniasis, 86
Tricyclic antidepressants
for chronic pelvic pain, 161
for generalized anxiety disorder, 524
hypertension caused by, 587
for mood disorders, 103
for obsessive-compulsive disorder, 521
for panic disorders with or without agoraphobia, 523
Trifluridine for herpes simplex virus prophylaxis, 503
Trigeminal neuralgia, 581
Trimethadione, teratogenic effects of, 249
Trimethobenzamide for migraine headache, 585
Trimethoprim/sulfamethoxazole
for prophylaxis in HIV-infected woman, 502
teratogenic effects of, 248
for urinary tract infections, 560, 562
"Triple analyte profile" to screen for birth defects, 241-243
Triple screening profile to screen for birth defects, 241-243
Triploidy, 251
Trisomy, 13, 251
Trisomy 16, 251
Trisomy 18, 251
Trisomy 21, 251, 252
Trophoblastic disease, gestational, 55-63; *see also* Gestational trophoblastic disease
causing hyperthyroidism, 316
Trophoblastic tumor, placental site, 60
Truncal varicose veins, 645
Tubal factors in infertility evaluation, 77-78
Tubal occlusion, 184-185
causing infertility, therapy for, 80
Tubal sterilization as risk factor for ectopic pregnancy, 45
Tube feeding, enteral, 613
Tuberculosis
during pregnancy, 300-302
prophylaxis for, 502
Tubes, feeding, 613-614
Tuboovarian abscess, 145; *see also* Pelvic inflammatory disease
Tumor(s)
adrenal rest, hirsutism with, 67
androgen-producing, hirsutism caused by, 64
germ cell
of ovary, 131-132
uterine bleeding in childhood and adolescence caused by, 200
granulosa cell, 132
causing uterine bleeding in childhood and adolescence, 200
hepatic, 346-347
hilus cell
hirsutism with, 67
therapy for, 72
hormone-producing, causing uterine bleeding in childhood and adolescence, 200
hypothalamic, amenorrhea caused by, 6
Krukenberg, of ovary, 133, 154
of larynx causing hoarseness, 604
ovarian, androgen-producing
evaluation to rule out, 68
hirsutism with, 67
phyllode, of breast, 22
pituitary
amenorrhea caused by, 6
as cause of amenorrhea, 4, 6
headache with, 585
hyperprolactinemia caused by, 6
treatment of, 8
prolactin-secreting, treatment of, 8

Tumor(s)–cont'd
  Sertoli-Leydig cell, 132
    hirsutism with, 67
    therapy for, 72
    uterine bleeding in childhood and adolescence caused by, 200
  sex cord–stromal, 132-133
  trophoblastic, placental site, 60
Turner's syndrome, ovarian failure caused by, 9
Twin, vanishing, 462
Twin-twin transfusion syndrome, 464
Twinning
  dizygotic, 459
  monozygotic, 459
Type A gastritis, 579
Type AB gastritis, 579
Type B gastritis, 579
Type C gastritis, 579
TYVU, 400

U

U sign in spina bifida, 277
Ulcer(s)
  peptic; *see* Peptic ulcer disease
  stress, 578
Ulcer collar, 620
Ulcer mound, 620
Ulcerative colitis, 349-350, 566
  therapy for, 569
Ulcerative infections of vulva, 83-86
Ultram; *see* Tramadol
Ultrasonographic and fetoscopic fetal sampling to screen for birth defects, 244
Ultrasound/ultrasonography
  abnormal, 272-282
  for alloimmunization, 415, 417
  to diagnose intrauterine growth restriction, 427-428
  to diagnose placenta previa, 409
  to diagnose polycystic ovarian disease, 66
  to diagnose varicose veins, 644
  Doppler, 266-271
    to diagnose thromboembolism, 421
  to evaluate chronic pelvic pain, 162
  to evaluate ovulatory bleeding, 202-203
  first trimester, 259-260
  guidelines for fetal anatomy evaluation using, 261
Ultrasound/ultrasonography–cont'd
  indications for, 258
  for multiple gestation, 464
  normal, 257-272
  ovarian, diagnosis of causes of hirsutism using, 70
  purposes for, 257
  safety of, 259
  second and third trimester, 260-266
  transvaginal, to diagnose ectopic pregnancy, 47
Umbilical cord, ultrasonographic evaluation of, 266
Umbilical blood sampling, percutaneous; *see* Percutaneous umbilical blood sampling
Unexplained infertility, 80
Uniparental disomy, 253
Urea for treatment of ectopic pregnancy, 48
Urethra, prolapsed, causing uterine bleeding in childhood and adolescence, 200
Urethral sphincter deficiency, intrinsic, 190
  surgery for, 192
Urethrocele, 165, 167
Urethropexy for stress incontinence, 192
Urge incontinence, 192-195
Uricosuric drugs for gout, 531
Urinary cortisol test, free, to diagnose Cushing's syndrome, 69
Urinary dysfunction, 186-198
Urinary dysfunction questionnaire, 188
Urinary incontinence, 186-189
  mixed, 195
Urinary tract infections, 558-563
  during pregnancy, 358-360
Urinary tract surgery, previous, pregnancy and, 362
Urine tests to diagnose cause of diarrhea, 568
Urine toxicology for substance abuse, 485
Urodynamics, 189
  to diagnose voiding dysfunction, 197
Urofollitropin to induce ovulation, 80, 81
Urokinase for thromboembolism during pregnancy, 423
Urolithiasis, 360
  pregnancy and, 362

Ursodeoxycholic acid for intrahepatic cholestasis of pregnancy, 343
Uterine anomalies, treatment of, 43
Uterine arteriovenous fistulas, bleeding caused by, symptoms and treatment of, 205
Uterine atony, treatment of, 448-449
Uterine bleeding
  abnormal, 199-208
  in childhood and adolescence, 200-201
  postmenopausal, 206
  in reproductive age women, 201-206
Uterine cancers, 209-216
Uterine factors in infertility evaluation, 77-78
Uterine inversion, treatment of, 449
Uterine leiomyoma, 153
Uterine massage for uterine atony, 448
Uterine myomas, treatment of, 43
Uterine polyps
  symptoms and treatment of, 204
  treatment of, 43
Uterine prolapse, 168-169
Uterine rupture causing third trimester bleeding, 412
Uterine sarcomas, 214-215
  bleeding from, 206
Uterine sepsis, pregnancy and, 364
Uterine suspension for uterine prolapse, 169
Uteroplacental insufficiency causing intrauterine growth restriction, 426-427
Uterosacral ligament division for dysmenorrhea, 43
Uterovaginal hemorrhage, severe, management of, 206, 207
Uterus
  anomalies of, dysmenorrhea caused by, 42
  Couvelaire, 405

V

V sign in idiopathic inflammatory myopathies, 552
V/Q scan; *see* Ventilation/perfusion scan
Vaccine(s)
  for adult immunization, guidelines for, 374
Vaccine(s)–cont'd
  for influenza, 598
Vagina
  examination of, 511, 515
  transverse septum of
    amenorrhea caused by, 7
    treatment of, 9
Vaginal cancer, 222-224
Vaginal cones for stress incontinence, 192
Vaginal delivery, anesthesia for, 472-473
Vaginal infections, 86-87
Vaginal pessary
  for stress incontinence, 192
  for vaginal prolapse, 164, 170
Vaginal prolapse, 163-171
Vaginal trauma, bleeding caused by, symptoms and treatment of, 205
Vaginal vault prolapse, 169
Vaginal vault suspension for vaginal vault prolapse, 169
Vaginal vault suspension procedures for cystocele, 167
Vaginectomy for vaginal cancer, 223-224
Vaginismus, 182-183
Vaginitis causing third trimester bleeding, 412
Vaginosis
  bacterial, 86-87
  wet mount to diagnose, 515
Valacyclovir for herpes simplex virus prophylaxis, 503
Valproic acid
  for migraine headache, 584
  teratogenic effects of, 249
Vanishing twin, 462
Variability, heart rate, fetal, 467
Variable decelerations in fetal heart rate, 467
Varicella pneumonia during pregnancy, 298, 299
Varicella titer, 517
Varicella zoster, congenital, 369-370
Varicella zoster immune globulin, 370
Varicose veins, 643-646
Vasa previa, 410
Vascular changes during pregnancy, 376
Vascular dissemination, theory of, to explain endometriosis, 53
Vascular headache, 582

Vascular resistance, systemic, maternal, changes in, during pregnancy, 293
Vasculitides, 555-557
Vasculitis
 hypersensitivity, 556
 necrotizing, systemic, 555
Vasectomy, 185
Veins, varicose, 643-646
Velamentous cord insertion, 410
Velocardiofacial syndrome, 256
Velocimetry, Doppler, for antenatal testing, 285
Venereal Diseases Reference laboratory (VDRL) test to diagnose syphilis, 84-85
Venlafaxine
 for mood disorders, 102-103
 use in pregnancy of, 106
Venography
 to diagnose thromboembolism, 421
 radiation exposure to fetus from, 421
Venous thrombosis, deep, 419; *see also* Thromboembolic disease
Ventilation, minute, maternal, changes in, during pregnancy, 294
Ventilation lung scan, radiation exposure to fetus from, 421
Ventilation/perfusion scan
 to diagnose thromboembolism, 421-422
 total, radiation exposure to fetus from, 421
Ventricular septal defects complicating pregnancy, 308
Ventriculomegaly, ultrasonography to detect, 273
Venulectases, 645
Verapamil
 for hypertension, 591
 for migraine headache, 584
Version, cephalic, external, 453-454
Vibroacoustic stimulation for nonstress testing, 283
Video endoscopy to diagnose peptic ulcer disease, 620
Videx; *see* Didanosine
Villus, chorionic, sampling of, to screen for birth defects, 243-244
Vincristine
 for ovarian germ cell tumors, 132
 for sex cord–stromal tumors, 133
Violence
 cycle of, 573
 domestic; *see* Domestic violence
VIPoma causing secretory diarrhea, 565, 566
Viral hepatitis
 acute, during pregnancy, 345-346
 chronic, pregnancy and, 346
Viral laryngitis, treatment of, 606
Viral pharyngitis, 602-603
Viral pneumonia, 627-633
Virilizing adrenal adenomas, hirsutism with, 69
Virus(es)
 Epstein-Barr, pharyngitis and, 602
 herpes simplex, congenital infection with, 368-369
 human immunodeficiency; *see* Human immunodeficiency virus
 influenza, 594
 pneumonia caused by, 633
Vistaril; *see* Hydroxyzine
Vitamin B_6 supplements for nausea/vomiting during pregnancy, 238
Vitamin B_{12} deficiency, 322
Vitamin D for osteoporosis, 120
Vitamin deficiency, 609
Vitamins, 609
Vocal cord
 paralysis of, causing hoarseness, 604-605
 trauma to, causing hoarseness, 605
Voiding diary for stress incontinence, 190
Voiding dysfunction, 195-197
Volume, blood, maternal, changes in, during pregnancy, 293, 294
Vomiting during pregnancy, 347-348
 management of, 238
von Willebrand's disease, symptoms and treatment of, 205
Vulva, ulcerative infections of, 83-86
Vulvar cancer, 216-222
Vulvar melanoma, 221-222
Vulvectomy
 for vulvar cancer, 218
 for vulvar melanoma, 222
Vulvitis, focal, causing chronic pelvic pain, 161

Vulvovaginitis causing uterine bleeding in childhood and adolescence, 200

W

Warfarin for thromboembolism during pregnancy, 423
Warts, genital, 90, 134; *see also* Papillomavirus infections
Weaning, 481
Wegener's granulomatosis, 555, 556
  pregnancy and, 362
Weight, birth, low or very low, 384
Weight gain during pregnancy
  excessive, management of, 239
  inadequate, management of, 239
  recommendations for, 236-237
Weight loss
  amenorrhea caused by, 6
  malnutrition and, 610
Wellbutrin; *see* Bupropion
Wet mount, procedure for, 515
Whiplash, headache with, 582
White classification of diabetes in pregnancy, 311
Whole-blood clotting time to screen for coagulopathy, 405
Williams syndrome, 256
Wolf-Hirschhorn syndrome, 256
Woman(women)
  battered, characteristics of, 573
  leading causes of death of, 507
  leading causes of morbidity among, 507
  urinary tract infections in, 558-559
Wound infections after cesarean delivery, 234
WR-2721 for advanced pelvic disease, 32

X

Xanax; *see* Alprazolam
Xanthine oxidase inhibitors for gout, 531
X-linked chromosomal abnormalities, 252, 253
X-rays
  to diagnose cause of backache, 539
  to diagnose cause of diarrhea, 568
  to diagnose pneumonia, 628-629
  radiation exposure to fetus from, 421

Y

Yeast infection, wet mount to diagnose, 515
Yohimbine for mood disorders, 103
Yolk sac, ultrasonographic visualization of, 259-260

Z

Zalcitabine for HIV therapy, 503, 504
ZDV; *see* Zidovudine
Zerit; *see* Stavudine
Zidovudine
  for HIV therapy, 503, 504
  to prevent perinatal HIV infection, 372
Zinc supplements during pregnancy, 238
Zoloft; *see* Sertraline
Zygote intrafallopian transfer for infertility, 81-82